# THE JOH...
# MANUAL OF GYNEC...
# AND OBSTETRICS

## Fifth Edition

# THE JOHNS HOPKINS MANUAL OF GYNECOLOGY AND OBSTETRICS

**Fifth Edition**

Department of Gynecology and Obstetrics
The Johns Hopkins University School of Medicine
Baltimore, Maryland

*Editors*

**Clark T. Johnson,** MD, MPH

**Jennifer L. Hallock,** MD

**Jessica L. Bienstock,** MD, MPH

**Harold E. Fox,** MD, MSc

**Edward E. Wallach,** MD

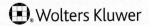

Philadelphia • Baltimore • New York • London
Buenos Aires • Hong Kong • Sydney • Tokyo

*Acquisitions Editor:* Jamie M. Elfrank
*Product Development Editor:* Ashley Fischer
*Production Product Manager:* David Saltzberg
*Manufacturing Manager:* Beth Welsh
*Marketing Manager:* Stephanie Kindlick
*Design Coordinator:* Teresa Mallon
*Production Service:* Absolute Service, Inc.

9 8 7 6 5 4 3 2 1

Printed in China

Library of Congress Cataloging-in-Publication Data

The Johns Hopkins manual of gynecology and obstetrics. — Fifth edition / Department of Gynecology and Obstetrics, The Johns Hopkins University School of Medicine ; editors, Clark T. Johnson, Jennifer L. Hallock, Jessica L. Bienstock, Harold E. Fox, Edward E. Wallach.
   p. ; cm.
  Manual of gynecology and obstetrics
  Includes bibliographical references and index.
  ISBN 978-1-4511-8880-6
  I. Johnson, Clark T., editor. II. Hallock, Jennifer L., editor. III. Bienstock, Jessica L., editor. IV. Fox, Harold E. (Harold Edward), 1945- , editor. V. Wallach, Edward E., 1933- , editor. VI. Johns Hopkins University. Department of Gynecology and Obstetrics, issuing body. VII. Title: Manual of gynecology and obstetrics.
  [DNLM: 1. Genital Diseases, Female—Handbooks. 2. Obstetrics—Handbooks. 3. Pregnancy Complications—Handbooks. 4. Women's Health—Handbooks. WQ 39]
  RG110
  618—dc23

                                                                              2015000034

LWW.com

CCS0315

With appreciation to all who have supported the residency training program in Gynecology and Obstetrics at the Johns Hopkins University School of Medicine.

This book is dedicated:

To the families of the house officers,
    without whose support and sacrifices none of us would be
        where we are today.

To the faculty,
    whose advocacy and efforts have affirmed a training
        program as strong as it is.

And to the mentors,
    the giants on whose shoulders we stand.

# Contents

# Introduction

We are currently in the midst of an era of incredible change. New means of communications and technologic advances have taken over the worlds of medicine and education. The growth of innovative electronics and computer science has paved the way for methods for diagnosis and therapy that would never have been considered earlier. Not only has this burst of energy contributed to extended longevity and quality of life, but it has also had a major influence on the need for rapid and highly effective transmission of knowledge. In the field of obstetrics and gynecology, we have witnessed the introduction of new minimally invasive surgical techniques. Sophisticated robotic equipment is now standard in the operating room. New diagnostic tools have changed our management of abnormal cervical cytology and focused on a sexually transmittable virus as the cause of cervical cancer. The development of in vitro fertilization 35 years ago has led to our ability to cryopreserve not only embryos but eggs as well, opening new avenues for conception and family building. Many men formerly thought to be hopelessly infertile now have the opportunity to father their own offspring, thanks to direct intracytoplasmic sperm injection. Prenatal diagnosis currently can be carried out for certain inheritable diseases by delicate genetic studies on an individual cell removed from an embryo prior to its transfer into the uterus and implantation. All of the examples alluded to as well as many others have either been refined or developed since publication of the previous (fourth) edition of *The Johns Hopkins Manual of Gynecology and Obstetrics* in 2011. Such new information is included in the fifth edition.

The first edition of *The Johns Hopkins Manual of Gynecology and Obstetrics* was published in 1999. The original concept for the Hopkins manual arose during informal discussions with Timothy Johnson, then a faculty member at Johns Hopkins and currently Chair of the Department of Obstetrics and Gynecology at the University of Michigan. The plan was to place responsibility for the preparation of each chapter in the hands of a resident physician who would partner together with a faculty member whose field of expertise matched the material covered in that particular chapter. Over the years, this team effort has resulted in a book which continues to serve as a trusted companion for house officers, medical students, and practitioners. The "manual," combining the skills of our faculty and residents, has also contributed markedly to the camaraderie in the Department of Gynecology and Obstetrics at Johns Hopkins.

It is exciting and most fitting that one of the senior residents assigned to serve as coeditor is Clark Johnson, Tim Johnson's son. Clark recently completed his residency and currently serves as a fellow in Maternal–Fetal Medicine at Johns Hopkins. The tradition of the manual and of the Johnson family thus continues into the fifth edition.

Edward E. Wallach, MD
Harold E. Fox, MD, MSc
Jessica L. Bienstock, MD, MPH

# Acknowledgments

The editors wish to acknowledge the role of our ancillary staff at Johns Hopkins for their assistance in ensuring that each chapter is prepared in a timely fashion and in suitable condition for publication. We are also grateful to Ashley Fischer, product development editor at Wolters Kluwer Health: Lippincott Williams & Wilkins, for her professionalism and encouragement.

# Contributors

**Abimbola Aina-Mumuney**, MD
*Assistant Professor of Gynecology and Obstetrics*
*Johns Hopkins University School of Medicine*
*Baltimore, Maryland*

**Janyne E. Althaus**, MD, MA
*Assistant Professor*
*Perinatal Outreach Director*
*Department of Gynecology and Obstetrics*
*Johns Hopkins University School of Medicine*
*Baltimore, Maryland*

**Kristiina Altman**, MD, PhD
*Assistant Professor*
*Department of Gynecology and Obstetrics*
*Johns Hopkins University School of Medicine*
*Baltimore, Maryland*

**Hannah Anastasio**, MD
*Resident Physician*
*Department of Gynecology and Obstetrics*
*Johns Hopkins University School of Medicine*
*Baltimore, Maryland*

**Cynthia Holcroft Argani**, MD
*Assistant Professor*
*Department of Gynecology and Obstetrics*
*Johns Hopkins University School of Medicine*
*Director, Labor and Delivery*
*Johns Hopkins Bayview Medical Center*
*Baltimore, Maryland*

**Jill Berkin**, MD
*Resident Physician*
*Department of Gynecology and Obstetrics*
*Johns Hopkins University School of Medicine*
*Baltimore, Maryland*

**Jessica L. Bienstock**, MD, MPH
*Professor*
*Residency Program Director*
*Vice-Chair for Education*
*Department of Gynecology and Obstetrics*
*Johns Hopkins University School of Medicine*
*Baltimore, Maryland*

**Meredith L. Birsner**, MD
*Clinical Fellow, Maternal Fetal Medicine*
*Department of Gynecology and Obstetrics*
*Johns Hopkins University School of Medicine*
*Baltimore, Maryland*

**Karin J. Blakemore**, MD
*Professor*
*Director, Maternal Fetal Medicine*
*Department of Gynecology and Obstetrics*
*Johns Hopkins University School of Medicine*
*Baltimore, Medicine*

**Irina Burd**, MD, PhD
*Assistant Professor*
*Department of Gynecology and Obstetrics*
*Johns Hopkins University School of Medicine*
*Baltimore, Maryland*

**Anne E. Burke**, MD, MPH
*Associate Professor*
*Director, Family Planning*
*Department of Gynecology and Obstetrics*
*Johns Hopkins University School of Medicine*
*Baltimore, Maryland*

**Dayna Burrell**, MD
*Assistant Professor*
*Department of Gynecology and Obstetrics*
*Johns Hopkins University School of Medicine*
*Baltimore, Maryland*

**Chi Chiung Grace Chen**, MD
*Assistant Professor*
*Department of Gynecology and Obstetrics*
*Johns Hopkins University School of Medicine*
*Baltimore, Maryland*

**Diana Cholakian**, MD
*Resident Physician*
*Department of Gynecology and Obstetrics*
*Johns Hopkins University School of Medicine*
*Baltimore, Maryland*

**Betty Chou, MD**
*Assistant Professor*
*Department of Gynecology and Obstetrics*
*Johns Hopkins University School of Medicine*
*Baltimore, Maryland*

**Veena Choubey, MD**
*Resident Physician*
*Department of Gynecology and Obstetrics*
*Johns Hopkins University School of Medicine*
*Baltimore, Maryland*

**Lauren Cobb, MD**
*Resident Physician*
*Department of Gynecology and Obstetrics*
*Johns Hopkins University School of Medicine*
*Baltimore, Maryland*

**Jenell Coleman, MD, MPH**
*Assistant Professor*
*Department of Gynecology and Obstetrics*
*Johns Hopkins University School of Medicine*
*Baltimore, Maryland*

**Mindy S. Christianson, MD**
*Assistant Professor*
*Department of Gynecology and Obstetrics*
*Johns Hopkins University School of Medicine*
*Baltimore, Maryland*

**Abigail E. Dennis, MD**
*Assistant Professor*
*Department of Gynecology and Obstetrics*
*Johns Hopkins University School of Medicine*
*Baltimore, Maryland*

**Christopher C. DeStephano, MD, MPH**
*Resident Physician*
*Department of Gynecology and Obstetrics*
*Johns Hopkins University School of Medicine*
*Baltimore, Maryland*

**Teresa P. Díaz-Montes, MD, MPH**
*Assistant Professor*
*Department of Gynecology and Obstetrics*
*Johns Hopkins University School of Medicine*
*Baltimore, Maryland*

**Cindy M. P. Duke, MD**
*Resident Physician*
*Department of Gynecology and Obstetrics*
*Johns Hopkins University School of Medicine*
*Baltimore, Maryland*

**Sonia Dutta, MD**
*Resident Physician*
*Department of Gynecology and Obstetrics*
*Johns Hopkins University School of Medicine*
*Baltimore, Maryland*

**Jill Edwardson, MD, MPH**
*Assistant Professor*
*Department of Gynecology and Obstetrics*
*Johns Hopkins University School of Medicine*
*Baltimore, Maryland*

**Robert M. Ehsanipoor, MD**
*Assistant Professor*
*Department of Gynecology and Obstetrics*
*Johns Hopkins University School of Medicine*
*Baltimore, Maryland*

**Amanda Nickles Fader, MD**
*Associate Professor*
*Director, The Kelly Gynecologic Oncology Service*
*Department of Gynecology and Obstetrics*
*Johns Hopkins University School of Medicine*
*Baltimore, Maryland*

**William Fletcher, MD**
*Resident Physician*
*Department of Gynecology and Obstetrics*
*Johns Hopkins University School of Medicine*
*Baltimore, Maryland*

**Harold E. Fox, MD, MSc**
*University Distinguished Service Professor*
*Director Emeritus*
*Department of Gynecology and Obstetrics*
*Johns Hopkins University School of Medicine*
*Baltimore, Maryland*

**Robert L. Giuntoli II, MD**
*Associate Professor*
*Department of Gynecology and Obstetrics*
*Johns Hopkins University School of Medicine*
*Baltimore, Maryland*

**Ernest M. Graham,** MD
*Associate Professor*
*Department of Gynecology and Obstetrics*
*Johns Hopkins University School of Medicine*
*Baltimore, Maryland*

**Isabel Green,** MD
*Assistant Professor*
*Department of Gynecology and Obstetrics*
*Johns Hopkins University School of Medicine*
*Baltimore, Medicine*

**Reinou S. Groen,** MD, MPH
*Resident Physician*
*Department of Gynecology and Obstetrics*
*Johns Hopkins University School of Medicine*
*Baltimore, Maryland*

**Amy H. Gueye,** MD, MPH
*Resident Physician*
*Department of Obstetrics and Gynecology*
*Johns Hopkins University School of Medicine*
*Baltimore, Maryland*

**Edith Gurewitsch Allen,** MD
*Associate Professor*
*Department of Gynecology and Obstetrics*
*Johns Hopkins University School of Medicine*
*Baltimore, Maryland*

**Jennifer L. Hallock,** MD
*Clinical Fellow, Female Pelvic Medicine and*
*  Reconstructive Surgery*
*Department of Gynecology and Obstetrics*
*Johns Hopkins University School of Medicine*
*Baltimore, Maryland*

**Janice Henderson,** MD, MA
*Assistant Professor*
*Director of Fetal Assessment Unit—High-Risk*
*  Obstetrics*
*Department of Gynecology and Obstetrics*
*Johns Hopkins University School of Medicine*
*Baltimore, Maryland*

**Nancy A. Hueppchen,** MD, MSc
*Associate Professor*
*Director, Medical Student Education*
*Department of Gynecology and Obstetrics*
*Assistant Dean for Clinical Curriculum*
*Johns Hopkins University School of Medicine*
*Baltimore, Maryland*

**Roxanne Marie Jamshidi,** MD
*Assistant Professor*
*Director, Johns Hopkins Women's Services at*
*  Odenton*
*Department of Gynecology and Obstetrics*
*Johns Hopkins University School of Medicine*
*Baltimore, Maryland*

**Amelia M. Jernigan,** MD
*Resident Physician*
*Department of Gynecology and Obstetrics*
*Johns Hopkins University School of Medicine*
*Baltimore, Maryland*

**Clark T. Johnson,** MD, MPH
*Clinical Fellow, Maternal Fetal Medicine*
*Department of Gynecology and Obstetrics*
*Johns Hopkins University School of Medicine*
*Baltimore, Maryland*

**Dipa Joshi,** MD
*Resident Physician*
*Department of Gynecology and Obstetrics*
*Johns Hopkins University School of Medicine*
*Baltimore, Maryland*

**Jean M. Keller,** PAC
*Assistant Professor*
*Codirector, Johns Hopkins HIV Women's*
*  Program*
*Department of Gynecology and Obstetrics*
*Johns Hopkins University School of Medicine*
*Baltimore, Maryland*

**Lisa Kolp,** MD
*Assistant Professor*
*Department of Gynecology and Obstetrics*
*Johns Hopkins University School of Medicine*
*Baltimore, Maryland*

**Katherine Latimer, MD**
*Resident Physician*
*Department of Gynecology and Obstetrics*
*Johns Hopkins Hospital*
*Baltimore, Maryland*

**Shari Lawson, MD**
*Assistant Professor*
*Medical Director, Johns Hopkins Women's*
  *Services at Bayview*
*Department of Gynecology and Obstetrics*
*Johns Hopkins University School of Medicine*
*Baltimore, Maryland*

**Stephen Martin, MD**
*Resident Physician*
*Department of Gynecology and Obstetrics*
*Johns Hopkins University School of Medicine*
*Baltimore, Maryland*

**Virginia Mensah, MD**
*Resident Physician*
*Department of Gynecology and Obstetrics*
*Johns Hopkins University School of Medicine*
*Baltimore, Maryland*

**Lorraine A. Milio, MD**
*Assistant Professor*
*Department of Gynecology and Obstetrics*
*Johns Hopkins University School of Medicine*
*Baltimore, Medicine*

**Jamie Murphy, MD**
*Assistant Professor*
*Director of Obstetric Anesthesia*
*Department of Anesthesiology and Critical*
  *Care Medicine*
*Johns Hopkins University School of Medicine*
*Baltimore, Maryland*

**Donna Neale, MD**
*Assistant Professor*
*Department of Gynecology and Obstetrics*
*Johns Hopkins University School of Medicine*
*Director*
*Center for Maternal and Fetal Medicine at*
  *Howard County General Hospital*
*Baltimore, Maryland*

**Sarah Oman, MD**
*Resident Physician*
*Department of Gynecology and Obstetrics*
*Johns Hopkins University School of Medicine*
*Baltimore, Maryland*

**Lauren Owens, MD, MPH**
*Resident Physician*
*Department of Gynecology and Obstetrics*
*Johns Hopkins Hospital*
*Baltimore, Maryland*

**Silka Patel, MD, MPH**
*Assistant Professor*
*Department of Gynecology and Obstetrics*
*Johns Hopkins University School of Medicine*
*Baltimore, Maryland*

**Meghan E. Pratts, MD**
*Resident Physician*
*Department of Gynecology and Obstetrics*
*Johns Hopkins University School of Medicine*
*Baltimore, Maryland*

**Nina Resetkova, MD, MBA**
*Resident Physician*
*Department of Gynecology and Obstetrics*
*Johns Hopkins University School of Medicine*
*Baltimore, Maryland*

**Linda Rogers, CRNP**
*Nurse Practitioner*
*Department of Gynecology and Obstetrics*
*Johns Hopkins Bayview Medical Center*
*Baltimore, Maryland*

**Melissa L. Russo, MD**
*Clinical Fellow, Maternal Fetal Medicine*
*Clinical Fellow, Medical Genetics*
*Department of Gynecology and Obstetrics*
*Johns Hopkins University School of Medicine*
*Baltimore, Maryland*

Andrew J. Satin, MD
*The Dorothy Edwards Professor in
    Gynecology and Obstetrics*
*Director, Department of Gynecology and
    Obstetrics*
*Department of Gynecology and Obstetrics*
*Johns Hopkins University School of Medicine*
*Baltimore, Maryland*

Stacey A. Scheib, MD
*Assistant Professor of Gynecology and
    Obstetrics*
*Department of Gynecology and Obstetrics*
*Johns Hopkins University School of Medicine*
*Baltimore, Maryland*

Sara Seifert, MD
*Resident Physician*
*Department of Gynecology and Obstetrics*
*Johns Hopkins University School of Medicine*
*Johns Hopkins Hospital*
*Baltimore, Maryland*

Wen Shen, MD, MPH
*Assistant Professor*
*Department of Gynecology and Obstetrics*
*Johns Hopkins University School of Medicine*
*Baltimore, Maryland*

Sangini Sheth, MD, MPH
*Resident Physician*
*Department of Gynecology and Obstetrics*
*Johns Hopkins University School of Medicine*
*Baltimore, Maryland*

Khara M. Simpson, MD
*Resident Physician*
*Department of Gynecology and Obstetrics*
*Johns Hopkins University School of Medicine*
*Baltimore, Maryland*

Julie S. Solomon, MD
*Resident Physician*
*Department of Gynecology and Obstetrics*
*Johns Hopkins University School of Medicine*
*Baltimore, Maryland*

Katherine Ikard Stewart, MD
*Resident Physician*
*Department of Gynecology and Obstetrics*
*Johns Hopkins University School of Medicine*
*Baltimore, Maryland*

Linda M. Szymanski, MD, PhD
*Assistant Professor*
*Department of Gynecology and Obstetrics*
*Johns Hopkins University School of Medicine*
*Baltimore, Maryland*

Edward J. Tanner III, MD
*Assistant Professor*
*Department of Gynecology and Obstetrics*
*Johns Hopkins University School of Medicine*
*Baltimore, Maryland*

Kyle J. Tobler, MD
*Clinical Fellow, Reproductive Endocrinology
    and Infertility*
*Department of Gynecology and Obstetrics*
*Johns Hopkins University School of Medicine*
*Baltimore, Maryland*

Cornelia Liu Trimble, MD
*Associate Professor*
*Department of Gynecology and Obstetrics*
*Johns Hopkins University School of Medicine*
*Baltimore, Maryland*

Jill H. Tseng, MD
*Resident Physician*
*Department of Gynecology and Obstetrics*
*Johns Hopkins Hospital*
*Baltimore, Maryland*

Berendena I. M. Vander Tuig, MD,
    MPH
*Resident Physician*
*Department of Gynecology and Obstetrics*
*Johns Hopkins University School of Medicine*
*Baltimore, Maryland*

**Edward E. Wallach,** MD
*University Distinguished Service Professor*
*Emeritus*
*Director Emeritus*
*Department of Gynecology and Obstetrics*
*Johns Hopkins University School of Medicine*
*Baltimore, Medicine*

**Chantel Washington,** MD
*Resident Physician*
*Department of Gynecology and Obstetrics*
*Johns Hopkins University School of Medicine*
*Baltimore, Maryland*

**Erika F. Werner,** MD, MS
*Assistant Professor*
*Department of Gynecology and Obstetrics*
*Johns Hopkins University School of Medicine*
*Baltimore, Maryland*

**Sarahn M. Wheeler,** MD
*Resident Physician*
*Department of Gynecology and Obstetrics*
*Johns Hopkins University School of Medicine*
*Baltimore, Maryland*

**Maryann B. Wilbur,** MD
*Resident Physician*
*Department of Gynecology and Obstetrics*
*Johns Hopkins University School of Medicine*
*Baltimore, Maryland*

**Abigail D. Winder,** MD
*Resident Physician*
*Department of Gynecology and Obstetrics*
*Johns Hopkins University School of Medicine*
*Baltimore, Maryland*

**Frank R. Witter,** MD
*Professor*
*Department of Gynecology and Obstetrics*
*Johns Hopkins University School of Medicine*
*Baltimore, Maryland*

**Irene Woo,** MD
*Resident Physician*
*Department of Gynecology and Obstetrics*
*Johns Hopkins University School of Medicine*
*Baltimore, Maryland*

**Emily S. Wu,** MD
*Resident Physician*
*Department of Gynecology and Obstetrics*
*Johns Hopkins University School of Medicine*
*Baltimore, Maryland*

**John L. Wu,** MD
*Resident Physician*
*Department of Gynecology and Obstetrics*
*Johns Hopkins University School of Medicine*
*Baltimore, Maryland*

**Melissa Yates,** MD
*Assistant Professor*
*Department of Gynecology and Obstetrics*
*Johns Hopkins University School of Medicine*
*Baltimore, Maryland*

**Howard A. Zacur,** MD, PhD
*Theodore and Ingrid Baramki Professor*
*Director, Reproductive Endocrinology*
*Department of Gynecology and Obstetrics*
*Johns Hopkins University School of Medicine*
*Baltimore, Maryland*

# Women's Health Care

# 1

# Primary and Preventive Care

Hannah Anastasio and Silka Patel

Obstetrician-gynecologists are in a unique position to interact with women across the reproductive and age spectrum and are seen by many patients as the sole provider of **primary and preventive health care**. The responsibilities of a primary care physician include screening and treatment of selected diseases, counseling, and providing immunizations. Additionally, common nongynecologic conditions that the obstetrician-gynecologist (ObGyn) should be familiar with include asthma, allergic rhinitis, respiratory tract infections, gastrointestinal disorders, urinary tract disorders, headache, low back pain, and skin disorders.

## SCREENING AND TREATMENT

- The majority of deaths among women younger than the age of 65 years are preventable or have modifiable risk factors (Table 1-1).
- **Primary prevention** is identification and control of risk factors before disease occurs
- **Secondary prevention** is early diagnosis of disease to reduce morbidity/mortality
- A condition which is a good target for screening should have the following:
  - A significant effect on the quality and quantity of life
  - An acceptable and available treatment
  - An asymptomatic period during which detection and treatment significantly reduce the risk for morbidity and mortality
  - An incidence sufficient to justify the cost of the screening
  - An asymptomatic phase during which treatment yields therapeutic results superior to those obtained by delaying treatment until symptoms develop
- The screening test should be:
  - Acceptable to patients and available at a reasonable cost
  - Reasonably accurate with acceptable sensitivity and specificity
    - ○ Test sensitivity: percentage of patients with the disease who test positive
    - ○ Test specificity: percentage of patients without disease who test negative

**TABLE 1-1** Leading Causes of Death among Females of All Races in the United States (2010)

| | 15–24 | 25–34 | 35–44 | 45–54 | 55–64 | 65+ |
|---|---|---|---|---|---|---|
| 1 | Unintentional injury | Unintentional injury | Malignant neoplasm | Malignant neoplasm | Malignant neoplasm | Heart disease |
| 2 | Suicide | Malignant neoplasm | Unintentional injury | Heart disease | Heart disease | Malignant neoplasm |
| 3 | Homicide | Suicide | Heart disease | Unintentional injury | Chronic respiratory disease | Cerebrovascular |
| 4 | Malignant neoplasm | Heart disease | Suicide | Liver disease | Cerebrovascular | Chronic respiratory disease |
| 5 | Heart disease | Homicide | Cerebrovascular | Cerebrovascular | Diabetes mellitus | Alzheimer disease |

Adapted from the Centers for Disease Control and Prevention. Web-based injury statistics query and reporting system (WISQARS). Centers for Disease Control and Prevention Web site. http://webappa.cdc.gov/saweb/ncipc/leadcause/0.html. Accessed February 10, 2013.

# CANCER

## Screening for Breast Cancer

- See Chapter 2.
- Breast cancer is the most common cancer in women, with a lifetime incidence of 12%. For those at average risk, the American College of Obstetricians and Gynecologists (ACOG), the American Cancer Society (ACS), and the National Comprehensive Cancer Network (NCCN) recommend routine mammography annually beginning at age 40 years. The U.S. Preventive Services Task Force (USP-STF), in contrast, recommends biennial screening between ages 50 and 74 years. In addition, ACOG recommends regular clinical breast examinations in all women as well as breast self-examination in high-risk women.
- ACOG and the Society of Gynecologic Oncology recommend referral for genetic counseling and BRCA testing in patients with 20% or greater chance of having an inherited predisposition to developing breast or ovarian cancer. This includes women with the following family history:
  - Women with a personal history of both breast and ovarian cancer
  - Women with ovarian cancer and a close relative with ovarian cancer or premenopausal breast cancer
  - Women with breast cancer at age 50 years or younger as well as either a close relative with ovarian cancer or breast cancer in a man at any age
  - Women of Ashkenazi Jewish ancestry with a diagnosis of breast cancer at age 40 years or younger or with ovarian cancer at any age
  - Women with close relative with known BRCA1 or BRCA2 mutation
- Additionally, further genetic risk assessment may be helpful in the following women (estimated to have between 5% and 10% risk of having an inherited predisposition toward developing breast or ovarian cancer):
  - Breast cancer at age 40 years or younger
  - Primary peritoneal, ovarian, or fallopian tube cancer at any age
  - Breast cancer at age 50 years or younger and a close relative with breast cancer at age 50 years or younger
  - Ashkenazi Jewish ancestry with breast cancer at or before age 50 years
  - Breast cancer at any age in addition to two close relatives with breast cancer (any age)
  - Unaffected women with a close relative that meets any of the previous criteria
- Women at high risk for breast cancer, such as those with BRCA1 or BRCA2 mutations, may undergo prophylactic mastectomies to reduce their risk of breast cancer.

## Screening for Lung Cancer

- Lung cancer, the second most common cancer in women, is the leading cause of cancer-related death. In 2009, in the United States, 95,784 women were diagnosed and 70,387 died from lung cancer.
- Risk factors include cigarette smoking (associated with 90% of lung cancers), radiation therapy, environmental toxins such as asbestos, and pulmonary fibrosis.
- The majority of studies examining screening modalities for lung cancer (via chest x-ray, sputum cytology, or computed tomography [CT] scan) have failed to show a mortality benefit from early detection of lung cancer. In 2011, the National Lung Screening Trial was the first to show approximately a 20% mortality benefit in asymptomatic heavy smokers (>30 pack-year history) screened with low-dose CT scans. The 2013 ACS recommendation (in abstract form) is that providers discuss lung cancer screening with a low-dose helical CT of the chest for patients between

ages 55 and 74 years with at least a 30 pack-year smoking history. At this time, the recommendation is that providers and patients have an informed discussion about the current data regarding lung cancer screening and use shared decision making to decide whether to initiate lung cancer screening.

- Smoking may confer a greater relative risk for women than men; however, many of the early studies on lung cancer screening did not include women. It is theorized that screening in women may have different outcomes due to higher rates of peripherally located adenocarcinoma.
- Smoking cessation, as well as continued abstinence in nonsmokers, is the single most important modifiable risk factor for lung cancer.

## Screening for Colorectal Cancer

- Colorectal cancer is the third most commonly diagnosed cancer and the third leading cause of cancer in women, with an annual incidence of 38.9 per 100,000. Most colorectal cancers have a long latency period and are curable or easily treatable if detected at an early stage.
- Risk factors include a family history of colorectal cancer, a personal history of colon polyps or cancer, a personal history of inflammatory bowel disease, and the genetic syndromes familial adenomatous polyposis and hereditary nonpolyposis colon cancer (HNPCC). High-risk individuals should be screened with colonoscopy beginning at earlier ages depending on risk.
- Women with a diagnosis of HNPCC should initiate screening at age 20 to 25 years or 10 years before the youngest age of colon cancer diagnosis in the family.
- The USPSTF recommends screening for colorectal cancer for all persons aged 50 years and older. The American College of Gastroenterology recommends beginning screening at age 45 years in African Americans due to higher incidence and earlier age of onset.
- Many screening protocols exist, including flexible sigmoidoscopy every 5 years, colonoscopy every 10 years, double-contrast barium enema every 5 years, CT colonography every 5 years, guaiac-based fecal occult blood test annually (two samples from each of three consecutive stools), fecal immunochemical test annually, and stool DNA test. The 2008 U.S. Multi-Society Task Force on Colorectal Cancer guidelines support any of the aforementioned regimens; ACOG encourages colonoscopy but ultimately recommends shared decision making to determine which screening modality the patient is most likely to comply with.

## Screening for Endometrial Cancer

- See Chapter 47.
- No routine screening is recommended for asymptomatic women. Certain high-risk groups (those with known or prior endometrial hyperplasia or patients with HNPCC) may undergo screening, such as endometrial biopsy, pelvic ultrasound, dilation and curettage, or a combination of these. All episodes of postmenopausal bleeding should be investigated. Additionally, in premenopausal obese women with a significant change in bleeding pattern, endometrial sampling should be considered.

## Screening for Skin Cancer

- Melanoma is the seventh leading cancer in women; risk factors include light skin tone and ultraviolet ray exposure, particularly childhood sunburns. People with between 50 and 100 typical nevi or large congenital nevi are also at increased risk (relative risk of 5 to 17 and >100, respectively).

- Although there are no consensus guidelines for total skin examination, ACOG recommends evaluation in those patients at high risk. All patients should be educated regarding sunscreen use and ultraviolet ray avoidance. In particular, all atypical vulvar lesions should be thoroughly investigated (see Chapter 44.)
- Guidelines regarding suspicious lesions are as follows:
  - **A**symmetry
  - **B**order irregularities
  - **C**olor variegation
  - **D**iameter >6 mm
  - **E**nlargement/**E**volution of color change, shape, or symptoms

## Screening for Ovarian Cancer

- See Chapter 48.
- No North American expert group recommends routine screening for ovarian cancer. Instead, a careful family history and an annual pelvic exam are recommended for all women.
- Women at high risk for ovarian cancer, such as those with BRCA1 or BRCA2 mutations, may undergo prophylactic bilateral salpingo-oophorectomy to reduce their risk of ovarian cancer.

## Screening for Cervical Cancer

- See Chapter 46.
- Routine screening for cervical cancer with either liquid-based or conventional Papanicolaou (Pap) testing is recommended starting at age 21 years, regardless of age of first sexual activity. The ACS and ACOG have suggested that women between the ages of 21 and 30 years should be screened with cytology alone every 3 years, provided the patient does not have a history of cervical intraepithelial neoplasia grade 2 (CIN 2) or worse, is not HIV positive or immunocompromised, and has no history of diethylstilbestrol exposure. Routine human papillomavirus (HPV) testing is not recommended in this age group given the high incidence of transient asymptomatic infection. Women ages 30 to 65 years should be screened every 5 years with cotesting (cytology and HPV testing). Alternatively, Pap screening with cytology alone (without HPV testing) every 3 years may be performed, but cotesting is preferable. After age 65 years, no further screening is recommended if the patient has had adequate negative screening for the past 10 years. Women with prior loop electrosurgical excision procedure/cryotherapy should continue age-based screening for at least 20 years from procedure.
- ACOG and the USPSTF both agree that cervical cancer screening may be discontinued for women who have had a total hysterectomy for benign indications and no history of CIN 2 or worse.
- Women with abnormal Pap smears should be managed per the American Society for Colposcopy and Cervical Pathology guidelines.
- There are currently two U.S. Food and Drug Administration–approved vaccines for the primary prevention of cervical cancer. Cervarix protects against high-risk HPV strains 16 and 18 known to cause cervical cancer, and Gardasil protects against HPV 6, 11, 16 and 18 conferring additional benefit against HPV strains known to cause genital warts. ACOG recommends universal vaccination of women against these HPV strains before initiation of sexual activity (as early as age 9 years) as well as in sexually active women up to age 26 years. Women who have received HPV vaccination should be screened for cervical cancer using the same schedule as unvaccinated women.

## HEART AND VASCULAR CONDITIONS

### Screening for Coronary Heart Disease

- Rates of coronary heart disease (CHD) in women increase with age, ranging between 5% and 15%. Risk factors include hypertension, dyslipidemia, diabetes, smoking, and family history of premature CHD (age <55 years in first-degree male relative or age <65 years in first-degree female relative).
- Validated risk stratification models include the Framingham risk score that predicts 10-year risk of a CHD event. The Framingham model was updated by the National Cholesterol Education Program (NCEP) Adult Treatment Panel III (ATP III) and adjusts for the following variables: age, gender, low-density lipoprotein cholesterol, high-density lipoprotein (HDL) cholesterol, blood pressure, diabetes, and smoking. The USPSTF recommends against routine screening of asymptomatic low-risk patients (defined as <10% 10-year risk) for CHD using resting electrocardiogram (ECG), ambulatory ECG, or exercise ECG.

### Aspirin for Primary Prevention of Cardiovascular Events

- The USPSTF *strongly* recommends that physicians consider aspirin prophylaxis in women ages 55 to 79 years at high risk for CHD based on ATP III and Framingham risk stratifications. Benefits of prevention of CHD should be weighed against the risks of gastrointestinal and intracranial bleeding (level A recommendation).
- Low-dose aspirin (75 to 100 mg/day) appears as effective as higher doses.

### Screening for Dyslipidemia

- Dyslipidemia is a direct and modifiable risk factor for CHD, and the USPSTF *strongly* recommends screening with fasting lipid profile for women aged >45 years if they are at increased risk of CHD (level A evidence). Screening of high-risk women aged 20 to 45 years is recommended (level B evidence), and screening of low-risk women is neither recommended nor discouraged (level C evidence). Recommended screening interval is every 5 years, but a shorter interval should be considered in patients at increased risk for dyslipidemia or with previous borderline results.
- Table 1-2 summarizes NCEP/ATP III treatment recommendations. Goal cholesterol level depends on number and severity of risk factors for CHD. CHD equivalents include peripheral arterial disease, abdominal aortic aneurysm, diabetes mellitus, and symptomatic carotid artery disease. Other risk factors (non-CHD equivalents) include smoking, hypertension (>140/90 mm Hg or requiring antihypertensive), low HDL (<40 mg/dL), family history of premature CHD, and age (men >45 years, women >55 years).
- Lifestyle changes include limiting fat intake (particularly *trans* and saturated fat), increasing dietary fiber and plant sterol intake, weight loss, and increasing physical activity.
- The most commonly used pharmacologic treatment for dyslipidemia include bile acid–binding resins, statins, nicotinic acid, fibric acid derivatives, and cholesterol absorption inhibitors. Treatment choice depends on the particular lipid profile; however, statins are the drug of choice for cardioprotection.

### Screening for Hypertension

- Hypertension (defined as blood pressure >140/90 mm Hg or requiring antihypertensive medication) is a leading risk factor for CHD, congestive heart failure,

**TABLE 1-2    NCEP/ATP III Cholesterol Treatment Guidelines (2002)**

| Risk Group | LDL Goal (mg/dL) | LDL Level to Start Lifestyle Changes (mg/dL) | LDL Level to Start Drug Therapy (mg/dL) |
|---|---|---|---|
| CHD or risk equivalent | <100 | ≥100 | ≥130 |
| 2+ Risk factors | <130 | ≥130 | 130–160 |
| 0–1 Risk factors | <160 | ≥160 | ≥190 |

NCEP, National Cholesterol Education Program; ATP III, Adult Treatment Panel III; LDL, low-density lipoprotein; CHD, coronary heart disease.
Adapted from ATPIII Guidelines and Grundy SM, Cleeman JI, Bairey Merz CN, et al. Implications of recent clinical trials for national cholesterol education program adult treatment panel III guidelines. *Circulation* 2004;110:227–239.

stroke, ruptured aortic aneurysm, renal disease, and retinopathy. Suboptimal blood pressure has been reported as the number one risk factor for death worldwide.

• Essential or primary hypertension may result from excess salt intake, obesity, low fruit/vegetable intake, low potassium, or excessive alcohol use. Secondary causes of hypertension may include chronic renal disease, aortic coarctation, pheochromocytoma, Cushing disease, primary aldosteronism, renovascular disease, sleep apnea, or thyroid disease.

• The 2003 Joint National Committee on Prevention, Detection, Evaluation, and Treatment of High Blood Pressure (JNC-7) guidelines for treatment are summarized in Table 1-3.

• Lifestyle modifications are encouraged in all patients with suboptimal blood pressure and include weight loss, reduction in dietary sodium intake, moderate alcohol consumption, increased physical activity, and using Dietary Approaches to Stop Hypertension (DASH).

• Drug choice is determined by comorbid conditions and contraindications and may include single-agent or combination therapy using thiazide diuretics, angiotensin-converting enzyme inhibitors, angiotensin II receptor blockers, beta-blockers, or calcium channel blockers.

• Compelling indications for pharmacologic treatment of prehypertension include diabetes and chronic kidney disease, with goal blood pressure <130/80 mm Hg.

## INFECTIOUS DISEASES

Women at highest risk for sexually transmitted disease include those with a history of multiple sexual partners, sexually transmitted diseases, inconsistent condom use, commercial sex work, and drug use. Preventive strategies such as abstinence, reduction in number of sexual partners, and barrier contraceptive methods should be discussed with all patients.

### Screening for HIV

• The 2006 Centers for Disease Control and Prevention (CDC) guidelines recommend routine screening in the United States of all adults and adolescents aged 13 to 64 years and all pregnant women, regardless of risk factors, using opt-out screening protocols.

**TABLE 1-3** JNC-7 Treatment Guidelines for Hypertension (2003)

| Blood Pressure Classification | Blood Pressure (mm Hg) | Drug Therapy |
|---|---|---|
| Normal | <120/80 | None |
| Prehypertension | (120–139)/(80–89) | Only for compelling indications |
| Stage I hypertension | (140–159)/(90–99) | |
| Stage II hypertension | ≥160/≥100 | |

JNC-7, Joint National Committee on Prevention, Detection, Evaluation, and Treatment of High Blood Pressure.
Adapted from Chobanian AV, Bakris GL, Black HR, et al.; National High Blood Pressure Education Program Coordinating Committee. The seventh report of the Joint National Committee on Prevention, Detection, Evaluation, and Treatment of High Blood Pressure: the JNC 7 report. *JAMA* 2003;289: 2560–2572. Accessed February 18, 2013.

## Screening for Chlamydia

- The 2006 CDC Sexually Transmitted Diseases Treatment Guidelines support chlamydia screening (with cervical/vaginal swab or urine testing) annually in all sexually active women younger than age 25 years and in older women with new/multiple sex partners or high-risk behavior. See Chapter 28.
- The USPSTF and CDC recommend against routine screening in asymptomatic individuals for hepatitis B, hepatitis C, gonorrhea, syphilis, herpes simplex virus, and trichomoniasis in low-risk nonpregnant patients.

## METABOLIC, ENDOCRINE, AND NUTRITIONAL CONDITIONS

### Screening for Diabetes

- See Chapter 13.
- The USPSTF recommends screening for type 2 diabetes in asymptomatic adults with sustained blood pressure >135/80 mm Hg.
- Screening normotensive adults for type 2 diabetes should be considered in some cases, such as age older than 45 years, obesity, family history of diabetes in first-degree relative, non-Caucasian ethnicity, history of gestational diabetes or delivering a baby >9 pounds, inactivity, dyslipidemia, polycystic ovarian syndrome, and vascular disease.
- Screening tests: fasting plasma glucose (FPG) or a 2-hour, 75-g glucose challenge test (GCT), and hemoglobin A1C.
- Diabetes = FPG ≥126 mL/dL *OR*
  GCT ≥200 mg/dL *OR*
  random plasma glucose >200 mg/dL with symptoms *OR*
  hemoglobin A1C ≥6.5
  classic symptoms include polyuria, polydipsia, and weight loss
- Impaired glucose tolerance = FPG 100 to 125 mg/dL *OR*
  GCT 140 to 199 mg/dL *OR*
  hemoglobin A1C 5.7 to 6.4

- Patients with impaired glucose tolerance should be referred for counseling on weight loss, diet, and exercise; medical therapy may be initiated in high-risk obese patients.
- Upon diagnosis of diabetes, screening should be performed to evaluate for retinopathy, nephropathy, neuropathy, CHD, cerebrovascular disease, peripheral artery disease, and dental disease.

## Screening for Thyroid Disorders

- See Chapter 13.
- The USPSTF does not recommend screening asymptomatic people for hypothyroidism. ACOG recommends screening women older than 50 years with thyroid-stimulating hormone levels every 5 years. This should also be considered in younger patients with autoimmune disease or strong family history of thyroid disease.

## Counseling on Nutrition

- The 2010 United States Department of Agriculture Dietary Guidelines recommend consumption of a variety of nutrient-dense foods and beverages (such as fruits, vegetables, whole grains, and fat-free or low-fat dairy products and seafood). Additionally, they recommend limiting the intake of saturated and *trans* fats, sodium, cholesterol, added sugars, and refined grains. Specific recommendations include:
  - Adults older than age 50 years should consume supplemental vitamin $B_{12}$ either in the form of fortified foods or dietary supplements.
  - Pregnant women and women of childbearing age should consume foods high in iron and folic acid. At least 400 µg of supplemental folic acid per day is recommended in women capable of or considering becoming pregnant. Preferably, iron-rich foods should be taken with vitamin C to enhance absorption.
  - Older adults, people with darker skin tones, and those with minimal exposure to sunlight should consume at least 600 to 800 IU/day of supplemental vitamin D. Recommended daily for postmenopausal women is 1,200 mg of calcium, either in the form of calcium-rich foods or dietary supplements.
- Estimated caloric requirement for nonpregnant adult women varies between 1,800 and 2,400 kcal based on level of activity.

## Counseling on Obesity

- The 2007–2008 National Health and Nutrition Examination Survey reported that 35.5% of adult women are obese (body mass index [BMI] $\geq$30 kg/m$^2$). It is estimated that 64.1% of American women are either overweight (BMI $\geq$25 kg/m$^2$) or obese.
- Obesity is associated with an increased risk of morbidity including type 2 diabetes, hypertension, infertility, heart disease, gallbladder disease, uterine cancer, and colon cancer.
- Screening for obesity should include calculation of BMI, measurement of waist circumference, and evaluation of overall risk due to comorbid conditions.
- BMI is a measure of obesity which correlates with body fat content.
- Underweight = BMI <18.5 kg/m$^2$
- Overweight = BMI 25 to 29.9 kg/m$^2$
- Obese = BMI $\geq$30 kg/m$^2$
  - Class I obesity = BMI 30 to 34.9 kg/m$^2$
  - Class II obesity = BMI 35 to 39.9 kg/m$^2$
  - Class III (morbid) obesity = BMI $\geq$40 kg/m$^2$

• The USPSTF recommends that all patients identified as obese be referred for intensive counseling and behavioral interventions to improve diet and physical activity. Medications, such as orlistat and sibutramine, or bariatric surgery may be appropriate for some women.

## SCREENING FOR OTHER MEDICAL CONDITIONS

### Screening for Osteoporosis

• See Chapter 43.
• Bone mineral density examinations should be performed routinely at age 65 years (or age 60 years for women with risk factors) or in any postmenopausal woman with a fracture. Dual energy x-ray absorptiometry (DEXA) is the standard of care for measurement of bone density. The most important measurement to consider is the patient's T score, which reflects the patient's bone density compared to a healthy 30-year-old of the same age and sex.
  • Risk factors for low bone mineral density include low body weight (<70 kg), smoking, family history of osteoporosis, chronic corticosteroid use, sedentary lifestyle, alcohol or caffeine use, immobilization, use of antiepileptic medications, endocrine disorders (such as hyperparathyroidism, hyperthyroidism, hypogonadism, Cushing syndrome), low calcium or vitamin D intake, or a fragility fracture.
  • A T score of −1.0 to −2.5 indicates osteopenia.
  • A T score of less than −2.5 indicates osteoporosis.
• Minimal intervals between successive bone mineral density examinations should be >2 years.
• Treatment of low bone density consists of pharmacologic intervention with calcium, vitamin D, and bisphosphonates as well as weight-bearing exercise.
• Total daily calcium intake should be 1,200 mg and total daily vitamin D intake should be 800 IU for postmenopausal women.
• The Fracture Risk Assessment Tool (FRAX) is a model used to predict 10-year risk of fracture based on DEXA results, as well as other risk factors for decreased bone density. FRAX can be used to guide clinical decision making regarding pharmacologic intervention.

### Screening for Depression

• Depression affects over 30 million American adults yearly. The lifetime risk for women of developing a major depressive disorder is 10% to 25%, two to three times higher than for men.
• Factors that may predispose women to depression include perinatal loss, infertility, or miscarriage; physical or sexual abuse; socioeconomic deprivation; lack of support, isolation, and feelings of helplessness; family history of mood disorders; loss of a parent during childhood (before age 10 years); history of substance abuse; and menopause.
• The symptoms of depression are summarized by the mnemonic SIG EM CAPS (five out of nine symptoms must be present for over 2 weeks to fulfill the definition of major depression, including either depressed mood or loss of interest).
  • **S**leep: insomnia or hypersomnia
  • **I**nterest: markedly decreased interest or pleasure in activities
  • **G**uilt: feelings of worthlessness or inappropriate guilt nearly every day
  • **E**nergy: fatigue or loss of energy

- **M**ood: depressed mood most of the day
- **C**oncentration: diminished ability to think, concentrate, or make decisions
- **A**ppetite: significant appetite or weight change
- **P**sychomotor: observable psychomotor retardation or agitation
- **S**uicide: recurrent thoughts of death or suicide
- Dysthymic disorder is characterized by chronically depressed mood on most days for 2 or more years plus at least two of the symptoms from the list defining a major depressive episode.
- The USPSTF recommends screening adults for depression. Many patient questionnaires for self-reporting exist. Additionally, in patients who report feelings of depression, direct questioning about suicidal or homicidal ideation is essential.
- **Psychosocial treatment** may be used alone or in conjunction with antidepressant medication. For patients with mild to moderate depression, psychosocial therapies have been found to be as effective as pharmacologic treatment. Commonly used methods include behavioral therapy, cognitive behavioral therapy, and interpersonal therapy.
- **Pharmacologic treatment** for depression includes selective serotonin reuptake inhibitors, selective norepinephrine reuptake inhibitors, and tricyclic antidepressants. Patients with severe or chronic depression or failure to respond after 12 weeks of psychotherapy should be started on medication. A large percentage of women experience significant improvement or even complete remission with medical treatment.

## Screening for Domestic Violence

- See Chapter 33.
- Health maintenance visits should include assessment for domestic violence using direct interview, patient questionnaires, or both (preferably while the patient is alone).

## Screening and Counseling for Substance Abuse

- The 2011 National Survey on Drug Use and Health found that 8% of Americans use illicit drugs, 27% engage in binge drinking, and 28% use tobacco products.
- All patients should be questioned on substance abuse; a number of screening tools exist (e.g., the CAGE questions, AUDIT-C, TWEAK, and CRAFFT questionnaires).
- The CAGE questionnaire has been shown to lack sensitivity among women and minorities. Therefore, ACOG recommends modified version, the TACE questionnaire, with a positive screen being 2 or more points:
  - Tolerance: How many drinks does it take to feel high? (more than two drinks = 2 points)
  - Annoyed: Have people annoyed you by criticizing your drinking? (positive response = 1 point)
  - Cut down: Have you ever felt you ought to cut down your drinking? (positive response = 1 point)
  - Eye opener: Have you ever had a drink first thing in the morning to steady your nerves or get rid of a hangover? (positive response = 1 point)
- The USPSTF recommends counseling for reducing alcohol abuse; brief 15-minute counseling interventions have been shown to reduce hazardous drinking.
- The USPSTF *strongly* recommends screening for tobacco use and counseling for cessation as it has been shown that 1 to 3 minutes of counseling significantly increases abstinence rates.
- Medical interventions include nicotine replacement therapy, bupropion, and varenicline.

## COUNSELING

- The routine health maintenance visit is an ideal time to counsel patients regarding many health-related behaviors.
- Several techniques for brief physician counseling have been developed, including the five *a*'s model:
  - *Assess* for problem.
  - *Advise* making a change.
  - *Agree* on action to be taken.
  - *Assist* with self-care support to make the change.
  - *Arrange* follow-up to support the change.
- It is important to recognize a patient's state of readiness, as an estimated 80% of people are unprepared to commit to a lifestyle change at initial encounter. The Stages of Change Model includes the following:
  - Precontemplation: no intention of changing behavior. Goal of counseling = introduce ambivalence.
  - Contemplation: considering making a change. Goal of counseling = explore both sides of the patient's attitude and help resolve behavior.
  - Preparation: resolved to make a change. Goal of counseling = identify successful strategies for change.
  - Action: making a change in behavior. Goal of counseling = provide solutions to deal with specific relapse triggers.
  - Maintenance: committed to change. Goal of counseling = solidify the patient's commitment to a continued change.

## IMMUNIZATIONS

Immunizations are an integral component of primary and preventive health care. A patient's vaccination history should be reviewed at regular intervals and updated as appropriate (see Figs. 1-1 and 1-2).

## OTHER PRIMARY CARE PROBLEMS

- **Urinary tract infections:** For uncomplicated cystitis, a 3-day course of trimethoprim-sulfamethoxazole is generally the first-line recommendation. Alternatives include fluoroquinolones or nitrofurantoin. Empiric antibiotic treatment without urine culture is appropriate in the nongravid patient if the patient displays dysuria and has urine leukocytes and nitrites present on urinalysis. The presence of fever or costovertebral angle tenderness is suggestive of an upper tract infection which requires more aggressive treatment. See Chapter 16.
- **Upper respiratory infections:** Typically viral in origin, mild upper respiratory infections should be treated supportively with rest, hydration, humidifier, and over-the-counter pharmacologic interventions (cough suppressants and decongestants). Antibiotics are not recommended as first line for treatment of uncomplicated upper respiratory illnesses. The presence of secondary bacterial infection is suggested by persistence of rhinosinusitis symptoms for 7 to 10 days and purulent nasal discharge, unilateral tooth, facial or maxillary sinus pain, or worsening symptoms after initial improvement. Patients with severe pain, fever, and failure of improvement

## Recommended Adult Immunization Schedule—United States - 2013

**Note: These recommendations must be read with the footnotes that follow containing number of doses, intervals between doses, and other important information.**

| VACCINE ▼ / AGE GROUP ► | 19-21 years | 22-26 years | 27-49 years | 50-59 years | 60-64 years | ≥ 65 years |
|---|---|---|---|---|---|---|
| Influenza [2,*] | 1 dose annually | | | | | |
| Tetanus, diphtheria, pertussis (Td/Tdap) [3,*] | Substitute 1-time dose of Tdap for Td booster; then boost with Td every 10 yrs | | | | | |
| Varicella [4,*] | 2 doses | | | | | |
| Human papillomavirus (HPV) Female [5,*] | 3 doses | | | | | |
| Human papillomavirus (HPV) Male [5,*] | 3 doses | | | | | |
| Zoster [6] | | | | | 1 dose | |
| Measles, mumps, rubella (MMR) [7,*] | 1 or 2 doses | | | | | |
| Pneumococcal polysaccharide (PPSV23) [8,9] | 1 or 2 doses | | | | | 1 dose |
| Pneumococcal 13-valent conjugate (PCV13) [10,*] | 1 dose | | | | | |
| Meningococcal [11,*] | 1 or more doses | | | | | |
| Hepatitis A [12,*] | 2 doses | | | | | |
| Hepatitis B [13,*] | 3 doses | | | | | |

*Covered by the Vaccine Injury Compensation Program

For all persons in this category who meet the age requirements and who lack documentation of vaccination or have no evidence of previous infection; zoster vaccine recommended regardless of prior episode of zoster

Recommended if some other risk factor is present (e.g., on the basis of medical, occupational, lifestyle, or other indication)

No recommendation

Report all clinically significant postvaccination reactions to the Vaccine Adverse Event Reporting System (VAERS). Reporting forms and instructions on filing a VAERS report are available at www.vaers.hhs.gov or by telephone, 800-822-7967.

Information on how to file a Vaccine Injury Compensation Program claim is available at www.hrsa.gov/vaccinecompensation or by telephone, 800-338-2382. To file a claim for vaccine injury, contact the U.S. Court of Federal Claims, 717 Madison Place, N.W., Washington, D.C. 20005; telephone, 202-357-6400.

Additional information about the vaccines in this schedule, extent of available data, and contraindications for vaccination is also available at www.cdc.gov/vaccines or from the CDC-INFO Contact Center at 800-CDC-INFO (800-232-4636) in English and Spanish, 8:00 a.m. - 8:00 p.m. Eastern Time, Monday - Friday, excluding holidays.

Use of trade names and commercial sources is for identification only and does not imply endorsement by the U.S. Department of Health and Human Services.

**The recommendations in this schedule were approved by the Centers for Disease Control and Prevention's (CDC) Advisory Committee on Immunization Practices (ACIP), the American Academy of Family Physicians (AAFP), the American College of Physicians (ACP), American College of Obstetricians and Gynecologists (ACOG) and American College of Nurse-Midwives (ACNM).**

**Figure 1-1.** Recommended U.S. adult immunization schedule by vaccine and age group, 2013. (Adapted from Centers for Disease Control and Prevention. Recommended U.S. adult immunization schedule by vaccine and age group, 2013. Centers for Disease Control and Prevention Web site. http://www.cdc.gov/vaccines/schedules/index.html. Accessed February 10, 2013.)

| VACCINE ▼ INDICATION ▶ | Pregnancy | Immuno-compromising conditions (excluding human immunodeficiency virus [HIV])[4,6,7,10,13] | HIV infection CD4+ T lymphocyte count[3,4,6,7,10,13] < 200 cells/μL | HIV infection CD4+ T lymphocyte count[3,4,6,7,10,13] ≥ 200 cells/μL | Men who have sex with men (MSM) | Heart disease, chronic lung disease, chronic alcoholism | Asplenia (including elective splenectomy and persistent complement component deficiencies)[10,14] | Chronic liver disease | Kidney failure, end-stage renal disease, receipt of hemodialysis | Diabetes | Healthcare personnel |
|---|---|---|---|---|---|---|---|---|---|---|---|
| Influenza[2,*] | 1 dose Tdap each pregnancy | 1 dose IIV annually | | | 1 dose IIV or LAIV annually | | | 1 dose IIV annually | | 1 dose IIV or LAIV annually | 1 dose IIV or LAIV annually |
| Tetanus, diphtheria, pertussis (Td/Tdap)[3,*] | | Substitute 1-time dose of Tdap for Td booster; then boost with Td every 10 yrs | | | | | | | | | |
| Varicella[4,*] | Contraindicated | | | 2 doses | | | | | | | |
| Human papillomavirus (HPV) Female[5,*] | | 3 doses through age 26 yrs | | | | | | | | | |
| Human papillomavirus (HPV) Male[5,*] | | 3 doses through age 26 yrs | | | 3 doses through age 21 yrs | | | | | | |
| Zoster[6] | Contraindicated | | | 1 dose | | | | | | | |
| Measles, mumps, rubella (MMR)[7,*] | Contraindicated | | | 1 or 2 doses | | | | | | | |
| Pneumococcal polysaccharide (PPSV23)[8,9] | | | | | 1 or 2 doses | | | | | | |
| Pneumococcal 13-valent conjugate (PCV13)[10,*] | | | | | 1 dose | | | | | | |
| Meningococcal[11,*] | | | | | 1 or more doses | | | | | | |
| Hepatitis A[12,*] | | | | | 2 doses | | | | | | |
| Hepatitis B[13,*] | | | | | 3 doses | | | | | | |

*Covered by the Vaccine Injury Compensation Program

For all persons in this category who meet the age requirements and who lack documentation of vaccination or have no evidence of previous infection; zoster vaccine recommended regardless of prior episode of zoster

Recommended if some other risk factor is present (e.g., on the basis of medical, occupational, lifestyle, or other indications)

No recommendation

These schedules indicate the recommended age groups and medical indications for which administration of currently licensed vaccines is commonly indicated for adults aged 19 years and older, as of January 1, 2013. For all vaccines being recommended on the Adult Immunization Schedule: a vaccine series does not need to be restarted, regardless of the time that has elapsed between doses. Licensed combination vaccines may be used whenever any components of the combination are indicated and when the vaccine's other components are not contraindicated. For detailed recommendations on all vaccines, including those used primarily for travelers or that are issued during the year, consult the manufacturers' package inserts and the complete statements from the Advisory Committee on Immunization Practices (www.cdc.gov/vaccines/pubs/acip-list.htm). Use of trade names and commercial sources is for identification only and does not imply endorsement by the U.S. Department of Health and Human Services.

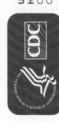

U.S. Department of Health and Human Services
Centers for Disease Control and Prevention

**Figure 1-2.** Recommended vaccinations indicated for adults based on medical and other indications schedule, 2013. (Adapted from Centers for Disease Control and Prevention. Recommended U.S. adult immunization schedule by vaccine and age group, 2013. Centers for Disease Control and Prevention Web site. http://www.cdc.gov/vaccines/schedules/index.html. Accessed February 10, 2013.)

after a period of observation should be treated with narrow-spectrum antibiotics such as amoxicillin, trimethoprim-sulfamethoxazole, or a macrolide for 10 to 14 days. See Chapter 15.

- **Asthma:** In addition to monitoring lung function and reducing exposure to triggers, pharmacologic treatment is conducted in a stepwise fashion. Mild intermittent asthma may be treated with quick-acting inhaled beta-agonists such as albuterol. For mild persistent asthma, add a low-dose inhaled glucocorticoid or leukotriene blocker. Patients with moderate persistent asthma may be treated with medium-dose inhaled glucocorticoid plus long-acting inhaled beta-agonist or a high-dose inhaled glucocorticoid. Severe, acute asthma exacerbations may necessitate oral or intravenous corticosteroids or inpatient admission. In addition to vital signs and physical examination, measurement of peak flow can help direct changes in pharmacologic therapy in patients with asthma. Patients with severe asthma should be referred to a pulmonologist or allergist for further management. See Chapter 15.

## SUGGESTED READINGS

American College of Obstetricians and Gynecologists. Practice bulletin no. 122: breast cancer screening. *Obstet Gynecol* 2011;118:372–382.

American College of Obstetricians and Gynecologists Committee on Gynecologic Practice. Committee opinion no. 482: colonoscopy and colorectal cancer screening strategies. *Obstet Gynecol* 2011;177:766–771.

American College of Obstetricians and Gynecologists Committee on Gynecologic Practice. Committee opinion no. 534: well-woman visit. *Obstet Gynecol* 2012;120:421–424.

American College of Obstetricians and Gynecologists Committee on Practice Bulletins— Gynecology. ACOG practice bulletin number 129: osteoporosis. *Obstet Gynecol* 2012;120:718–734.

American College of Obstetricians and Gynecologists; Society of Gynecologic Oncologists. ACOG practice bulletin no. 103: hereditary breast and ovarian cancer syndrome. *Obstet Gynecol* 2009;113:957–966.

American Diabetes Association. Diagnosis and classification of diabetes mellitus. *Diabetes Care* 2012;35(suppl 1):S64–S71.

American Gastroenterological Association. American Gastroenterological Association medical position statement on obesity. *Gastroenterology* 2002;123:879.

Centers for Disease Control and Prevention web site: http://www.cdc.gov/. Accessed February 10, 2013.

Chobanian AV, Bakris GL, Black HR, et al. The seventh report of the Joint National Committee on Prevention, Detection, Evaluation, and Treatment of High Blood Pressure. *JAMA* 2003;289:2560–2572.

Flegal KM, Carroll MD, Ogden CL, et al. Prevalence and trends in obesity among US adults, 1999–2008. *JAMA* 2010;303(3):235–241.

Levin B, Lieberman DA, McFarland B, et al. Screening and surveillance for the early detection of colorectal cancer and adenomatous polyps, 2008: a joint guideline from the American Cancer Society, the US Multi-Society Task Force on Colorectal Cancer, and the American College of Radiology. *Gastroenterology* 2008;134(5):1570–1595.

National Cholesterol Education Program Expert Panel on Detection, Evaluation, and Treatment of High Blood Cholesterol in Adults (Adult Treatment Panel III). Third Report of the National Cholesterol Education Program (NCEP) expert panel on detection, evaluation, and treatment of high blood cholesterol in adults (Adult Treatment Panel III) final report. *Circulation* 2002;106(25):3143–3421.

U.S. Department of Health and Human Services, Agency for Healthcare Research and Quality. U.S. Preventive Services Task Force (USPSTF): an introduction. Agency for Healthcare Research and Quality Web site. http://www.ahrq.gov/professionals/clinicians-providers/guidelines-recommendations/uspstf/index.html. Accessed February 10, 2013.

U.S. Department of Health and Human Services; U.S. Department of Agriculture. *Dietary Guidelines for Americans, 2010.* 7th ed. Washington, DC: U.S. Government Printing Office. http://www.dietaryguidelines.gov. Accessed February 10, 2013.

Wender R, Fontham ET, Barrera E Jr, et al. American Cancer Society lung cancer screening guidelines. *CA Cancer J Clin* 2013;63(2):107–117.

World Health Organization Collaborating Centre for Metabolic Bone Diseases. WHO Fracture Risk Assessment Tool (FRAX). World Health Organization Collaborating Centre for Metabolic Bone Diseases Web site. http://www.shef.ac.uk/FRAX/tool.jsp. Accessed February 10, 2013.

# 2

# Breast Diseases

Abigail D. Winder and Jill Edwardson

**Breast cancer** is a common and devastating health issue for many women. One in eight women will develop breast cancer in her lifetime. Benign breast disease can be difficult to differentiate from malignant breast disease, and it is crucial that the gynecologist be able to evaluate and treat breast disease (Fig. 2-1).

## ANATOMY

- The borders of the adult breast are the second and sixth ribs in the vertical axis and the sternal edge and midaxillary line in the horizontal axis. A small portion of breast tissue also projects into the axilla, forming the *axillary tail of Spence*.
- The breast is composed of three major tissues: skin, subcutaneous tissue, and breast tissue. The breast tissue, in turn, consists of parenchyma and stroma. The parenchyma is divided into 15 to 20 segments that converge at the nipple in a radial arrangement. There are between 5 and 10 collecting ducts that open into the nipple. Each duct gives rise to buds that form 15 to 20 lobules, and each lobule consists of 10 to 100 alveoli, which constitute the gland.
- The breast is enveloped by fascial tissue. The superficial pectoral fascia envelops the breast and is continuous with the superficial abdominal fascia of Camper. The undersurface of the breast lies on the deep pectoral fascia, covering the pectoralis major and serratus anterior muscles. Connecting the two fascial layers are fibrous bands (Cooper suspensory ligaments) that are the natural support of the breast.
- The principal blood supply to the breast is the *internal mammary artery*, constituting two thirds of the total blood supply. The additional third, which supplies primarily the upper outer quadrant, is provided by the *lateral thoracic artery*. Nearly all of the lymphatic drainage of the breast is to the axillary nodes. The internal mammary nodes also receive drainage from all quadrants of the breast and are an unusual, but potential, site of metastasis.
- The majority of abnormalities in the breast that result in biopsy are due to benign breast disease. Benign abnormalities can result in pain, a mass, calcifications, and nipple discharge. Similar findings can be present in malignant disease.

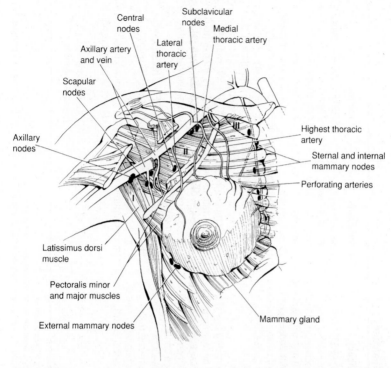

**Figure 2-1.** Anatomy of the breast. Roman numerals (I, II, III) indicate axillary lymph node levels. (From Green VL. Breast diseases: benign and malignant. In Rock JA, Jones HW, eds. *TeLinde's Operative Gynecology*, 10th ed. Philadelphia, PA: Lippincott Williams & Wilkins, 2008, with permission.)

- For the purposes of delineating metastatic progression, the axillary lymph nodes are categorized into levels. Level I lymph nodes lie lateral to the outer border of the pectoralis minor muscle, level II nodes lie behind the pectoralis minor muscle, and level III nodes are located medial to the medial border of the pectoralis minor muscle.

## SCREENING AND DIAGNOSIS

The main screening modalities include clinical breast exam, breast self-exam, and screening mammography (Table 2-1). Diagnostic modalities include diagnostic mammography and breast biopsy (including fine needle, core, and excisional). Additional diagnostic modalities include ultrasound and magnetic resonance imaging (MRI).

### Breast Exam

- The clinical breast examination (CBE) should be part of the gynecologic examination (Fig. 2-2) and is best for detecting tumors greater than 2 cm in size. The National Breast and Cervical Cancer Early Detection Program found that CBE detects approximately 5% of cancers that are not visible on mammography. Also, it

**TABLE 2-1** Breast Cancer Screening Techniques and Guidelines

| | Application | Sensitivity/Efficacy | Limitations | Guidelines[a] |
|---|---|---|---|---|
| Mammography | Detects microcalcifications, abnormal shadowing, or soft tissue distortion | Sensitivity 74%–95%<br>Specificity 89%–99%<br>Sensitivity is decreased in women younger than age 50 years and in women with dense breasts.<br>Reduces risk of cancer-related mortality by 16%–35% | Less sensitive for faster growing tumors (young women)<br>Breast density<br>Hormone therapy<br>Breast implants | USPSTF: ≥50–74, every 2 years<br>ACOG: 40–49, every 1–2 years, then ≥50–75 years, annually<br>ACS: 40–69, annually<br>NCI: ≥40, every 1–2 years |
| Clinical breast exam | Inspection and palpation in the supine and sitting positions, including axillary and supraclavicular lymph nodes as well as nipple and areola<br>Recommended 6–10 min | Sensitivity 54%<br>Specificity 94%<br>Detects approximately 5% of cancers missed by mammography<br>Most studies show efficiency in conjunction with mammography—likely that each contributes | Examiner dependent<br>Less specificity than mammography—higher rate of biopsy for benign disease<br>Limited in obese women | USPSTF: insufficient evidence<br>ACOG: 20–39, every 1–3 years, then annually<br>ACS: 20–39, every 3 years, then annually |
| Breast self-examination | Monthly exams, during approximately 10th day of cycle | Sensitivity 20%–30%<br>Very few randomized trials<br>Failed to show benefit in rate of diagnosis, cancer death, or tumor size | Examiner dependent<br>Higher rate of biopsy for benign disease<br>Studies limited | USPSTF: do not support teaching self-breast exams<br>ACS: Inform women regarding benefits and limitations.<br>ACOG: supports self-breast awareness |

Screening recommendations differ for patients with a family or personal history of breast cancer.

[a]A summary of guidelines can be found at the National Guideline Clearinghouse. Available at: http://www.guideline.gov.
USPSTF, U.S. Preventive Services Task Force; ACOG, American College of Obstetricians and Gynecologists; ACS, American Cancer Society; NCI, National Cancer Institute.

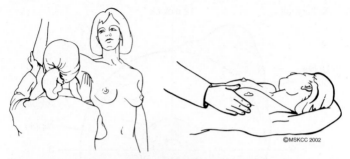

©MSKCC 2002

**Figure 2-2.** Breast examination. (From Scott JR, Gibbs RS, Karlan BY, et al. *Danforth's Obstetrics and Gynecology*, 9th ed. Philadelphia, PA: Lippincott Williams & Wilkins, 2003:892–893, with permission.)

offers an opportunity to demonstrate the technique of breast self-examination and to encourage women to perform this examination on a regular basis. The examination consists of:

- Inspection and palpation of the breasts in the supine and sitting positions, with hands above the head and then on the hips. The supine position flattens the breast tissue against the chest, allowing for a more thorough exam.
- Observation of the contour, symmetry, and vascular pattern of the breasts for signs of skin retraction, edema, or erythema in each of the previously mentioned positions
- Systematic palpation of each breast, the axilla, and supraclavicular areas in a circular motion using light, medium, and deep pressures. Use the pads of the three middle fingers to palpate for masses. A vertical strip pattern appears more thorough than concentric circles. To ensure that all breast tissue is examined, cover a rectangular area bordered superiorly by the clavicle, laterally by the midaxillary line, and inferiorly by the bra line.
- Evaluation for nipple discharge, crusting, or ulceration
- For the anatomic location and description of tumors or disease, the surface of the breast is divided into four quadrants and the numbers of the face of a clock are used as reference points (Fig. 2-3). A finding may be described as "a hard mass palpated in the upper inner quadrant of the right breast at the 2 o'clock position, approximately 2 cm from the nipple."
- The clinical use of **breast self-examination** is controversial (see Table 2-1). **Breast self-awareness** is a woman's awareness of the normal appearance and feel of her breasts and may or may not include breast self-examination. She is encouraged to discuss any changes in her breasts with her health care provider.

## Mammography

- Although mammography remains the primary screening modality for breast cancer, <40% of women actually undergo annual mammography. Breast cancers detected by mammography tend to be smaller and have more favorable histologic and biologic features. Limitations to mammography include patient age, rate of tumor growth, density of breast tissue, use of hormone replacement therapy (HRT), and breast implants. Approximately 5% to 15% of cancers are not apparent on mammography, and all palpable lesions require biopsy.

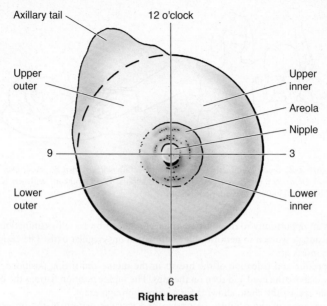

**Right breast**

Figure 2-3. Breast quadrants. For the anatomic location and description of tumors, the surface of the breast is divided into four quadrants. (From Moore KL, Dalley AF. *Clinically Oriented Anatomy*, 4th ed. Baltimore, MD: Lippincott Williams & Wilkins, 1999:74, with permission.)

- **Screening mammography** is for women with no signs or symptoms of breast disease and consists of bilateral two-view images. Mammography can potentially detect lesions as small as 1 mm. Digital mammography is more effective than film mammography, especially for women younger than 60 years or with dense breasts.
- **Diagnostic mammography** presents various views (e.g., spot compression, magnification) and localization techniques and is usually used after the discovery of an abnormal finding on clinical exam, self-exam, or screening mammography. Mammography is an essential part of the evaluation of a patient with clinically evident breast cancer. In this situation, mammography is useful for evaluating other areas of the breast as well as the contralateral breast.

## Abnormal Mammogram

- Suspicious radiologic findings require surgical consultation and consideration of breast biopsy, even with an unremarkable physical examination.
- **Radiologic findings of concern on mammography:**
  - Soft tissue density, especially if borders are not well defined
  - Clustered microcalcifications in one area
  - Calcification within or closely associated with a soft tissue density
  - Asymmetric density or parenchymal distortion
  - New abnormality compared with previous mammogram
- When a woman's screening mammography is ambiguous, diagnostic mammography should be performed with possible radiographically directed biopsy. Biopsy

techniques for radiographically identified nonpalpable lesions include needle localization, excisional biopsy, and stereotactic core biopsy. If the mammographic studies are inconclusive, a short-term follow-up study at 3 to 6 months can be considered (Table 2-2).

## Alternate Screening Modalities

• **Ultrasound:** Although ultrasound is not a substitute for mammography, it has become a common tool in the evaluation of breast lesions. Ultrasound is particularly useful in differentiating cystic from solid lesions and is most commonly used

| TABLE 2-2 | American College of Radiology Breast Imaging Reporting and Data System Mammography Assessment Categories | | |
|---|---|---|---|
| Category | Assessment | Definition | Likelihood Ratio for Breast Cancer Diagnosis[a] |
| 1 | Negative | Breasts appear normal. | 0.1 |
| 2 | Benign finding(s) | A negative mammogram result, but the interpreter wishes to describe a finding | 0.1 |
| 3 | Probably benign finding—short interval follow-up suggested | Lesion with a high probability of being benign | 1.2 |
| 0 | Needs additional imaging evaluation and/or previous mammograms for comparison | Lesion noted— additional imaging is needed; used almost always in a screening situation | 7.0 |
| 4 | Suspicious abnormality—biopsy should be considered | A lesion is noted for which the radiologist has sufficient concern to recommend biopsy. | 125 |
| 5 | Highly suggestive of malignancy—appropriate action should be taken | A lesion is noted that has a high probability of being cancer. | 2,200 |

[a]Likelihood ratio at first screening mammography: ratio of diseased to nondiseased persons for a given test result.
From Kerlikowske K, Smith-Bindman R, Ljung BM, et al. Evaluation of abnormal mammography results and palpable breast abnormalities. *Ann Intern Med* 2003;139:274–284, with permission.

in evaluating lesions in young women, especially those younger than age 40 years. It can also be used as an adjunctive screening tool in women with dense or cystic breasts or those with breast implants. Suspicious features include solid masses with ill-defined borders, acoustic shadowing, or complex cystic lesions. Ultrasound guidance also assists in diagnostic procedures, including biopsy or fine-needle aspiration.

- **MRI** has been shown in studies to be more sensitive but less specific and more expensive than mammography in the detection of breast cancers.
  - MRI screening is recommended for women with a greater than 20% lifetime risk of developing breast cancer. These include women with known BRCA1 or BRCA2 mutations, first-degree relatives of those with BRCA1 or BRCA2 mutations who have not undergone genetic testing, history of radiation therapy to the chest between ages 10 and 30 years, women with certain genetic syndromes (including Li-Fraumeni and Cowden syndromes), or a first-degree relative with one of those syndromes.
  - MRI screening is not recommended for women at average risk of developing breast cancer.

## COMMON BREAST DISORDERS AND COMPLAINTS

Approximately 16% of women ages 40 to 69 years seek a physician's advice over breast-related complaints in any 10-year period, with the most common complaint being a breast lump (40%). Other common complaints include nipple discharge and breast pain. Breast cancer will account for only 10% of these complaints and the failure to diagnose breast cancer is high on the list of malpractice claims in the United States. The most common reasons for breast-related lawsuits against obstetrician-gynecologists are "physical findings failed to impress" and "failure to refer to the specialist for biopsy." Physicians must be prepared to fully evaluate, address, and educate patients regarding their concerns.

### Mastalgia

- Breast pain may be cyclic or noncyclic. Cyclic breast pain is maximal premenstrually and is relieved with the onset of menses. It can be either unilateral or bilateral and may be associated with fibrocystic changes. Fibrocystic pain is primarily localized to the subareolar or upper outer regions of the breast. This pain is likely due to stromal edema, ductal dilation, and some degree of inflammation. Microcysts in fibrocystic disease can progress to form palpable macrocysts.
- Noncyclic pain can have various causes, including hormonal fluctuations, firm adenomas, duct ectasia, and macrocysts. It may also arise from musculoskeletal structures, such as soreness in the pectoral muscles from exertion or trauma, stretching of the Cooper ligaments, or costochondritis. Mastitis and hidradenitis suppurativa may present with breast pain. With most noncyclic breast pain, no definite cause is determined. Carcinoma can present with breast pain (<10%), but this is uncommon. The evaluation of breast pain includes a careful history and physical, as well as mammography for women older than age 35 years. The primary value of mammography is to provide reassurance. Patients with no dominant mass can be reassured.
- In most cases, mastalgia resolves spontaneously, although sometimes only after months or years. Restriction of methylxanthine-containing substances (e.g., coffee, tea) has not been shown to be superior to placebo, but some patients may note relief.

Pain from a macrocyst may be relieved with aspiration. Symptomatic relief may be achieved with a supportive brassiere, acetaminophen, or a nonsteroidal anti-inflammatory drug (NSAID). Finally, cyclic pain may be partially relieved with oral contraceptives, thiazide diuretic, danazol, or tamoxifen.

## Breast Mass

- Evaluation of a palpable breast mass requires a careful personal history, family history, physical examination, and radiographic examination. A breast mass reported by the patient should undergo the same evaluation, even if it fails to be appreciated on physical exam.

- In general, breast tissue can be lumpy and irregular. The following are characteristics concerning for cancerous lesions: single, hard, immobile, irregular margins, and >2 cm. In the majority of cases, cancerous masses are painless, but 10% of patients with cancer present with some symptoms of breast discomfort. Symptoms that may be associated with breast cancer include nipple discharge, nipple rash or ulceration, diffuse erythema of the breast, adenopathy, or symptoms associated with metastatic disease.

- Diagnostic mammography is recommended in the evaluation of any woman older than age 35 years with a palpable breast mass. Findings suspicious for cancer on mammography include increased density, irregular margins, spiculation, or an accompanying cluster of microcalcifications (Fig. 2-4).

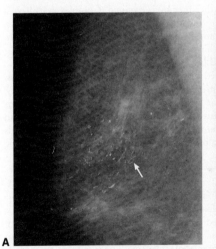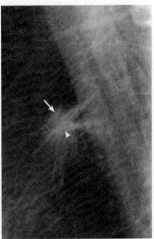

**A**          **B**

**Figure 2-4.** (**A**) A 53-year-old woman with bloody discharge from the nipple. Mediolateral view of the right breast demonstrates casting calcifications involving a large part of the breast extending to the nipple. The calcifications are nonuniform, irregular, and branched (*arrow*), and they form a dot–dash linear pattern. They are aligned with the ductal system. (**B**) A 60-year-old woman with a palpable mass and no other pertinent history. Mediolateral view of the right breast reveals a spiculated mass (*arrow*) with architectural distortion. Within the center of the mass, irregular (pleomorphic) microcalcifications are present (*arrowhead*). The diagnosis is carcinoma, largely DCIS, of comedo type (**A**) and invasive ductal carcinoma, not otherwise specified (**B**). (From Pope TL Jr. *Aunt Minnie's Atlas and Imaging Specific Diagnosis*, 2nd ed. Philadelphia, PA: Lippincott Williams & Wilkins, 2003:329, with permission.)

- In women younger than age 35 years, ultrasonography may be used to distinguish a simple cyst from a more worrisome complex cyst, solid mass, or tumor.
- Fine-needle aspiration, core needle biopsy, or excisional biopsy can be used for ultimate tissue diagnosis of the palpable mass. Bloody fluid yielded on aspiration or persistence of a mass after aspiration should prompt excisional biopsy or surgical consultation.
- The combination of physical examination, mammography, and fine-needle aspiration biopsy is referred to as *triple diagnosis*. Fewer than 1% of breast cancers are missed using this diagnostic approach.
- **Benign breast masses** include fibroadenomas, breast cysts, or fat necrosis.
  - **Fibroadenoma** is the most common mass lesion found in women younger than 25 years of age. Growth is gradual, and occasional cystic tenderness may be present. If the lesion is palpable, increasing in size, or psychologically disturbing, core or excisional biopsy should be considered. Conservative treatment may be appropriate for small lesions that are not palpable and have been identified as fibroadenomas. Carcinoma within a fibroadenoma is a rare occurrence. A rare malignant tumor that can be confused with fibroadenoma is *cystosarcoma phyllodes*, which is treated by wide resection with negative margins. Local recurrence is uncommon, and distant metastasis is very rare.
  - **Breast cysts** can be found in premenopausal or postmenopausal women. Physical examination cannot distinguish cysts from solid masses. Ultrasonography and cyst aspiration are diagnostic. Simple cysts have a thin wall with no internal echoes and are benign. In these cases, no further therapy is required. Complex cysts have a thickened wall or internal septation and are considered suspicious. Complex cysts generally undergo some form of biopsy. If a cyst does not resolve with aspiration, yields a bloody aspirate, recurs within 6 weeks, or is complex on ultrasound evaluation, surgical consultation should be obtained.
  - **Fat necrosis** is frequently associated with breast trauma resulting in a breast mass. It can occur after breast biopsy, infection, duct ectasia, reduction mammoplasty, lumpectomy, and radiotherapy for breast carcinoma. Fat necrosis is most common in the subareolar region. This process can be difficult to distinguish from breast cancer on both physical examination and mammography. The lesion needs to be evaluated like any other palpable breast lesion. Only a benign histologic appearance affords reassurance.

## Breast Infections

- **Puerperal mastitis** is an acute cellulitis of the breast in a lactating woman. Mastitis usually occurs in the early weeks of breast-feeding. On inspection, cellulitis is often present in a wedge-shaped pattern over a portion of the breast skin, and tissue is warm, red, and tender. The infection is around rather than within the duct system, leading to the absence of purulent discharge from the nipple. Patients may present with high fevers, chills, flu-like malaise, and body aches. The most common causal organism is *Staphylococcus aureus*. Prompt initiation of antibiotic therapy, usually with dicloxacillin (500 mg by mouth four times a day for 10 days), reduces the risk of abscess formation. Aggressive emptying of the affected breast is an important treatment. The patient should be encouraged to continue breast-feeding or pumping to promote drainage. Warm compresses and manual pressure are also beneficial. Microbiologic culture is indicated if the mastitis does not resolve or if an abscess develops. The latter case also warrants incision and drainage.

- **Nonpuerperal mastitis** is an uncommon, subareolar infection. In contrast to puerperal mastitis, nonpuerperal mastitis is usually a polymicrobial infection and the woman is generally not systemically ill. Antibiotic coverage typically includes clindamycin or metronidazole, in addition to a beta-lactam antibiotic. All breast inflammation must raise concern for inflammatory breast cancer, and the threshold for performing a skin biopsy should be low, particularly in the elderly population. Failure to respond to antibiotic treatment should prompt biopsy in any patient. Finally, the patient should be up-to-date with mammography screening.

## NIPPLE DISCHARGE

- **Nipple discharge** is a common complaint and finding on examination of the breast. Nipple discharge is usually benign (95% of cases). The causes of discharge range from physiologic to endocrine-related to pathologic. See Figure 2-5 for an algorithm for evaluation of nipple discharge.
- **Physiologic secretion** from the nipple during examination or nipple stimulation is a common occurrence. As many as 50% to 80% of women in their reproductive years can express one or more drops of fluid. This benign discharge is usually non-spontaneous, bilateral, and serous in character. If the remainder of the breast exam is normal, reassurance is sufficient, and no further workup is necessary.
- **Galactorrhea** is milk production unrelated to nursing or pregnancy and is typically a bilateral, multiductal discharge. Several endocrine abnormalities give rise to galactorrhea, such as dopamine inhibitors, hypothalamic/pituitary disease, hypothyroidism, postthoracotomy syndrome, and chronic renal failure. Chronic breast stimulation or exogenous estrogen via oral contraceptive pills may cause galactorrhea. One third of cases are idiopathic. Evaluation includes a careful history reviewing medications and recent trauma/stimulation of the breast and physical exam. Questioning includes symptoms of amenorrhea, hypothyroid disease, visual field changes, or new-onset headaches which may suggest the underlying cause of the galactorrhea. Further evaluation includes a prolactin level, thyroid function tests, and brain MRI if the prolactin level is elevated. Prolactin levels may be falsely elevated after meals, after breast examination, or based on diurnal variation.

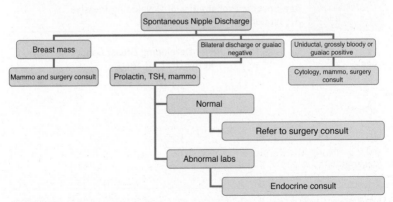

**Figure 2-5.** Algorithm for evaluation of nipple discharge. Mammo, mammogram; TSH, thyroid-stimulating hormone.

- **Pathologic discharge** is typically unilateral and spontaneous. It may be greenish gray, serous, or bloody. Causes of pathologic discharge are carcinoma, intraductal papilloma (straw-colored), duct ectasia, and fibrocystic changes. Only 5% of pathologic discharge is caused by carcinoma. A physical exam should attempt to identify the area of the breast and the specific duct from which the discharge is expressed. Skin lesions or an associated mass may be identified. If the fluid is not grossly bloody, guaiac testing may be performed to identify subtle bloody fluid. If grossly bloody or guaiac positive, cytology is performed; otherwise, the sensitivity of cytology is very low for malignancy. In addition, imaging with bilateral mammography is required. If the patient is younger than 35 years, ultrasound may also be used.

## BREAST CANCER

Breast cancer is the most common cancer affecting women in the United States and second only to lung cancer in cancer mortality for women. Median ages of diagnosis and of death are 61 and 69 years, respectively. Primarily due to improved screening, the prevalence of breast cancer has doubled in the past 50 years. The lifetime risk of breast cancer for a woman is 12.7% (about one in eight).

### Risk Factors

- The most commonly used model to determine breast cancer risk is the **Gail model**. The number of first-degree relatives with breast cancer, age at menarche, age at first live birth, number of breast biopsies, and presence of atypical hyperplasia on a breast biopsy are its components. Its accuracy is limited as it omits a detailed family history of breast and ovarian cancers and underestimates the risk in African American women and overestimates the risk in Asian American women. *This model should not be used in women who have a personal history of breast cancer or women who are known gene mutation carriers.*
- **Age** is the primary risk factor for breast cancer (Table 2-3). Approximately 95% of breast cancers occur in women older than 40 years of age.

| TABLE 2-3 | Age-Specific Probabilities of Developing Invasive Breast Cancer |
|---|---|
| Age | Probability of Developing Breast Cancer in the Next 10 Years |
| 20 | 1:1,681 |
| 30 | 1:232 |
| 40 | 1:69 |
| 50 | 1:42 |
| 60 | 1:29 |
| 70 | 1:27 |
| Lifetime | 1:8 |

From American Cancer Society. *Breast Cancer Facts and Figures 2011–2012.* Atlanta, GA: American Cancer Society, 2012.

- **Family history and genetic predisposition:** Family history confers an increased risk for breast cancer, specifically with a history of premenopausal breast cancer in a first-degree relative, male breast cancer, bilateral breast cancer, or a combination of breast and ovarian cancers within a family.
- BRCA1 and BRCA2 are tumor suppressor genes with autosomal dominant inheritance. Inheriting BRCA1 or BRCA2 confers a 40% to 85% lifetime risk of breast cancer, yet these cases account for <10% of all diagnoses. In addition, BRCA1 confers a 40% risk of ovarian cancer and BRCA2 a 20% risk for ovarian cancer. Both mutations are more common in the Ashkenazi Jewish population (1 in 40). Women with these mutations have a 35% to 43% chance of developing a second primary breast cancer within the first 10 years of her first breast cancer diagnosis and are at increased risk of pancreatic cancer (see Chapter 48).
- Patients with Li-Fraumeni syndrome, Cowden syndrome (multiple hamartoma syndrome), and Peutz-Jeghers syndrome are also at increased risk of developing breast cancer.
- **Hormone exposure:** Early menarche (<12 years), late natural menopause (>55 years), older age at first full-term pregnancy, and fewer pregnancies increase a woman's risk of developing breast cancer. Breast-feeding is associated with a lower risk of breast cancer. In addition, moderate alcohol use, which is related to an increase in estrogen, carries a higher risk. Finally, the role of exogenous estrogen use in the development of breast cancer remains controversial. Long-term oral contraceptive use (>10 years) and current hormone therapy use are associated with a nonsignificant increased risk of breast cancer.
- **Diet and lifestyle:** Significant differences in the incidence of breast cancer in different geographic and cultural areas have long raised the suspicion of dietary risk factors. High-fat diets have been implicated, but data are insufficient to support firm dietary advice for reduction in breast cancer risk. Lifestyle activities with protective effects include physical activity and weight control.
- **Personal history:** Women with a history of breast cancer are at a 0.5% to 1% risk per year of developing cancer in the contralateral breast, in addition to the risk of recurrence in the treated breast. The majority of recurrences occur within the first 5 years after diagnosis. A personal history of a benign breast biopsy or atypical hyperplasia also yields an increased risk, as does prior radiation therapy to the chest wall.

## Premalignant Conditions

- **Atypical hyperplasia** is a proliferative lesion of the breast that possesses some of the features of carcinoma in situ and should be considered premalignant. It carries a four- to fivefold increased risk of breast cancer, usually in the ipsilateral breast. Complete excision is recommended. Proliferative lesions, such as sclerosing adenosis, ductal epithelium hyperplasia, and intraductal papillomas, also carry an increased risk of cancer.
- **Lobular carcinoma in situ (LCIS)**, sometimes called *lobular neoplasia*, is a nonpalpable, noninvasive lesion arising from the lobules. LCIS is more common in premenopausal women and is often an incidental finding on biopsy. It is often multicentric and bilateral, and it is considered an indicator lesion or marker that identifies women at increased risk of subsequent invasive cancer. Absolute risk of developing invasive cancer is approximately 1% per year. Management is controversial and includes observation, tamoxifen administration, or prophylactic mastectomy to reduce the risk of developing subsequent breast cancer.

## Pathology

- Breast cancer most commonly arises in the upper outer quadrant of the breast, taking an average of 5 years to become palpable. It arises in the terminal duct-lobular unit of the breast and can be invasive or noninvasive (in situ). The growth pattern is described as comedo or noncomedo (solid, cribriform, micropapillary, and papillary).
- **Ductal carcinoma in situ (DCIS)**, also called *intraductal cancer*, refers to a proliferation of cancer cells within the ducts without invasion through the basement membrane into the surrounding stroma. Histologically, DCIS can be divided into multiple subtypes: solid, micropapillary, cribriform, and comedo. DCIS can also be graded as low, intermediate, or high. DCIS is an early, noninfiltrating form of breast cancer with minimal risk of metastasis and an excellent prognosis with surgical therapy with or without radiation therapy. The goal of treatment of DCIS is to prevent the development of invasive breast cancer. With the increased use of mammography, DCIS is being diagnosed more often.
- **Invasive cancer:** The two most common types of invasive cancers are lobular and ductal. **Infiltrating lobular** carcinoma is a variant associated with microscopic lobular architecture. These carcinomas account for 10% to 15% of invasive breast cancers, are often multifocal, have a higher incidence of bilaterality, and are less evident on mammography. **Infiltrating ductal** carcinoma accounts for 60% to 75% of all tumors. These cancers account for a group of tumors classified by cell type, architecture, and pattern of spread. These include mucinous, tubular, and medullary carcinomas.

## Staging and Prognostic Factors

- The tumor-node-metastasis (TNM) staging system for breast cancer from the American Joint Committee on Cancer uses tumor size, axillary node status (incorporating sentinel nodes), and metastasis status (Tables 2-4 and 2-5). Prognosis is strongly correlated with tumor size and node status. Expression of estrogen and progesterone receptors in tumor tissue is associated with a better prognosis and can assist in systemic treatment. Other prognostic factors include tumor grade, tumor size, and expression of the *human epidermal growth factor receptor 2 (HER2/neu)* oncogene.
- **HER2/neu** is a gene encoding transmembrane receptors for growth factors, thus regulating cellular growth and differentiation. Overexpression of this oncogene leads to a more aggressive subtype of breast cancer, which tends to be poorly differentiated and high grade. They have high rates of lymph node involvement and are more resistant to conventional chemotherapy. All newly diagnosed invasive breast cancer patients should have HER2 status checked.

## Treatment

Early detection is the key to improved survival (Table 2-6). In general, clinical stage I, IIA, or IIB, and certain patients with clinical stage IIIA disease (T3N0) are considered early stages of breast cancer. These patients are generally treated with surgery to the breast and regional lymph nodes with or without radiation therapy. Systemic therapy may be offered based on primary tumor characteristics, such as hormone and HER2 receptor status, lymph node involvement, and tumor size and grade. Treatment for locally advanced breast cancers (clinical stage IIIA with T0 to T3, N2 disease, or T4 disease) includes multimodal therapy.

| TABLE 2-4 | TNM Classification of Breast Cancer |
|---|---|

| Notation | Description |
|---|---|
| **Tumor size** | |
| TX | Primary tumor cannot be assessed |
| T0 | No evidence of primary tumor |
| Tis | Carcinoma in situ: intraductal carcinoma, LCIS, or Paget disease of the nipple with no tumor |
| T1 | Tumor 2 cm in greatest dimension |
| T1a | Tumor 0.5 cm in greatest dimension |
| T1b | Tumor >0.5 cm but 1 cm in greatest dimension |
| T1c | Tumor >1 cm but 2 cm in greatest dimension |
| T2 | Tumor >2 cm but 5 cm in greatest dimension |
| T3 | Tumor >5 cm in greatest dimension |
| T4 | Tumor of any size with direct extension to the chest wall or skin |
| T4a | Extension to the chest wall |
| T4b | Edema (including *peau d'orange*) or ulceration of the skin of the breast or satellite skin |
| T4c | Both T4a and T4b |
| T4d | Inflammatory carcinoma |
| **Lymph node metastases** | |
| NX | Regional lymph nodes cannot be assessed (e.g., previously removed) |
| N0 | No regional lymph node metastasis |
| N1 | Metastasis to movable ipsilateral axillary lymph node(s) |
| N2 | Metastasis to ipsilateral axillary lymph node(s), fixed to one another or other structures |
| N3 | Metastasis to ipsilateral internal mammary lymph node(s) |
| **Distant metastases** | |
| M | Presence of distant metastasis cannot be assessed |
| M0 | No distant metastasis |
| M1 | Distant metastasis (including metastasis to ipsilateral supraclavicular lymph node[s]) |

TNM, tumor-node-metastasis.
From American Cancer Society. How is cancer staged? http://www.cancer.org/Cancer/BreastCancer/DetailedGuide/breast-cancer-staging. Accessed May 13, 2013.

*Surgical or Local Treatment*

- **Mastectomy** involves the complete surgical removal of breast tissue. Mastectomy is recommended if the disease is multicentric, invades skin and chest wall, or has inflammatory features or if negative margins cannot be achieved with breast preservation. **Radical** mastectomy includes removal of the breast, overlying skin, pectoralis major and minor, and the entire axillary contents. The **modified radical**

| TABLE 2-5 | TNM Staging System for Breast Cancer | | |
|---|---|---|---|
| **Stage** | **Tumor Size** | **Lymph Node Metastases** | **Distant Metastases** |
| 0 | Tis | N0 | M0 |
| I | T1 | N0 | M0 |
| IIa | T0 | N1 | M0 |
| | T1 | N1 | M0 |
| | T2 | N0 | M0 |
| IIb | T2 | N1 | M0 |
| | T3 | N0 | M0 |
| IIIa | T0 | N2 | M0 |
| | T1 | N2 | M0 |
| | T2 | N2 | M0 |
| | T3 | N1, N2 | M0 |
| IIIb | T4 | Any N | M0 |
| | Any T | N3 | M0 |
| IV | Any T | Any N | M1 |

TNM, tumor-node-metastasis.
From American Cancer Society. How is cancer staged? http://www.cancer.org/Cancer/BreastCancer/DetailedGuide/breast-cancer-staging. Accessed May 13, 2013.

**mastectomy** includes removal of the entire breast and underlying fascia of the pectoralis major muscle and levels I and II of the axillary lymph nodes. A total or **simple mastectomy** removes the breast with the nipple areolar complex but without lymph nodes. "Skin-sparing" mastectomy provides superior cosmetic results and may be appropriate for patients with DCIS; stage I, II, or III breast cancer; or for prophylactic mastectomy. Nipple-sparing mastectomy is controversial in the treatment of breast cancer. Any type of mastectomy can be performed with or without immediate reconstruction.

| TABLE 2-6 | Prognosis by Stage: 10-Year Breast Cancer Survival Based on the National Cancer Database[a] |
|---|---|
| **Stage** | **10-Year Survival Rates** |
| Stage 0 | 95% |
| Stage I | 88% |
| Stage II | 66% |
| Stage III | 36% |
| Stage IV | 7% |

[a]The National Cancer Database is a joint project of the Commission on Cancer of the American College of Surgeons and the American Cancer Society. It collects and analyzes data from a wide variety of sources throughout the United States, including small community hospitals.
From Fremgen AM, Bland KI, McGinnis LS Jr, et al. Clinical highlights from the National Cancer Database, 1999. *CA Cancer J Clin* 1999;49:145–158.

- In **breast-conserving therapy (BCT)**, a wide local excision or lumpectomy is performed to achieve a 1- to 2-mm negative histologic margin. Adjuvant radiation therapy (RT) is required. Radiation is delivered to the entire breast with a possible boost dose to the lumpectomy bed. Trials comparing BCT + RT and mastectomy show comparable survival rates.
- Assessing **axillary lymph node** status is important in prognosis, staging, and treatment planning. However, potential complications of axillary dissection include lymphedema (10% to 15%), pain, numbness, or weakness of the affected arm.
- Evaluation of the clinically suspicious axillary node can be accomplished with ultrasound plus fine-needle aspiration or core biopsy.
- **Sentinel lymph node biopsy** has evolved into the method of choice for axillary node staging in the clinically negative axilla. The sentinel lymph node is identified using radioactive tracer or dye injected into the periareolar region of the breast. When the isotope and dye are used in combination, the positive predictive value of sentinel node biopsy approaches 100%.
- **RT**, although most often administered as part of BCT, can also be used for other indications.

## Systemic Therapy

- Systemic therapy given before surgery is termed *neoadjuvant therapy* and is often recommended for patients with locally advanced disease. **Adjuvant therapy**, which is given after surgery, is typically recommended to patients with hormone receptor–positive breast cancer, positive lymph node findings, or other high-risk characteristics.
- **Hormonal therapy** is the most frequently recommended adjuvant systemic therapy and is aimed at targeting estrogen receptor– and/or progesterone receptor–positive breast cancer. Tamoxifen, a **selective estrogen receptor modulator**, has been used most commonly. Hormone therapy results in a 26% annual reduction in the risk of recurrence and a 14% annual reduction in the risk of death from breast cancer. Tamoxifen is administered at 20 mg/day for at least 5 years. It is associated with a twofold increased risk of endometrial cancer. Therefore, abnormal uterine bleeding in a premenopausal woman or any postmenopausal bleeding in a woman taking tamoxifen should be assessed with endometrial sampling. However, routine imaging or endometrial sampling is not recommended for tamoxifen users.
- **Aromatase inhibitors** (e.g., letrozole, anastrozole, and exemestane) are potent inhibitors of estrogen synthesis and are therefore only used in postmenopausal women. They have been shown to be more effective than tamoxifen in treating breast cancer, with virtually no risk of endometrial hyperplasia and a reduced risk of thromboembolic events when compared to tamoxifen. Side effects include osteoporosis, myalgias, elevated cholesterol, and joint pain. These agents are effective as first-line agents or as second-line agents in patients whose cancer has progressed during or after tamoxifen therapy.
- **Biologic therapy:** Trastuzumab (Herceptin) is a genetically engineered monoclonal antibody to the *HER2 protein*. Its use concurrently with chemotherapy in HER2-positive breast cancers results in significant improvement in disease-free and overall survival. There is, however, an increased risk of congestive heart failure and decreased left ventricular ejection fraction in patients receiving trastuzumab, so routine cardiac monitoring is recommended.

- **Chemotherapy** has been shown to improve overall survival and reduce the odds of death by 25% in selected patients. The decision to use cytotoxic chemotherapy depends on tumor histology, tumor size, nodal status, genomic profiling, and benefit–risk calculators.

### Metastatic or Advanced Disease

- Although breast cancer is uncommonly found to be metastatic at the time of presentation, approximately one third of patients subsequently develop distant metastatic disease. Median survival for patients with metastatic disease is 18 to 24 months, but fewer than 5% live beyond 5 years. Breast cancer metastasizes to the bone, liver, and brain. The goal of therapy in metastatic disease is prolongation of survival and palliation of symptoms. Treatments typically include endocrine therapy, chemotherapy, or biologic therapy. Surgery or radiation could be considered for recurrence limited to one organ.

## Prevention

- **Chemoprevention** includes treatment with tamoxifen and raloxifene. Appropriate candidates for prophylactic endocrine therapy include women older than age 35 years with a history of LCIS, DCIS, or atypical ductal or lobular hyperplasia; women older than age 60 years; women between ages 35 and 59 years with Gail model risk of breast cancer ≥1.66% over 5 years; or women with known BRCA1 or BRCA2 mutations who do not undergo prophylactic mastectomy. **Prophylactic tamoxifen** reduces the risk for estrogen receptor–positive breast cancer in women without previous breast cancer but does not impact overall survival.

  - **Raloxifene** is a selective estrogen receptor modulator that reduces the incidence of hormone-positive breast cancer in postmenopausal women but like tamoxifen has no effect on survival. It is slightly less effective than tamoxifen in preventing breast cancer but has lower risks of uterine cancer/hyperplasia and thromboembolic disease. Its use has not been studied in premenopausal women.

- **Aromatase inhibitors** are currently being evaluated in clinical trials for the primary prevention of breast cancer.

- **Surgical prevention** can be considered in two groups of women: (a) patients positive for BRCA1 or BRCA2 and (b) patients with a strong family history suggestive of hereditary breast cancer but negative for BRCA1 or BRCA2. Surgical prevention includes contralateral mastectomy, prophylactic bilateral mastectomy, and bilateral salpingo-oophorectomy. Prophylactic bilateral mastectomies have been shown to reduce the risk of breast cancer by 90%. This is increased to 95% if combined with a bilateral salpingo-oophorectomy.

## Pregnancy and Breast Cancer

- Pregnancy-associated breast cancer is diagnosed during pregnancy, in the first postpartum year, or any time during lactation. Breast cancer is the most common cancer in pregnancy, with an incidence of 1 in 3,000 gestations. The average patient age is 32 to 38 years. Breast cancer can be especially difficult to diagnose during pregnancy and lactation (secondary to increased glandular breast tissue), which may lead to a delay in diagnosis. Thus, cancers are often found at a later stage in pregnant women or immediately postpartum. Mammograms may be performed safely during pregnancy. Pregnant patients do as well as their nonpregnant counterparts at a similar disease stage.

• Treatment during pregnancy is generally the same as that for nonpregnant patients. The tumor can usually be fully excised or mastectomy performed during pregnancy. The agents used to identify the sentinel lymph node are not approved in pregnancy and therefore, axillary dissection is commonly performed. Initiation of chemotherapy is generally considered safe after the first trimester. Radiotherapy should be avoided until after delivery. No evidence has been reported that aborting the fetus or interrupting the pregnancy leads to improved outcome.

## SUGGESTED READINGS

American College of Obstetricians and Gynecologists. Practice bulletin no. 122: breast cancer screening. *Obstet Gynecol* 2011;118:372–382.
American College of Obstetricians and Gynecologists. Practice bulletin no. 103: hereditary breast and ovarian cancer syndrome. *Obstet Gynecol* 2009;113:957–966.
Leach MO. Breast cancer screening in women at high risk using MRI. *NMR Biomed* 2009;22:17–27.
Speroff L, Fritz MA, eds. The breast. In *Clinical Gynecologic Endocrinology and Infertility*. Philadelphia, PA: Lippincott Williams & Wilkins, 2005:573–620.

# Critical Care

Emily S. Wu and Meredith L. Birsner

## INTRODUCTION

Intensive care unit (ICU) admission is indicated for patients requiring intensive monitoring and physiologic support for organ failure. Indications for intensive care include hemodynamic instability, single- or multisystem organ failure, active or potential requirement for ventilator support or vasoactive medications, severe medical illness, and postoperative care after major surgery.

## CARDIOVASCULAR CRITICAL CARE

**Cardiovascular function** in critical care can be assessed with **invasive hemodynamic monitoring** that provides information on the cardiac performance, fluid status, tissue perfusion, and arterial pressure.
• **Intra-arterial lines**, most commonly placed in the radial or femoral artery, are used to accurately and continuously assess arterial blood pressure and facilitate blood gas analysis. These lines are vital when monitoring and titrating vasoactive medications for hemodynamically unstable patients.
• A **pulmonary artery (PA) catheter (Swan-Ganz PA catheter)** can be used to measure or calculate hemodynamic parameters. It is placed via the subclavian or internal jugular vein (preferred) and has two lumens. The proximal lumen is

positioned in the superior vena cava or right atrium, whereas the other opens at the tip of the catheter and contains a balloon that can be "floated" through the right atrium and ventricle into the PA. Indications include distinguishing cardiogenic from other causes of pulmonary edema; managing perioperative fluids in high-risk patients with severe cardiac, pulmonary, or renal disease; guiding fluid resuscitation in patients with shock, renal failure, or unexplained acidosis; and calculating oxygen consumption and intrapulmonary shunt fraction in patients with acute respiratory failure. Despite its potential usage, clinical trials have demonstrated limited patient benefit. The **hemodynamic parameters** that can be measured with a PA catheter are central venous pressure, pulmonary capillary wedge pressure, cardiac index, right ventricular end-diastolic volume, right ventricular stroke work index, stroke volume index, left ventricular stroke work index (LVSWI), systemic vascular resistance index, pulmonary vascular resistance index, arterial oxygen delivery ($DO^2$), mixed venous oxygen saturation ($SvO^2$), and oxygen extraction ratio ($O_2ER$). A parameter that is expressed relative to body surface area (BSA) is called an *index*.

- **Central venous pressure (CVP)** is recorded from the proximal lumen of the catheter and reflects **right atrial pressure (RAP)**. A normal value is 1 to 6 mm Hg. When there is no obstruction between the right atrium and ventricle, CVP = RAP = right ventricular end-diastolic pressure. It exhibits a complex waveform that can be affected by various pathologic processes and is most often interpreted as a proxy for fluid status and therefore used to guide fluid management. However, CVP can be misleading and vary based on patient position, changes in thoracic pressure (from respiration or ventilation settings), and cardiac disease.

- **Pulmonary capillary wedge pressure (PCWP)** is recorded with the PA catheter balloon inflated and wedged in a branch of the PA. A normal value is 6 to 12 mm Hg. When there is no obstruction between the left atrium and ventricle, PCWP = left atrial pressure = left ventricular end-diastolic pressure. As with CVP, PCWP values can be misleading. Left ventricular end-diastolic pressure reflects left ventricular preload only with normal ventricular compliance, which often is not the case in critically ill patients.

- **Cardiac index (CI)** is cardiac output (stroke volume × heart rate)/BSA. A normal value is 2.4 to 4 $L/m^2$. Cardiac output is measured with a PA catheter using a thermodilution technique. A thermistor located near the end of the PA catheter tip detects the flow of a cold fluid injected via the proximal port to calculate blood flow rate (equivalent to cardiac output).

- **$SvO^2$** is the oxygen saturation in pulmonary arterial blood and measures overall oxygen extraction from the blood. A decrease in this variable implies decreased oxygen delivery or increased oxygen use. A normal value is **70% to 75%**.

## Heart Failure

Heart failure is classified by right-sided versus left-sided and diastolic versus systolic failure. **Systolic heart failure** occurs due to impaired ventricular contraction. **Diastolic heart failure** is a disorder of ventricular relaxation and therefore inadequate filling. The two can be distinguished by the end-diastolic volume, which increases in systolic heart failure and decreases in diastolic heart failure. Although ejection fraction is decreased in systolic heart failure, it is often maintained in diastolic heart failure.

- Common **etiologies** of heart failure include cardiac ischemia, hypertensive heart disease, cardiac arrhythmias, pulmonary embolism, and cardiomyopathy.

- In acute decompensated heart failure, patients most commonly exhibit dyspnea, orthopnea, tachypnea, tachycardia, and anxiety. Decreased peripheral perfusion, pulmonary crackles, wheezing, elevated jugular venous pressure, and peripheral edema may be noted on physical exam.
- The **workup** for heart failure should include ECG, cardiac enzymes, echocardiography, and chest radiography. Although there is no consensus on the role of brain natriuretic peptide (BNP) and diagnosing and monitoring heart failure in the ICU setting, it can be useful because of its high negative predictive value. In severe cases, invasive hemodynamic monitoring may be used to manage treatment.
- In addition to correcting any precipitating factors such as hypertension, myocardial ischemia, and cardiac arrhythmias, **treatment** should be aimed at improving symptoms, optimizing volume status, and restoring oxygenation. After the patient recovers from the acute phase, chronic heart failure therapy should be optimized.
- In the presence of hypoxia, patients should receive **supplemental oxygen** and be positioned upright. Noninvasive positive pressure ventilation (NIPPV) should be considered in patients with severe dyspnea and pulmonary edema.
- If there is evidence of fluid overload, **loop diuretics** should be administered while monitoring daily weights, strict intake and output, and electrolytes.
- Afterload reduction with intravenous (IV) **vasodilators** such as nitroglycerin, nitroprusside, or nesiritide can be considered in patients with left-sided **systolic heart failure** without hypotension. If these patients exhibit hypotension, **inotropes** such as milrinone or dobutamine are more appropriate.
- In general, inotropes and diuretics are considered counterproductive in **diastolic heart failure**. Rather, vasodilators are more frequently employed.

## Acute Coronary Syndrome

Acute coronary syndrome (ACS) is composed of **unstable angina** and myocardial infarction with and without associated ST segment elevation (non–ST segment elevation myocardial infarction [**NSTEMI**] and ST-segment elevation myocardial infarction [**STEMI**]). Factors that cause coronary artery obstruction including thrombus formation or vasospasm lead to myocardial ischemia, hypoxia, and acidosis. Diagnosis is based on patient symptoms, ECG findings, and cardiac biomarker values.

- Patients with suspected myocardial ischemia should be treated with oxygen, sublingual nitroglycerin, and chewable aspirin (162 to 325 mg) as soon as possible. Opiates should be administered for pain and to reduce anxiety, which in turn may help reduce myocardial demand.
- Patients with **STEMI** symptom onset within the last 12 hours should receive immediate reperfusion therapy.
- Depending on risk factors and eligibility criteria, primary percutaneous coronary intervention (PCI), rather than fibrinolytic therapy, is recommended.
- Patients undergoing reperfusion therapy should receive a loading dose of a thienopyridine such as clopidogrel as early as possible. Anticoagulation, with unfractionated heparin or other agents depending on the type of reperfusion therapy to be performed, should also be administered.
- Depending on the situation, other medications such as beta-blocker and angiotensin-converting enzyme (ACE) inhibitors should be administered within 24 hours of an STEMI.
- In the absence of contraindications, patients with **unstable angina** and **NSTEMI** should be treated with aspirin, a second antiplatelet agent such as clopidogrel,

beta-blockade, anticoagulant therapy, and a glycoprotein IIb/IIIa inhibitor until a revascularization decision is made.

- If a patient experiences **cardiac arrest**, code team activation, early and proficient provision of cardiopulmonary resuscitation, and early defibrillation for ventricular fibrillation (VF) or pulseless ventricular tachycardia (VT) should occur immediately.

## Cardiac Arrhythmias

- **Tachycardia** is defined as a heart rate >100 beats per minute (bpm). In pregnancy, a higher threshold, typically 120 bpm, is used. Tachycardias can be classified by the site of origin and regularity of rhythm. Typically, tachycardias that originate above the atrioventricular (AV) node are narrow complex, whereas those that originate below the AV node are wide complex. Patients with rate-related cardiovascular compromise should proceed to immediate synchronized cardioversion per advanced cardiac life support protocol; adenosine can be considered in patients with narrow complex regular tachycardia with monomorphic QRS complexes.
- **Narrow complex, regular rhythm** tachycardias include sinus tachycardia, atrial flutter, and AV nodal reentry tachycardia (AVNRT). The atrial rate with **atrial flutter** is typically 250 to 350 bpm, most often with a 2:1 ventricular conduction ratio. Treatment is similar to that in atrial fibrillation, as described in the following text. Acute episodes of **AVNRT** can be terminated with vagal maneuvers, adenosine, or calcium channel blockers.
- **Narrow complex, irregular rhythm** tachycardias include atrial fibrillation, multifocal atrial tachycardia (MAT), and atrial flutter with variable AV block. Medical management for **atrial fibrillation** involves rate control and prevention of thromboembolic events. Rhythm control with chemical or electrical cardioversion is generally a second-line treatment. In patients with atrial fibrillation with rapid ventricular response, IV beta-blockers and nondihydropyridine calcium channel blockers (e.g., diltiazem) are the drugs of choice.
- **Wide complex, regular rhythm** tachycardias include monomorphic VT or supraventricular tachycardia with aberrancy. Preferred treatment for stable patients with likely VT are elective cardioversion or antiarrhythmics.
- **Wide complex, irregular rhythm** tachycardias include VF, polymorphic VT, and atrial fibrillation with aberrancy.
- **Bradycardia** is defined as a heart rate <60 bpm. Common causes include electrolyte abnormalities, increased vagal tone, myocardial ischemia, myocarditis, cardiomyopathy, and medications. Initial therapy for persistent bradyarrhythmia in an unstable patient is atropine. If this fails, transcutaneous pacing, dopamine, or epinephrine can be attempted.

## Hypotension and Shock

**Shock** is a clinical syndrome in which decreased perfusion causes cellular injury due to inadequate delivery of oxygen. This triggers an inflammatory cascade that leads to symptoms of vital organ dysfunction, including tachycardia, hypotension, oliguria, and altered mentation. In patients with gynecologic malignancy, common postoperative causes include hemorrhage, pulmonary embolism, myocardial infarction, and sepsis.

- No absolute criteria for hypotension define shock, but systolic blood pressure (SBP) <90 mm Hg or a decrease of >40 mm Hg from baseline deserves further evaluation.

| TABLE 3-1 | Hemodynamic Profiles for Critical Care Diagnosis |
| --- | --- |

| | PCWP or CVP | CO | SVR | $SvO^2$ |
| --- | --- | --- | --- | --- |
| Hypovolemic | ↓ | ↓ | ↑ | ↓ |
| Cardiogenic | ↑ | ↓ | ↑ | ↓ |
| Obstructive | | | | |
|   Tamponade | ↑ | ↓ | ↑ | ↓ |
|   Pulmonary embolus | nl or ↓ | ↓ | ↑ | ↓ |
| Distributive | | | | |
|   Early septic shock | ↑↓ | ↑ | ↓ | ↑ |
|   Late septic shock | ↑↓ | ↓ | ↑ | ↑↓ |
|   Neurogenic shock | ↓ | ↓ | ↓ | ↓ |

↑, increased; ↓, decreased; ↑↓, either decreased or increased; nl, normal; PCWP, pulmonary capillary wedge pressure; CVP, central venous pressure; CO, cardiac output; SVR, systemic vascular resistance; $SvO^2$, mixed venous oxygen saturation.

- The Weil-Shubin classification scheme defines four categories of shock: **hypovolemic**, **cardiogenic**, **obstructive**, and **distributive**. See Table 3-1 for a comparison of hemodynamic parameters in various shock states. Because a patient may exhibit multiple types of shock, strict classification can be difficult.
- Management starts with determining and correcting the etiology of the underlying disease process. Ensuring sufficient perfusion and adequate oxygenation is the primary goal.

**Hypovolemic shock** is due to intravascular fluid loss (e.g., bleeding, nasogastric [NG] suction, diarrhea). **Hemorrhagic shock** is a type of hypovolemic shock classified by the volume of blood loss and physiologic response (Table 3-2). Expedient volume resuscitation is required when blood loss exceeds 30% to 40%. The mainstay of treatment in hypovolemic shock is volume replacement.

- It is important to **replace blood products** in patients with significant bleeding or anemia. Patient core temperature should be closely monitored during massive transfusion. Hematologic critical care is further addressed later in this chapter.

| TABLE 3-2 | Classification of Hemorrhage by Extent of Blood Loss |
| --- | --- |

| Parameter | Class I | Class II | Class III | Class IV |
| --- | --- | --- | --- | --- |
| Blood loss (mL) | 750 | 750–1,500 | 1,500–2,000 | >2,000 |
| Blood volume lost (%) | <15 | 15–30 | 30–40 | >40 |
| Pulse rate (beats/min) | <100 | >100 | >120 | >140 |
| Supine blood pressure | Normal | Normal | Decreased | Decreased |
| Urine output (mL/hr) | >30 | 20–30 | 5–15 | <5 |
| Mental status | Anxious | Agitated | Confused | Lethargic |

From Gutierrez G, Reines HD, Wulf-Guterrez ME. Clinical review: hemorrhagic shock. *Crit Care* 2004;8:373–381.

- **Crystalloid** is typically available on any unit, inexpensive, and carries less risk than colloid administration, therefore making it a common first choice for volume resuscitation. Ringer lactate is less acidic than normal saline and can ameliorate the hyperchloremic metabolic acidosis that results from large volume saline infusion, although there is no important physiologic difference in the degree of resuscitation provided by Ringer versus normal saline.
- **Colloid** therapy is more costly but may provide better short-term volume expansion, although it has not been shown to confer a survival benefit. **Albumin 5%** is generally considered safe in ICU patients; however, **hetastarch** has been shown to increase the risk of renal failure and death in ICU patients and should therefore be avoided.
- **Vasoactive pharmacotherapy** may be required along with fluid resuscitation. Intensive care and possibly invasive monitoring are required. Norepinephrine is often employed in the treatment of severe hypotensive shock (Table 3-3).

**Cardiogenic shock** occurs with decreased myocardial contractility and function. Common etiologies include myocardial infarction, congestive heart failure, cardiac arrhythmias, and valvular disease.

- Treatment is targeted at improving myocardial function. For example, inotropes may be used to improve contractility, and vasopressor agents may be used to increase aortic diastolic pressure in order to improve myocardial perfusion. Where these fail, a mechanical assist device such as an intra-aortic balloon pump should be considered.
- Fluid administration in patients with cardiogenic shock should be approached with caution.

**Obstructive shock** occurs secondary to mechanical obstruction of blood flow (e.g., cardiac tamponade, tension pneumothorax, massive pulmonary embolism [PE], prosthetic valve thrombosis) rather than primary cardiac disease.

**Distributive shock** results from loss of peripheral vascular tone resulting in relative hypovolemia. It encompasses a wide range of conditions including septic shock, other systemic inflammatory response syndrome (SIRS) responses (e.g., trauma, surgery, pancreatitis, hepatic failure), anaphylaxis, neurogenic shock (e.g., spinal cord injury), acute adrenal insufficiency, and toxic shock syndrome.

- The initial approach to treatment is similar in hypovolemic shock. The goal is to restore and maintain adequate intravascular volume and add vasoactive agents as needed.
- In addition, adjunctive agents should be added depending on etiology. Epinephrine should be administered in anaphylaxis. Corticosteroids should be provided in acute adrenal insufficiency. Underlying conditions should be addressed.
- Sepsis and toxic shock syndrome are discussed later in this chapter.

## RESPIRATORY CRITICAL CARE

**Respiratory support** is frequently required for critical care patients.

- **Hypoxic respiratory failure** is characterized by decreased arterial partial pressure of oxygen ($Pa_{O_2}$) <60 mm Hg and/or arterial oxygen saturation ($Sa_{O_2}$) <90% and is typically associated with tachypnea and hypocapnia. Initially, the $Sa_{O_2}$ may be normal or elevated from baseline.
  - The differential diagnosis includes drug-induced hypoventilation, acute neuromuscular dysfunction, PE, heart failure, chronic obstructive pulmonary disease (COPD), pulmonary edema, pneumonia, atelectasis, and acute respiratory distress syndrome.

**TABLE 3-3** Selected Vasoactive Agents in Critical Care

| Drug | Main Effects | Dose | Mechanism | Use | Warnings |
|---|---|---|---|---|---|
| Dobutamine | Increased inotropy and systemic vasodilation | 3–15 µg/kg/min | Potent β₁ agonist, weak β₂ agonist | Primarily for decompensated heart failure | Adverse effects include tachycardia, ventricular ectopy. Contraindicated with hypertrophic cardiomyopathy. |
| Dopamine | Low-dose: renal and splanchnic vasodilation and natriuresis; medium dose: increased inotropy and systemic vasodilation; high dose: systemic vasoconstriction | 1–3 µg/kg/min; or 3–10 µg/kg/min; or >10 µg/kg/min | Dose-dependent agonist for dopamine receptors (low), β-adrenergic receptors (medium), and peripheral α-adrenergic receptors (high) | May be useful for cardiogenic or hypotensive shock where both cardiac stimulation and peripheral vasoconstriction are needed | Low-dose dopamine is not appropriate for acute renal failure. Adverse effects include tachyarrhythmia, ischemic limb necrosis, increased intraocular pressure, and delayed gastric emptying. |
| Epinephrine | Dose-dependent increase in cardiac output, increased systemic vascular resistance, relaxation of bronchial smooth muscle | 0.3–0.5 µg IM; 2–8 µg/min infusion | β-Adrenergic receptor agonist (low dose) and α agonist (high dose) | Drug of choice for anaphylaxis. Used in ACLS protocols for cardiac arrest. Nebulized racemic epimer used for laryngospasm and severe asthma exacerbation. | Contraindicated with narrow angle glaucoma, ischemic cardiac disease. Local infiltration can cause tissue necrosis. |

(Continued)

**TABLE 3-3** Selected Vasoactive Agents in Critical Care *(Continued)*

| Drug | Main Effects | Dose | Mechanism | Use | Warnings |
|------|------|------|------|------|------|
| Norepinephrine | Dose-dependent increase in systemic vascular resistance | 0.2–5 μg/kg/min | α-Adrenergic receptor agonist and cardiac β agonist | Preferred vasopressor for septic shock or refractory hypotension | Extreme vasoconstriction can exacerbate end-organ damage. Extravasation can produce local tissue necrosis. |
| Nitroglycerin | Low-dose: venodilation; high-dose: arteriodilation | 1–50 μg/min; or >50 mg/min | Metabolized in endothelial cells to produce nitric oxide (NO) that stimulates cGMP production, causing smooth muscle relaxation. Dose-dependent vasodilator. | Used for unstable angina and to augment cardiac output in decompensated heart failure. | Rapid onset and metabolism. Tolerance develops quickly. Contraindicated for patients taking phosphodiesterase inhibitors. |
| Nitroprusside | Systemic vasodilation | 0.3–2 μg/kg/min | Releases NO in bloodstream; similar mechanism to nitroglycerin. | Used for rapid control of severe hypertension and for decompensated heart failure. | Risk for accumulation of cyanide metabolite |

IM, intramuscular; ACLS, advanced cardiac life support; cGMP, cyclic guanosine monophosphate. Adapted from Marino PL. *The ICU Book*, 3rd ed. Philadelphia, PA: Lippincott Williams & Wilkins, 2007.

- **Hypercapnic respiratory failure** is characterized by increased arterial partial pressure of carbon dioxide ($Pa_{CO2}$) >46 mm Hg and pH <7.35 and is associated with hypoventilation. $Sa_{O2}$ may be normal.
- The differential diagnosis includes infection, seizures, overfeeding, shock, chronic neuromuscular disorder, electrolyte abnormalities, cardiac surgery, obesity, and drug-induced respiratory depression. Consider hypercapnia as a cause of hypertension in somnolent, tachycardic postoperative patients who may be overmedicated, and avoid administering additional narcotics.
- A stepwise **evaluation of respiratory failure** (i.e., hypoxemia or hypercapnia) begins with an arterial blood gas and calculation of the alveolar–arteriolar (A-a) oxygen gradient.
- The **A-a gradient** = $FiO_2$ ($P_{atmosphere} - P_{H2O}$) − $Pa_{CO2}$/RQ − $Pa_{O2}$. It is the difference in the partial pressure of oxygen between the alveolus and the arterial blood. $FiO_2$ is the fraction of inspired oxygen and RQ is the respiratory quotient. A patient at sea level breathing room air ($FiO_2$ = 21%) would therefore have an A-a gradient of 148 − 1.2 ($Pa_{CO2}$) − $Pa_{O2}$. The **expected A-a gradient** can be estimated using the formula: age/4 + 4. Supplemental oxygen increases the normal gradient by 5 to 7 mm Hg for every 10% increase in $FiO_2$.
  - *If the A-a gradient is normal/unchanged*, the culprit is hypoventilation. To distinguish central hypoventilation versus a neuromuscular disorder, maximum inspiratory effort ($PI_{max}$) is evaluated. $PI_{max}$ is measured by having the patient inspire maximally against a closed valve. For most adults, $PI_{max}$ should be >80 cm $H_2O$ but varies with age and sex.
  - If the $PI_{max}$ is normal, drug-induced central hypoventilation should be considered.
  - If the $PI_{max}$ is low, neuromuscular cause of hypoventilation should be considered.
  - *If the A-a gradient is increased with hypoxemia*, measure the mixed venous oxygen pressure ($Pv_{O2}$) to assess for ventilation-perfusion (V/Q) abnormalities. $Pv_{O2}$ is ideally measured from pulmonary arterial blood using a PA catheter, but superior vena caval blood can be used. Normal values from the PA are 35 to 45 mm Hg.
  - If the $Pv_{O2}$ is normal, consider a V/Q abnormality.
    - *V/Q* >1 indicates increased dead space ventilation and occurs with PE, congestive heart failure, emphysema, and alveolar overdistension from positive pressure ventilation.
    - *V/Q* <1 indicates intrapulmonary shunt and occurs with asthma, bronchitis, pulmonary edema, pneumonia, and atelectasis. The portion of cardiac output in an intrapulmonary shunt is called the *shunt fraction* and is normally <10%. Shunt fractions >50% will not improve with oxygen supplementation.
  - If the $Pv_{O2}$ is low, consider an imbalance in oxygen delivery/uptake ($D_{O2}$/$V_{O2}$) such as anemia, low cardiac output, or hypermetabolism.
  - *If the A-a gradient is increased with hypercapnia*, measure the rate of $CO_2$ production ($V_{CO2}$) to assess metabolic versus other disorders. $V_{CO2}$ is evaluated by a metabolic cart using infrared light to measure $CO_2$ in expired gas. Normal $V_{CO2}$ is 90 to 130 mL/min/m$^2$.
  - If the $V_{CO2}$ is increased, consider overfeeding (especially with carbohydrate load), fever, sepsis, and seizures.
  - If the $V_{CO2}$ is normal, consider increased dead space ventilation (see earlier text) and hypoventilation from respiratory weakness (e.g., shock, multisystem organ failure, prolonged neuromuscular blockade, electrolyte imbalances, cardiac surgery) or central hypoventilation (e.g., opiate or benzodiazepine depression, obesity).

## Acute Respiratory Distress Syndrome

- Acute respiratory distress syndrome (ARDS) is a leading cause of acute respiratory failure, resulting from inflammatory lung injury. The pathophysiology involves activation of diffuse pulmonary inflammation and endothelial damage producing inflammatory alveolar exudates, microvascular thrombosis, pulmonary fibrosis, and high mortality rates exceeding 50% to 60%. Predisposing conditions include sepsis, blood product transfusion, aspiration or chemical pneumonitis, pneumonia, pancreatitis, multiple or long bone fractures, intracranial hypertension, cardiopulmonary bypass, amniotic fluid embolism, and pyelonephritis in pregnancy. Clinically, ARDS is characterized by severe early hypoxemia, normal pulmonary capillary hydrostatic pressures, and diffuse pulmonary infiltrates.
- **Diagnosis** is by clinical criteria: acute onset, bilateral infiltrates on chest radiograph, $Pa_{O_2}/FiO_2$ ratio <200, and PCWP <18 mm Hg or no clinical evidence of left atrial hypertension. In cases where the $Pa_{O_2}/FiO_2$ ratio is <300, the patient has **acute lung injury**. Only careful evaluation distinguishes ARDS from severe pneumonia, PE, and cardiogenic pulmonary edema. ARDS may be confirmed with bronchoalveolar lavage demonstrating an increased lavage/serum protein ratio (>0.7) and florid neutrophil invasion.
- **Management** of ARDS is essentially supportive. The underlying disorder should be corrected while respiratory support is provided. Multiple clinical trials have demonstrated the value of low tidal volume (TV) "lung protective" ventilation (<6 mL/kg ideal body weight) with low-level positive end-expiratory pressure (PEEP), permissive hypercapnia, and limitation of plateau pressure (<30 mm Hg) to avoid the destructive proinflammatory effects of ventilator-induced barotrauma. Lower $Sa_{O_2}$ (>88%) and $Pa_{O_2}$ (>55 mm Hg) can be tolerated. Additional supportive measures that are sometimes used include prone positioning, conservative fluid management, and steroid treatment. Protocols for and studies regarding ARDS management can be accessed online at http://www.ardsnet.org.

## Oxygen Therapy

- **Oxygen therapy** can be used in many patients to improve oxygenation of peripheral tissues but should be applied judiciously. Oxygen can contribute directly to cellular injury and pathophysiology: It increases toxic-free radical metabolites, stimulates peripheral vasoconstriction which decreases systemic blood flow, directly injures pulmonary tissues at high concentrations, and has a negative cardiac inotropic effect which reduces cardiac output. An $FiO_2$ of >60% for longer than 48 hours is generally considered toxic. In critically ill patients, even an $FiO_2$ of >21% may be toxic. Therefore, oxygen supplementation should only be used when there is evidence or risk of inadequate tissue oxygenation such as $Pa_{O_2}$ <60 mm Hg, venous oxygen saturation <50%, serum lactate >4 mmol/L, or CI <2 L/min/m². Respiratory treatments should be assessed and optimized frequently.
  - **Oxygen delivery systems** are classified as low flow (e.g., nasal cannula, face mask with and without bags) and high flow.
  - **Nasal cannulas** use the patient's oro-nasopharynx as an oxygen reservoir (about 50 mL capacity). A patient with normal ventilation (i.e., TV 500 mL; respiratory rate 20 breaths/min; inspiratory/expiratory ratio 1:2) increases their $FiO_2$ by 3% to 4% for each additional volume (L/min) of oxygen flow. The increase in $FiO_2$ is significantly reduced with hyperventilation when minute ventilation exceeds the system flow rate, and as the oxygen reservoir is drained, the patient inspires

only room air. Above the maximum flow rate of 6 L/min, there is no increase in $FiO_2$ (~45%).

- **Face masks without bags** have an oxygen reservoir of 100 to 200 mL. In order to clear exhaled gases, a minimum flow rate of 5 L/min is required. The maximum flow rate of 10 L/min provides an $FiO_2$ of 60%.
- **Face masks with bags** have an oxygen reservoir of 600 to 1,000 mL. There are two types of reservoir mask devices:
  - A **partial rebreather** has a maximum $FiO_2$ of 70% to 80%. It "captures" initial exhaled air containing a higher proportion of $O_2$ from the upper airway (anatomic dead space) in the reservoir bag and releases the terminal exhaled air containing more $CO_2$. The reservoir bag maintains a high $O_2$ content.
  - A **nonrebreather** has a maximum $FiO_2$ of 100%. It requires a tight seal during use and can be used to administer nebulizer treatments but does not allow easy oral feeding. The reservoir bag maintains 100% $O_2$ content.
- **High-flow oxygen masks** deliver a constant $FiO_2$ at a flow rate that exceeds the peak inspiratory rate, preventing the variability seen with low flow systems. They may be useful in patients with chronic hypercapnia who require a constant $FiO_2$ to avoid increased $CO_2$ retention. The maximum $FiO_2$ is 50%.
- **Noninvasive positive pressure ventilation (NIPPV)** can be a useful alternative to invasive (i.e., endotracheal or tracheostomy) intubation. It has been used to successfully manage obstructive sleep apnea in general medical patients but is also appropriate for critical care patients with moderate respiratory compromise due to mild neuromuscular weakness, congestive heart failure/cardiogenic pulmonary edema, and decompensated COPD.
  - A cooperative patient with no risk for emergent intubation and moderate dyspnea, tachypnea, increased work of breathing, hypercapnia, or hypoxemia can be considered for NIPPV.
  - Contraindications include cardiac or respiratory arrest or severe cardiopulmonary compromise, coma, status epilepticus, potential airway obstruction, patient inability to protect her airway, and emergent conditions.
  - NIPPV can be supplied via mouthpiece, nasal pillows, face mask, or helmet; the device must fit properly to avoid air leaks. $FiO_2$ is titrated to the necessary minimum and the backup rate, pressure support, and PEEP are adjusted to maintain an appropriate TV (5 to 7 mL/kg/breath).
  - Complications with NIPPV include facial or nasal pressure sores, gastric distension, aspiration, and inspissated uncleared secretions.
- **Mechanical ventilation** should be instituted for patients who cannot be adequately managed with the aforementioned systems, are in respiratory distress, or are at risk for cardiopulmonary collapse. Indicators for endotracheal intubation include tachypnea >35 breaths/min, $Pa_{O2}$ <60 mm Hg, $Pa_{CO2}$ >46 mm Hg with pH <7.35, and absent gag reflex. Standard positive pressure ventilation is delivered with a preset volume-cycled device; additional modes of ventilation such as high-frequency and proportional assist ventilation are not discussed here. Selection of ventilation modes is tailored to the patient and is largely selected by provider preference.
  - In **assist-control ventilation (ACV)**, the patient initiates breaths and the ventilator delivers a set TV. If the patient fails to initiate, the ventilator "assists" at a preset "controlled" rate and TV. Tachypnea is not well tolerated in this mode and can lead to overventilation, respiratory alkalosis, and hyperinflation. Patients with respiratory muscle weakness are appropriately ventilated with ACV.

○ In **intermittent mandatory ventilation (IMV)**, a breath is delivered at a preset rate and volume, but the patient can breathe spontaneously between machine breaths without assistance. In **synchronized IMV**, machine breaths are coordinated with spontaneous respirations to avoid respiratory alkalosis and "stacking" breaths. Asynchronous IMV is not ideal because it can deliver a breath at any time during the patient's spontaneous breaths (i.e., during expiration).

○ In **pressure-controlled ventilation (PCV)**, regardless of how or when breaths are delivered, a constant pressure is provided by regulating the inspiratory flow rate throughout each breath. This may result in variable inflation volumes, especially as lung compliance changes. PCV is well suited to patients with neuromuscular disease with stable lung mechanics.

○ In **inverse-ratio ventilation (IRV)**, PCV is delivered with a prolonged inspiratory phase. A normal inspiratory:expiratory ratio is 1:2 to 1:4. In IRV, the ratio is reversed to 2:1, which prevents alveolar collapse and provides auto-PEEP but may lead to reduced cardiac output. The main use of IRV is for ARDS with hypoxemia or hypercapnia that is refractory to conventional ventilation modes.

○ In **pressure support ventilation (PSV)**, the patient breathes spontaneously and the machine adds extra support to maintain inspiratory pressures. It is a common weaning mode of ventilation.

• **Ventilator management** is a continuous and dynamic process, ideally leading to weaning from mechanical ventilation and extubation. The following basic parameters can be adjusted: mode, $FiO_2$, TV, PEEP, and pressure support.

○ $FiO_2$ is initially set to 100% and then titrated to the minimum needed to maintain $Pa_{O2}$ above 60 mm Hg or $Sa_{O2}$ above 90%. Although oxygen can be toxic, in acute respiratory distress, treatment of hypoxemia takes precedence.

○ Normal **minute ventilation** (respiratory rate × TV) is 6 to 8 L/min. Infection, inflammation, and acid–base disorders can effect large variation in the required ventilation.

○ PEEP is the positive airway pressure at the end of respiration (i.e., alveolar pressure higher than atmospheric pressure) that prevents alveolar collapse.

  ○ **Extrinsic PEEP** is created by a device that stops exhalation at a preselected pressure. PEEP reduces the risk of oxygen toxicity by improving gas exchange, increasing lung compliance, and increasing the $Pa_{O2}$, which allows reduced $FiO_2$.

  ○ **Intrinsic PEEP** (auto-PEEP) is created by increasing minute ventilation or shortening the expiratory phase. It is common in patients with prolonged expiration such as during an asthma exacerbation.

  ○ PEEP can progress to the point of sudden cardiovascular collapse; elevated auto-PEEP requires immediate disconnection from the ventilator to allow the patient to fully exhale. This may take 30 to 60 seconds, but it is life-saving.

• **Weaning from mechanical ventilation** is the gradual process of reducing ventilation to minimum settings (i.e., $FiO_2$ <50%, IMV, with PEEP and pressure support <5 cm $H_2O$ each) or T-piece ventilation, followed by extubation. Duration of mechanical ventilation is directly related to complications, so extubation should be performed as soon as feasible. A daily sedation break and spontaneous breathing trial should be performed on all eligible patients. Criteria for extubation include progressive clinical recovery from illness, intact neurologic status (i.e., alert, oriented) with ability to follow commands, patent airway without concern for occlusion (see the following discussion on cuff test), and normal arterial blood gas on minimal supplemental oxygen.

○ Assessment of airway patency and **respiration mechanics** helps assess whether a patient is ready for extubation. Patients who cannot meet minimum criteria or are neurologically impaired and unable to cooperate with the evaluation may not be ready for unassisted respiration.

○ The **"cuff test"** can be used to assess the airway. The endotracheal tube cuff is deflated and the patient is asked to breathe while the tube is occluded. A positive cuff leak demonstrates tracheal edema is not to the point that the endotracheal tube is required, and extubation can be considered.

○ **Forced vital capacity** should be at least 10 mL/kg and is typically at least 1,000 mL.

○ **Negative inspiratory force (NIF)** should be $-25$ to $-30$ cm $H_2O$. When performed as an "occlusion NIF," the test is not effort-dependent. A normal person can generate NIF of $-80$ cm $H_2O$.

○ **Rapid shallow breathing index (RSBI or Tobin index)** should be <80 and predicts the patient's ability to remain extubated for 24 hours. It is measured by switching from any ventilator mode to continuous positive airway pressure and assessing the patient's respiratory rate (f) and TV over 1 minute. The RSBI = f/TV.

  • Patients with RSBI <80 are eight- to ninefold more likely to remain extubated.
  • Patients with RSBI >100 are eight- to ninefold more likely to require reintubation.
  • Patients with RSBI between 80 and 100 require clinical judgment regarding suitable timing for extubation.

○ After extubation, **secretions** should be cleared and humidified oxygen should be supplied by face mask. The patient should be encouraged to cough and breathe deeply at regular intervals. If reintubation is necessary, perform a complete assessment of the reasons for failure and attempt extubation again within 24 to 72 hours.

## FLUIDS AND ELECTROLYTES

**Fluid and electrolyte disorders** are common for critically ill patients and for women with obstetric morbidity or undergoing major gynecologic surgery. Some of the most common issues are addressed here.

### Hyponatremia

• **Hyponatremia** is defined as serum sodium <136 mEq/L. It can be classified on the basis of volume status and further diagnosed with urine sodium and osmolality (Fig. 3-1). Management includes treating the underlying condition and replacing the sodium deficit if present.

• Rapid **correction of chronic or severe hyponatremia** can cause cerebral edema and increased intracranial pressure leading to a demyelinating encephalopathy or central pontine myelinolysis. Hyponatremia can be corrected as follows:

  • **Step 1:** Calculate the sodium deficit. Sodium deficit = total body water (TBW) × (desired Na − actual Na). In women, **TBW** in liters = 50% of lean body weight in kilograms.

  • **Step 2:** Calculate the volume of crystalloid needed to correct the deficit. This volume is the (sodium deficit)/(mEq of sodium found in replacement fluid in Na/L). Three percent NaCl contains 513 mEq Na/L.

  • **Step 3:** Calculate the infusion rate to correct the Na at no more than 0.5 mEq/L/hr. Use serial serum sodium measurements to assess response.

    ○ For example, a 60-kg woman with a sodium level of 120 mEq/L with a goal sodium of 130 mEq/L has a calculated sodium deficit of 300 mEq that should be corrected by total infusion of 585 mL of 3% NaCl over 20 hours at a rate of 29 mL/hr.

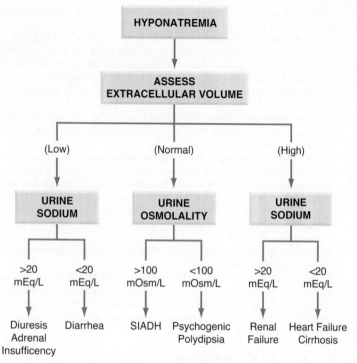

**Figure 3-1.** Classification and diagnosis of hyponatremia. SIADH, syndrome of inappropriate antidiuretic hormone secretion. (From Marino PL. *The ICU Book*, 3rd ed. Philadelphia, PA: Lippincott Williams & Wilkins, 2007:606, with permission.)

## Hypernatremia

Hypernatremia is defined as serum sodium >145 mEq/L. It reflects a relative deficiency of free water as occurs with vomiting, diarrhea, overdiuresis, diabetes mellitus with nonketotic hyperglycemia, and diabetes insipidus (see Chapter 13). Iatrogenic hypernatremia from hypertonic saline or sodium bicarbonate infusion is also possible. Clinical findings can vary from tachycardia and decreased urine output to encephalopathy, seizures, and coma.

- **Management** is generally directed toward volume replacement with crystalloid or colloid and maintenance of cardiac output. It is based on accurate assessment of extracellular volume by invasive monitoring or clinical evaluation.
  - **Hypovolemic hypernatremia** should be corrected by replacing the free water deficit over 24 to 72 hours. The serum sodium should be lowered at a rate less than 0.5 mEq/L/hr in order to avoid cerebral edema. The free water deficit is TBW × (serum sodium − 140)/140.
  - **Euvolemic hypernatremia** is treated with isotonic saline to slowly replace the water deficit.
  - **Hypervolemic hypernatremia** will be corrected by the kidneys via renal sodium excretion. In some cases, diuresis may be helpful but care must be taken to avoid hypovolemia and exacerbating the problem.

## Hypokalemia

**Hypokalemia** is defined as serum potassium <3.5 mEq/L. It can be caused by artifactual dilution (i.e., drawn near an IV infusion site), decreased potassium intake, insufficient replacement of NG tube output, diuretic therapy, diarrhea, and laxative abuse.

- **Clinical findings** of severe hypokalemia include muscle weakness and mental status changes. ECG changes can be seen, such as flattened T waves, prolonged QT intervals, and U waves. Chronic hypokalemia can result in renal tubular disorders with concentrating abnormalities, phosphaturia, and azotemia.
- **Management** includes correcting the underlying cause (e.g., alkalosis) and replacing the potassium deficit to a level of 4 mEq/L. Typically, potassium repletion is not an emergency, except in the most severe cases with active arrhythmias or in patients who are on digoxin therapy.
- For each 10 mEq oral or IV KCl, the serum potassium rises by about 1 mEq/L.
- Rapid increases in serum potassium can predispose to cardiac arrest, so the maximum rate of IV KCl infusion is 20 mEq/L via central catheter or 10 mEq/L via peripheral IV.
- Hypomagnesemia can cause refractory hypokalemia and should be replaced along with potassium. Serum magnesium levels are not generally helpful unless the patient is receiving magnesium infusion (e.g., for preeclampsia) or the patient has impaired renal function.
- Patients with significant kidney disease (i.e., glomerular filtration rate [GFR] <25 mL/min) should have potassium therapy titrated using serial serum potassium levels. Patients taking potassium-sparing diuretics may also require close monitoring.

## Hyperkalemia

**Hyperkalemia** is defined as serum potassium >5.0 mEq/L. It is not as well tolerated and can be life-threatening. It can be caused by laboratory artifact (i.e., hemolyzed specimen), cellular redistribution associated with acidosis (e.g., diabetic ketoacidosis, sepsis), renal insufficiency, adrenal insufficiency, and tissue injury (e.g., hemolysis, rhabdomyolysis, crush injury, burns).

- **Clinical findings** in the majority of patients are unimpressive. ECG changes are seen when serum potassium approaches 6 mEq/L; the earliest findings include peaked T waves, especially in precordial leads, flattened P waves, and prolonged PR intervals. This progresses to absent P waves, wide QRS complexes, and ultimately VF and asystole.
- **Management** in an asymptomatic patient with unexpected hyperkalemia starts with repeating the measurement and discontinuing any potassium supplementation. If the abnormal value is confirmed, acute management as described in the following text is guided by serum potassium and ECG findings, if any.
  - **Calcium gluconate** stabilizes the myocardium, but response lasts only 20 to 30 minutes.
  - **Insulin/glucose** facilitates movement of potassium into cellular compartment and can reduce serum concentrations by 1 mEq/L for 1 to 2 hours.
  - **Kayexalate** is a cation exchange resin that facilitates removing potassium from the body but may require time and multiple doses to take effect.
  - **Loop diuretics** enhance urinary potassium secretion but should be avoided in renal failure and hemodynamically unstable patients.
  - **Urgent hemodialysis** is necessary in cases of life-threatening hyperkalemia.

## Hypocalcemia

**Hypocalcemia** is defined as total serum calcium <8.5 mg/dL or ionized serum calcium <1.1 mmol/L. A "normal" plasma calcium is lower in patients with hypoalbuminemia, due to decreased protein binding. Causes of hypocalcemia include hypoparathyroidism, hypomagnesemia, alkalosis, blood transfusion, chronic renal failure, pancreatitis, some drugs (e.g., aminoglycosides, heparin), and sepsis.

- **Clinical findings** include hyperreflexia, paresthesias, tetany, seizures, hypotension, cardiac arrhythmias, heart block, and VT.
- **Management** is directed toward diagnosis and correction of the underlying condition. Symptomatic hypocalcemia or ionized calcium <0.65 mmol/L should be immediately corrected with calcium chloride or calcium gluconate IV, preferably through a central vein.

## Hypercalcemia

- **Hypercalcemia** is defined as total serum calcium >10.5 mg/dL or ionized serum calcium >1.3 mmol/L. In 90% of cases, the underlying cause is hyperparathyroidism or malignancy; severe hypercalcemia (i.e., total calcium >14 mg/dL or ionized calcium >3.5 mmol/L) is associated with neoplasm. Other causes include thyrotoxicosis, thiazide diuretics, and lithium treatment. The most common mechanism of hypercalcemia in gynecologic oncology patients is increased osteoclastic bone resorption without direct bone metastases.
- **Clinical findings** are nonspecific but can include gastrointestinal (GI) (e.g., nausea, constipation, ileus, abdominal pain, pancreatitis), cardiovascular (e.g., hypovolemia, hypotension, hypertension, shortened QT interval), renal (e.g., polyuria, nephrolithiasis), and neurologic (e.g., lethargy, confusion, coma) abnormalities. Symptoms are usually present when total serum calcium exceeds 12 mg/dL.
- **Acute management** aims to increase excretion and storage of calcium.
  - Hydration with **isotonic saline** promotes renal natriuresis and thereby increases calcium excretion.
  - Diuresis with **furosemide** (40 to 80 mg IV every 2 hours) with a goal of 100 to 200 mL urine output per hour further promotes urinary calcium excretion. Urine output, stimulated by hydration or pharmacologic diuresis, should be replaced with isotonic saline to prevent hypovolemia.
  - **Calcitonin** (salmon calcitonin 4 U/kg subcutaneously or intramuscularly every 12 hours) rapidly inhibits bone resorption and may decrease serum calcium levels, although the effect is not profound.
  - **Hydrocortisone** (200 mg IV daily divided into three doses) inhibits some lymphoid neoplastic growth, decreasing bone calcium release.
  - **Pamidronate disodium** (90 mg IV over 2 hours) or zoledronate are effective for severe hypercalcemia, with peak effect in 2 to 4 days.
  - **Dialysis** is appropriate for patients with severe renal failure.

## Acid–Base Disorders

Evaluation of acid–base disorders requires arterial blood gas interpretation. A stepwise approach for basic analysis is outlined here.

- **Step 1: Determine the primary disorder.** Assess the pH and $Pa_{CO2}$. If either the pH or $Pa_{CO2}$ is abnormal, a disorder is present.
  - If the pH is <7.36, the patient is acidemic. A **respiratory acidosis** is present if the $Pa_{CO2}$ >44 and a **metabolic acidosis** is present if the $HCO_3$ <22.

- If the pH is >7.44, the patient is alkalemic. A **respiratory alkalosis** is present if the $Pa_{CO2}$ <36 and a **metabolic alkalosis** is present if $HCO_3$ >26.
  - ○ A mixed disorder is present if either the pH or the $Pa_{CO2}$ is normal. Compensatory responses never completely correct the primary acid–base disturbance, so equal and opposite processes are occurring.
- **Step 2: Determine the expected compensatory response.** See Table 3-4.
- In metabolic disorders, if the measured $Pa_{CO2}$ is higher than expected, there is a **superimposed respiratory acidosis**. If the measured $Pa_{CO2}$ is lower than expected, there is a **superimposed respiratory alkalosis**.
- In respiratory disorders, if the change in pH is more than 0.008 times the change in $P_{CO2}$, then a superimposed metabolic disorder is present.
- **Step 3: Calculate the anion gap.** The anion gap = $Na^+ - [Cl^- + HCO_3^-]$. For every 1 g/dL reduction of **albumin** from 4 g/dL, add another 2.5 to the anion gap. The normal range is 10 to 14 mEq/L. If an anion gap is present, the patient has an anion gap metabolic acidosis, regardless of what other disturbances are present.
- **Causes of normal anion gap acidosis** (mnemonic **USEDCAR**) include **U**rinary diversion (ureterosigmoidostomy), **S**aline administration (in the face of renal dysfunction), **E**ndocrine disorder (Addison disease, primary hyperparathyroidism), **D**iarrhea/**D**rugs (spironolactone, triamterene, amiloride, amphotericin), **C**arbonic anhydrase inhibitors (acetazolamide, methazolamide, topiramate), **A**mmonium chloride/hyper**A**limentation, and **R**enal tubular acidosis.
- **Causes of increased anion gap acidosis** (mnemonic **MUDPILES**) include Methanol, Uremia, Diabetes (ketoacidosis)/Drugs (metformin), Paraldehyde, Isoniazid/Infection/Ischemia, Lactic acidosis, Ethylene glycol, Salicylates/Starvation.

| TABLE 3-4 | Normal Values and Expected Changes in Various Acid–Base Disorders |
|---|---|
| **Primary Disorder** | **Expected Result** |
| Metabolic acidosis | Expected $Pa_{CO2} = (1.5 \times HCO_3) + (8 \pm 2)$ |
| Metabolic alkalosis | Expected $Pa_{CO2} = (0.7 \times HCO_3) + (21 \pm 2)$ |
| Acute respiratory acidosis | $DpH = 0.008 \times DPa_{CO2}$<br>Expected pH = $7.40 - [0.008 \times (Pa_{CO2} - 40)]$ |
| Acute respiratory alkalosis | $DpH = 0.008 \times DPa_{CO2}$<br>Expected pH = $7.40 + [0.008 \times (40 - Pa_{CO2})]$ |
| Chronic respiratory acidosis | $DpH = 0.003 \times DPa_{CO2}$<br>Expected pH = $7.40 - [0.003 \times (Pa_{CO2} - 40)]$ |
| Chronic respiratory alkalosis | $DpH = 0.003 \times DPa_{CO2}$<br>Expected pH = $7.40 - [0.003 \times (40 - Pa_{CO2})]$ |

Normal values: pH = 7.36–7.44; $P_{CO2}$ = 36–44 mm Hg; $HCO_3$ = 22–26 mEq/L
Normal in pregnancy: pH = 7.40–7.45; $P_{CO2}$ = 27–32 mm Hg;
   $HCO_3$ = 19–25 mEq/L

DpH, change in arterial pH; $DPa_{CO2}$, change in arterial $CO_2$; $HCO_3$, serum bicarbonate.
Adapted from Marino PL. *The ICU Book*, 3rd ed. Philadelphia, PA: Lippincott Williams & Wilkins, 2007:535.

- **Step 4: If there is an anion gap, calculate the delta gap.** The delta gap = $(25 - HCO_3)$ − (anion gap − 12). If this is >5, there is a coexisting nonanion gap metabolic acidosis.
- **Step 5: Calculate the osmolar gap in patients with unexplained anion gap metabolic acidosis.** Osmolar gap = measured OsM − calculated OsM. Calculated OsM = 2 × Na + glucose/18 + blood urea nitrogen [BUN]/2.8.
  - Increased osmolar gap is seen in ingestion of ethylene glycol, alcohol, methanol, isopropyl alcohol, mannitol, sorbitol, and paraldehyde.
- **Treatment** is based on the severity and diagnosis. Typically it is only necessary to treat the underlying cause(s). In patients with profound disturbances (i.e., pH <7.2 or bicarbonate levels <10 mEq/L), bicarbonate infusion may be warranted.

## RENAL FAILURE

- **Acute kidney injury** (AKI) is characterized by an abrupt decrease in the GFR and resulting disruption in fluid and electrolyte homeostasis. Severity is classified by the RIFLE criteria (risk, injury, failure, loss, end-stage kidney disease), which correlates well with overall mortality.
- The **differential diagnosis** of AKI is classified by anatomic location of the problem.
  - A **prerenal disorder** causing decreased kidney perfusion is the etiology in approximately 40% of AKI cases.
  - In obstetrics and gynecology, the most common causes are intravascular volume depletion from hemorrhage, third spacing of fluids (e.g., with preeclampsia), or inadequate fluid resuscitation. Other common causes include hypotension, heart failure, renal vasoconstriction (e.g., from nonsteroidal anti-inflammatory drugs), and reduced glomerular filtration pressure (e.g., from ACE inhibitors).
  - A prerenal disorder is suggested by elevated urine specific gravity, decreased fractional excretion of sodium ($FE_{Na}$) of <1%, BUN:creatinine ratio >20, and urine sodium <20 mEq/L.
  - An **intrinsic renal disorder** from direct injury to the kidney is the etiology in up to 50% of AKI cases in ICU patients. Causes include ischemia/hypoperfusion injury, inflammation, sepsis, radiocontrast dye, myoglobinuria, and other drugs/toxins. These can result in three types of renal pathology: acute tubular necrosis (ATN), acute glomerulonephritis, and acute interstitial nephritis (AIN).
    - **ATN** is the most common cause of intrinsic renal dysfunction and is typically the result of any process that leads to renal hypoperfusion. The renal tubules and parenchyma are damaged, but glomeruli are usually intact. Injured tubular epithelial cells are shed, blocking the proximal tubular lumen and reducing net GFR. ATN is suggested by $FE_{Na}$ >2%, fractional excretion of urea >50%, urine sodium >40 mmol/L, urine osmolarity <350 mOsm/L, and granular casts on microscopy.
    - **AIN** is the result of inflammatory injury to the renal interstitium and can often present as AKI without oliguria. It is classically precipitated by antibiotics such as penicillins, aminoglycosides, and vancomycin. AIN is suggested by eosinophils and leukocyte casts on urine microscopy.
  - A **postrenal disorder** results from obstruction of the urinary tract distal to the kidney and rarely leads to oliguria unless there is a single kidney or the condition is bilateral (e.g., advanced cervical cancer).
    - The obstruction may occur in the collecting system (e.g., papillary necrosis), ureters (e.g., compression, calculus, tumor, papillary sloughing, clot/hematoma),

bladder (e.g., calculus, neurogenic bladder, carcinoma, clot/hematoma), and urethra (e.g., calculus, stricture, clot/hematoma).

- ○ Assessment includes bladder catheterization, urinary tract ultrasound/imaging, and laboratory evaluation for prerenal and intrarenal diseases.
- ○ Early treatment can prevent permanent kidney damage. Significant postobstructive diuresis occurs with resolution of bilateral obstruction, leading to electrolyte abnormalities and volume contraction. Decompression of an overly distended bladder can reveal capillary bleeding with hematuria or even frank hemorrhage.
- ○ Particularly after major abdominal surgery or advanced gynecologic cancers, **abdominal compartment syndrome** can lead to AKI. Acute oliguria can result from reduced perfusion by increasing outflow pressure, direct renal parenchymal compression, and compromised cardiac output due to impaired venous return.

- **Clinical assessment** should include review of strict intake and output and medications administered; identifying problems with urinary drainage such as an obstructed catheter; and evaluating for signs and symptoms of hypovolemia, cardiac dysfunction, and infection.
- **Laboratory assessment** includes the following:
  - The **urine specific gravity** (range: 1.003 to 1.030) is elevated in the setting of dehydration. False elevations can occur with mannitol, glucose, and radiocontrast dye.
  - **Urine microscopy** helps distinguish intrinsic disorders; it is not useful for prerenal diagnoses. Tubular epithelial cells and granular casts are pathognomonic for ATN. Leukocyte casts suggest interstitial nephritis (pyelonephritis). Red cell casts suggest glomerulonephritis. Pigmented casts suggest myoglobinuria. Sloughed papillae from papillary necrosis may be seen in postrenal disorders involving the renal collecting system.
  - The **urine sodium level (urine$_{Na}$)** is best assessed with a 24-hour urine specimen, but a random 10-mL specimen may also be used. Urine$_{Na}$ <20 mEq/L suggests a prerenal disorder; renal hypoperfusion leads to increased sodium reabsorption and decreased excretion. Urine$_{Na}$ >40 mEq/L suggests impaired sodium reabsorption from an intrinsic renal disorder, although it does not rule out coexisting prerenal disorders and may not be useful if diuretics have been administered or in elderly patients with obligatory urinary sodium loss.
  - **Fractional excretion of sodium (FE$_{Na}$)** is the fraction of sodium filtered at the glomerulus that is ultimately excreted in the urine. FE$_{Na}$ <1% suggests a prerenal disorder and a FE$_{Na}$ >2% suggests an intrinsic renal disorder. It is not a useful test for nonoliguric renal dysfunction. Calculation of this value in the setting of oliguria is one of the most reliable tests for distinguishing prerenal causes from intrarenal causes of AKI. FE$_{Na}$ is calculated by the formula:

$$[(\text{urine}_{Na}/\text{plasma}_{Na})/(\text{urine}_{Cr}/\text{plasma}_{Cr})] \times 100$$

  - **Fractional excretion of urea (FE$_{urea}$)** may be useful in patients on diuretics. A value <35% indicates prerenal disorders, whereas FE$_{urea}$ >50% suggests an intrarenal cause. It is calculated by the formula:

$$[(\text{urine}_{urea} \times \text{plasma}_{creatinine})/(\text{urine}_{creatinine} \times \text{plasma}_{urea})] \times 100$$

  - **Creatinine clearance (Cl$_{Cr}$)** is best assessed with a 24-hour urine collection. Normal Cl$_{Cr}$ for women is 72 to 110 mL/min at our institution. Renal impairment is considered at a Cl$_{Cr}$ level of 50 to 70 mL/min, renal insufficiency at a level of 20 to 50 mL/min, and renal failure at a level of 4 to 20 mL/min. Note that serum creatinine level of 1.2 mg/dL in a pregnant patient indicates >50% reduction in GFR. $Cl_{Cr}$ is calculated by the formula:

$$Cl_{Cr} \text{ (mL/min)} = [Cr_{urine} \text{ (mg/dL)} \times \text{volume of urine (mL)}]/ [Cr_{serum} \text{ (mg/dL)} \times \text{time (minutes)}]$$

- **Management** of acute oliguria should optimize central hemodynamics and increase glomerulotubular flow. Precipitating factors should be identified and corrected. Nephrotoxic agents should be minimized and all medications renally dosed. Electrolytes should be monitored and repleted.
  - If there is evidence for volume depletion, a fluid challenge should first be administered and volume infused until cardiac output is restored. In patients with invasive hemodynamic monitoring, base the management on cardiac filling pressures (CVP and PCWP), cardiac output (using CI), and blood pressure (BP).
  - There is no evidence that low "renal dose" dopamine or furosemide treatments are beneficial. Dopamine may increase risk for bowel ischemia.
  - Low-dose dopamine (5 mg/kg/min) has traditionally been used to improve inotropy in oliguric renal failure. However, recent studies have shown that dopamine has little benefit in these situations and may increase risk for bowel ischemia.
  - Similarly, loop diuretics are often used to treat oliguric renal failure, but multiple studies have suggested that not only is there no benefit, but their use may cause harm to critically ill patients. If loop diuretics are used, it should be as a continuous infusion. Rarely, a "Lasix-dependent" patient is encountered who requires diuretic to maintain adequate urine output. This is very uncommon, however, and most postoperative patients with oliguria are simply hypovolemic. Volume status and cardiac output should be optimized before proceeding with pharmacologic management.
  - Special attention should be given to urine output in postoperative gynecologic oncology patients who have had malignant ascites removed. The fluid tends to reaccumulate in the abdominal cavity quickly after drainage and may require massive ongoing fluid replacement.
  - Patients who fail conservative management of AKI may require **renal replacement therapy**. Indications include volume overload, uremia, hyperkalemia, severe acidosis, and rapidly increasing serum creatinine.

## HEMATOLOGIC CRITICAL CARE

### Anemia

- **Anemia** is defined as a hemoglobin level of less than 12 g/dL in women and 14 g/dL in men. Levels of 7 g/dL, or even lower, are typically well tolerated in patients without cardiovascular disease.
- The decision to transfuse depends on the clinical situation and should balance the potential risks of a blood transfusion with patient symptoms, comorbidities, and risk of further bleeding. A landmark study that compared a conservative transfusion threshold (<7 g/dL) with a liberal threshold (<10 g/dL) demonstrated a lower complication rate and 28-day mortality in the conservative group.
- However, higher hemoglobin levels may be desired in preoperative patients in whom blood loss is anticipated; patients with cardiac ischemia who need better oxygen delivery; and in patients undergoing radiation therapy, where availability of oxygen to form free radicals may contribute to better treatment outcomes.

- Adverse effects include hypocalcemia due to citrate anticoagulant in banked blood, hyperkalemia in patients with circulatory shock, hemolytic reactions, transmission of infectious diseases, and transfusion-related acute lung injury (TRALI).
- Due to the risk of developing coagulopathy during **massive hemorrhage**, resuscitation should include transfusing a combination of red blood cells (RBCs), fresh frozen plasma (FFP), and platelets. There does not yet exist consensus regarding the optimal ratio, but some institutions have proposed a 1:1:1 ratio of RBC:FFP:platelets.

## Thrombocytopenia

- **Thrombocytopenia** is defined as a platelet count of less than 140,000/$\mu$L. Bleeding complications typically do not occur until levels fall below 50,000/$\mu$L.
- Drugs that may cause thrombocytopenia include trimethoprim-sulfamethoxazole, penicillins, thiazide diuretics, chemotherapeutic agents, and heparin. **Heparin-induced thrombocytopenia** (HIT) is an antibody-mediated reaction that most often occurs 4 to 10 days after initiating heparin treatment. The diagnosis should be considered in patients receiving heparin in whom platelet count drops >50%. After HIT is diagnosed, heparin should immediately be discontinued and an alternative anticoagulant such as lepirudin, bivalirudin, and argatroban should be initiated.

## Disseminated Intravascular Coagulation

- **Disseminated intravascular coagulation** is a disorder of hemostasis in which intravascular activation of both clotting and fibrinolytic systems leads to consumption of coagulation factors and platelets. Widespread endothelial damage causes release of **tissue factor** that activates these systems. Clinically, a patient will experience systemic hemorrhage concurrent with widespread microvascular thrombosis.
- **Lab abnormalities** include increased prothrombin time, partial thromboplastin time, and fibrin split products (D-dimer). Platelet counts and fibrinogen are decreased. Peripheral blood smears show fragmented RBCs (i.e., schistocytes) and thrombocytopenia with large platelets.
- Risk factors include **sepsis, trauma, obstetric complications, malignancy, liver failure**, and **renal failure**.
- **Treatment** is supportive and difficult. Any inciting factors should be addressed. **Transfusion therapy** with platelets, FFP, and/or cryoprecipitate may be provided. However, this rarely helps and may feed the consumption of platelets and coagulation factors, leading to further microvascular thrombosis.

# INFECTIOUS DISEASES

## Sepsis

- **Sepsis** is a clinical syndrome characterized by a host's inflammatory response to infection including vasodilation, complement activation, loss of hemostatic balance, and increased microvascular permeability. This results in widespread microvascular and cellular injury, which causes further inflammation, multiorgan dysfunction, and ultimately organ failure. Table 3-5 lists definitions for the SIRS, sepsis, severe sepsis, and septic shock. Early septic shock is **distributive**, whereas later stages of septic shock can produce **cardiogenic** shock when hypotension, acidosis, and ischemia suppress myocardial function. Additionally, infection, tissue trauma, or obstetric accidents can activate the intrinsic coagulation pathway with subsequent intravascular thrombosis and fibrinolysis, causing disseminated intravascular coagulation and massive bleeding.

| TABLE 3-5 | Criteria for Sepsis and Related Disorders |
|---|---|
| SIRS | At least two of: <br> Temperature >38°C or <36°C <br> Heart rate >90 beats/min <br> Respiratory rate >20 breaths/min or $Pa_{CO2}$ <32 mm Hg <br> WBC >12,000 cells/mm$^3$ or <4,000 cells/mm$^3$ or <br> >10% bands |
| Sepsis | SIRS that is the result of an infection |
| Severe sepsis | Sepsis resulting in organ dysfunction |
| Septic shock | Severe sepsis with hypotension refractory to volume resuscitation |

SIRS, systemic inflammatory response syndrome; WBC, white blood cell.

- Successful management of sepsis includes early recognition, aggressive but appropriate fluid replacement, broad-spectrum antibiotics, source identification and control, and ongoing supportive care. Table 3-6 contains the sepsis bundle proposed by the Surviving Sepsis Campaign. This and guidelines for managing sepsis can be found at http://www.survivingsepsis.org.
- Goals for **initial resuscitation** during the first 6 hours in patients with sepsis-induced hypotension (hypotension despite initial fluid challenge or a lactate >4 mmol/L) include CVP 8 to 12 mm Hg, mean arterial pressure ≥65 mm Hg, urine output 0.5 mL/kg/hr, central venous or mixed oxygen saturation of 70% or 65% respectively, and normalizing lactate.

| TABLE 3-6 | Surviving Sepsis Campaign Bundles |
|---|---|
| To be completed within 3 hr | 1. Measure lactate levels. <br> 2. Obtain cultures prior to antibiotic administration. <br> 3. Administer broad-spectrum antibiotics. <br> 4. Administer 30 mL/kg crystalloid for hypotension or lactate >4 mmol/L. |
| To be completed within 6 hr | 5. Apply vasopressors (for hypotension that does not respond to initial fluid resuscitation) to maintain a mean arterial pressure (MAP) ≥65 mm Hg. <br> 6. In the event of persistent arterial hypotension despite volume resuscitation (septic shock) or initial lactate 4 mmol/L: <br> • Measure central venous pressure (CVP).[a] <br> • Measure central venous oxygen saturation (ScvO$_2$).[a] <br> 7. Remeasure lactate if initial lactate was elevated.[a] |

[a]Targets for quantitative resuscitation included in the guidelines are CVP of ≥8 mm Hg, ScvO$_2$ of 70%, and normalization of lactate.
Adapted from Dellinger RP, Levy MM, Rhodes A, et al. Surviving sepsis campaign: international guidelines for management of severe sepsis and septic shock: 2012. *Crit Care Med* 2013;41:580–637.

- Crystalloids are the initial fluids of choice. Albumin can be considered if significant amounts of fluids are required. Current evidence argues against the use of hydroxyethyl starches.
- If vasopressors are required, norepinephrine is generally used first line. Epinephrine is the adjunctive agent of choice.
- If none of these measures successfully restore hemodynamic stability, IV hydrocortisone 200 mg/day can be considered.
- **Diagnosis** should include cultures as long as collection does not delay antimicrobial therapy >45 minutes and imaging studies if this will help confirm the source of infection.
- Broad-spectrum antibiotics should be initiated within 1 hour of recognizing severe sepsis or septic shock. Regimens should be assessed daily, and empiric therapy should not be continued beyond 3 to 5 days. Early source control should be pursued aggressively and should involve removal of nonessential intravascular devices.
- Adjunctive therapies that include immunoglobulin and selenium are no longer recommended. There has been conflicting evidence regarding recombinant activated protein C; however, the drug has recently been withdrawn from the market.
- **Toxic shock syndrome** occurs in <5 per 100,000 reproductive age women. Staphylococcal toxic shock syndrome (STSS) results from toxin 1 produced by *Staphylococcus aureus*. Toxic shock–like syndrome (TSLS) results from pyrogenic exotoxin produced by group A *Streptococcus* (GAS). Both can cause dramatic and rapid critical illness including fever, hypotension, malaise, mucosal hyperemia, erythroderma and desquamation, and diarrhea. There is an association with extended or superabsorbent tampon use, surgical wounds, skin infection, and abscesses. STSS can occur in otherwise healthy individuals, whereas TSLS typically presents with a prior infection. Blood cultures can be negative.
- The **diagnostic criteria** for STSS are the following: fever >39.9°C; diffuse blanching erythroderma progressing to desquamation at 10 to 14 days, especially on the palms and soles; hypotension with systolic BP <90 mm Hg or orthostasis; and involvement of three or more organ systems such as GI (diarrhea, vomiting), musculoskeletal (severe myalgia, creatine kinase greater than twice upper limit of normal), mucous membrane hyperemia (oropharynx, conjunctiva, vagina), renal dysfunction (BUN or creatinine greater than twice upper limit of normal), liver dysfunction (bilirubin, aspartate aminotransferase, or alanine aminotransferase greater than twice the upper limit of normal), hematologic abnormalities (platelets <100,000/mL), or mental status changes without focal findings. Diagnostic criteria for TSLS are similar but require isolation of GAS and dysfunction in at least two organ systems.
- The **differential diagnosis** includes Rocky Mountain spotted fever, Stevens-Johnson syndrome, scarlet fever, viral exanthems, drug reaction, meningococcemia, leptospirosis, and heat stroke.
- **Treatment** includes early recognition, elimination/debridement of infectious source if identified, antibiotics, and ICU supportive care with fluids, oxygen, and vasopressors if needed. Mortality ranges from 5% to 60% depending on the bacterial strain and severity of illness.
  - Beta-lactam agents, including penicillin G, are effective against GAS, whereas STSS requires vancomycin, nafcillin, or oxacillin.
  - Clindamycin is given for its inhibitory action on protein synthesis including toxin suppression.
  - In patients who do not show rapid clinical response, immunoglobulins may be administered to neutralize superantigens and potentially shorten the disease course.

## NEUROLOGIC CRITICAL CARE

- In addition to patient comfort, **sedation** and **pain control** in the ICU can serve to minimize stress-mediated activation of neuroendocrine pathways and increase in sympathetic tone. Presence of pain, anxiety, and delirium should be evaluated in an acutely agitated patient.
- The most commonly used medications for sedation are haloperidol, opioid analgesics, midazolam, propofol, diazepam, and lorazepam. Midazolam and diazepam are most appropriate for rapid sedation of acutely agitated patients but should be used with caution in elderly patients. Propofol is most useful when the ability to rapidly awaken a patient is needed; however, if greater than 2 days of infusion are administered, triglyceride levels should be monitored.
- To minimize prolonged sedative effects, systematic tapering or daily interruptions in sedative doses is recommended. Sedation goals should be established and regularly reviewed for each patient.
- There exist several scales to assess a patient's level of sedation, including the sedation-analgesia scale (SAS), Richmond Agitation Sedation Scale (RASS), Vancouver Interaction and Calmness Scale (VICS), Motor Activity Assessment Scale (MAAS), and the Ramsay Scale for Scoring Sedation. These scales are subjective, but RASS, MAAS, and VICS have been validated for critically ill patients.
- **Delirium** is an acute, transient, fluctuating state of confusion characterized by impairment in maintaining attention. Recent studies have suggested an association between presence of delirium and risk of dying. Delirium can be hypoactive (decreased physical and mental activity, inattention), hyperactive (combativeness, agitation), or mixed.
- The mnemonic **DELIRIUM** can be used to remember risk factors: **d**rugs, **e**lectrolyte abnormalities, **l**ack of drugs (withdrawal), **i**nfection, **r**educed sensory input, **i**ntracranial problems, **u**rinary retention and fecal impaction, and **m**yocardial problems.
- Tools to assess delirium include the Confusion Assessment Method for the ICU (CAM-ICU), the Intensive Care Delirium Screening Checklist (ICDSC), and the Neelon and Champagne (NEECHAM) Confusion Scale.
- **Treatment** should include identifying and treating the underlying cause. Concurrent strategies include reorienting patients, restoring normal sleep-wake cycles, removing medications that exacerbate delirium, providing hearing aids/glasses, and removing invasive devices whenever possible. If pharmacologic therapy is used, benzodiazepines should be avoided in favor of antipsychotics such as haloperidol (2 to 5 mg every 6 to 12 hours).

## SPECIAL OBSTETRIC CONSIDERATIONS IN CRITICAL CARE

Hypertension, hemorrhage, sepsis, and cardiopulmonary conditions account for the majority of intensive care admissions in the antepartum and postpartum period. Physiologic alterations in pregnancy can continue into the postpartum period and are important to account for when interpreting critical care data.

- Profound **hemodynamic alterations** occur during pregnancy, including a 40% to 50% increase in blood volume, 30% to 50% increase in cardiac output, decrease in systemic vascular resistance, and increase in heart rate. Little data exists to determine the use of invasive hemodynamic monitoring in obstetric patients.

- Although the need for **cardiopulmonary resuscitation** is rare, left lateral uterine displacement is essential to maximizing cardiac output generated during chest compressions.
- In addition to etiologies typically seen outside of pregnancy, chorioamnionitis, pyelonephritis, tocolytic therapy, and preeclampsia should be considered when an obstetric patient presents with **ARDS**. In this condition, pregnancy-induced respiratory alkalosis may be exacerbated by hyperventilation. Otherwise, management with supportive care and lung protective ventilation is similar to that for nonobstetric patients.
- Colloid osmotic pressure is decreased by up to 20% in pregnancy, thereby increasing the risk of developing cardiogenic and noncardiogenic pulmonary edema, especially in women with underlying cardiac conditions. Careful fluid management in these patients is paramount.
- In critically ill obstetric patients, the decision to move toward delivery should be evaluated as a patient's clinical course evolves. If a condition is exacerbated by pregnancy and is refractory to all conservative interventions, delivery can be considered. The risks of prematurity should be carefully balanced with the risks to the mother of maintaining her pregnancy.

## SUGGESTED READINGS

American Society of Anesthesiologists Task Force on Pulmonary Artery Catheterization. Practice guidelines for pulmonary artery catheterization: an updated report. *Anesthesiology* 2004;99:988–1014.

Anderson JL, Adams CD, Antman EM, et al. ACC/AHA 2007 guidelines for the management of patients with unstable angina/non–ST-elevation myocardial infarction: a report of the American College of Cardiology/American Heart Association Task Force on Practice Guidelines (Writing Committee to Revise the 2002 Guidelines for the Management of Patients With Unstable Angina/Non–ST-Elevation Myocardial Infarction). *Circulation* 2007;116:e148–e304.

Deakin CD, Morrison LJ, Morley PT, et al; Advanced Life Support Chapter Collaborators. Part 8: advanced life support: 2010 International Consensus on Cardiopulmonary Resuscitation and Emergency Cardiovascular Care Science with Treatment Recommendations. *Resuscitation* 2010;81(suppl 1):e93–e174.

De Backer D, Biston P, Devriendt J, et al. Comparison of dopamine and norepinephrine in the treatment of shock. *N Engl J Med* 2010;362(9):779–789.

Dellinger RP, Levy MM, Rhodes A, et al; Surviving Sepsis Campaign Guidelines Committee including the Pediatric Subgroup. Surviving Sepsis Campaign: international guidelines for management of severe sepsis and septic shock: 2012. *Crit Care Med* 2013;41:580–637.

Fan E, Needham DM, Stewart TE. Ventilator management of acute lung injury and acute respiratory distress syndrome. *JAMA* 2005;294:2889–2896.

Hébert PC, Wells G, Blajchman MA, et al. A multicenter, randomized, controlled clinical trial of transfusion requirements in critical care. *N Engl J Med* 1999;340(6):409–417.

Jaax ME, Greinacher A. Management of heparin-induced thrombocytopenia. *Expert Opin Pharmacother* 2012;13(7):987–1006.

Jacobi J, Fraser GL, Coursin DB, et al; Task Force of the American College of Critical Care Medicine of the Society of Critical Care Medicine, American Society of Health-System Pharmacists, American College of Chest Physicians. Clinical practice guidelines for the sustained use of sedatives and analgesics in the critically ill adult. *Crit Care Med* 2002;30(1):119–141.

Kellum JA. The use of diuretics and dopamine in acute renal failure: a systematic review of the evidence. *Crit Care* 1997;1(2):53–59.

Lappin E, Ferguson AJ. Gram-positive toxic shock syndromes. *Lancet Infect Dis* 2009;9(5):281–290.

Lindenfeld J, Albert NM, Boehmer JP, et al. Executive summary: HFSA 2010 comprehensive heart failure practice guideline. *J Card Fail* 2010;16:475–539.

National Heart, Lung, and Blood Institute ARDS Clinical Network. Higher versus lower positive end-expiratory pressures in patients with acute respiratory distress syndrome. *N Engl J Med* 2004;351:327–336.

O'Gara PT, Kushner FG, Ascheim DD, et al; American College of Cardiology Foundation/ American Heart Association Task Force on Practice Guidelines. 2013 ACCF/AHA guideline for the management of ST-elevation myocardial infarction: a report of the American College of Cardiology Foundation/American Heart Association Task Force on Practice Guidelines. *Circulation* 2013;127(4):e362–e425.

Ricci Z, Cruz D, Ronco C. The RIFLE criteria and mortality in acute kidney injury: a systematic review. *Kidney Int* 2008;73(5):538–546.

SAFE Study Investigators. A comparison of albumin and saline for fluid resuscitation in the intensive care unit. *N Engl J Med* 2004;350:2247–2256.

Shafiee MAS, Bohn D, Hoorn EJ, et al. How to select optimal maintenance intravenous fluid therapy. *Q J Med* 2003;96:601–610.

Weil MH, Shubin H. Proposed reclassification of shock states with special reference to distributive defects. *Adv Exp Med Biol* 1971;23:13–23.

Yeomans ER, Gilstrap LC III. Physiologic changes in pregnancy and their impact on critical care. *Crit Care Med* 2005;33(10)(suppl):S256–S258.

Zeeman GG. Obstetric critical care: a blueprint for improved outcomes. *Crit Care Med* 2006;34(9)(suppl):S208–S214.

# 4 Preconception Counseling and Prenatal Care

William Fletcher and Melissa L. Russo

## PRECONCEPTION CARE AND COUNSELING

**Preconception care and counseling** are important to identify any medical, pharmacologic, behavioral, or social risks to a woman's health and initiate an intervention prior to pregnancy in an effort to reduce the risk of maternal–fetal morbidity and mortality. The preconception evaluation offers a unique opportunity to inform women of potential infertility or pregnancy issues. Preconception care is especially useful for women who have underlying medical conditions (e.g., diabetes mellitus, phenylketonurics, renal disease), exposure to potential teratogens (e.g., warfarin, isotretinoin), or high-risk behaviors (e.g., smoking or cocaine use). Preconception counseling should emphasize healthy preconception habits and confirm that vaccines are up-to-date. This should be incorporated into routine health care visits for women of childbearing age because approximately half of pregnancies in the United States are unplanned. The following sections will highlight the main areas to address during a preconception evaluation.

## Medical Assessment

- Preconception care (Table 4-1) should include a thorough assessment of an individual's medical problems. This is becoming increasingly important as the incidence of obesity-related comorbidities, such as diabetes mellitus and hypertension, increases. These conditions should be as well-controlled as possible prior to conception because they can have significant adverse effects on the developing fetus and adverse effects in the mother. For example, the risk of birth defects increases with hemoglobin A1C level in diabetic patients, with an A1C greater than 10.6% conferring eight times the risk of having a birth defect compared to women with an A1C of less than 8%.
- With maternal medical issues, it is important to discuss the impact on the fetus and the potential for the pregnancy to exacerbate the underlying medical condition.
- With any complex medical condition, expertise from a maternal–fetal medicine specialist is advised and ongoing collaboration with other specialists may be indicated.

## Gynecologic and Reproductive History

- The gynecologic and obstetric history may reveal potential factors contributing to infertility or complications in a future pregnancy.
- Discussion of menstrual and contraceptive history provides an educational opportunity for conception counseling and to discuss optimal timing of a pregnancy in a medically complex patient.
- Past history of sexually transmitted infections is important to note because these women may be at increased risk of these infections in a future pregnancy. These infections include *Neisseria gonorrhea*, *Chlamydia trachomatis*, *Treponema pallidum*, genital herpes simplex virus (HSV), and HIV.

| TABLE 4-1 | Preconception Risk Assessment: Laboratory Testing |
|---|---|
| **Recommended for All Women** | **Recommended for Some Women** |
| Hemoglobin level or hematocrit<br>Rh factor<br>Urine dipstick testing (protein and sugar)<br>Pap smear test (for cervical cancer)<br>Gonococcal/chlamydial screen<br>Syphilis test<br>Hepatitis B surface antigen<br>Rubella IgG<br>HIV screen<br>Illicit drug screen (offer) | Tuberculosis screen<br>Hepatitis C<br>Lead level<br>Varicella IgG screen<br>Toxoplasmosis IgG screen<br>CMV IgG screen<br>Parvovirus B19 IgG screen<br>Genetic carrier screening for hemoglobinopathies, Tay-Sachs disease, Canavan disease, cystic fibrosis, or other genetic diseases<br>Screening for parental karyotype for habitual spontaneous abortion |

IgG, immunoglobulin G; CMV, cytomegalovirus. Adapted from U.S. Department of Health and Human Services. *Caring for our Future: The Content of Prenatal Care. A Report of the PHS Export Panel.* Washington, DC: U.S. Department of Health and Human Services, 1989, with permission.

- With prior poor pregnancy outcomes, the recurrence risk of an adverse outcome should be discussed. In some cases, there are interventions to reduce these risks in a future pregnancy.
- Known congenital uterine malformations are important to identify because these conditions can be associated with recurrent pregnancy loss, malpresentation, or preterm birth.

## Age

- Advanced maternal age (older than 35 years at time of delivery) is associated with increased risks that include infertility, fetal aneuploidy, gestational diabetes, preeclampsia, and stillbirth.
- Prior to pregnancy, it is important to educate women about these risks and discuss aneuploidy screening and diagnostic tests that are available, as well as management options, if available.

## Family History

- A patient's family history can identify genetic risks to a future pregnancy.
- A preconception history includes evaluation for family history of congenital anomalies; chromosomal abnormalities (e.g., Down syndrome); mental retardation/developmental delay; inherited diseases such as hemoglobinopathies, cystic fibrosis, and hemophilia; recurrent pregnancy loss/stillbirth/early infant death in the family; ethnicity; and consanguinity.
- **Carrier screening** for hereditary disease is traditionally based on ethnic background of the couple and allows counseling before the first potentially affected pregnancy. Early recognition of carrier status informs patients of their risks outside of the emotional context of pregnancy and facilitates educated decisions about reproductive goals and testing during or after pregnancy. Expanded carrier screening is an option for patients, in which over 100 diseases are screened in a single test. Family history can identify those at increased risks for specific diseases, such as muscular dystrophy, fragile X syndrome, or Down syndrome, for which genetic counseling should be offered. Information about diagnostic tests, such as chorionic villus sampling (CVS) or amniocentesis, can be explained. In some instances, genetic counseling may result in a decision to forgo pregnancy or to use assisted reproductive technologies that can decrease this risk.

## Medications

Both over-the-counter and prescription drugs, herbs, and supplements should be reviewed. In general, U.S. Food and Drug Administration (FDA) pregnancy categories X and D medications should be avoided or discontinued. For other medications, maternal and fetal risk–benefit should be assessed, with appreciation that in cases maternal risk of not using a specific medicine may outweigh fetal risks of administration. Assistance in answering questions about reproductive toxicology is available through the online database **REPROTOX** (http://www.reprotox.org). The Reproductive Toxicology Center at Columbia Hospital for Women Medical Center, one of the sponsors of REPROTOX, also offers a clinical inquiry program. Many states have teratogen hotlines or state-funded programs; the Organization of Teratology Information Specialists (OTIS) is a good source for information about these programs and offers other resources (http://www.otispregnancy.org).

- **Isotretinoin (Accutane):** An oral treatment for severe cystic acne, it is highly teratogenic, causing craniofacial defects (microtia, anotia). It should be discontinued prior to pregnancy.

- **Warfarin (Coumadin) and vitamin K antagonists:** Such anticoagulants have been associated with warfarin embryopathy. Because heparins (both unfractionated and low-molecular-weight) do not cross the placenta, women requiring anticoagulation should be encouraged to switch to heparin therapy prior to conception, except in rare cases.
- **Antiepileptic drugs (AED):** Children born to mothers treated with certain AEDs are at increased risk for congenital malformations, particularly when these drugs are used in the first trimester. **Valproic acid** is associated with neural tube defects (NTDs); adverse neurocognitive effects; and craniofacial, limb, and cardiac abnormalities. **Carbamazepine** exposure has been associated with facial dysmorphism and fingernail hypoplasia. Data on newer AEDs are still limited. For women with seizure disorders, it is important to have them on AED regimens with less teratogenicity. Notably, a patient with an unintended pregnancy using an AED should not abruptly discontinue her medication but rather be switched to another medication where possible, due to risk of seizure recurrence. A detailed fetal anatomy sonogram, maternal serum alpha-fetoprotein (MSAFP), and fetal echocardiogram may provide useful information for these patients.
- **Lithium** has been associated with increased incidence of heart defects and should only be continued based on the severity and frequency of illness. Fetal echocardiogram is recommended for women taking lithium in the first trimester. **Lamotrigine** is a mood stabilizer with a significantly better reproductive safety profile than lithium. It should be considered as an alternative in women with bipolar disorder.
- **Selective serotonin reuptake inhibitors (SSRIs)** are considered safe; however, paroxetine early in pregnancy has been associated with increased risk of heart defects, and an FDA advisory notes an association between late-term SSRI use and persistent pulmonary hypertension in the newborn. SSRI use in pregnancy should be individualized, balancing the risks of maternal depression and potential fetal effects.

## Nutritional Assessment

- **Folic acid** supplementation reduces the risk of NTDs. The U.S. Public Health Service recommends daily supplementation with 0.4 mg of folic acid for all women capable of becoming pregnant. Unless contraindicated by the presence of pernicious anemia, women who have previously had a fetus with an NTD should take 4.0 mg of folic acid daily.
- The body mass index (BMI), defined as (weight in kilograms/[height in meters]$^2$), is the preferred indicator of nutritional status. Very overweight (BMI above 30) and very underweight women (BMI <20) are at risk for poor pregnancy outcomes.
- Eating habits (fasting, pica, eating disorders, and the use of megavitamin supplementation) should be discussed.
- Excess use of multivitamin supplements containing **vitamin A** should be avoided because the estimated dietary intake of vitamin A for most women in the United States is sufficient. Vitamin A is teratogenic in humans at dosages of more than 20,000 to 50,000 IU daily, producing fetal malformations like those seen with isotretinoin.
- Women with a history of anorexia or bulimia may benefit from both nutritional and psychological counseling before conception.
- Women with history of gastric bypass must see a nutritional specialist in addition to their obstetrician to ensure they are getting adequate caloric and nutritional needs in a pregnancy.

## Substance Use Assessment

All patients should be asked about alcohol, tobacco, and illicit drug use. Alcohol is a known teratogen, and a clear dose-response relationship exists between alcohol use and fetal effects, including fetal alcohol syndrome. Tobacco use has been identified as the leading preventable cause of low birth weight. Cocaine has been identified as a teratogen, as well as a cause of prematurity, abruptio placentae, and intrauterine growth restriction (IUGR). If substance addiction is present, structured recovery programs are needed to effect behavioral change. The preconception interview allows timely education about drug use and pregnancy, informed decision making about the risks of using these substances at the time of conception, and the introduction of interventions for women who need treatment.

- **Smoking:** Approximately 11% of pregnant women in the United States smoke. Carbon monoxide and nicotine are believed to be the main ingredients in cigarette smoke that are responsible for adverse fetal effects. Smoking is associated with increases in the following:
  - Spontaneous abortion (1.2 to 1.8 times greater in smokers than in nonsmokers)
  - Abortion of a chromosomally normal fetus (39% more likely in smokers than in nonsmokers)
  - Abruptio placentae, placenta previa, and premature rupture of membranes
  - Preterm birth (1.2 to 1.5 times greater in smokers than in nonsmokers)
  - Low infant birth weight
  - Sudden infant death syndrome
- **Smoking cessation** should be encouraged prior to conception. However, cessation during pregnancy still improves the birth weight of the infant, especially if use stops before 16 weeks' gestation. Prospective randomized controlled clinical trials have shown that **intensive smoking reduction programs**, with frequent patient contact and close supervision, aid in smoking cessation and result in increased infant birth weights.
- Successful interventions emphasize ways to stop smoking rather than merely providing mandates to stop smoking.
- **Nicotine replacement therapy** (chewing gum or transdermal patch) carry warnings about the adverse effects of nicotine on mother and fetus. However, nicotine is only one of the toxins in tobacco smoke. Smoking cessation with nicotine replacement reduces fetal exposure to carbon monoxide and other toxins and may improve outcomes. For women who are otherwise unable to reduce their smoking, it may be reasonable to advise nicotine replacement as an adjunct to counseling even during pregnancy. Use of nicotine replacement in a patient who is unable to reduce her smoking may impose greater fetal risk.
- **Alcohol:** Ethanol freely crosses the placenta and the fetal blood–brain barrier and is a known teratogen. Fetal ethanol toxicity is dose-related but without a defined lower threshold of exposure.
  - The exposure time of greatest risk is the first trimester. Nevertheless, fetal brain development may be affected throughout gestation.
  - Although an occasional drink during pregnancy has not been shown to be harmful, patients should be counseled that the threshold for adverse effects is unknown.
  - **Fetal alcohol syndrome** is characterized by growth retardation, facial abnormalities, and central nervous system (CNS) dysfunction. Facial abnormalities include shortened palpebral fissures, low-set ears, midfacial hypoplasia, a smooth philtrum, and a thin upper lip. CNS abnormalities of fetal alcohol syndrome include microcephaly, mental retardation, and behavioral disorders, such as attention

deficit disorder. Skeletal abnormalities and structural cardiac defects are also seen with greater frequency in the children of women who abuse alcohol during pregnancy than in those who do not. The most common cardiac structural anomaly is ventricular septal defect, but several others occur.

- **Illicit drug use:** Recent data show approximately 4% of pregnant women use some illicit substance in pregnancy.
  - **Marijuana:** Marijuana has been shown to alter brain neurotransmitters as well as brain chemistry. Marijuana can remain in the body for up to 30 days, thus prolonging fetal exposure. Smoking marijuana produces as much as five times the amount of carbon monoxide as does cigarette smoking, perhaps altering fetal oxygenation. Marijuana has been associated with deficits in problem-solving skills that require sustained attention and visual memory, analysis, and integration and with subtle deficits in learning and memory.
  - **Cocaine:** Adverse maternal effects include profound vasoconstriction, leading to malignant hypertension, cardiac ischemia, and cerebral infarction. Cocaine may have a direct cardiotoxic effect, leading to sudden death. Complications of cocaine use in pregnancy include spontaneous abortion, fetal death in utero, premature rupture of membranes, preterm labor and delivery, IUGR, meconium staining of amniotic fluid, and abruptio placentae. Cocaine is teratogenic, and its use has been associated with cases of in utero fetal cerebral infarction, microcephaly, and limb reduction defects. Genitourinary malformations have been reported with first-trimester cocaine use. Infants born to women who use cocaine are at risk for neurobehavioral abnormalities and impairment in orientation and motor function.
  - **Opiates:** Opiate use is associated with increased rates of stillbirth, fetal growth restriction, prematurity, and neonatal mortality, perhaps due to risky behaviors in opiate substance abusers. Methadone treatment is associated with improved pregnancy outcomes. Neonates born to narcotic addicts are at risk for a severe, potentially fatal, narcotic withdrawal syndrome. Although the incidence of clinically significant withdrawal is slightly lower among methadone-treated addicts, its course can be just as severe. Neonatal withdrawal is characterized by a high-pitched cry, poor feeding, hypertonicity, tremors, irritability, sneezing, sweating, vomiting, diarrhea, and, occasionally, seizures. Frequent sharing of needles has resulted in high rates of HIV infection (>50%) and hepatitis among intravenous narcotic addicts.
  - **Amphetamines:** Crystal methamphetamine, a potent stimulant that is inhaled, injected, or snorted, has been associated with decreased fetal head circumference and increased risk of abruptio placentae, IUGR, and fetal death in utero. However, no proven teratogenicity exists.
  - **Hallucinogens:** No evidence proves that lysergic acid diethylamide (LSD) or other hallucinogens cause chromosomal damage, as was once reported. Few studies exist on the possible deleterious effects of maternal hallucinogen use during pregnancy. No proven teratogenicity to LSD exists.

## Social History

A social and lifestyle history should be obtained to identify risky behaviors and exposures that may compromise reproductive outcome. Social, financial, and psychological issues that could affect pregnancy planning can also be identified.

- **Domestic violence:** Women are more likely to be abused during pregnancy than at other times. Approximately 37% of abused women are assaulted during their pregnancy, resulting in possible abruptio placentae, antepartum hemorrhage, fetal fractures, rupture of the internal organs, and preterm labor. Information about community, social, and legal resources should be made available to women who are abused and a plan devised for dealing with the abusive partner. See Chapter 33.

• **Insurance coverage and financial difficulties:** Many women and couples do not know the eligibility requirements or amount of maternity coverage provided by their insurance carriers or may lack medical insurance coverage altogether. Referral for medical assistance programs should be part of preconception planning as needed.

## GENETIC COUNSELING AND TESTING

### Genetic Counseling

Genetic counseling, risk assessment, and intervention are based on the family history of the biologic mother and father, maternal age, ethnicity, drug or environmental exposures, and medical and obstetric history (Tables 4-2 and 4-3). Information on hereditary birth defects is best assessed with a three-generation pedigree. Table 4-4 describes major modes of inheritance.

• Assisted reproductive technologies, such as donor egg and sperm, sperm sorting, and preimplantation genetic diagnosis (PGD), may obviate the risk in specific cases.

| TABLE 4-2 | Recommendations for Ethnicity-Based Carrier Screening |
|---|---|
| **Disease** | **Carrier Frequency** |
| *Ashkenazi Jewish* | |
| Tay-Sachs | 1/30 |
| Canavan | 1/40 |
| Cystic fibrosis | 1/29 |
| Familial dysautonomia | 1/30 |
| *Mediterranean* | |
| Thalassemia | 1/20–1/50 |
| Sickle cell anemia | 1/30–1/50 |
| *European Caucasian* | |
| Cystic fibrosis | 1/25–1/29 |
| *African American* | |
| Sickle cell anemia | 1/10 |
| Thalassemia | 1/30–1/75 |
| Cystic fibrosis | 1/65 |
| *Asian* | |
| Thalassemia | 1/20–1/50 |
| Cystic fibrosis | 1/90 |
| *Hispanic* | |
| Cystic fibrosis | 1/46 |
| Sickle cell anemia | 1/30–1/200 |
| Thalassemia | 1/30–1/75 |
| *French Canadian* | |
| Tay-Sachs | 1/15 |
| Cystic fibrosis | 1/29 |

| TABLE 4-3 | Indications for Genetic Counseling |
|---|---|

Mother 35 years or older at her estimated date of delivery
Fetal anomalies detected via ultrasonography
Abnormal first-trimester serum/nuchal translucency screening
Abnormal triple/quad screening or abnormal alpha-fetoprotein test results
Parental exposure to teratogens
  Drugs
  Radiation
  Infection
Family history of genetic disease (includes chromosome, single gene, and
  multifactorial disorders)
Birth defects
Mental retardation
Cancer, heart disease, hypertension, diabetes, and other common conditions
  (especially when onset occurs at an early age)
Membership in ethnic group in which certain genetic disorders are frequent
  when appropriate screening for or prenatal diagnosis of the disease is available
  (e.g., sickle cell anemia, Tay-Sachs disease, Canavan disease, thalassemia)
Consanguinity
Reproductive failure
Infertility
Repeated spontaneous abortions
Stillbirths and neonatal deaths
Infant, child, or adult with the following:
  Dysmorphic features
  Developmental and/or growth delay
  Ambiguous genitalia or abnormal sexual development

Adoption and avoidance of pregnancy represent other choices. CVS and amniocentesis permit early diagnosis, facilitate preparation for the care of an affected child, and give the option for pregnancy termination.

• In general, prenatal screening involves three groups: the general pregnant population, patients with a specific ethnic background or positive family history for a genetic disorder, and patients with a fetal anomaly. The National Society of Genetic Counselors (NSGC) urges caution regarding prenatal testing for adult-onset conditions unless there are treatments or preventive measures that can be initiated during pregnancy or in early childhood.

## Prenatal Genetic Screening

**Aneuploidy** refers to any condition in which there are an abnormal number of chromosomes. Normally, 46 chromosomes (23 pairs) are found in every somatic cell of the body. Regardless of the maternal age, aneuploidy screening (Table 4-5) should be offered to all women before 20 weeks' gestation. Women who do not seek prenatal care until the second trimester should be offered quadruple screening and ultrasound assessment. Women seen in the first trimester should be offered first-trimester serum and nuchal translucency screening or an integrated approach combining first- and second-trimester screening.

## TABLE 4-4 — Major Modes of Inheritance

| Inheritance | Risk of Recurrence | Properties | Conditions |
| --- | --- | --- | --- |
| Autosomal dominant | If parent has gene: 50% for child | Multiple generations<br>Both genders affected equally | Achondroplasia<br>Acute intermittent porphyria<br>Adult polycystic kidney disease<br>BRCA1–BRCA2 breast cancer<br>Familial hypercholesterolemia<br>Familial hypertrophic cardiomyopathy<br>Hemorrhagic telangiectasia<br>Hereditary spherocytosis<br>Huntington chorea<br>Marfan syndrome<br>Myotonic dystrophy<br>Neurofibromatosis type 1<br>Nonpolyposis colon cancer<br>Osteogenesis imperfecta<br>Polyposis of the colon<br>Tuberous sclerosis<br>von Willebrand<br>Waardenburg syndrome |
| Autosomal recessive | If both parents are carriers: 25% for child | Often seen in only one generation<br>Both genders affected equally<br>Consanguinity may be present between parents of an affected child<br>Parents of an affected child are asymptomatic carriers | Albinism<br>Canavan disease<br>Congenital adrenal hyperplasia<br>Cystic fibrosis<br>Galactosemia<br>Familial dysautonomia<br>Friedreich ataxia<br>Hemochromatosis<br>Homocystinuria<br>Maple syrup urine disease<br>Phenylketonuria<br>Sickle cell disease<br>Tay-Sachs disease<br>Thalassemia<br>Wilson disease |

*(Continued)*

| TABLE 4-4 | Major Modes of Inheritance (Continued) | | |
|---|---|---|---|
| Inheritance | Risk of Recurrence | Properties | Conditions |
| X-linked recessive | If mother is carrier: 50% affected sons, 50% carrier daughters | No male-to-male transmission Heterozygous females usually unaffected but may express | Duchenne muscular dystrophy Glucose-6-phosphate dehydrogenase deficiency Hemophilia A Hemophilia B |
| | If father is affected: 0% affected sons, 100% carrier daughters | Condition (variable severity) due to skewed X-inactivation A large proportion of isolated cases are due to new mutations. | Lesch-Nyan syndrome Menkes syndrome |
| X-linked dominant | If mother is affected: 50% of sons and 50% of daughters are affected. If father is affected: 0% affected sons, 100% affected daughters | No male-to-male transmission Often lethal in males Homozygous affected females may have more severe disease. | Hypophosphatemic rickets Incontinentia pigmenti, type 2 |
| Mitochondrial | Recurrence in males and females is variable due to heteroplasmy of mitochondria | Mitochondrial DNA inherited exclusively through females Variations in severity | Leber optic neuropathy MELAS Myoclonic epilepsy |

BRCA1, breast cancer 1 gene; BRCA2, breast cancer 2 gene; MELAS, mitochondrial myopathy, encephalopathy, lactic acidosis, and stroke syndrome.

| TABLE 4-5 | Summary of Prenatal Genetic Screening Tests | | |
|---|---|---|---|
| **Test** | **Components** | **Testing Time Frame** | **Comments** |
| First-trimester screen | • Maternal age<br>• Maternal serum free β-hCG<br>• PAPP-A<br>• Fetal ultrasound<br>  • Nuchal translucency<br>  • +/− fetal nasal bone | 11–14 wk | Provides risk for trisomies 21 and 13/18. Improved detection when fetal nasal bone is assessed. |
| Quad screen | • Maternal age<br>• MSAFP<br>• β-hCG<br>• Unconjugated estriol (uE3)<br>• Dimeric inhibin A (DIA) | 15–20 wk | Provides risk for trisomies 21 and 18 and open NTDs |
| Combined screening (integrated) | • Fetal nuchal translucency<br>• PAPP-A<br>• MSAFP<br>• β-hCG<br>• Unconjugated estriol (uE3)<br>• Dimeric inhibin A (DIA) | First and second trimester (as noted earlier) | Detects Down syndrome equally as effective as first-trimester screen with nasal bone is included (95% detection). |
| Combined screening (sequential) | • Patient given results of first-trimester screen and can then decide whether to undergo invasive testing (if positive) or quad screen (if negative) | First and second trimester (as noted earlier) | Allows patient to decide the extent of testing they wish to pursue |
| MSAFP | • Maternal serum alpha-fetoprotein | Second trimester | Provides risk for open neural tube defects |
| Cell-free fetal DNA analysis | • Maternal blood draw with analysis of fetal DNA | 10–20 wk | Only recommended for patients at high risk of aneuploidy |

β-hCG, beta-human chorionic gonadotropin; PAPP-A, pregnancy-associated plasma protein-A; MSAFP, maternal serum alpha-fetoprotein; NTD, neural tube defect.

• **Trisomy 21 (Down syndrome)**, the most common aneuploid condition in live borns, is the result of an extra chromosome 21. Trisomy 21 most often results from meiotic nondisjunction during maternal chromosomal replication and division. It is characterized by mental retardation, cardiac defects, hypotonia, and characteristic facial features. Although its incidence increases with maternal age (Table 4-6), 70% of cases occur in women younger than 35 years because most pregnancies occur in these younger women.

| TABLE 4-6 | Chromosomal Abnormalities in Liveborns[a] | |
|---|---|---|
| Maternal Age | Risk of Down Syndrome | Total Risk of Chromosomal Abnormalities[a] |
| 20 | 1:1,667 | 1:526 |
| 21 | 1:1,667 | 1:526 |
| 22 | 1:1,429 | 1:500 |
| 23 | 1:1,429 | 1:500 |
| 24 | 1:1,250 | 1:476 |
| 25 | 1:1,250 | 1:476 |
| 26 | 1:1,176 | 1:476 |
| 27 | 1:1,111 | 1:455 |
| 28 | 1:1,053 | 1:435 |
| 29 | 1:1,000 | 1:417 |
| 30 | 1:952 | 1:385 |
| 31 | 1:909 | 1:385 |
| 32 | 1:769 | 1:322 |
| 33 | 1:602 | 1:286 |
| 34 | 1:485 | 1:238 |
| 35 | 1:378 | 1:192 |
| 36 | 1:289 | 1:156 |
| 37 | 1:224 | 1:127 |
| 38 | 1:173 | 1:102 |
| 39 | 1:136 | 1:83 |
| 40 | 1:106 | 1:66 |
| 41 | 1:82 | 1:53 |
| 42 | 1:63 | 1:42 |
| 43 | 1:49 | 1:33 |
| 44 | 1:38 | 1:26 |
| 45 | 1:30 | 1:21 |
| 46 | 1:23 | 1:16 |
| 47 | 1:18 | 1:13 |
| 48 | 1:14 | 1:10 |
| 49 | 1:11 | 1:8 |

[a]Karyotype 47, XXX was excluded for ages 20 to 32 years (data not available).
Adapted from Hook EB, Cross PK, Schreinemachers DM. Chromosomal abnormality rates at amniocentesis and in live-born infants. *JAMA* 1983;249:2034–2038, with permission; Hook EB. Rates of chromosomal abnormalities at different maternal ages. *Obstet Gynecol* 1981;58:282–285, with permission.

- **Trisomy 13 (Patau syndrome) and 18 (Edward syndrome)** are more severe disorders that cause profound mental retardation and severe multiorgan birth defects. Few babies with trisomy 13 or 18 survive more than a few months. The risk of trisomy recurrence for a chromosomally normal couple is often cited to be 1%.

### First-Trimester Screening

- **First-trimester screening**, performed between 11 and 14 weeks, includes maternal age, nuchal translucency, maternal serum free beta-human chorionic gonadotropin (free β-hCG), and pregnancy-associated plasma protein-A (PAPP-A).
- The detection rate for Down syndrome and trisomy 18 is about 89% and 95%, respectively, with a 5% false-positive rate.
- First-trimester screening with ultrasound assessment of the nasal bone (absent in about 70% of trisomy 21 fetuses) improves the detection rate for Down syndrome to approximately 95% with a 5% false-positive rate.
- First-trimester screening does not screen for open NTDs.

### Second-Trimester Screening

- **Second-trimester quad screening** is performed between 15 and 20 weeks and estimates risk for Down syndrome, open NTDs, and trisomy 18. It uses MSAFP, β-hCG, unconjugated estriol (uE3), and dimeric inhibin A (DIA), combined with maternal age.
- The detection rate for trisomy 21 is approximately 75% for women younger than 35 years old and 90% for those older than 35 years. Additionally, abnormal values on this screening (elevated alpha-fetoprotein [AFP] and/or hCG) correlate with an increased risk of perinatal complications.

### Combined Screening

Combined screening uses combined first- and second-trimester screening to adjust a woman's age-related risk for a fetus with Down syndrome.

- **Integrated screening** uses nuchal translucency and PAPP-A from the first-trimester screening and MSAFP, estriol, hCG, and inhibin A from the second-trimester screening. Results are reported only after *both* screening tests are completed. The detection rate for this method is 94% to 96% with 5% false positives; this is equivalent to first-trimester screening when nasal bone is included in the risk assessment.
- **Sequential screening** is where the patient is given the first-trimester results. If at high risk, patients are given the option for invasive testing, whereas those at low risk can still undergo second-trimester screening to achieve a higher detection rate.

### Cell-Free Fetal DNA Screening

- **Cell-free fetal DNA** can be found in maternal circulation in increasing quantity as pregnancy progresses.
- Clinical testing of this DNA has recently become available and is currently **only recommended for patients at increased risk of aneuploidy** and should not be considered routine screening.
- Screening can be performed for trisomies 21, 13, and 18 as early as 10 weeks' gestation by determining the relative amount of fetal DNA from various fetal chromosomes.
- This form of screening has been found to detect over 98% of trisomies 21 and 18 pregnancies with a very low false-positive rate of less than 0.5%.
- High-risk patients include women with advanced maternal age, sonographic findings suggesting increased risk of aneuploidy, history of trisomy in a prior pregnancy, and a prior screening test suggesting an increased risk of aneuploidy.

- As with the other forms of prenatal genetic screening, patients with a result indicating an increased risk of aneuploidy should be offered diagnostic testing because results are not considered diagnostic due to screening imperfections.

*Screening for Neural Tube Defects*

- **NTDs** result from a failure of the neural tube to close or attain its normal musculo-skeletal coverings in early embryogenesis. Among the most common major congenital malformations with an incidence of 1 to 2 in 1,000 live births, NTDs include the fatal condition of anencephaly as well as spina bifida (meningomyelocele and meningocele); most have the potential for surgical correction.
  - Family history of NTD increases risk. If one partner has an NTD, the recurrence risk is 2% to 3%. In a couple with a previously affected child, the risk of recurrence is also 2% to 3%. Ninety percent of NTDs, however, occur in families without such histories. All pregnant women should be offered NTD screening.
  - MSAFP is a fetal glycoprotein synthesized sequentially in the embryonic yolk sac, gastrointestinal (GI) tract, and liver. Normally, AFP crosses the placenta to appear in the mother's blood. In addition, a small amount of AFP enters the amniotic fluid via fetal urination, GI secretions, and transudation from exposed blood vessels. The concentration of AFP in amniotic fluid (amniotic fluid alpha-fetoprotein [AFAFP]) is highest at the end of the first trimester and slowly declines during the remainder of pregnancy. MSAFP concentrations, on the other hand, rise until approximately 30 weeks' gestation.
  - With an open fetal NTD or an abdominal wall defect, increased AFP more than 2.5 multiples of the median (MoM) will be detected in amniotic fluid in over 95% of cases and in the mother's blood in about 80% of cases.
  - Elevated MSAFP levels can also occur with incorrect pregnancy dating, multiple pregnancies, congenital hereditary nephrosis, Turner syndrome with cystic hygroma, fetal bowel obstruction, teratomas, IUGR, and fetal death.
  - Women who elected to undergo first-trimester screening or have a normal result from CVS should still be offered NTD screening with an MSAFP in the second trimester.
  - Diagnostic ultrasonography should be performed on patients with elevated MSAFP screening results to confirm gestational age, as well as to visualize the placenta, detect multiple pregnancies, and detect any fetal anomalies.
  - Assignment of incorrect gestational age may lead to incorrect interpretation of AFP levels because both MSAFP and AFAFP levels change in relation to gestational age. Maternal smoking is also associated with false-positive elevations in MSAFP.

## Prenatal Diagnostic Testing

- In the United States, it is standard to offer CVS or amniocentesis to women who will be 35 years or older when they give birth, due to inherent age-associated risks.
- **CVS** uses either a catheter (transcervically) or a needle (transabdominally) to biopsy placental tissue derived from the same fertilized egg as the fetus.
  - CVS is usually performed at 10 to 13 weeks' gestation but transabdominal CVS may be performed throughout the second or third trimester.
  - CVS offers the psychological and medical advantages of early diagnosis and possibility for first-trimester termination.
  - When adjusted for confounding factors, such as gestational age and early spontaneous miscarriage rate, the CVS-related miscarriage rate is not statistically different from that for second-trimester amniocentesis.

- Unsensitized Rh-negative women should be given Rh immunoglobin after CVS.
- Cytogenetically ambiguous results caused by maternal cell contamination or mosaicism are reported more often after CVS than after amniocentesis. In such instances, follow-up amniocentesis may be required to clarify results, which increases both the total cost of testing and the risk of miscarriage.
- Reports of infants born with limb defects after CVS were first published in 1991. This outcome is associated with gestational age, and therefore, CVS is not generally recommended before 9 weeks' gestation.
- **Amniocentesis** aspirates a small amount of amniotic fluid, containing cells that are shed from the fetal bladder, skin, GI tract, and amnion, and these cells can be used for karyotyping or other genetic testing.
  - Amniocentesis is most commonly performed at 15 to 18 weeks' gestation.
  - Patients with an obstetric history of NTD should be counseled about their 2% to 3% risk of recurrence and offered second-trimester amniocentesis for AFP testing as well as detailed ultrasonographic evaluation of fetal anatomy at 18 to 20 weeks' gestation.
  - The amniocentesis site should be selected carefully, avoiding the placenta if possible, as contamination with fetal blood will falsely elevate the AFAFP. False-positive results due to contamination with fetal blood can be identified by acetylcholinesterase testing (absent in pregnancies for which the elevated AFAFP can be explained by contamination with fetal blood).
  - The miscarriage rate from midtrimester (16 to 20 weeks) amniocentesis is estimated to be 1 in 200 to 500. Other complications such as vaginal spotting or amniotic fluid leakage occur infrequently; most are transient.
  - Unsensitized Rh-negative women should be given Rh-immune globulin after amniocentesis.
- **Midtrimester ultrasonographic evaluation** at 18 to 22 weeks' gestation should include a systematic fetal anatomy survey and growth assessment.
  - Ultrasound screening for Down syndrome, also called **age-adjusted ultrasound risk assessment** (AAURA), uses likelihood ratios associated with specific markers to adjust a woman's a priori risk.
  - AAURA screening includes thickened nuchal fold, echogenicity of the fetal bowl, short humerus and femur lengths, dilated renal pyelectasis, and intracardiac echogenic focus.
  - Although helpful, an ultrasound cannot diagnose Down syndrome with certainty.
  - Ultrasonography is better at detecting aneuploidies other than Down syndrome, such as trisomy 18 or trisomy 13, which are associated with a higher incidence of major structural anomalies.

## ROUTINE PRENATAL CARE

### Establishment of Expected Date of Confinement

The gestational dating of a pregnancy is very important to establish at the first prenatal visit because this can later play an important role in management of a pregnancy and can impact plans for delivery. The average duration of human pregnancy is 280 days from the first day of the last menstrual period (LMP) until delivery. The 40-week gestational period is based on menstrual weeks (not weeks since conception), assuming ovulation and conception on the 14th day of a 28-day cycle.

- **Clinical dating using Naegele's rule:** The estimated date of delivery is calculated by subtracting 3 months from the first day of the LMP then adding 1 week.

| TABLE 4-7 | Accuracy of Pregnancy Dating by Ultrasonography According to Gestational Age | |
| --- | --- | --- |

| Gestational Age (wk) | Ultrasonographic Measurements | Accuracy |
| --- | --- | --- |
| <8 | Sac size | ±10 d |
| 8–12 | CRL | ±7 d |
| 12–14 | CRL or BPD | ±14 d |
| 15–20 | BPD/HC/Fl/AC | ±10 d |
| 20–28 | BPD/HC/Fl/AC | ±2 wk |
| >28 | BPD/HC/Fl/AC | ±3 wk |

CRL, crown-rump length; BPD, biparietal diameter; HC, head circumference; Fl, femur length. ; AC, abdominal circumference

- **Doppler ultrasonography** allows detection of fetal heart tones by 11 to 12 weeks' gestation.
- **Ultrasonographic dating** is most accurate from 7 to 11-6/7 weeks of gestation. If LMP dating is consistent with ultrasonographic dating within the established range of accuracy for ultrasonography (Table 4-7), the estimated date of delivery is based on LMP.
- A fetoscope can enable detection of heart tones at 19 to 20 weeks' gestation. Quickening (maternal detection of fetal movement) is noted at approximately 19 weeks in the first pregnancy; in subsequent pregnancies, it is usually noted approximately 2 weeks earlier.

## Nutrition and Weight Gain

- Pregnant women require 15% more **calories** than nonpregnant women, usually 300 to 500 kcal more per day, depending on the patient's weight and activity.
- Dietary allowances for most **vitamins and minerals** increase with pregnancy and are adequately supplied in a well-balanced diet.
- **Iron** is needed for both the fetus and the mother. Consumption of iron-containing foods should be encouraged, and iron supplements may be prescribed. The 30-mg daily elemental ferrous iron supplement is contained in approximately 150 mg of ferrous sulfate, 300 mg of ferrous gluconate, or 100 mg of ferrous fumarate.
- Prenatal **calcium** requirement is 1,200 mg/day.
- The **recommended weight gain** for pregnancy is based on the prepregnancy BMI and has been established by the Institute of Medicine.
  - The total weight gain recommended is 25 to 35 pounds for women with a normal BMI. Underweight women may gain 28 to 40 pounds, and overweight/obese women should limit weight gain to <25 pounds or less.
  - Three to 6 pounds are gained typically in the first trimester and 0.5 to 1.0 pound/week is gained in the last two trimesters of pregnancy. If a patient has not gained 10 pounds by midpregnancy, her nutritional status should be evaluated carefully.

## Exercise

- In the absence of obstetric or medical complications, moderate physical activity can maintain cardiovascular and muscular fitness throughout pregnancy and the postpartum period.

- Women who are moderately active prior to pregnancy should be encouraged to maintain their level of activity, as tolerated, during pregnancy. No data suggest that moderate aerobic exercise is harmful to the mother or fetus. The effect of regular, high-intensity exercise on pregnancy remains unclear.
- The following conditions are **contraindications** to exercise during pregnancy: gestational hypertension, preterm rupture of membranes, preterm labor during a previous pregnancy or the current pregnancy, incompetent cervix or cerclage, persistent second- or third-trimester bleeding, and IUGR.
- Women with certain other conditions, including chronic hypertension or active thyroid, cardiac, vascular, or pulmonary disease, should be carefully evaluated to determine whether an exercise program is appropriate.

## Immunizations

- No evidence of fetal risk exists from inactivated virus vaccines, bacterial vaccines, or tetanus immunoglobulin, and these agents should be administered, if appropriate. As noted, live vaccines should be administered outside the time of gestation.
- **Hepatitis B:** Pregnancy is not a contraindication to the administration of hepatitis B virus (HBV) vaccine or hepatitis B immune globulin.
  - Women at high risk of HBV infection who should be vaccinated during pregnancy include those with histories of the following: intravenous drug use, acute episode of any sexually transmitted disease, multiple sexual partners, occupational exposure in a health care or public safety environment, household contact with an HBV carrier, occupational exposure or residence in an institution for the developmentally disabled, occupational exposure or treatment in a hemodialysis unit, or receipt of clotting factor concentrates for bleeding disorders.
- Combined **tetanus**, **diphtheria**, and **pertussis** toxoids are the only immunobiologic agents routinely indicated for susceptible pregnant women. Current Centers for Disease Control and Prevention (CDC) guidelines recommend giving a Tdap vaccination to all pregnant women during pregnancy.
- **Measles**, **mumps**, and **rubella** single-antigen vaccines, as well as the combined vaccine, contain live attenuated antigen and should be given at a preconception or postpartum visit. Despite theoretic risks, no evidence has been reported of congenital rubella syndrome in infants born to women inadvertently given rubella vaccine while pregnant. Women who undergo immunization should be advised not to become pregnant for at least 4 weeks afterward. There is no evidence for transmission from vaccinated family members.
- Immune globulin or vaccination against **poliomyelitis**, **yellow fever**, **typhoid**, or **hepatitis** may be indicated for travelers to areas where these diseases are endemic or epidemic, using inactivated vaccines.
- **Influenza/H1N1 influenza** vaccination is indicated for all pregnant women during flu season, especially those who work at chronic care facilities that house patients with chronic medical conditions or who themselves have cardiopulmonary disorders, are immunosuppressed, or have diabetes mellitus.
- **Pneumococcal** vaccine is recommended for pregnant women with special conditions that put them at high risk of infection.
- **Varicella zoster** immune globulin (VZIG) should be administered to any newborn whose mother developed chickenpox within 5 days before or 2 days after delivery. No evidence shows that administration of VZIG to mothers reduces the rare occurrence of congenital varicella syndrome. VZIG can be considered for treating a pregnant woman to try to prevent the maternal complications of chickenpox. Varicella vaccine is a live attenuated vaccine that is contraindicated during pregnancy.

- Recombinant vaccine for HPV viruses is not currently recommended for use in pregnant women.

## Sexual Intercourse

- Generally, no restriction of sexual activity is necessary for pregnant women, and it is not an isolated risk factor for preterm delivery. Patients should be instructed that pregnancy may cause changes in physical comfort and sexual desire.
- Increased uterine activity after intercourse is common. For women at risk of pre-term labor, those with placenta previa that persists into the third trimester, or vasa previa, avoiding sexual activity may be advised.

## Employment

- Most patients are able to work throughout their entire pregnancy, although heavy lifting and excessive physical activity should be avoided.
- Modification of occupational activity is rarely needed, unless the job involves physical danger.
- Jobs that involve strenuous physical exercise, standing for prolonged periods, operating industrial machinery, or adverse environmental exposure should be modified.

## Travel

- Prolonged immobility (i.e., sitting) should be avoided because of the increased risk of venous thrombosis and thrombophlebitis during pregnancy.
- Patients should drive or stay seated a maximum of 6 hours a day if possible and should ambulate for 10 minutes at least every 2 hours to minimize vascular stasis.
- Support stockings should be worn for prolonged sitting in cars or airplanes.
- A seat belt should always be worn; the belt should be placed under the abdomen as the pregnancy advances.

## Nausea and Vomiting

- Nausea and vomiting is a common complaint in pregnancy and can affect up to 85% of pregnant women, most commonly in the first trimester. It is often not treated or undertreated, which can result in progression to hyperemesis gravidarum. This affects up to 2% of pregnancies and is a diagnosis of exclusion that can result in serious consequences for both mother and fetus and often necessitates hospitalization.
- First-line treatment should include vitamin $B_6$ and doxylamine. Refractory cases may warrant treatment with benzamides, phenothiazines, or 5-HT$_3$ receptor antagonists.
- Supplemental nutrition with feeding tube should be considered in patients with weight loss that is refractory to more conservative treatments.

## Carpal Tunnel Syndrome

- In pregnancy, weight gain and edema can compress the median nerve, producing carpal tunnel syndrome.
- The syndrome consists of pain, numbness, or tingling in the thumb, index finger, middle finger, and radial side of the ring finger on the palmar aspect.
- Compressing the median nerve and percussing the wrist and forearm with a reflex hammer (Tinel maneuver) often exacerbates the pain.
- The syndrome most often occurs in primigravidas older than age 30 years during the third trimester and usually resolves within 2 weeks of delivery.
- Conservative treatment with wrist splints at night or local steroid injections for more severe cases may be helpful.

## Back Pain

- Back pain may be aggravated by excessive weight gain.
- Exercises to strengthen back muscles and loosen the hamstrings can help alleviate back pain.
- Many pregnant women find pregnancy support belts or maternity girdles helpful in alleviating low back pain.
- Pregnant women should maintain good posture and wear low-heeled shoes.
- Physical therapy can be helpful.

## Round Ligament Pain

- These very sharp groin pains are caused by spasm of the round ligaments associated with movement. The spasms are generally unilateral and are more frequent on the right side than on the left because of the usual dextroversion of the uterus.
- Patients sometimes awaken at night with round ligament pain after having suddenly rolled over in their sleep.
- No treatment is necessary, and the patient should be reassured that they are a common and benign complaint in pregnancy.

## Hemorrhoids

- **Hemorrhoids** are varicose veins of the rectum and may become swollen and painful during pregnancy.
- Patients with hemorrhoids should avoid constipation because straining during bowel movements can aggravate hemorrhoids.
- Good hydration and increased fiber consumption may help soften the stool.
- Hemorrhoids often regress after delivery but usually do not resolve completely.

## LAB ASSESSMENT/INFECTION SCREENING

- Table 4-8 lists the routine prenatal testing through a pregnancy.
- Women are screened for various infections during initial prenatal care laboratory assessment or if they have certain environmental exposures.
- **Rubella:** Screening for antirubella immunoglobulin G (IgG) identifies nonimmune women who should then be offered vaccination preconception or in the postpartum period.
- **HBV:** Screening of pregnant women for hepatitis B surface antigen is recommended. Women with risks for exposure to HBV (i.e., HIV and certain immunocompromised populations) should be counseled and offered vaccination.
- **Tuberculosis (TB):** Patients at risk for TB should be tested with subcutaneous purified protein derivative (PPD) challenge; if the patient has a history of bacillus Calmette-Guerin (BCG) vaccination, the PPD screen should still be used unless they have known positive skin testing. Preconception treatment for latent TB infection can be ordered as indicated.
- **Cytomegalovirus (CMV):** Screening should be offered to women who work in neonatal intensive care units, child care facilities, or dialysis units.
- **Parvovirus B19:** IgG testing may be offered preconceptually to school teachers and child care workers.
- **Toxoplasmosis:** Cat owners and women who eat or handle raw meat are at increased risk, but routine testing without risk factors is not recommended. Routine toxoplasmosis screening to determine antibody status before conception mainly provides reassurance to those who are already immune; patients' cats can also be tested.

| TABLE 4-8 | Routine Prenatal Testing |
|---|---|
| **Timing** | **Tests** |
| Initial obstetric visit | Blood type, Rh type, antibody screen, CBC, rubella, STS/RPR, HBsAg, HIV, Hgb electrophoresis, urine culture and sensitivity, urine toxicology, Pap smear, gonorrhea, and chlamydia testing. Dating sonogram, if questionable dating criteria for first-trimester screening |
| 11–14 weeks' gestation | First-trimester screening |
| 16–20 weeks' gestation | MSAFP/quad screen |
| 18–22 weeks' gestation | Anatomy ultrasound to rule out fetal anomalies |
| 24–28 weeks' gestation | Blood type, Rh type, antibody screen, CBC, STS/RPR, glucose screen. If high-risk patient, repeat HBsAg, HIV, gonorrhea, and chlamydia testing |
| 36 weeks' gestation | Group B streptococci culture |

CBC, complete blood count; STS, serologic test for syphilis; RPR, rapid plasma reagin; HBsAg, hepatitis B surface antigen; Hgb, hemoglobin; MSAFP, maternal serum alpha-fetoprotein.

- **Varicella:** Screening for IgG should be performed if a positive history cannot be obtained. The varicella zoster virus vaccine is now recommended for all nonimmune adults. It is a live virus vaccine that should be given prior to conception. Nonimmune individuals can be counseled regarding postexposure prophylaxis during pregnancy.
- **HIV:** Counseling and testing should be offered routinely to all women. The CDC recommends an "opt-out" strategy to increase screening compliance.

## SUGGESTED READINGS

American College of Obstetricians and Gynecologists Committee on Genetics. Committee opinion no. 545: noninvasive prenatal testing for fetal aneuploidy. *Obstet Gynecol* 2012;120:1532–1534.

American College of Obstetricians and Gynecologists Committee on Practice Bulletins—Obstetrics. ACOG practice bulletin no. 92: clinical management guidelines for obstetrician-gynecologists: use of psychiatric medications during pregnancy and lactation. *Obstet Gynecol* 2008;111(4):1001–1020.

American College of Obstetricians and Gynecologists Committee on Practice Bulletins. ACOG practice bulletin no. 77: screening for fetal chromosomal abnormalities. *Obstet Gynecol* 2007; 109(1):217–227.

Behnke M, VC Smith. Prenatal substance abuse: short- and long-term effects on the exposed fetus. *Pediatrics* 2013;131(3):e1009–e1024.

Bennett RL, Motulsky AG, Bittles A, et al. Genetic counseling and screening of consanguineous couples and their offspring: recommendations of the National Society of Genetic Counselors. *J Gen Couns* 2002;11(2):97–119.

Jack B, Atrash HK, eds. Preconception health and health care: the clinical content of preconception care. *Am J Obstet Gynecol* 2008;199(6)(suppl B):257–395.

Spencer K. Aneuploidy screening in the first trimester. *Am J Med Genet C Semin Med Genet* 2007; 145C:18–32.

# II Obstetrics

# 5 Normal Labor and Delivery, Operative Delivery, and Malpresentations

John L. Wu and Betty Chou

Labor is defined as repetitive uterine contractions of sufficient frequency, intensity, and duration to cause progressive cervical effacement and dilation.

## STAGES AND PHASES OF LABOR

- The **first stage of labor** begins with the onset of labor and ends with full cervical dilation. It is divided into latent and active phases (Table 5-1).
  - The **latent phase** begins with regular contractions and ends when there is an increase in the rate of cervical dilation.
  - The **active phase** is characterized by an increased rate of cervical dilation and descent of the presenting fetal part, which may not occur until after 6 cm of dilation. It ends with complete cervical dilation and is further subdivided into:
    - **Acceleration phase:** A gradual increase in the rate of dilation initiates the active phase and marks a change to rapid dilation.
    - **Phase of maximum slope:** the period of active labor with the greatest rate of cervical dilation
    - **Deceleration phase:** the terminal portion of the active phase in which the rate of dilation may slow until full cervical dilation
- The **second stage of labor** is the interval between full cervical dilation and delivery of the neonate.
- The **third stage of labor** is the interval between delivery of the neonate and delivery of the placenta.
- The **fourth stage of labor**, or puerperium, follows delivery and concludes with resolution of the physiologic changes of pregnancy, usually by 6 weeks postpartum.

| TABLE 5-1 | Stages and Phases of Labor | |
|---|---|---|

| Parameter | Nulliparous | Multiparous |
|---|---|---|
| *Latent phase of first-stage labor* | | |
| Mean | 6 hr | 5 hr |
| Fifth percentile | 21 hr | 14 hr |
| *First stage of labor (total)* | | |
| Mean | 10 hr | 8 hr |
| Fifth percentile | 25 hr | 19 hr |
| *Second stage of labor* | | |
| Mean | | |
| Fifth percentile | 33 min | 9 min |
| Prolonged (without epidural) | 118 min | 47 min |
| Prolonged (with epidural) | 2 hr | 1 hr |
| Prolonged (with epidural) | 3 hr | 2 hr |
| *Third stage of labor* | | |
| Mean | 5 min | 5 min |
| Prolonged | 30 min | 30 min |
| *Rate of maximal dilation* | | |
| Mean | 3.0 cm/hr | 5.7 cm/hr |
| Fifth percentile | 1.2 cm/hr | 1.5 cm/hr |
| *Rate of descent* | | |
| Mean | 3.3 cm/hr | 6.6 cm/hr |
| Fifth percentile | 1.0 cm/hr | 2.0 cm/hr |

Adapted from Liao JB, Buhimschi CS, Norwitz ER. Normal labor: mechanism and duration. *Obstet Gynecol Clin North Am* 2005;32(2):145–164; American College of Obstetricians and Gynecologists Committee on Practice Bulletins—Obstetrics. Practice bulletin no. 49: dystocia and augmentation of labor. *Obstet Gynecol* 2003;102:1445–1454.

During this time, the reproductive tract returns to its nonpregnant state, and ovulation may resume.

## MECHANISM OF LABOR

The **cardinal movements of labor** refer to the changes in position of the fetal head during its descent through the birth canal in vertex presentation:
- **Descent** (lightening): movement of the fetal head through the pelvis toward the pelvic floor. The highest rate of descent occurs during the deceleration phase of the first stage and during the second stage of labor.
- **Engagement:** the descent of the widest diameter of the presenting fetal part below the plane of the pelvic inlet. The widest diameter in cephalic presentation is the biparietal diameter. In breech presentation, the bitrochanteric diameter determines the station.
- **Flexion:** a passive movement that permits the smallest diameter of the fetal head (suboccipitobregmatic diameter) to pass through the maternal pelvis
- **Internal rotation:** The fetal occiput rotates from its original position (usually transverse) toward the symphysis pubis (occiput anterior) or, less commonly, toward the hollow of the sacrum (occiput posterior).

- **Extension:** The fetal head is delivered by extension from the flexed position as it travels beneath the symphysis pubis.
- **External rotation:** The fetal head turns to realign with the long axis of the spine, allowing the shoulders to align in the anterior–posterior axis.
- **Expulsion:** The anterior shoulder descends to the level of the symphysis pubis. After the shoulder is delivered under the symphysis pubis, the remainder of the fetus is delivered.

## MANAGEMENT OF NORMAL LABOR AND DELIVERY

### Initial Assessment
*History*
- Age, parity (full-term deliveries [≥37 weeks], preterm deliveries [≥20 to <37 weeks], abortions [<20 weeks], and living children), estimated gestational age
- Labor-related symptoms including (a) onset, strength, and frequency of contractions; (b) leakage of fluid; (c) vaginal bleeding; and (d) fetal movement
- Maternal drug allergies
- Medications
- Last oral intake
- Review of prenatal labs and imaging studies including fetal ultrasounds
- Past medical and surgical history, gynecologic history including abnormal Pap smears and sexually transmitted infections, obstetric history including birth weight and method of delivery of previous children, social history including tobacco/alcohol/illicit drug use

*Physical Exam*
- Maternal vital signs (pulse, blood pressure [BP], respiratory rate, and temperature)
- Confirmation of gestational age, where appropriate, and confirmation of viability at approximately 24 weeks
- Assessment of fetal well-being (fetal heart rate)
- Frequency and intensity of contractions
- Fetal presentation
- Estimated fetal weight (may be performed via **Leopold maneuvers**, as noted in the following procedures)
  - Step 1: Palpate the fundus to ascertain a fetal pole and obtain fundal height.
  - Step 2: Palpate the lateral walls of the uterus to determine fetal lie (vertical vs. transverse) and the location of fetal spine and extremities.
  - Step 3: Grasp and palpate the upper and lower poles to determine presentation, to assess mobility and fetal weight, and to estimate the amniotic fluid volume.
  - Step 4: Palpate the presenting part from lateral to medial to assess engagement in the maternal pelvis, the location of the fetal brow, and the degree of flexion.
- **Sterile speculum exam**
  - Vulvar, vaginal, and cervical inspection (especially noting lesions or scars)
  - Evaluate for ruptured membranes (vaginal pooling of fluid in the posterior fornix, nitrazine test, and ferning seen on microscopic slide).
  - Wet mount, gonorrhea/chlamydia screening, group B *Streptococcus* (GBS) culture, if indicated
- **Sterile digital exam**—defer if estimated gestational age is <34 weeks with ruptured membranes. This exam can provide the following data:
  - **Cervical dilation** is the estimated diameter of the internal os in centimeters. Ten centimeters corresponds to complete dilation.

- **Cervical effacement** is the length of the cervix, expressed as the percentage change from full length, approximately 4 cm (0% or "long" means not shortened at all, whereas 100% means only a paper-thin rim of cervix is detected).
- **Fetal station** describes the distance in centimeters between the presenting *bony* part and the plane of the ischial spines. Station 0 defines the level of the ischial spines. Below the spines is +1 cm to +5 at the perineum. Station above the spines is −1 cm to −5 at the level of the pelvic inlet.
- **Clinical pelvimetry**: evaluation of the maternal pelvis by vaginal exam
  - **Diagonal conjugate**: The distance between the sacral promontory and the posterior edge of the pubic symphysis. A distance of at least 11.5 cm suggests a sufficiently adequate pelvic inlet for an average-weight fetus.
  - **Transverse diameter:** The distance between the ischial tuberosities, which can be approximated by placing a closed fist of known width at the perineum. An intertuberous diameter of at least 8.5 cm suggests an adequate pelvic outlet.
- The **pelvic type** can be classified into four types based on general shape and bony characteristics. Gynecoid and anthropoid types are most amenable to a successful vaginal birth.

### Standard Admission Procedures

- Standard admission labs include urine testing (for protein and glucose), complete blood count (CBC), and a type and screen.
- For patients without prenatal care, hepatitis B surface antigen, HIV, ABO blood group and antibody screen, urine culture and toxicology, rubella immunoglobulin G, CBC, and syphilis screening should be sent.
- Intravenous (IV) access (heplock or continuous infusion) is recommended.
- Informed consent for management of labor and delivery and for blood products should be obtained.

## Management of Labor

- The quality and frequency of uterine contractions should be assessed regularly by palpation, tocodynamometer, or intrauterine pressure catheter (if indicated).
- The fetal heart rate should be assessed by intermittent auscultation, continuous electronic Doppler monitoring, or fetal scalp electrode (if indicated).
- Cervical examinations should be kept to the minimum required to detect abnormalities in the progression of labor.
- The lithotomy position is the most frequently assumed position for vaginal delivery in the United States, although alternative birthing positions, such as the lateral or Sims position or the partial sitting or squatting positions, are preferred by some patients, physicians, and midwives.

## Induction of Labor

- **Indications:** Induction of labor is indicated when the benefits of delivery (for the mother or fetus) outweigh the benefits of continued pregnancy. Induction should not be initiated if vaginal delivery is contraindicated (Table 5-2). Consideration of **fetal lung maturity** is necessary before elective induction of labor prior to 39 weeks of gestation. Amniocentesis is not necessary if the induction is medically indicated and the risk of continuing the pregnancy is greater than the risk of delivering before lung maturity. The favorability of the cervix at the time of induction is related to the success of labor induction. When the Bishop score (Table 5-3) exceeds 8, the

| TABLE 5-2 | Induction of Labor: Indications and Contraindications |
|---|---|

**Indications**

- Abruptio placentae, chorioamnionitis, gestational hypertension
- Premature rupture of membranes, postterm pregnancy, preeclampsia, eclampsia
- Maternal medical conditions (e.g., diabetes mellitus, renal disease, chronic pulmonary disease, chronic hypertension)
- Fetal compromise (e.g., severe fetal growth restriction, isoimmunization)
- Fetal demise
- Elective inductions for gestational age >39 wk for logistical issues such as remote access to care, psychosocial reasons, and history of rapid deliveries. Typically only considered if cervix is favorable.

**Contraindications**

- Vasa previa or complete placenta previa
- Transverse fetal lie
- Infection—active HSV, high viral load HIV
- Pelvic structural deformities
- Umbilical cord prolapse
- Advanced cervical cancer

HSV, herpes simplex virus.
Adapted from American College of Obstetricians and Gynecologists—Obstetrics. ACOG practice bulletin no. 107: induction of labor. *Obstet Gynecol* 2009;114:386–397.

likelihood of vaginal delivery after induction is similar to that with spontaneous labor. Induction with a lower Bishop score has been associated with a higher rate of failure, prolonged labor, and cesarean delivery.
- **Cervical ripening** may be used to soften the cervix before induction if the Bishop score is low. Cervical ripening can be achieved using pharmacologic and mechanical methods.

| TABLE 5-3 | Components of the Bishop Score |
|---|---|

| | Rating | | | |
|---|---|---|---|---|
| **Factor** | **0** | **1** | **2** | **3** |
| Dilation | Closed | 1–2 cm | 3–4 cm | 5+ cm |
| Effacement | 0%–30% | 40%–50% | 60%–70% | 80%+ |
| Station | −3 | −2 | −1, 0 | >+1 |
| Consistency | Firm | Medium | Soft | — |
| Position | Posterior | Mid position | Anterior | — |

Adapted from Bishop EH. Pelvic scoring for elective induction. *Obstet Gynecol* 1964;24:267.

- **Pharmacologic methods of induction of labor and cervical ripening**
  - **Low-dose oxytocin** may be used with or without mechanical dilators.
  - **Prostaglandin E$_2$** is superior to placebo in promoting cervical effacement and dilation and may enhance sensitivity to oxytocin.
    - **Prepidil** gel contains 0.5 mg of dinoprostone in a 2.5-mL syringe; the gel is injected into the cervical canal every 6 hours for up to 3 doses in a 24-hour period.
    - **Cervidil** is a vaginal insert containing 10 mg of dinoprostone. It provides a lower rate of release (0.3 mg/hr) than the gel but has the advantage that it can be removed if uterine tachysystole occurs (>5 contractions in 10 minutes).
  - **Prostaglandin E$_1$** is also effective in stimulating cervical ripening.
    - **Cytotec (misoprostol)** is administered as 25 to 50 mg every 3 to 6 hours intravaginally. The use of misoprostol for cervical ripening is off-label.
  - **Side effects**: Any pharmacologic induction method includes a risk of uterine tachysystole. If oxytocin is being used, it can be titrated down or turned off with quick effect due to its short half-life. If Cervidil is being used, the insert can be removed. If indicated, a beta-adrenergic agonist (e.g., terbutaline sulfate) can be administered. Maternal systemic effects of prostaglandins may include fever, vomiting, and diarrhea.
  - **Contraindications**: A history of uterine scar or prior cesarean delivery, allergy to the medication, or active vaginal bleeding. Caution should be exercised when using prostaglandin E$_2$ in patients with glaucoma or severe hepatic or renal impairment.
- **Mechanical methods of labor induction and cervical ripening**
  - Membrane stripping
  - Amniotomy (artificial rupture of membranes): The risk of umbilical cord prolapse can be reduced by performing the amniotomy while the fetal presenting part is well applied to the cervix.
  - Balloon catheters placed transcervically: A single-balloon device such as a 24-French Foley catheter with 30-mL bulb inserted into the extra-amniotic space. Other options are to use larger volume bulb catheters or a double-balloon device.
  - Hygroscopic dilators (laminaria)

## OXYTOCIN ADMINISTRATION

- **Indications:** Oxytocin is used for both induction and augmentation of labor. Augmentation should be considered for protracted or arrest disorders of labor or the presence of a hypotonic uterine contraction pattern. A range of opinions regarding the dosage of oxytocin exist. A reasonable starting dosage is 0.5 to 4 mIU/min, with incremental increases of 1 to 2 mIU/min every 20 to 30 minutes. Cervical dilation of at least 1 cm/hr in the active phase indicates that oxytocin dosing is adequate. If an intrauterine pressure catheter is in place, 180 Montevideo units (MVU) per 10-minute period is considered adequate. However, some practitioners use a threshold of 250 to 275 MVU with increased success of induction and minimal adverse consequences.
- **Complications:** Adverse effects of oxytocin are primarily dose-related. The most common complication is uterine tachysystole, which may result in uteroplacental hypoperfusion and nonreassuring fetal heart tracing. Uterine tachysystole is usually reversible when oxytocin infusion is decreased or discontinued. If necessary, a beta-adrenergic agent may be administered. Rapid infusion of oxytocin can result in hypotension. Prolonged infusion can result in water intoxication and hyponatremia

because oxytocin structurally resembles antidiuretic hormone; it also increases the risk of postpartum uterine atony and hemorrhage.

## Labor Progress Assessment

- Dr. Emanuel Friedman's studies on normal labor resulted in widely used guidelines for normal labor progress (see Table 5-1, p. 79).
- Abnormal labor progression is identified when the patient falls below the fifth percentile of expected cervical change and fetal descent.
- **Latent phase prolongation** is somewhat controversial, as measurement of this phase is difficult and inexact. Generally speaking, without induction, this phase is considered prolonged if it exceeds 20 hours in a nulliparous patient and 14 hours in a multiparous patient.
- The **active phase** is considered protracted if the rate of cervical change is <1.2 cm/hr for the nulliparous patient and <1.5 cm/hr in the multiparous patient. **Arrest of dilation** occurs when there is no apparent cervical change over a 2-hour period despite adequate contractions (180 to 250 MVU).
- The **second stage of labor** is considered protracted after 2 hours of pushing in nulliparous patients or 1 hour in parous patients. An additional hour may be allowed if epidural anesthesia is used. Arrest of descent occurs when there is no apparent descent of the presenting part over a 1-hour period of pushing during the second stage.
- The **third stage of labor** averages 10 minutes and is considered prolonged if it lasts longer than 30 minutes.
- Patients undergoing induction or augmentation of labor may not necessarily follow the Friedman curve for normal labor progression. Their individual labor curves need to be evaluated and more liberal definitions of progress applied.
- **Abnormal labor** may be due to:
  - Power: inadequate uterine contractions or maternal expulsive effort
  - Passenger: size of fetus or abnormal proportions, presentation, or position
  - Passage: small pelvis or obstructed birth canal
- **Risk factors** for abnormal labor could be any medical condition or clinical situation that affects the aforementioned categories.
  - Risks for an abnormal first stage of labor: increased maternal age, diabetes, hypertension, premature rupture of membranes, macrosomnia (usually defined as ≥4,000 g or ≥4,500 g), epidural anesthesia, chorioamnionitis, a history of previous complications like perinatal death, and amniotic fluid abnormalities
  - Risks for an abnormal second stage of labor: a prolonged first stage, occiput posterior position, epidural anesthesia, nulliparity, short maternal stature, increased birth weight, and high station at complete cervical dilation

## Interventions for Abnormal Labor

- **Amniotomy:** Artificial rupture of membranes may enhance progress for a patient who is in active labor, although it may increase the risk of chorioamnionitis.
- **Augmentation of labor via oxytocin:** Oxytocin has been shown to decrease the time of active labor in nulliparous women. In addition, some studies have shown that it decreases the rate of cesarean section for failure to progress.
- **Uterine contraction monitoring:** Placement of an intrauterine pressure catheter provides information about the frequency and strength of contractions and may be useful for titrating oxytocin to maximize the chance for successful vaginal delivery.

# FETAL HEART RATE EVALUATION

Guidelines for fetal heart rate (FHR) or fetal heart tracing (FHT) interpretation are given in Table 5-4.

- **Baseline rate:** lasts for at least 2 minutes during a 10-minute section rounded to the nearest 5 beats per minute (bpm)
- **Normal rate: 110 to 160 bpm**
- **Bradycardia:** A baseline FHR <110 bpm. Causes of bradycardia include fetal head compression, hypoxemia, and maternal hypothermia. The clinical picture is as important as the heart rate in interpreting fetal bradycardia.
- **Tachycardia:** A baseline FHR >160 bpm. The most common cause is maternal fever or infection. Other less common causes of fetal tachycardia include fetal arrhythmias or maternal administration of parasympatholytic or sympathomimetic drugs.
- **Variability:** Beat-to-beat fluctuations in the FHR. It is most reliable when measured with a fetal scalp electrode.
  - **Absent:** absent variability
  - **Minimal:** detectable variability of <5 bpm
  - **Moderate:** variability of 6 to 25 bpm
  - **Marked:** variability of >25 bpm
- **Accelerations:** For gestational age (GA) >32 weeks, an acceleration is an increase in FHR of at least 15 bpm that lasts for at least 15 seconds. For GA <32 weeks, an acceleration is an increase in FHR >10 bpm for 10 seconds.
- FHT is **reactive** if it shows two accelerations within 10 minutes.
- A **sinusoidal** FHT is a persistent smooth undulating pattern with a frequency of 3 to 5 cycles/min. It is concerning and requires immediate evaluation. Fetal anemia; analgesic drugs such as morphine, meperidine, alphaprodine, and butorphanol; and chronic fetal distress should be considered.
- **Decelerations:** a decrease in FHR below the baseline. In some instances, the pattern of deceleration of the FHR can be used to identify the cause.
  - **Variable decelerations** may start before, during, or after the uterine contraction starts (hence the designation "variable"). They usually show an abrupt onset to nadir in <30 seconds and return, which gives them a characteristic V shape. The decrease is >15 bpm lasting >15 seconds but <2 minutes. Variable decelerations are commonly caused by umbilical cord compression.
  - **Early decelerations** are shallow, symmetric, and reach their nadir at the peak of the contraction. They are caused by vagus nerve–mediated response to fetal head compression.
  - **Late decelerations** are U-shaped decelerations of gradual onset to nadir in >30 seconds and gradual return, reach their nadir after the peak of the contraction, and do not return to the baseline until after the contraction is over. They may result from uteroplacental insufficiency and relative fetal hypoxia. Recurrent late decelerations can be an ominous sign.
  - **Prolonged deceleration:** a deceleration that lasts longer than 2 minutes but <10 minutes
  - **Recurrent decelerations:** occur with >50% of uterine contractions in any 20-minute span
  - **Intermittent decelerations:** occur with <50% of uterine contractions in any 20-minute span

| **TABLE 5-4** | Fetal Heart Tracing Interpretation, Categories, and Criteria |

**Three-Tiered Fetal Heart Rate Interpretation System**

### *Category I*
- Category I FHR tracings include all of the following:
  - Baseline rate: 110–160 beats/min
  - Baseline FHR variability: moderate
  - Late or variable decelerations: absent
  - Early decelerations: present or absent
  - Accelerations: present or absent

### *Category II*
Category II FHR tracings include all FHR tracings not categorized as category I or category III. Category II tracings may represent an appreciable fraction of those encountered in clinical care. Examples of category II FHR tracings include any of the following:

Baseline rate
- Bradycardia not accompanied by absent baseline variability
- Tachycardia

Baseline FHR variability
- Minimal baseline variability
- Absent baseline variability with no recurrent decelerations
- Marked baseline variability

Accelerations
- Absence of induced accelerations after fetal stimulation

Periodic or episodic decelerations
- Recurrent variable decelerations accompanied by minimal or moderate baseline variability
- Prolonged deceleration more than 2 min but less than 10 min
- Recurrent late decelerations with moderate baseline variability
- Variable decelerations with other characteristics such as slow return to baseline, overshoots, or "shoulders"

### *Category III*
Category III FHR tracings include either:
- Absent baseline FHR variability and any of the following:
  - Recurrent late decelerations
  - Recurrent variable decelerations
  - Bradycardia
- Sinusoidal pattern

---

FHR, fetal heart rate.
From Macones GA, Hankins GD, Spong CY, et al. The 2008 National Institute of Child Health and Human Development workshop report on electronic fetal monitoring: update on definitions, interpretation, and research guidelines. *Obstet Gynecol* 2008;112:661–666.

*Overall Assessment*

- **Category I FHT** must have a baseline FHR between 110 and 160 bpm and moderate variability; accelerations may be present or absent, with no late or variable decelerations.
- **Category II FHT** are those that cannot be classified as category I or III.
- **Category III FHT** have concerning findings such as minimal variability, recurrent variable or late decelerations, bradycardia, or sinusoidal pattern. Consideration for delivery should be given.

## Management of Nonreassuring Fetal Heart Rate Patterns

- Nonreassuring FHR patterns do not necessarily predict adverse events, and although electronic fetal heart monitoring has resulted in increased cesarean deliveries, there has not been a decrease in long-term adverse neurologic outcomes such as cerebral palsy. Nevertheless, the known relationships between fetal hypoxemia/acidemia and abnormal heart rate patterns make FHT interpretation a critical part of labor management.

*Noninvasive Management*

- **Oxygen:** Maternal supplemental oxygen often results in improved fetal oxygenation, assuming adequate placental exchange and circulation.
- **Maternal positioning:** Left lateral positioning releases vena cava compression by the gravid uterus, promoting increased venous return, increased cardiac output, increased BP, and improved uterine blood flow.
- **Discontinue oxytocin** until the FHR and uterine activity become normal.
- **Vibroacoustic stimulation (VAS)** or **fetal scalp stimulation:** Fetal stimuli may be used to induce accelerations when the FHR lacks variability for a long period of time. Heart rate acceleration in response to these stimuli indicates the absence of acidosis and correlates with a mean pH value of about 7.30. Conversely, a 50% chance of acidosis exists in a fetus that fails to respond to VAS in the setting of a nonreassuring heart rate pattern.

*Invasive Management*

- **Amniotomy:** If the FHR cannot be monitored adequately externally, an amniotomy should be performed to place internal monitors, unless these are contraindicated by the clinical situation.
- **Fetal scalp electrode (FSE):** Direct application of an FSE records the fetal electrocardiogram (fECG) waveform and may allow closer evaluation of the FHR. An FSE may be contraindicated in cases of fetal coagulopathy or maternal infections such as HIV, active herpes simplex virus, and hepatitis B or C.
- **Intrauterine pressure catheter and amnioinfusion:** A catheter is inserted into the chorioamnionic sac and attached to a pressure gauge. Pressure readings provide quantitative data on the strength and duration of contractions. Amnioinfusion of room temperature normal saline can be used to replace amniotic fluid volume to relieve recurrent variable decelerations in patients with oligohydramnios. Care should be used to avoid overdistention of the uterus.
- **Tocolytic agents:** Beta-adrenergic agonists (e.g., terbutaline, 0.25 mg subcutaneously or 0.125 to 0.25 mg IV) can be administered to decrease uterine activity in the presence of uterine tachysystole. Potential side effects of beta-adrenergic agonists include elevated serum glucose levels and increased maternal and fetal heart rates.
- **Management of maternal hypotension:** Maternal hypotension, as a complication of the sympathetic blockade associated with epidural anesthesia or from

compression of the vena cava, can lead to decreased placental perfusion and FHR decelerations. IV fluid bolus, left uterine displacement, and ephedrine or phenylephrine administration may be appropriate.
- **Fetal scalp blood pH:** Determination of fetal scalp blood pH can clarify the acid–base state of the fetus. A pH value of 7.25 or higher is normal. A pH range of 7.20 to 7.24 is a preacidotic. A pH of <7.20 on two measurements 5 to 10 minutes apart may indicate sufficient fetal acidosis to warrant immediate delivery.

## ASSISTED SPONTANEOUS VAGINAL DELIVERY

The goals of assisted spontaneous vaginal delivery are reduction of maternal trauma, prevention of fetal injury, and initial support of the newborn.
- **Episiotomy** is an incision into the perineal body to enlarge the outlet area and facilitate delivery. Episiotomy may occasionally be necessary in cases of vaginal soft tissue dystocia or as an accompaniment to forceps- or vacuum-assisted vaginal delivery. Prophylactic episiotomy increases the risk of higher degrees of perineal tears.
  - An incision is made vertically in the perineal body (midline episiotomy) or at a 45-degree angle off the midline (mediolateral episiotomy). The incision should be approximately half the length of the perineal body and extend into the vagina 2 to 3 cm. Excessive blood loss can result from performing the episiotomy too early. The episiotomy can be performed either before or after the application of forceps or a vacuum.
  - Midline episiotomies are associated with increased risk of extension to third- or fourth-degree laceration when compared with mediolateral episiotomy or no episiotomy. Mediolateral episiotomies may require more postpartum analgesia.
- **Delivery of the head:** The goal is to prevent excessively rapid delivery by controlling the expulsion of the head. If extension of the head does not occur easily, a modified Ritgen maneuver can be performed by palpating the fetal chin through the perineum and applying pressure upward. After delivery of the head, external rotation is possible, which brings the occiput in line with the fetal spine. If a nuchal cord is present, it is reduced over the head or double-clamped and cut. Mucous and amniotic fluids are aspirated from the infant's mouth and nose using bulb suction.
- **Delivery of the shoulders and body:** The fetus is directed posteriorly with gentle downward pressure until the anterior shoulder has passed beneath the symphysis pubis. The fetus is then directed anteriorly until the posterior shoulder passes the perineum. After the shoulders are delivered, the fetus is grasped with one hand supporting the head and neck and the other hand along the spine.

## OPERATIVE VAGINAL DELIVERY

Operative vaginal delivery can be an effective alternative to cesarean section for women in the second stage of labor who meet specific criteria.

### Forceps Delivery
- Classification is by station of the fetal head at the time that the forceps are applied.
  - **Mid forceps:** Head is engaged but higher than +2 station.
  - **Low forceps:** Station is +2 or lower.
  - **Outlet forceps:** Scalp is visible without separating the labia, skull has reached pelvic floor, head is at or on perineum, and the occiput is either directly anterior-posterior in alignment or does not require more than 45 degrees of rotation.

- **Indications:** None are absolute, but they include:
  - Prolonged second stage of labor
  - Maternal exhaustion
  - Inadequate maternal expulsive effort
  - Fetal intolerance of labor
  - A maternal condition requiring a shortened/passive second stage
- **Prerequisites:** Before operative vaginal delivery with forceps is attempted, the following criteria should be met:
  - The fetal head must be engaged in the pelvis.
  - The cervix must be fully dilated.
  - The bladder should be empty.
  - The exact station and position of the fetal head should be known.
  - Maternal pelvis must be adequate.
  - If time permits, the patient should be given adequate anesthesia.
  - If forceps delivery is done for nonreassuring fetal status, someone who is able to perform neonatal resuscitation should be available.
  - The operator should have knowledge about, and experience with, the appropriate instrument, its proper application, and the possible complications.
- **Maternal complications:** uterine, cervical, or vaginal lacerations, extension of the episiotomy, bladder or urethral injuries, and hematomas
- **Fetal complications:** cephalohematoma, bruising, lacerations, facial nerve injury, and, rarely, skull fracture and intracranial hemorrhage

### Soft Cup Vacuum Delivery

- Indications, contraindications, and complications are largely the same as for forceps delivery.
- The suction cup is applied in the midline on the sagittal suture about 2 cm anterior to the posterior fontanelle (the "flexion point").
- Maximum vacuum suction of 0.7 to 0.8 kg/cm$^2$ (500 to 600 mm Hg) is applied and then one hand maintains fetal flexion and supports the vacuum cup while the other applies sustained traction to assist delivery of the fetal head, without rocking or twisting, only during contractions.
- Vacuum pressure can be released between contractions and should not be maintained for longer than 30 minutes.
- Vacuum use should be avoided in fetuses <34 weeks' GA or with known thrombocytopenia, hemophilia, or von Willebrand disease.

## SHOULDER DYSTOCIA

**Shoulder dystocia** occurs in 0.15% to 1.70% of all vaginal deliveries and is defined as an impaction of the fetal shoulder after delivery of the head. It is associated with increased fetal morbidity and mortality secondary to brachial plexus injuries and asphyxia. The diagnosis should be considered when the application of gentle, downward pressure of the fetal head fails to accomplish delivery.

- **Macrosomia** is strongly associated with shoulder dystocia. Compared to average-sized infants, the risk of shoulder dystocia is 11 and 22 times greater for infants weighing more than 4,000 and 4,500 g, respectively. Up to 50% of cases, however, occur in infants weighing <4,000 g. Postterm (≥42 weeks' gestation) and macrosomic infants are at risk because the trunk and shoulder growth is disproportionate to growth of the head in late pregnancy.

• Other **risk factors** include maternal obesity, previous macrosomic infant, diabetes mellitus, and gestational diabetes. Shoulder dystocia should be suspected in cases of prolonged second stage of labor or prolonged deceleration phase of first stage of labor.

## Management

• Anticipation and preparation are important. Help should be available as extra hands may be needed during the delivery. A pediatrician should be notified. If available, an anesthesiologist should also be informed.

• The time should be marked when the dystocia is called and the total time until delivery recorded in the notes. Once the shoulder dystocia is identified, no significant pressure should be applied to the head until the shoulders are delivered. Fundal pressure should *never* be applied as it only exacerbates the shoulder impaction.

• **McRoberts maneuver** is performed by hyperflexion and abduction of the maternal hips, flattening the lumbar spine, and rotating the pelvis to increase the anterior–posterior outlet diameter.

• **Suprapubic pressure** is applied in a vector chosen to anteriorly rotate the anterior fetal shoulder and dislodge the shoulder from the symphysis.

• Other measures in combination are chosen for the specific clinical situation based on clinician experience. There is no "right order" in which the maneuvers described in the following text should be performed, and maneuvers can and should be used more than once, as needed.

  • **Delivery of the posterior arm: By grabbing the posterior hand**, the posterior arm can be flexed and swept across the fetal chest, delivered first, thereby creating more room for the anterior shoulder.

  • **Episiotomy:** Incision of the perineum provides additional room and should be considered if it might facilitate delivery or additional maneuvering.

  • **Rubin maneuver:** The anterior fetal shoulder is rotated obliquely with a vaginal hand. This maneuver may also be performed in a posterior manner.

  • **Wood corkscrew:** The posterior shoulder is rotated over 180 degrees with a vaginal hand to assist delivery of the shoulders.

  • **Gaskin maneuver:** Facilitated in the unanesthetized patient, she is turned over on "all fours," inverting the anterior and posterior shoulders.

• Delivery that does not occur following the aforementioned maneuvers may require some of the more invasive and traumatic procedures noted in the following text for the sake of fetal viability.

  • **Neonatal clavicular fracture:** Palpate the clavicles and apply outward pressure with the thumb to avoid lung or subclavian artery injury.

  • In extreme cases, the **Zavanelli maneuver** (in which the fetal head is flexed and pushed back up into the uterus as preparations for emergent cesarean section are made) or **symphysiotomy** (performed by laterally displacing the urethra using the index and middle fingers placed against the posterior aspect of the symphysis and incising the cartilaginous portion of the symphysis) could be performed.

## CESAREAN SECTION

• **Fetal indications** for cesarean delivery include:
  • Nonreassuring FHT
  • Nonvertex presentation (malpresentation)
  • Fetal anomalies, such as hydrocephalus, that would make successful vaginal delivery unlikely

- Umbilical cord prolapse
- Conjoined twins
- **Maternal indications** for cesarean delivery include:
  - Obstruction of the lower genital tract (e.g., large condyloma)
  - Previous cesarean section (if vaginal birth after cesarean [VBAC] is declined or not appropriate)
  - Previous uterine surgery involving the contractile portion of the uterus (i.e., classical cesarean, transmural myomectomy)
  - History of severe pelvic floor injury from a prior vaginal delivery
  - Abdominal cerclage
- **Maternal and fetal indications** include:
  - Abruptio placentae
  - Active maternal herpes simplex virus infection
  - Labor dystocia or cephalopelvic disproportion
  - Placenta previa or known vasa previa (absolute indication)
- The patient should be counseled regarding standard **risks of surgery**, such as pain, bleeding that may require transfusion, infection, damage to nearby organs, and a small but increased risk of death when compared to vaginal delivery.

## VAGINAL BIRTH AFTER CESAREAN SECTION

- Provided there are no contraindications to vaginal delivery, a patient may be counseled and offered a trial of labor after previous cesarean delivery (TOLAC). Success rates of VBAC are higher for patients with nonrecurring conditions, such as malpresentation or fetal intolerance of labor (60% to 85%), than for those with a prior diagnosis of dystocia (15% to 30%). Patients should be counseled regarding the risk of uterine rupture (0.9% to 3.7%), failed trial of labor, and need for cesarean delivery. Someone with a history of two prior C-sections may consider a TOLAC, depending on prior indications, although some providers may choose not to offer it.
- **Contraindications** include previous classical or inverted T-shaped uterine incision, transfundal uterine surgery, history of uterine rupture, contracted pelvis, and medical or obstetric contraindications to vaginal delivery.
- Epidural anesthesia and oxytocin may be used with VBAC. The delivery hospital must have facilities and staffing for emergency cesarean delivery. Blood products should be readily available. The most common sign of uterine rupture is a nonreassuring FHR pattern with variable decelerations evolving into late decelerations, bradycardia, and undetectable FHR. Other findings include uterine or abdominal pain, loss of station of the presenting part, vaginal bleeding, and hypovolemia.

## MALPRESENTATIONS

Normal presentation is defined by longitudinal lie, cephalic presentation, and flexion of the fetal neck. All other presentations are malpresentations. Occurring in approximately 5% of all deliveries, malpresentations may lead to abnormalities of labor and increased risk for mother or fetus.

- **Risk factors** for malpresentation are conditions that decrease the polarity of the uterus, increase or decrease fetal mobility, or block the presenting part from the pelvis.
  - **Maternal factors** include grand multiparity, pelvic tumors, uterine fibroids, pelvic contracture, and uterine malformations.

- **Fetal factors** include prematurity, multiple gestation, polyhydramnios or oligohydramnios, macrosomia, placenta previa, hydrocephaly, trisomy, anencephaly, and myotonic dystrophy.
- **Breech** presentation occurs when the cephalic pole is in the uterine fundus. Major congenital anomalies occur in 6.3% of term breech presentation infants compared to 2.4% of vertex presentation infants.
  - The incidence of breech presentation is 25% of pregnancies at <28 weeks' gestation, 7% of pregnancies at 32 weeks' gestation, and 3% to 4% of term pregnancies in labor.
  - The three types of breech presentation are:
    - **Frank breech** (48% to 73%) occurs when both hips are flexed and both knees are extended.
    - **Complete breech** (5% to 12%) occurs when the fetus is flexed at the hips and flexed at the knees.
    - **Incomplete, or footling breech** (12% to 38%), occurs when the fetus has one or both hips extended (Fig. 5-1).
- **Risks** of breech presentation include cord prolapse (15% in footling breech, 5% in complete breech, and 0.5% in frank breech), head entrapment, and spinal cord injury (with neck hyperextension).
- Fetuses in a complete or frank breech presentation may occasionally be considered for vaginal delivery with appropriate selection and counseling.
- Cesarean delivery poses risk of increased maternal morbidity and mortality.
- Vaginal breech delivery poses increased risk of fetal asphyxia, cord prolapse, birth trauma, spinal cord injury, and mortality. Planned vaginal breech delivery is not routinely offered but with careful selection and evaluation may be permitted.
- For patients in advanced labor with a breech fetus for whom delivery is imminent, a trial of labor may be attempted if:
  - The breech is frank or complete.
  - The estimated fetal weight is <3,800 g.
  - Pelvimetry suggests an adequate pelvis.
  - The fetal head is flexed.
  - Anesthesia is immediately available.
  - The fetus is continuously monitored.

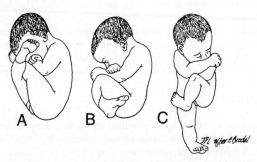

**Figure 5-1.** Breech presentations. (**A**) Frank breech. (**B**) Complete breech. (**C**) Incomplete breech, single footling. (From Beckmann CR, Ling FW, Herbert WN, et al. *Obstetrics and Gynecology*, 2nd ed. Baltimore, MD: Lippincott Williams & Wilkins, 1995:194, with permission.)

- A pediatrician is available.
- An obstetrician is available who is experienced with vaginal breech delivery.
- In breech presentation, the fetus usually emerges in the sacrum transverse or oblique position. As crowning occurs (the bitrochanteric diameter passes under the symphysis), an episiotomy can be considered.
- When the umbilicus appears, place fingers medial to each thigh and press out laterally to deliver the legs (Pinard maneuver). The fetus should then be rotated to the anterior sacrum position, and the trunk can be wrapped in a towel for traction.
- When the infant's scapulas appear, the arms can be delivered. The shoulders can be grasped posteriorly, the humerus followed down, and each arm rotated across the chest and out (Lovsett maneuver). To deliver the *right* arm, the fetus is turned in a *counterclockwise* direction; to deliver the *left* arm, the fetus is turned in a *clockwise* direction.
- If the head does not deliver spontaneously, the head may be flexed by placing downward traction and pressure on the maxillary ridge (Mauriceau-Smellie-Veit maneuver). Direct vertical suprapubic pressure may also be applied. Piper forceps may be used to assist in delivery of the head.
- For delivery of a breech second twin, ultrasonography should be available in the delivery room. The operator reaches into the uterus and grasps both feet, trying to keep the membranes intact. The feet are brought down to the introitus, then amniotomy is performed. The body is delivered to the scapula by applying gentle traction on the feet. The remainder of the delivery is the same as that described earlier for a singleton breech.
- **Head entrapment** during breech vaginal delivery may be managed by one or more of the following procedures:
  - **Dührssen incisions** are made in the cervix at the 2, 6, and 10 o'clock positions. Up to three incisions may be needed to facilitate delivery of the fetal head through the cervix. The 3 and 9 o'clock positions should be avoided due to the risk of dividing the cervical vessels with resultant hemorrhage.
  - Relaxation agents (nitric oxide or nitroglycerine) may release the entrapped head, enabling proper head flexion and vaginal delivery.
  - Cephalocentesis can be performed if the fetus is not viable. The procedure is performed by perforating the base of the skull and suctioning the cranial contents.
- **External cephalic version**
  - **Indication** is persistent breech presentation at term. The version is performed to avoid breech presentation in labor.
  - **Risks** include compromised umbilical blood flow, placental separation, fetal distress, fetal injury, premature rupture of membranes, and fetomaternal bleeding (overall incidence is 0% to 1.4%). The most common "risk" is failed version.
  - **Success rate** for external cephalic version ranges from 35% to 86%, but in 2% of cases, the fetus reverts back to breech presentation.
  - **Technique:** A GA of at least 36 weeks, reactive nonstress test, and informed consent must be obtained. Version is generally accomplished by applying a liberal amount of lubrication then transabdominally grasping the fetal head and fetal breech and manipulating the fetus through a forward or backward roll. Ultrasonographic guidance is an important adjunct to confirm position and monitor FHR. Tocolysis and spinal or epidural anesthesia may improve success rates. After the procedure, the patient should be monitored continuously until the FHR is reactive, no decelerations are present, and no evidence of regular contractions exists. Rh-negative patients should receive $Rh_o$ (D) immunoglobulin (RhoGAM) after the procedure because of the potential for fetomaternal bleeding.

- **Factors associated with failure** include obesity, oligohydramnios, deep engagement of the presenting part, a partial uterine septum, and fetal back posterior. Nulliparity and an anterior placenta may also reduce the likelihood of success.
- **Contraindications** to external cephalic version include conditions in which labor or vaginal delivery would be contraindicated. Version is not generally recommended in cases of ruptured membranes, third-trimester bleeding, oligohydramnios, multiple gestations, or after labor has begun.
- **Abnormal lie**
  - Lie refers to the alignment of the fetal spine in relation to the maternal spine. Longitudinal lie is normal, whereas oblique and transverse lies are abnormal. Abnormal lie is associated with multiparity, prematurity, pelvic contraction, and disorders of the placenta.
  - **Incidence** of abnormal lie is 1 in 300 term pregnancies. At 32 weeks' gestation, the incidence is <2%.
  - **Risk:** The greatest risk of abnormal lie is cord prolapse because the fetal parts do not fill the pelvic inlet.
  - **Management:** If abnormal lie persists beyond 35 to 38 weeks, external version may be attempted. An ultrasonographic examination should be performed to rule out major anomalies and abnormal placentation. If an abnormal axial lie persists, mode of delivery should be cesarean section. An intraoperative cephalic version may be attempted. A vertical uterine incision may be prudent in cases with back down transverse or oblique lie with ruptured membranes or poorly developed lower uterine segment.
- **Abnormal attitude and deflexion:** Full flexion of the fetal neck is considered normal. Abnormalities range from partial deflexion to full extension.
  - **Face presentation** results from extension of the fetal neck. The chin is the presenting part.
    - ○ **Incidence** is between 0.14% and 0.54%. In 60% of cases, face presentation is associated with a fetal malformation. Anencephaly accounts for 33% of all cases.
    - ○ **Diagnosis:** Face presentation may be diagnosed by vaginal examination, ultrasonography, or palpation of the cephalic prominence and the fetal back on the same side of the maternal abdomen when performing Leopold maneuvers.
    - ○ **Risk:** Perinatal mortality ranges from 0.6% to 5.0%.
    - ○ **Management:** The fetus must be mentum (chin) anterior for a vaginal delivery to be successful.
  - **Brow presentation** results from partial deflexion of the fetal neck.
    - ○ **Incidence** is 1 in 670 to 1 in 3,433 pregnancies. Causes of brow presentation are similar to those of face presentation.
    - ○ **Risks:** Perinatal mortality ranges from 1.28% to 8.00%.
    - ○ **Management:** The majority of cases spontaneously convert to a flexed attitude. A vaginal delivery should be considered only if the maternal pelvis is large, the fetus is small, and labor progresses adequately.
- **Compound presentation** occurs when an extremity prolapses beside the presenting part.
  - **Incidence** is 1 in 377 to 1 in 1,213 pregnancies and is associated with prematurity.
  - **Risks:** Fetal risks are cord prolapse in 10% to 20% of cases and birth trauma including neurologic and musculoskeletal damage to the involved extremity.
  - **Management:** The prolapsing extremity should not be manipulated. Continuous fetal monitoring is recommended because compound presentation can be

associated with occult cord prolapse. Spontaneous vaginal delivery occurs in 75% of vertex/upper extremity presentations. Cesarean section is indicated in cases of nonreassuring FHT, cord prolapse, and failure of labor to progress.

## SUGGESTED READINGS

American College of Obstetricians and Gynecologists. Practice bulletin no. 115: vaginal birth after previous cesarean delivery. *Obstet Gynecol* 2010;116(2)(pt 1):450–463.

Cunningham FG, Leveno KJ, Bloom SL, et al. (Normal labor and delivery) and 18 (intrapartum assessment). *Williams Obstetrics*, 23rd ed. New York, NY: McGraw-Hill, 2009.

Hale RW, Dennen EW. *Dennen's Forceps Deliveries*, 4th ed. Washington, DC: American College of Obstetricians and Gynecologists, 2001.

Halpern SH, Leighton BL, Ohlsson A, et al. Effect of epidural versus parenteral opioid analgesia on the progress of labor: a meta-analysis. *JAMA* 1998;280(24):2105–2110.

Zhang J, Landy HJ, Branch DW, et al; Consortium on Safe Labor. Contemporary patterns of spontaneous labor with normal neonatal outcomes. *Obstet Gynecol* 2010;116(6):1281–1287.

# 6 Fetal Assessment

Sarahn M. Wheeler and Edith Gurewitsch Allen

**Antenatal fetal surveillance** is performed using various modalities that allow care providers to closely monitor fetuses at risk for uteroplacental insufficiency. Its purpose is to detect signs of fetal compromise related to poor uteroplacental perfusion in order to circumvent fetal hypoxemia, acidemia, and death. Performed serially at regular intervals, antenatal fetal testing is used to assess ongoing fetal well-being, guide antenatal management, and determine possible need for imminent delivery or other acute obstetric management. It is therefore important that providers of obstetric care be well versed in the different modalities of fetal testing, including their limitations and implications.

## METHODS OF FETAL ASSESSMENT

There are numerous methods to assess fetal well-being, and no single test is superior to another method. Each test has its own individual merits (as well as limitations) and often are used in combination to create an overall picture of the fetal state and help identify fetal compromise (Table 6-1).

### Fetal Movement
- **Maternal assessment of fetal movement (kick counts)**
  - Least expensive and least invasive fetal assessment test
  - Requires neither equipment nor hospital setting

| TABLE 6-1 | Comparison of Antenatal Fetal Tests | | |
|---|---|---|---|
| **Antenatal Tests** | **Strengths** | **Limitations** | **Influential Factors** |
| **Kick counts** | • Inexpensive<br>• Noninvasive<br>• Simple | • Need maternal participation<br>• No supervision of physician | |
| **Nonstress test (NST)** | • Noninvasive<br>• Simple | • Limited value <32 wk<br>• Low sensitivity<br>• High false-positive rate | • Smoking<br>• Maternal medications<br>• Illicit drug use<br>• Magnesium sulfate<br>• Sleep cycle<br>• Prematurity |
| **Vibroacoustic stimulation (VAS)** | • Noninvasive<br>• Prevents some false-positive results from NST | • Limited value <32 wk<br>• Low sensitivity | |
| **Contraction stress test (CST)** | • Highest specificity | • Contraindications: preterm labor, ruptured membranes, placenta previa, extensive uterine surgery<br>• Cannot be used in premature infants<br>• Labor-intensive | |
| **Biophysical profile (BPP)** | • Useful in premature fetuses | • High false-positive rate | • Betamethasone<br>• Maternal hypoglycemia |
| **Uterine artery Doppler ultrasound** | • Predicts fetal compromise earlier than other tests | • Only useful in specific conditions | |

- **Purpose:** Kick counts can be used for routine screening and reassurance in low-risk pregnancies when a patient perceives decreased fetal movement. It can also be used as a method of surveillance in some higher risk pregnancies, for example, in women with a prior history of stillbirth.
- **Method of testing:** The patient counts the number of fetal movements in a finite period of time. While performing this test, the woman should lie on her left side to improve blood flow to the fetus and eat prior to starting the test to

stimulate the fetus. Multiple testing strategies have been described, all with equal efficacy.

- ○ To perform the Cardiff technique, the patient counts fetal movements when she first gets up in the morning and records the time required for the fetus to move 10 times. Lack of 10 movements over 3 hours should prompt the patient to call her physician for further fetal testing.
- ○ Using the Sadovsky technique, the patient counts fetal movements over the course of 1 hour. To be considered "reassuring," four or more fetal movements should be felt over the course of the hour. However, a second hour of monitoring to attain four movements is permissible. If four fetal movements have not been felt after 2 hours, the patient should contact her doctor for further recommendations.
- **Management after abnormal results:** After the observation of decreased fetal movement, the follow-up test to evaluate fetal well-being is a nonstress test (NST).

## Fetal Heart Monitoring

- **Nonstress test**
- In the absence of acidosis or neurologic impairment, the fetal heart rate normally rises temporarily and randomly during fetal movement.
- These increases in heart rate or accelerations are detectable using cardiotocography.
- **Method of testing:** The NST is a noninvasive assessment that records the fetal heart rate simultaneously with uterine activity. The fetal heart rate is monitored with an external cardiotachometer, which uses ultrasound to evaluate fetal heart motion, giving an average of fetal heart beats. Uterine activity is monitored with an external tocodynamometer.
- **Criteria for test results:** A "reactive" NST demonstrates at least two accelerations of the fetal heart rate over a 20-minute period. Prior to 32 weeks' gestation, accelerations must be 10 seconds in duration and reach a peak 10 beats above the baseline to qualify as reactive. As the sympathetic and parasympathetic nervous systems mature, more stringent criteria are applied. In a fetus 32 weeks' gestation or greater, each of the two accelerations must be 15 seconds in duration and must reach a peak of 15 beats above the baseline level (Fig. 6-1). If the fetal heart rate

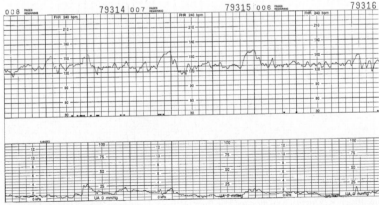

**Figure 6-1.** Reactive nonstress test. Fetal monitor strip records fetal heart rate (**top**) and uterine contractile activity (**bottom**). Several accelerations are evident.

is "nonreactive" after 20 minutes, the fetal heart rate should be observed for an additional 20 minutes to account for the possibility that the fetus may have been in quiet sleep during the initial observation period. There are many other factors that can influence the fetal heart rate tracing (see the following text).

- **Strengths and limitations:** A reactive NST is highly predictive of a low risk of fetal mortality in the subsequent 72 hours, 96 hours, or a week depending on the indication for fetal testing. The negative predictive value of an NST is >90%. The positive predictive value is only 50% to 70%. Therefore, the NST is better suited to rule out rather than predict fetal compromise. Given the high false-positive rate, a nonreactive NST should be followed by more extensive testing such as biophysical profile, vibroacoustic stimulation, or contraction stress test.

- **Contraction stress test (CST)** or **oxytocin challenge test (OCT)**
  - **Purpose:** The CST is designed to assess fetal response to the stress of induced uterine contractions causing transient uteroplacental insufficiency.
  - **Method of testing:** The mother is placed in the left lateral tilt position, and external monitors are applied. If three contractions of 40 seconds duration or greater are noted, a "spontaneous" CST can be performed without stimulation. In the absence of spontaneous contractions, uterine activity can be induced either by nipple stimulation or with a dilute solution of oxytocin until three contractions occur in a 10-minute time period.
  - **Criteria for test results:** A "positive" CST demonstrates late decelerations with more than 50% of contractions (Fig. 6-2). Late decelerations reach their nadir after the peak of the contraction. A "negative" CST demonstrates no late decelerations. A CST with intermittent late decelerations is considered equivocal, and further evaluation of the pregnancy is warranted. An "inadequate" or "unsatisfactory" CST is one in which adequate contractions are not achieved.

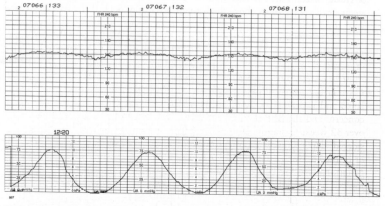

**Figure 6-2.** Fetal heart tracing with late decelerations. Following each contraction (**bottom tracing**) is a slight depression of the fetal heart rate (**top tracing**), suggesting uteroplacental insufficiency. (Original fetal monitor strip from Dr. Janice Henderson, Johns Hopkins Hospital, Department of Gynecology and Obstetrics, Division of Maternal Fetal Medicine.)

If hyperstimulation occurs, an abnormal fetal response may be the result of the testing technique alone and should be repeated or another form of testing should be done.

- **Strengths and limitations:** CST is one of the most labor-intensive methods of fetal surveillance but has the highest specificity for detecting the compromised fetus. It has a negative predictive value of >99%. Relative contraindications to CST include preterm labor, preterm premature rupture of membranes (PPROM), placenta previa, and high risk for uterine rupture. Previous low transverse cesarean section is not a contraindication.
- **Vibroacoustic stimulation test (VAS)**
  - **Purpose:** VAS is a useful adjunct to a nonreactive NST. This test will decrease false-positive results of nonreactive NST if the cause of the abnormal test is fetal sleep and potentially decrease testing.
  - **Method of testing:** VAS is performed by placing a vibrating auditory source, such as an artificial larynx, on the maternal abdomen. The sound device is placed halfway between the pubic symphysis and umbilicus, and it delivers a short burst of sound to the fetus for 5 seconds. The procedure stimulates the fetus to move and shortens the time necessary to produce fetal heart rate accelerations. It is important to avoid stimulating the fetus when it is experiencing stress from a contraction because this may cause the fetus to have a drop in heart rate.
  - **Criteria for test results:** The VAS is used in conjunction with the NST and is interpreted similarly to the NST as discussed earlier.

## Fetal Heart Monitoring with Ultrasonography

- **Biophysical profile (BPP)**
  - **Purpose:** The BPP uses ultrasound observations in conjunction with the NST to help predict acute and chronic tissue hypoxia. It has excellent negative predictive value for fetal mortality in the 72 to 96 hours after the test. It has been shown to reduce perinatal morbidity and mortality.
  - **Method of testing:** The BPP has five components: fetal breathing, fetal movement, fetal tone, and amniotic fluid assessment determined by ultrasound along with the NST. Two points are awarded for each observed parameter. No points are awarded for a nonreactive NST or the absence of any parameter. Therefore, only even number scores are possible, with a maximum score of 10. The specific criteria of these components are listed in Table 6-2. All of the sonographic criteria must be observed within a 30-minute period.
  - **Criteria for test results:** A score of 8 or 10 is reassuring, and routine surveillance and expectant obstetric management may continue. A score of 6 raises concern, and the BPP should be repeated in 6 to 24 hours, especially in fetuses over 32 weeks' gestation. If the score does not improve, delivery should be considered, depending on gestational age and individual circumstances. Scores of 4 or below are worrisome, and delivery should be considered, again depending on gestational age and clinical context. It is important to consider that fetal breathing can be reduced in preterm fetuses <34 weeks' gestation, and this may affect interpretation.
- **Modified BPP**
  - **Purpose:** This test combines the **NST and amniotic fluid index (AFI)**. In the third trimester, an AFI and NST are often used together to assess fetal well-being. The AFI is the sum of the maximum vertical pockets of umbilical cord–free

**TABLE 6-2**    Biophysical Profile

| Biophysical Variable | Normal (Score = 2) | Abnormal (Score = 0) |
|---|---|---|
| Fetal breathing movements | One episode of fetal breathing 30 s | Less than 30 s of fetal breathing; absent breathing |
| Fetal movements | Three discrete body/limb movements | Two or fewer body/limb movements |
| Fetal tone | One episode of active extension, with return to flexion of fetal limbs or trunk | Extended position with no or slow return to flexion; absent movement |
| Nonstress test | Reactive | Nonreactive |
| Amniotic fluid volume | One pocket of fluid at least 2 cm in two perpendicular planes | No amniotic fluid or pocket <2 cm in size |

amniotic fluid in each of the four quadrants of the uterus. In general, the AFI reflects fetal perfusion and, if decreased, raises suspicion for uteroplacental insufficiency.

- **Criteria for test results:** A normal test includes a reactive NST and an AFI >5. An abnormal test lacks one or both of these findings and should be further evaluated.
- **Doppler velocimetry**
  - **Purpose:** Doppler velocimetry is a noninvasive method of assessing fetal vascular impedance (Fig. 6-3).
  - **Method of testing:** Umbilical artery flow can be documented using real-time sonography. A free-floating loop of umbilical cord is identified, and continuous or pulsed wave Dopplers are used to identify arterial flow. The waveform pattern is recorded and analyzed. The most common method of analysis is the systolic/diastolic (S/D) ratio. The presence of diastolic flow has greater clinical significance than the S/D ratio. The normal values vary depending on gestational age. Significant elevations in the S/D ratio have been associated with intrauterine growth restriction (IUGR), fetal hypoxia, fetal acidosis, and thus with higher rates of perinatal morbidity and mortality. Absent and reversed end-diastolic flow are the more extreme examples of abnormal S/D ratio and may prompt delivery in some situations.
  - **Strengths and limitations:** Abnormal umbilical artery blood flow patterns are reported to precede abnormal fetal heart rate patterns by a median of 7 days. For this reason, it is used in conjunction with other tests for pregnancies complicated by IUGR, preeclampsia, or chronic hypertension.
  - **Indications for use:** Umbilical artery Doppler velocimetry should not be used as a screening tool in the general population of normally grown fetuses. It has been shown to be useful in pregnancies complicated by IUGR, hypertension, or preeclampsia. The use of Doppler studies in a normally grown fetus in an otherwise uncomplicated pregnancy continue to be investigated.

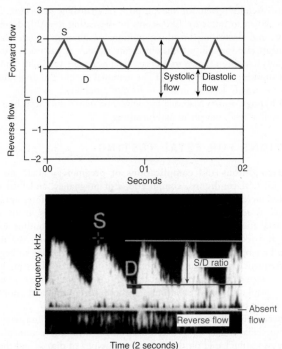

**Figure 6-3.** Evaluation of umbilical artery flow by Doppler velocimetry. **Top panel** illustrates the findings for a normal umbilical artery. **Bottom image** is a typical normal Doppler recording. Ratio of flow during systole and diastole (S/D ratio) reflects placental bed resistance. S, systole; D, diastole. (Adapted from Druzin ML, Gabbe SG, Reed KL. Antepartum fetal evaluation. In Gabbe SG, Niebyl JR, Simpson JL, eds. *Obstetrics: Normal and Problem Pregnancies*, 4th ed. New York, NY: Churchill Livingstone, 2001:334; MacDonald MG, Mullet MD, Seshia MMK. *Avery's Neonatology Pathophysiology & Management of the Newborn*, 6th ed. Philadelphia, PA: Lippincott Williams & Wilkins, 2005.)

## CONFOUNDING FACTORS IN FETAL ASSESSMENT

- **Sleep cycles:** The fetus may have sleep cycles 20 to 80 minutes in duration. During these periods, the long-term variability of the fetal heart rate is decreased, and the tracing is likely to be nonreactive. To rule out sleep cycle as a cause for a nonreactive NST, prolonged monitoring (longer than 80 minutes at times) or VAS may be required.
- **Medications:** Certain maternal medications cross the placenta and can have an effect on the fetal heart rate, movement, and amniotic fluid volume. There are a number of medications administered in the management of labor and complications of labor that can have an influence on the tests for fetal well-being.

Glucocorticosteroids given for the purpose of maturing premature fetal lungs have been shown to influence BPP scores by decreasing the AFI, decreasing fetal movement, and decreasing breathing motion. Magnesium sulfate can decrease the fetal heart rate variability. Other medications such as narcotics, sedatives, and beta-blockers have been shown to decrease fetal heart rate variability and reactivity.

• **Maternal smoking and illicit drugs:** The maternal use of illicit drugs and smoking results in a transient decrease in fetal heart rate variability.

• **Maternal hypoglycemia:** Maternal hypoglycemia may reduce fetal heart rate variability as well as fetal movement and breathing.

## INDICATIONS FOR FETAL TESTING

• **Maternal conditions and complications of pregnancy:** There are numerous maternal medical conditions, complications of pregnancy, and fetal conditions that confer increased risk of adverse fetal outcomes. Therefore, antenatal fetal surveillance is recommended in these high-risk pregnancies in an attempt to decrease fetal morbidity and mortality. Tables 6-3 and 6-4 outline some of the maternal and fetal indications for antenatal fetal surveillance, the methods of testing to be employed for fetal assessment, the gestational age to begin testing, and the frequency of monitoring. Other indications for fetal testing are chronic hypertension, preeclampsia, maternal renal disease, lupus, maternal hemoglobin-opathies, antiphospholipid syndrome, chronic abruption, and monoamnionic monochorionic twins.

• **Commencement and frequency of testing:** Each maternal and fetal indication for fetal surveillance has its own recommendations for the commencement and frequency of testing based on the underlying etiology of disease and the perceived risk to the fetus.

| TABLE 6-3 | Recommendations for Antenatal Fetal Assessment: Diabetes | | |
|---|---|---|---|
| Indication | Recommended Tests | Suggested Gestational Age for Commencement | Frequency of Testing |
| Pregestational diabetes | US and fetal echo | 18–20 wk | Once |
| | Kick counts | 26–28 wk | Daily |
| | US fetal growth | 28 wk | q4wk |
| | NST/BPP | 32 wk | Twice weekly |
| Gestational diabetes class A1 | Kick counts | 28 wk | Daily |
| Gestational diabetes class A2 | Kick counts | 26–28 wk | Daily |
| | US fetal growth | 28 wk | q4–6wk |
| | NST/BPP or modified BPP | 32 wk | Once or twice weekly |

US, ultrasound; NST, nonstress test; BPP, biophysical profile.

**TABLE 6-4** Recommendations for Antenatal Fetal Testing: Fetal Conditions

| Indication | Recommended Tests | Suggested Gestational Age for Commencement | Frequency of Testing |
|---|---|---|---|
| Intrauterine growth restriction | Umbilical Dopplers | Time of diagnosis | Weekly or twice weekly |
| | NST | | Weekly to daily |
| | AFI | | Weekly |
| | BPP | | Weekly to daily |
| Postterm pregnancy | NST | 41 wk | Twice or thrice weekly |
| Isoimmunization | MCA Doppler for fetal anemia | 16–18 wk | Weekly |
| Preterm premature rupture of membranes (PPROM) | NST | At time of PPROM | Daily to twice weekly |
| | BPP | | |
| Cholestasis of pregnancy | NST | 28–32 wk. | Twice weekly |
| | AFI | Time of diagnosis | Weekly |
| Oligohydramnios | Kick counts | 26–28 wk | Daily |
| History of prior stillbirth | NST, AFI, BPP | 32 wk or 1–2 wk prior to GA of previous stillbirth | Weekly to twice weekly |

NST, nonstress test; AFI, amniotic fluid index; BPP, biophysical profile; MCA, middle cerebral artery; GA, gestational age.

## SUGGESTED READINGS

American College of Obstetricians and Gynecologists. Practice bulletin no. 9: antepartum fetal surveillance. *Int J Gynaecol Obstet* 2000;68(2):175–185.

Devoe LD. Antenatal fetal assessment: contraction stress test, nonstress test, vibroacoustic stimulation, amniotic fluid volume, biophysical profile, and modified biophysical profile—an overview. *Semin Perinatol* 2008;32:247–252.

Nageotte M. Antenatal testing: diabetes mellitus. *Semin Perinatol* 2008;32:269–270.

Turan S, Miller J, Baschat A. Integrated testing and management in fetal growth restriction. *Semin Perinatol* 2008;32:194–200.

# 7 Complications of Labor and Delivery

Veena Choubey and Erika F. Werner

## UTERINE DEHISCENCE OR RUPTURE

**Dehiscence** is defined as lower uterine scar separation that does not breach the serosa; it rarely causes significant bleeding. **Rupture** is defined as complete separation of the uterine wall and may lead to fetal distress and significant maternal hemorrhage.

### Incidence

- Uterine rupture occurs in 0.2% to 1.8% of patients with one or more previous low-segment transverse cesarean sections and in 4% to 9% of patients with a prior uterine active segment incision (classical cesarean or T-incision). One third of prior classical cesarean scar rupture occurs before the onset of labor.

### Etiology

- Significant risk factors include:
  - Cesarean section
  - Prior uterine perforation
  - Previous resection of cornual ectopic pregnancy
  - Prostaglandin induction of labor with history of prior cesarean
- Other situations that may increase the risk of uterine rupture but not as significantly include:
  - Collagen disorders
  - Abdominal myomectomies in which the endometrial cavity was invaded

### Diagnosis and Management

- Fetal bradycardia is clinically manifested in 33% to 70% of cases. Fetal distress may be the initial presentation in catastrophic uterine rupture. In more subtle cases, the initial presentation may be a simple rise in fetal station or change in the position for fetal heart monitor placement. Maternal signs and symptoms include hypotension, uterine tenderness, a change in uterine shape, or constant abdominal pain.

- When uterine rupture is suspected, it is important to proceed emergently to laparotomy with delivery of the infant and repair of the uterine rupture. Rates of recurrent rupture in subsequent pregnancies carried to term approach 22%. Recommendations are for early delivery via cesarean section by 36 weeks.

## UMBILICAL CORD PROLAPSE

- **Umbilical cord prolapse** occurs when the umbilical cord slips beyond the presenting fetal part and passes through the open cervical os (overt) or descends alongside the presenting part (occult). The fetal blood supply is effectively compromised when the cord is compressed. The overall incidence is 1 to 6 per 1,000 births. The incidence in breech deliveries is slightly higher than 1%, and in footling breech or rupture of membranes with transverse lie may be as high as 10% to 15%.

### Etiology

- Risk factors include ruptured membranes, unengaged fetal presenting part (including disengagement), malpresentation (breech, transverse, oblique), prematurity, multiple gestation (second twin), multiparity, and polyhydramnios.

### Diagnosis

- Cord prolapse usually causes severe prolonged fetal bradycardia or persistent moderate to severe variable decelerations. Vaginal exam may confirm overt prolapse; the cord will be palpable.

### Management

- If the cord is felt on vaginal examination, elevate the presenting part to relieve pressure on the cord, call for help, and move to the operating room for emergent cesarean section.
- Appropriate anesthesia should be administered in the operating room and the viability of the fetus confirmed before proceeding with cesarean section.
- Placing the patient in Trendelenburg or knee-chest position may relieve cord compression with prolapse, but the vaginal hand should continue to elevate the presenting part. This should not delay transportation to the operating room.
- The interval between cord prolapse and delivery is the major predictor of newborn status. If delivered expeditiously, the neonatal outcomes are generally favorable. A cord gas should be obtained at the delivery to assess the degree of hypoxia.

## AMNIOTIC FLUID EMBOLISM

**Amniotic fluid embolism (AFE)** is a rare complication. Fetal fluid, tissue, or debris enters the maternal circulation via the placental bed and triggers acute anaphylaxis.

### Incidence

- Approximately 1 in 20,000 singleton pregnancies is complicated by AFE.
- Mortality is around 25% in the United States, much lower than the typically reported 60% to 80%. AFE accounts for 10% of maternal deaths in the United

States. Severe neurologic deficits occur in a high percentage of survivors. Neonatal survival is reported at 70%.

## Etiology and Diagnosis

- The term *embolism* is a misnomer because the clinical findings are probably a result of anaphylactic shock rather than pulmonary embolism. Amniotic fluid has been shown to cause vasospasm of the pulmonary vasculature in animal models.
- Risk factors include induced labor, advanced maternal age, multiparity, uterine rupture, abdominal trauma, placental abruption, diabetes, cervical lacerations, and operative delivery.
- AFE is primarily a clinical diagnosis of exclusion, made when a woman acutely presents with profound hypoxia, shock, and cardiovascular collapse during or immediately after labor. Cyanosis, hemorrhage, coma, and disseminated intravascular coagulation rapidly ensue.
- The differential diagnosis includes other acute events such as pulmonary embolism, hemorrhage, drug reaction, anaphylaxis, sepsis, and myocardial infarction.
- Useful laboratory data include arterial blood gas, serum electrolytes, calcium and magnesium levels, coagulation profile, and complete blood count.
- Definitive diagnosis is made only at autopsy, when amniotic fluid debris (e.g., fetal squamous cells or hair) are found in the maternal pulmonary vasculature. This debris may be present in the maternal circulation of women without AFE, however, so this finding is not pathognomonic.

## Management

- Approximately 65% of AFE occurs before delivery. Emergent delivery is required for both fetal and maternal benefits.
- The patient should be intubated and aggressively resuscitated.
- Administer intravenous (IV) fluids, inotropic agents, and pressors to maintain adequate blood pressure. Packed red blood cells (PRBC) and fresh frozen plasma (FFP) should be available, as there is a high risk for disseminated intravascular coagulation (DIC). Factor VII has been used in cases of severe DIC. Despite all efforts, significant maternal morbidity and mortality remain high.

## POSTPARTUM HEMORRHAGE

**Postpartum hemorrhage (PPH) is defined as:**
- Estimated blood loss (EBL) >500 mL for a vaginal delivery or >1,000 mL for a cesarean delivery; or
- Ten percent drop in hematocrit between admission and the postpartum period; or
- Any bleeding sufficient to cause symptoms or require erythrocyte transfusion (Table 7-1).

## Incidence

- PPH is the leading cause of maternal death, accounting for at least 25% of maternal deaths worldwide. It is the second leading cause of pregnancy-related death in the United States, accounting for 17% of maternal mortality.

## Etiology and Management

- Patients often tolerate loss of up to 20% of blood volume before symptoms of hypovolemia develop (see Chapter 3). Prompt, even anticipatory, action is crucial.

| TABLE 7-1 | Etiology of Postpartum Hemorrhage |
| --- | --- |

| Early (<24 hr Postpartum) | Late (24 hr to Several Months Postpartum) |
| --- | --- |
| Uterine atony | Infection |
| Retained placental fragments | Placental site subinvolution |
| Lower genital tract lacerations | Retained placental fragments |
| Uterine rupture | Hereditary coagulopathy |
| Uterine inversion | Preexisting uterine pathology |
| Hereditary coagulopathy | |
| Placenta accreta | |

Adapted from American College of Obstetricians and Gynecologists. Practice bulletin no. 76: postpartum hemorrhage. *Obstet Gynecol* 2006;108:1039–1047, with permission.

Blood flow to the gravid uterus is 600 to 900 mL/min; patients can become unstable rapidly.

- Establish large-bore IV access. Initiate IV fluid resuscitation. Administer supplemental oxygen and order cross-matched blood. After these initial steps, examine the patient to determine the underlying cause and address the problem expeditiously.
- Blood transfusion should be considered after 1 to 2 L EBL and may be initiated earlier if bleeding is expected to continue or the patient is symptomatic.
- Coagulation factors (FFP and cryoprecipitate) and platelets should be repleted with massive blood loss. Historically, one unit of FFP was given for every 4 to 6 units of PRBC to reduce dilutional and citrate coagulopathy as every 500 mL red cells is expected to dilute coagulation factors by 10%. Additionally, platelets were transfused when the platelet count dropped below 50,000/mL or after 6 to 10 units of red cell transfusion. More recent evidence suggests better outcomes with a protocol of 1:1:1 repletion of PRBC, FFP, and platelets when bleeding is ongoing or massive transfusion (>8 units of PRBC) is needed. In the operative setting, direct manual aortic compression can decrease pulse pressure and slow active bleeding to allow hemodynamic stabilization before proceeding with definitive management.
- Factor VII infusion may be considered in extreme cases of hemorrhage with DIC.

*Uterine Atony*

- **Uterine atony** (postpartum uterine contraction inadequate for hemostasis) is the most common cause of PPH.
- Normally, uterine contraction after delivery compresses uterine vessels, thereby reducing blood loss. Atony permits continuous brisk bleeding.
- Risk factors include uterine overdistention (as with fetal macrosomia, polyhydramnios, or multiple gestation); prolonged, augmented, or precipitous labor; chorioamnionitis; grand multiparity; and use of tocolytic agents.
- Initial management is **bimanual massage** of the uterus to stimulate contraction and evacuation of clot from the lower uterine segment to remove a distending mass. Along with oxytocin administration, this is sufficient in most cases.
- Procontractile agents can be administered if atony persists (Table 7-2). Oxytocin, methylergonovine, and prostaglandins are appropriate. Rectal misoprostol (800 to 1,000 μg) is often used to stimulate sustained uterine contraction.

**TABLE 7-2  Medical Management of Postpartum Hemorrhage with Uterotonic Agents**

| Agent | Dose | Comments and Contraindications |
| --- | --- | --- |
| Oxytocin (*Pitocin*) | 10–40 U/L IV at 120 mL/hr or 10 units IM | Do not give undiluted IV bolus. Antidiuretic effect with prolonged infusion or high dose; can cause volume overload |
| Methylergonovine maleate (*Methergine*) | 0.2 mg IM every 2–4 hr or 0.2 mg PO every 6 hr<br>Do not start PO until 4 hr after last parenteral dose. | Avoid in patients with hypertension, preeclampsia, or Raynaud phenomenon<br>May cause nausea and vomiting |
| 15-Methyl prostaglandin F$_2\alpha$ analogs (carboprost tromethamine [*Hemabate*]) | 0.25 mg IM (skeletal or myometrium) every 15–90 min to a maximum of 8 doses | Avoid in patients with asthma<br>Renal, hepatic, and cardiac diseases are relative contraindications.<br>May cause nausea/vomiting, tachycardia, diarrhea, pyrexia |
| Prostin E$_2$ (dinoprostone)<br>Prostaglandin E$_1$ analog (misoprostol [*Cytotec*]) | 20 mg vaginal or rectal suppository every 2 hr<br>800–1,000 µg rectal suppository | Avoid in hypotensive patients.<br>Commonly causes fever<br>Caution in renal disease and cardiac disease |

Adapted from American College of Obstetricians and Gynecologists. Practice bulletin no. 76: postpartum hemorrhage. *Obstet Gynecol* 2006;108:1039–1047.

- Selective **uterine arterial embolization** may also be considered for continued post-partum atony if the patient is stable for transport to a fluoroscopy suite.
- When these more conservative interventions are unsuccessful, **surgical exploration** through a vertical midline incision should be considered. Depending on the patient's desire for future childbearing, the extent of hemorrhage, and the experience of the surgeon, several approaches may be used:
  - **Uterine compressive sutures** can be effective for uterine atony. The B-Lynch suture was the original technique described (Fig. 7-1). Since then, multiple compressive sutures have been proposed including combinations of vertical and horizontal sutures to transfix the anterior and posterior uterine walls. All have similar efficacy in achieving hemostasis.
  - **O'Leary bilateral uterine artery ligation** effectively reduces blood loss (Fig. 7-2). After identifying the ureter, ascending branches of the uterine arteries are ligated at the level of the vesicouterine peritoneal reflection. The suture is placed through the lateral lower uterine segment, close to the cervix and then passed through an avascular area of the broad ligament lateral to the uterine vessels. Utero-ovarian vessels (near the cornua) and infundibulopelvic vessels may also be ligated if needed.
  - **Internal iliac artery ligation** (anterior division of the internal iliac/hypogastric artery) significantly decreases uterine pulse pressure, promoting hemostasis. The artery is carefully isolated and ligated with permanent suture such as silk approximately 2 cm distal to the origin of the posterior branch; this placement prevents gluteal ischemia and improves hemostasis by limiting collateral flow to the uterus.

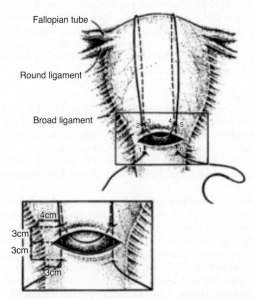

**Figure 7-1.** B-Lynch suture. (From Dildy GA. Postpartum hemorrhage: new management options. *Clin Obstet Gynecol* 2002;45:330–344.)

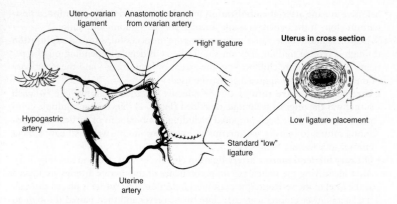

**Figure 7-2.** O'Leary uterine artery ligation. (From Rock JA, Jones HW, eds. *TeLinde's Operative Gynecology*, 10th ed. Philadelphia, PA: Lippincott Williams & Wilkins, 2008. With permission from *Contemp Obstet Gynecol* 1984;24:70 and *Surgical Obstetrics*. Philadelphia, PA: WB Saunders, 1992:272.)

Care should be taken to avoid injuring the fragile hypogastric vein, ligating the nearby external iliac artery or damaging the ureter. This procedure is not always successful (<50% effective), carries significant risk of morbidity, and requires a high level of surgical expertise which may preclude its use to some circumstances.

- **Hysterectomy** is the definitive procedure for intractable uterine bleeding and should not be delayed when needed. Delay to hysterectomy is associated with increased mortality. Intensive care monitoring may be required after peripartum hysterectomy due to massive blood loss, large postoperative fluid shifts, and potential need for ventilatory support.

*Lacerations and Hematomas*

- **Uterine**, **vaginal**, or **cervical laceration** should be suspected if the uterine fundus is well contracted but bleeding persists, particularly if operative delivery or episiotomy was performed. Adequate visualization (light and exposure) is mandatory to investigate a laceration. Adequate analgesia is also valuable.
- The cervix, entire vagina, and perineum should be evaluated systematically. Moving to the operating room often facilitates this process with adequate exposure and instrumentation.
- Occult bleeding in **vulvar and vaginal hematomas** is identified mainly by hypotension and pelvic pain. Stable hematomas may be managed conservatively, but expanding hematomas should be evacuated by performing a generous incision, copiously irrigating, and ligating the bleeding vessels. Layered closure is recommended to assist hemostasis and eliminate dead space. Vaginal packing (for 12 to 18 hours) may be helpful. Broad-spectrum antibiotics should be administered. Arterial embolization may be helpful if unable to be managed surgically.
- **Retroperitoneal hematoma** is potentially life-threatening due to the volume of blood that can develop in that space. Definitive diagnosis is made via computed tomography (CT) with IV contrast. It may present as hypotension, cardiovascular shock, or flank pain. Stable retroperitoneal bleeding can be managed conservatively.

The pressure from the expanding hematoma will tamponade vessels and stop blood loss. Continued expansion necessitates surgical exploration or interventional radiology embolization.

### Retained Products of Conception
- Retained products of conception can cause PPH.
- Risk factors include accessory placental lobes, abnormal placentation, *placenta accreta*, chorioamnionitis, and very preterm delivery.
- If retained products are suspected, blunt curettage may be performed. Using large "banjo" curettes with a broad tip under ultrasound guidance may reduce the risk of uterine perforation.
- In *placenta accreta*, the normal plane of separation between uterus and placenta is absent (see Chapter 10). If the third stage of labor lasts longer than 30 minutes, abnormal placentation should be considered. Manual extraction and uterine exploration are performed. Blunt curettage may be required. It may be impossible to remove the entire placenta without damaging the uterus. If bleeding is controlled with uterotonic agents, conservative management may be sufficient.
- Balloon catheter (Bakri balloon) can be placed in the uterus and inflated to tamponade bleeding from abnormal placentation. It may provide complete hemostasis or simply give time to stabilize the patient and arrange additional care, such as uterine artery embolization. The balloon catheter may be left in place for 12 to 24 hours.
- Laparotomy and peripartum hysterectomy are the definitive procedures for bleeding due to *placenta accreta*.

### Coagulopathy
- **Coagulopathy** can cause or contribute to PPH.
- Risk factors include severe preeclampsia, abruptio placentae, idiopathic/autoimmune thrombocytopenia, AFE, DIC, intrauterine fetal demise, and hereditary coagulopathies (e.g., von Willebrand disease).
- If bleeding is due to coagulopathy, surgical treatment will only increase the hemorrhage. Replete coagulation factors and platelets as needed.

## UTERINE INVERSION

In **uterine inversion**, the uterus is turned inside out, with the fundus protruding through the cervical os into or out of the vagina. It is classified as *incomplete* if the corpus travels partially through the cervix, *complete* if the corpus travels entirely through the cervix, and *prolapsed* if the corpus travels beyond the vaginal introitus.

### Incidence
- Occurs in approximately 1 in 2,500 deliveries, usually with a fundal placenta

### Etiology and Management
- Risk factors include multiparity, long labor, short umbilical cord, abnormal placentation (i.e., accreta), connective tissue disorders, and excessive traction on the cord.
- Establishment of additional IV access with aggressive fluid resuscitation, anticipating massive PPH. Uterotonics including oxytocin should be discontinued.
- An attempt to replace the uterus manually should be made.
  - In the *Johnson maneuver*, the inverted fundus is grasped and replaced cephalad through the cervix into the normal position. Leaving the placenta in place may

reduce blood loss; it can be removed manually after normal anatomy is restored. However, if the placenta prevents replacement of the uterus, it should be removed quickly before attempting to push the fundus into place.

- If the maneuver is unsuccessful or a contracted ring of uterine tissue prevents access, uterine-relaxing agents can be administered. The preferred agent is nitroglycerin (up to three doses of 50 to 100 mg IV or sublingual spray); it has a rapid onset of about 30 seconds and a short half-life. Other uterine relaxants such as terbutaline sulfate or halogenated general anesthetics (e.g., halothane, isoflurane) can also be used.
- Uterotonics should be implemented as soon as normal uterine anatomy is restored.
- Laparotomy is indicated if manual restoration fails. Vaginal elevation, upward traction on the round ligaments, or a posterior vertical incision on the lower uterine segment and cervical ring can all facilitate replacement of the fundus.

## CHORIOAMNIONITIS

**Chorioamnionitis** is infection/inflammation of the placenta, chorion, and amnion.

### Incidence
- Occurs in 1% to 2% of term and 5% to 10% of preterm deliveries

### Etiology and Diagnosis
- Risk factors include nulliparity, prolonged labor, prolonged ruptured membranes, use of internal monitors, maternal bacterial vaginosis, untreated infection, and multiple vaginal examinations.
- Chorioamnionitis is an ascending polymicrobial infection. The most common pathogens are *Ureaplasma urealyticum*, *Mycoplasma hominis*, *Bacteroides bivius*, *Gardnerella vaginalis*, group B streptococci, and *Escherichia coli*.
- The diagnosis is clinical. Signs and symptoms include maternal fever 38.0°C or higher without other obvious infection, maternal or fetal tachycardia, uterine tenderness, foul-smelling amniotic fluid or frankly purulent discharge, and leukocytosis (typically >15,000 with a left shift).
- If the diagnosis is uncertain and the clinical situation warrants, amniocentesis may be performed. Positive amniotic fluid culture gives definitive diagnosis. An amniotic fluid white blood cell count >30 cells/$\mu$L, glucose level <15 mg/dL, interleukin-6 $\geq$11.2 ng/mL, or a positive Gram stain also suggest infection.

### Management
- Definitive treatment is delivery and evacuation of uterine contents. Antibiotics are administered during labor for fetal benefit. When the diagnosis of chorioamnionitis is made, delivery is indicated. Often, a rapidly progressing preterm delivery will ensue without assistance. Vaginal delivery should be considered unless contraindicated.
- Acceptable antibiotic regimens include:
  - Ampicillin (2 g IV every 6 hours) plus gentamicin sulfate (2 mg/kg IV to load then 1.5 mg/kg IV every 8 hours) until delivery. If cesarean delivery is performed, clindamycin or metronidazole may be added for anaerobic coverage postpartum.

- For nonanaphylactic penicillin allergy, substitute cefazolin (1 g IV every 8 hours) for ampicillin.
- For severe penicillin allergy, substitute clindamycin (900 mg IV every 8 hours) or vancomycin (500 mg every 6 hours) for ampicillin.
- Single-drug regimens have also been used: ampicillin/sulbactam (Unasyn, 3 g IV every 6 hours), piperacillin/tazobactam (Zosyn, 3.375 g IV every 6 hours), and ticarcillin/clavulanate (Timentin, 3.1 g every 6 hours).
- No data suggest that one regimen is better than another.
- At delivery, the pediatrician should be notified as the neonate may be affected.
- The placenta should be sent to pathology for histologic examination. Membrane culture can be obtained by carefully peeling the amnion and chorion apart and swabbing between the layers. Cord blood may also be sent for culture.
- Unless the patient remains febrile, maternal antibiotics are not indicated beyond one dose after vaginal delivery.
- After cesarean section with chorioamnionitis, broad coverage should be continued for at least one additional dose of antibiotics (8 hours). It may be reasonable to continue antibiotics for as long as 48 hours after the last recorded temperature of 38.0°C or higher. Gentamicin and clindamycin is the typical regimen, but ampicillin can be added to achieve broader coverage (especially for enterococcus).

## POSTPARTUM ENDOMYOMETRITIS

**Postpartum endomyometritis** is infection of the endometrium, myometrium, and parametrial tissues.

### Incidence
- About 5% of vaginal deliveries and 10% of cesarean deliveries are affected by postpartum uterine infection. Rates are significantly higher in women of lower socioeconomic status.

### Etiology and Diagnosis
- Risk factors include cesarean section, maternal diabetes mellitus, manual removal of the placenta, and all of the risks for chorioamnionitis.
- Endomyometritis, like chorioamnionitis, is an ascending polymicrobial infection often caused by normal vaginal flora.
- May develop immediately to several days after delivery
- Diagnosis is clinical: fever 38.0°C or greater on two separate occasions >2 to 4 hours apart or single temperature >39.0°C, uterine tenderness, tachycardia, purulent vaginal discharge, and associated findings such as dynamic ileus, pelvic peritonitis, pelvic abscess, and bowel obstruction.
- Endometrial cultures are unnecessary; they are typically contaminated by normal flora and yield results much later than clinically required. Blood culture is indicated only for the most severe cases with concern for sepsis.

### Management
- Acceptable broad-spectrum antibiotic regimens include:
  - Therapy with gentamicin and clindamycin +/− ampicillin until 24 to 48 hours afebrile.

- Alternate single-agent therapies include ertapenem, ceftriaxone, cefotetan, Unasyn, Zosyn, or Timentin. The aim is broad polymicrobial coverage.
- Gentamicin is administered every 8 hours before delivery. For postpartum treatment, however, several studies show 5 to 7 mg/kg daily dosing is safe, efficacious, and cost-effective. Drug levels are not monitored for daily dosing.
- Endomyometritis typically resolves with 48 hours of antibiotic treatment. Oral antibiotics are not required after completion of IV course.
- If fever persists or patient develops sepsis, additional workup should be considered. This may include urine and blood cultures; chest and abdominal radiographs; pelvic examination; and pelvic/abdominal ultrasound, CT, or magnetic resonance imaging (MRI).
- Infections with clostridia, group A streptococci, and staphylococci should be suspected in patients presenting with sepsis. Group A streptococcal septicemia is the leading cause of peripartum sepsis worldwide but relatively rare in the United States. Toxic shock syndrome may be suspected when there is high fever, desquamation, diffuse macular rash, and multisystem organ failure. In rare cases, postpartum hysterectomy has been reported for uterine myonecrosis.

## SEPTIC PELVIC THROMBOPHLEBITIS

**Septic pelvic thrombophlebitis (SPT)** exists in two forms: **ovarian vein thrombosis/thrombophlebitis** and **deep pelvic septic thrombophlebitis**. SPT occurs in 1 in 2,000 to 1 in 3,000 deliveries, most commonly after cesarean section.

### Diagnosis and Etiology

- SPT should be considered in patients with persistent spiking fevers despite 3 days of antibiotic treatment for endometritis. The patient usually appears well between febrile episodes, and pain is minimal. Thrombi form in the deep pelvic veins as a result of pregnancy-induced hypercoagulability and venous congestion. These may become infected, releasing septic emboli which travel to the lungs. Less than 2% of cases have pulmonary emboli by imaging. When other causes of postpartum fever have been excluded, pelvic ultrasound and pelvic/abdominal CT or MRI help diagnose abscess or large thrombus. A negative result, however, does not rule out SPT, which is largely a diagnosis of exclusion. Blood cultures are typically negative.

### Management

- As SPT is often a diagnosis of exclusion in patients with persistent fever, most are already being treated with broad-spectrum antibiotics, which also cover the typical pathogens of endomyometritis. Once the diagnosis is suspected, anticoagulation with heparin or enoxaparin is initiated.
- Heparin theoretically terminates embolic showers that may cause the spiking fever. Therapeutic IV heparin infusion may be initiated with a 5,000-unit heparin bolus, then a continuous infusion (usually 16 to 18 mm/kg/hr) with an activated partial thromboplastin time ratio (aPTTr) goal of 1.5 to 2.0 times normal. Low molecular weight heparin at a dose of 1 mg/kg every 12 hours is also acceptable.
- Antibiotics may be continued until the patient is 24 to 48 hours afebrile. The duration of anticoagulation is somewhat controversial, with recommendations ranging from 24 hours to 2 weeks after the last fever. If imaging clearly detects a deep vein

or pulmonary thrombus, 6 months of anticoagulation with warfarin or enoxaparin are indicated.

## MECONIUM ASPIRATION

**Meconium** staining of the amniotic fluid complicates 7% to 20% of all live births. It increases the risk of neonatal respiratory disorders. Of infants born through meconium-stained fluid, 2% to 10% are subsequently diagnosed with **meconium aspiration syndrome**, with a mortality rate of up to 12%.

### Etiology and Complications

- Fetal acidosis, fetal heart rate abnormalities, and low Apgar scores are associated with meconium-stained fluid. Fetal stress and hypoxia stimulate meconium passage. The majority of pregnancies complicated by meconium-stained amniotic fluid, however, result in normal healthy newborns.
- Aspiration has three major pulmonary effects: (a) airway obstruction, (b) surfactant dysfunction, and (c) chemical pneumonitis.
- Risk factors for meconium aspiration syndrome include moderate or thick meconium, nonreassuring fetal heart rate tracing, meconium below the cords, and low Apgar scores.

### Management

- **Amnioinfusion** is no longer used for all cases of meconium. A large multicenter trial showed that amnioinfusion for thick meconium did not reduce the risk of moderate or severe meconium aspiration syndrome, perinatal death, or other major neonatal complications.
- The most recent Neonatal Resuscitation Program guidelines advise against routine intrapartum suctioning for infants with meconium-stained fluid. A large multicenter trial showed that deep suctioning before delivery of the shoulders did not reduce the rate of intubation, meconium aspiration syndrome, the need for mechanical ventilation, or overall mortality. After delivery, the infant should be passed to the pediatric team with minimal stimulation, with endotracheal suctioning performed for nonvigorous infants.

## SUGGESTED READINGS

Conde-Agudelo A, Romero R. Amniotic fluid embolism: an evidence-based review. *Am J Obstet Gynecol* 2009;201:445.e1–e13.

French LM, Smaill FM. Antibiotic regimens for endometritis after delivery. *Cochrane Database Syst Rev* 2004;(4):CD001067.

Mousa HA, Alfirevic Z. Treatment for primary postpartum haemorrhage. *Cochrane Database Syst Rev* 2007;(1):CD003249.

Tomacruz RS, Bristow RE, Montz FJ. Management of pelvic hemorrhage. *Surg Clin North Am* 2001;81(4):925–948.

Vain NE, Szyld EG, Prudent LM, et al. What (not) to do at and after delivery? Prevention and management of meconium aspiration syndrome. *Early Hum Dev* 2009;85:621–626.

Xu H, Hofmeyr J, Roy C, et al. Intrapartum amnioinfusion for meconium-stained amniotic fluid: a systematic review of randomised controlled trials. *BJOG* 2007;114:383–390.

You WB, Zahn CM. Postpartum hemorrhage: abnormally adherent placenta, uterine inversion, and puerperal hematomas. *Clin Obstet Gynecol* 2006;49:184–197.

# 8 Gestational Complications

Meghan E. Pratts and Janice Henderson

This chapter reviews several common **antenatal complications**:
* Amniotic fluid disorders (including oligohydramnios, polyhydramnios)
* Intrauterine growth restriction
* Cervical insufficiency
* Multiple gestation
* Postterm pregnancy
* Fetal demise in utero (FDIU)

## AMNIOTIC FLUID DISORDERS

* **Amniotic fluid volume** (**AFV**) represents the balance between production and removal of fetal fluids.
  * In early gestation, fluid is produced from the fetal surface of the placenta, from transfer across the amnion, and from embryonic surface secretions.
  * In mid to late gestation, fluid is produced by fetal urination and alveolar transudate. By 16 weeks, there is about 250 mL of fluid, increasing to approximately 800 mL by 34 to 36 weeks' gestation.
  * Fluid is removed by fetal swallowing and absorption at the amnion-chorion interface.
  * The most accurate measurement of AFV is by dye dilution techniques or direct measurement at the time of hysterotomy. Ultrasound provides a standard noninvasive tool to estimate AFV (Table 8-1).
* **Polyhydramnios** is the pathologic accumulation of amniotic fluid defined as more than 2,000 mL at any gestational age, more than the 95th percentile for gestational age, or an amniotic fluid index (AFI) >25 cm at term.
  * The incidence of polyhydramnios in the general population is about 1%.
  * Implications: Mildly increased AFV is usually clinically insignificant. Markedly increased AFV is associated with increased perinatal morbidity due to preterm labor, cord prolapse upon membrane rupture, underlying comorbidities, and congenital malformations. Abruptio placentae is associated with polyhydramnios and rupture of membranes due to rapid decompression of the overdistended uterus. Increased maternal morbidity also results from postpartum hemorrhage due to uterine overdistention leading to atony. If polyhydramnios is severe, uterine distention can cause venous and ureteral compression causing severe lower extremity edema and hydronephrosis.
  * The most common **etiology** of polyhydramnios is idiopathic (Fig. 8-1); however, in severe cases, a cause is more often apparent and likely to be associated with a detectable fetal anomaly. Specific causes include:
    o **Fetal structural malformations:** In cases of acrania or anencephaly, polyhydramnios occurs from an impaired swallowing mechanism, low antidiuretic

| TABLE 8-1 | Methods of Amniotic Fluid Assessment |
| --- | --- |

| Diagnostic Method | Interpretation | Clinical Value |
| --- | --- | --- |
| Maximum vertical pocket (MVP) | Oligo ≤2 cm<br>Normal = 2.1–8 cm<br>Poly ≥8 cm | • 94% concordant with dye-determined normal pregnancies<br>• Less accurate for low AFV<br>• Useful predictor of adverse events |
| Amniotic fluid index (AFI)— measurement and summation of deepest pocket in each of four quadrants | Oligo <5 cm<br>Normal = 5.1–25 cm<br>Poly ≥25 cm | • 71%–78% concordant with dye-determined normals<br>• Abnormal not highly predictive of adverse events<br>• High false-positive rate |
| Subjective assessment— performed by experienced sonographer | Subjective result | • 65%–70% concordant with dye-determined normals<br>• Very poorly identifies abnormal volumes |
| 2 × 2 cm pocket— sonographic survey to verify at least one 2 × 2 cm fluid pocket | Evaluates for presence or absence of 2 × 2 cm pocket | • 98% concordant with dye-determined normals<br>• Found in <10% of oligohydramnios |

AFV, amniotic fluid volume.
Adapted and expanded from Moore TR. Clinical assessment of amniotic fluid. *Clin Obstet Gynecol* 1997;40(2):303–313.

hormone causing polyuria, and possibly transudation across the exposed fetal meninges. Gastrointestinal tract anomalies may also lead to polyhydramnios by either direct physical obstruction or decreased absorption. Ventral wall defects increase AFV from transudation across the peritoneal surface or bowel wall.

o **Chromosomal and genetic abnormalities:** As many as 35% of fetuses with polyhydramnios have chromosomal abnormalities. The most common are trisomies 13, 18, and 21.

o **Neuromuscular disorders:** Impaired fetal swallowing can increase AFV.

o **Diabetes mellitus:** Maternal diabetes mellitus is a common cause of polyhydramnios, especially with poor glycemic control or associated fetal malformations. Fetal hyperglycemia can increase fluid transudation across the placental interface and cause fetal polyuria.

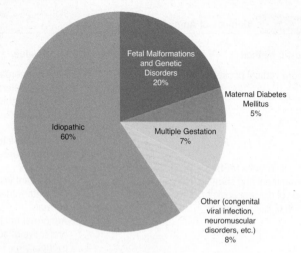

**Figure 8-1.** Causes of polyhydramnios.

- ○ **Alloimmunization:** *Hydrops fetalis* can increase AFV.
- ○ **Congenital infections:** In the absence of other factors, polyhydramnios warrants screening for congenital infections, such as toxoplasmosis, cytomegalovirus (CMV), and syphilis. These are, however, rare causes of polyhydramnios.
- ○ **Twin-to-twin transfusion syndrome (TTTS):** The recipient twin develops polyhydramnios and occasionally *hydrops fetalis*, whereas the donor twin develops growth restriction and oligohydramnios.
- **Ultrasound** estimates AFV, identifies multiple gestations, and may detect fetal abnormalities. **Amniocentesis** for karyotype is offered if any anomalies are diagnosed.
- **Treatment** is aimed at the underlying cause. Mild to moderate polyhydramnios can be managed expectantly until the onset of labor or spontaneous rupture of membranes. If the patient develops significant dyspnea, abdominal pain, or difficulty ambulating, treatment becomes necessary.
  - ○ **Amnioreduction** can alleviate significant maternal symptoms. Amniocentesis is performed, and fluid is removed. Frequent removal of smaller volumes (total 1,500 to 2,000 mL or until the AFI is <8 cm) will result in a lower risk of preterm labor compared with removal of larger volumes. Amnioreduction is repeated every 1 to 3 weeks as needed. Antibiotic prophylaxis is unnecessary.
  - ○ **Pharmacologic treatment** with indomethacin reduces fetal urine production. Fetal renal blood flow and glomerular filtration rate (GFR) are sensitive to prostaglandins. The cyclooxygenase inhibitor indomethacin (25 mg orally every 6 hours) can decrease fetal renal blood flow and urination. Premature closure of the fetal ductus arteriosus is a potential complication of indomethacin that requires close AFV and ductus diameter monitoring. Discontinue therapy if there is any suggestion of ductus closure. The risk of complications is low if the total daily dose of indomethacin is <200 mg, the treatment is limited to pregnancies <32 weeks, and the duration of therapy is <48 hours. In contrast, diuretics are ineffective as a treatment of polyhydramnios.

- **Oligohydramnios** has multiple definitions, most commonly as a gestation with an AFI of <5 cm. Alternative definitions include less than the fifth percentile for gestational age or with a single maximum vertical pocket (MVP) of amniotic fluid of <2 cm. It is associated with increased perinatal morbidity and mortality at any gestational age, but the risks are particularly high during the second trimester when perinatal mortality approaches 80% to 90%. Pulmonary hypoplasia can result from insufficient fluid filling the terminal air sacs. Prolonged oligohydramnios in the second and third trimester leads to cranial, facial, or skeletal abnormalities in 10% to 15% of cases. Cord compression leads to increased incidence of fetal heart rate decelerations in labor.

- The **etiology** of oligohydramnios includes ruptured membranes, fetal urinary tract malformations, postterm pregnancy, placental insufficiency, and medications reducing fetal urine production. Rupture of membranes must be considered at any gestational age. Renal agenesis or urinary tract obstruction often becomes apparent during the second trimester of pregnancy, when fetal urine flow begins to contribute significantly to AFV. Placental insufficiency can cause both oligohydramnios and intrauterine growth restriction. The cause of oligohydramnios in postterm pregnancies may be deteriorating placental function (Fig. 8-2).

- **Ultrasound** is used to diagnose oligohydramnios. Rupture of membranes should be evaluated, and in cases of preterm gestation with uncertain membrane status, a tampon dye test can be performed (see Chapter 9).

- **Treatment** for oligohydramnios is limited. Maternal intravascular fluid status appears to be closely tied to that of the fetus; maternal hydration (intravenous or oral) may improve the AFV depending on the etiology of oligohydramnios. In cases of obstructive genitourinary defects, in utero surgical diversion has produced

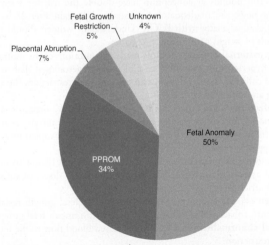

**Figure 8-2.** Causes of oligohydramnios. PPROM, preterm premature rupture of membranes. (Adapted from Shipp TD, Bromley B. Outcome of singleton pregnancies with severe oligohydramnios in the second and third trimesters. *Ultrasound Obstet Gynecol* 1996;7[2]:108–113.)

some promising results. For optimal benefit, urinary diversion must be performed before renal dysplasia develops and early enough in gestation to permit normal lung development. Until near term, oligohydramnios is managed with frequent fetal surveillance. Indications for induction of labor include term gestation or nonreassuring fetal testing after 34 weeks. Oligohydramnios is not a contraindication to labor. There is no consensus as to which of the measurements of AFV is most recommended when deciding if induction for oligohydramnios is indicated. MVP may be a superior option to AFI, as AFI measurement has a higher rate of false positives for oligohydramnios and thus increases induction and cesarean section rates without evidence of improvement in neonatal outcomes.

## INTRAUTERINE GROWTH RESTRICTION

**Intrauterine growth restriction (IUGR)** is suggested when the estimated fetal weight falls below the 10th percentile for gestational age. Approximately 70% of so-called IUGR is merely constitutional, although underlying etiology may be difficult to elucidate. The incidence of pathologic IUGR is between 4% to 8% of gestations in developed countries and 6% to 30% in developing countries. Fetuses with IUGR have a two- to sixfold increase in perinatal morbidity and mortality. Asymmetric versus symmetric IUGR may suggest etiology. In symmetric IUGR, the fetus is proportionally small, whereas in asymmetric IUGR, abdominal growth lags behind head circumference. Symmetric growth restriction implies an early insult such as chemical exposure, infection, or aneuploidy. Asymmetric growth is more associated with a late pregnancy insult such as placental insufficiency.

- The **etiology** of IUGR includes both maternal and fetal causes:
  - **Constitutionally small mothers and inadequate weight gain:** Women who weigh <100 pounds at conception have double the risk for a small-for-gestational-age newborn. Inadequate or arrested weight gain after 28 weeks of pregnancy is also associated with IUGR. Underweight women should have a 28 to 40 pounds of weight gain during pregnancy.
  - **Chronic maternal disease:** Multiple medical conditions of the mother, including chronic hypertension, cyanotic heart disease, pregestational diabetes, malnutrition, and collagen vascular disease, can cause growth restriction. Preeclampsia and smoking are associated with IUGR.
  - **Fetal infection:** Viral causes including rubella, CMV, hepatitis A, parvovirus B19, varicella, and influenza are among the best known infectious antecedents of IUGR. In addition, bacterial (listeriosis), protozoal (toxoplasmosis), and spirochetal (syphilis) infections may be causative.
  - **Chromosomal abnormalities**, such as trisomies 13 and 18 and Turner syndrome, are often associated with IUGR. Trisomy 21 usually does not cause significant growth restriction.
  - **Teratogen exposure:** Any teratogen can produce fetal growth restriction. Anticonvulsants, tobacco, illicit drugs, and alcohol can impair fetal growth.
  - **Placental abnormalities** that lead to decreased blood flow to the fetus can cause growth restriction.
  - **Multiple gestation** is complicated by growth impairment of at least one fetus in 12% to 47% of cases.
- **Diagnosis** is made by sonographic assessment (Table 8-2). Gestational age must be established with certainty, preferably in the first trimester, to assess fetal growth

| TABLE 8-2 | Sonographic Measurements Used to Assess Fetal Growth |
| --- | --- |

| Sonographic Measurement | Advantages | Disadvantages |
| --- | --- | --- |
| Abdominal circumference | • Best correlates with fetal weight<br>• High sensitivity for IUGR | • Cannot determine asymmetric vs. symmetric IUGR<br>• Subject to variability due to sonographer and fetal position changes |
| Transverse cerebellar diameter | • Correlates with gestational age up to 24 wk<br>• Not significantly affected by growth restriction | • Correlates best up to 24 wk<br>• Status as a predictor is variable |
| HC:AC ratio (head circumference:abdominal circumference) | • More accurate at diagnosing growth restriction related to placental insufficiency | • Not specific<br>• Not all scans with increased HC/AC ratio are confirmed to have IUGR |
| Umbilical artery Dopplers | • Can help distinguish between constitutionally small vs. IUGR<br>• Useful for evaluating pregnancies at risk for adverse events | • Not beneficial in low-risk pregnancies<br>• Not useful as a screening tool |

IUGR, intrauterine growth restriction.
For additional information, see Platz E, Newman R. Diagnosis of IUGR: traditional biometry. *Semin Perinatol* 2008;32:140–147; and Turan S, Miller J, Baschat AA. Integrated testing and management in fetal growth restriction. *Semin Perinatol* 2008;32:194–200.

accurately. A lag in fundal height of more than 3 cm from gestational age after 20 weeks should prompt sonographic evaluation. Oligohydramnios is often associated with fetal growth restriction.

• **Management** generally depends on gestational age. In general, growth restriction less than the third percentile diagnosed before 32 weeks prompts offering amniocentesis or fetal blood sampling for karyotype and viral studies. Even when termination is not considered, the information gained from these tests may be important for parents, obstetricians, and pediatricians planning the delivery and newborn care. Other management includes:
  • **IUGR ≥37 weeks**: delivery
  • **IUGR at 34 to 36 weeks:** Deliver if no fetal growth has been documented in the preceding weeks (over an appropriate interval for ultrasound to demonstrate growth).

- **IUGR remote from term:** Attempt conservative management. Restrict physical activity, ensure adequate nutrition, and initiate fetal surveillance. Fetal assessment includes daily kick counts, serial fetal growth ultrasounds every 3 to 4 weeks, and nonstress testing or biophysical profile twice per week. Umbilical artery Doppler velocimetry showing elevated systolic-to-diastolic ratio or absent or reversed end-diastolic flow suggests fetal compromise (see Chapter 6).
- The decision to **deliver** an IUGR infant remote from term weighs the risk of preterm birth against continued exposure to the intrauterine environment. Vaginal delivery is not contraindicated, but there is an increased risk of fetal intolerance of labor. Growth-restricted newborns are susceptible to hypothermia and other metabolic abnormalities, such as hypoglycemia. Some data show that fetal growth restriction has long-term negative effects on cognitive function, independent of other variables.

## CERVICAL INSUFFICIENCY

**Cervical insufficiency (CI)**, or cervical incompetence, occurs in 1 in 50 to 1 in 2,000 gestations. Risk factors include prior cervical laceration, history of cervical conization, multiple terminations with mechanical cervical dilation, intrauterine diethylstilbestrol exposure, and congenital cervical anomaly.

- The epidemiology is as imprecise as the various, sometimes controversial, criteria used to diagnose CI. One reasonable definition is recurrent painless cervical dilation in the absence of infection, placental abruption, uterine contractions, or uterine anomaly. Because CI is a diagnosis of exclusion, alternate diagnoses must be rigorously sought. *Although prophylactic cervical cerclage has only been shown to be beneficial after **three or more** second-trimester pregnancy losses due to CI*, patient concerns and provider judgment rarely tolerate waiting so long before proceeding with elective preventive treatment (i.e., cerclage). Cervical funneling on ultrasound is not adequate justification for cerclage placement, although serial cervical ultrasound of *high-risk* women starting at 16 to 20 weeks may identify those pregnancies requiring additional management (see Chapter 11).
- Admittedly, diagnosis of CI and selection of patients for elective cervical cerclage are as much art as science.
- Pelvic rest, pessary placement, and cervical cerclage have been suggested to prevent repeated pregnancy loss from CI, but the evidence for their effectiveness is mixed. A careful review of maternal history and prior pregnancy losses, complete counseling on the risks and benefits of cerclage (e.g., preterm premature rupture of membrane, chorioamnionitis, preterm birth, cervical laceration), and early screening for aneuploidy and congenital anomalies (see Chapter 12) should be offered *before* proceeding with cerclage placement. Ideally, cerclage placement should occur before the onset of cervical dilation. Once dilation occurs, a rescue cerclage may be placed.
  - McDonald or Shirodkar cerclages are placed vaginally, usually at 12 to 14 weeks' gestation; selection of technique depends on the available cervical length and surgeon experience/preference. Prophylactic antibiotics and postoperative tocolysis have not been shown to affect outcome but are often employed. The risk of iatrogenic pregnancy loss ranges from 1% to nearly 20% for elective cases. Rescue cerclage for CI/bulging membranes is associated with >50% risk of complications.

Abdominal cerclage is placed at laparotomy in rare instances for women who have minimal to no residual cervical length (often due to large cone biopsies or trachelectomy). Subsequent cesarean section is necessary.
- Cerclage is removed when the patient begins to labor, when membranes rupture, if there is evidence of uterine infection, or if the patient reaches 36 weeks' gestation.

## MULTIPLE GESTATION

**Multiple gestation** occurs in approximately 3% of all births in the United States and is increasing annually due to assisted reproductive technologies (ART). The incidence of monozygotic twins is constant at approximately 4 in 1,000 gestations. The incidence of dizygotic twins varies widely and is higher in some families; in individuals of African descent; with ovulation induction and in vitro fertilization; and with increasing maternal age, parity, weight, and height. In the absence of fertility drugs, triplet pregnancies occur in approximately 1 in 8,000 gestations. Higher order births are much rarer. Multiple gestation increases morbidity and mortality for both mother and fetus. Perinatal mortality rates in developed countries range from 50 to 100 per 1,000 births for twins and from 100 to 200 per 1,000 births for triplets.

- **Diagnosis** is confirmed by sonogram most accurately in the first trimester when separate gestational sacs are easily seen to determine chorionicity. In later gestations, sonogram can detect the "twin-peak" sign also known as the "lambda sign" for dichorionic twins and the *T sign* for monochorionic diamnionic twins. Multiple gestation is suspected if uterine size is greater than expected for gestational age, multiple fetal heart rates are detected, multiple fetal parts are felt, the human chorionic gonadotropin (hCG) and maternal serum alpha-fetoprotein levels are elevated for gestational age, or the pregnancy is a result of ART.
- **Zygosity, placentation, and mortality**
  - **Dizygotic dichorionic/diamnionic twins** (70% to 80% of all twins) result from the fertilization of two ova. Each fetus has its own placenta and a complete and separate amnion-chorion membrane.
  - **Monozygotic twins** (20% to 30% of all twins) result from cleavage of a single, fertilized conceptus. The timing of cleavage determines the placentation.
    - **Dichorionic/diamnionic monozygotic twins** (8% of all twins) are produced by cleavage in the first 3 days after fertilization. They will have separate amnions and chorions, just like dizygotic twins. They have the lowest perinatal mortality rate (<10%) of all monozygotic twins.
    - **Monochorionic/diamnionic twins** (14% to 20% of all twins) are produced by cleavage between days 4 and 8 after fertilization. They share a single placenta but have separate amnionic sacs. The mortality rate for monochorionic/diamnionic twins is approximately 25%.
    - **Monochorionic/monoamnionic twinning** (<1% of cases) occurs after the eighth day. The fetuses share a single placenta and a single amnionic sac because both amnion and chorion were formed before cleavage. Later, cleavage is even rarer and results in conjoined fetuses. Monoamnionic gestations have a 50% to 60% mortality rate, usually occurring before 32 weeks.
  - **Higher order multiples** have more frequent placental anomalies. Monochorionic and dichorionic placentation may both be present.

- **Complications** are more common in multiple gestations.
  - **Miscarriage** is at least twice as common in multiple gestations, compared with singleton pregnancies. Fewer than 50% of twin pregnancies diagnosed by ultrasonography in the first trimester result in live birth of twins.
  - **Congenital anomalies and malformations** are about twice as common in dizygotic twins and three times more common in trizygotic triplets compared to singletons. Monozygotic twins have a 2% to 10% risk of developmental defects, about twice the rate for dizygotic twins. Because the risk of chromosomal anomalies increases with each additional fetus, we offer amniocentesis at 33 years for twins and at 28 years for triplets.
  - **Nausea and vomiting** are often worse in multiple gestations. Although the etiology is unclear, higher levels of hCG may be the cause.
  - **Preeclampsia** is more common, occurs earlier, and is more severe in multiple gestations. Approximately 40% of twin pregnancies and 60% of triplet pregnancies are affected.
  - **Polyhydramnios** occurs in 5% to 8% of multiple pregnancies, particularly with monoamnionic twins. Acute polyhydramnios before 28 weeks' gestation has been reported in 1.7% of twin pregnancies. The perinatal mortality in those cases approaches 90%.
  - **Preterm delivery** approaches 50% in twin gestations. The average gestational age at delivery is 36 to 37 weeks for twins and 32 to 33 weeks for triplets. Twin gestations account for 10% of all preterm deliveries and 25% of all preterm perinatal deaths. Most neonatal deaths in multiple premature births are associated with gestations <32 weeks and birth weight under 1,500 g (see Chapter 9).
  - **IUGR** is common, and low birth weight has an additive effect with prematurity on neonatal morbidity and mortality.
  - **Discordant twin growth** is defined as a discrepancy of more than 20% in the estimated fetal weights. It is calculated as a percentage of the larger twin's weight. Causes include TTTS, chromosomal or structural anomalies in either twin, discordant viral infection, and unequal division of the placenta mass. When discordance exceeds 25%, the fetal and neonatal death rates increase 6.5-fold and 2.5-fold, respectively.
  - The risk of uterine atony and **postpartum hemorrhage** is significantly increased in multiple pregnancies.
  - **Intrapartum complications** including malpresentation, cord prolapse, cord entanglement, dysfunctional labor, fetal distress, and urgent cesarean delivery are more common for multiple gestations compared with singletons.
  - **TTTS** occurs in 20% to 25% of monochorionic twin pregnancies. Fifty percent to 75% of monochorionic twin placentae have vascular anastomoses. When anastomoses are not balanced, one fetus "donates" blood to the other, leading to hypervolemia, heart failure, and hydrops in the recipient twin and hypovolemia, oligohydramnios, and growth restriction in the donor twin.
    - Rapid uterine growth between 20 and 30 weeks' gestation from polyhydramnios of the recipient twin is common. TTTS can be diagnosed when sonography suggests a single chorion, discordant fetal growth, polyhydramnios around the larger twin, and oligohydramnios around the smaller fetus ("stuck twin" sign or "poly-oli" syndrome). The severity and timing of growth discrepancy depend on the degree of arteriovenous shunting. Fetal hydrops is an ominous sign.

○ If extreme prematurity prevents immediate delivery, management includes serial amnioreduction for the recipient twin, intrauterine blood transfusion for the donor twin, selective fetal reduction, or fetoscopic laser ablation of placental anastomoses.

- **Antenatal management of multiple gestations** includes adequate nutrition (300 additional calories per day per fetus), more frequent prenatal visits, periodic ultrasound assessment of fetal growth and well-being, and prompt hospital admission for preterm labor or obstetric complications. No evidence supports bed rest or prophylactic tocolytics in multiple gestations. In addition, neither prophylactic cerclage or progesterone therapy have been shown to reduce preterm birth rates in multiples and cerclage specifically may worsen outcomes.

  - **Ultrasonographic assessments** should be conducted every 3 to 4 weeks from 23 weeks' gestation to monitor fetal growth and detect discordance. Monochorionic placentation may warrant ultrasonography every 2 weeks to evaluate for evidence of TTTS.

  - **Fetal surveillance** with nonstress testing (NST) is not indicated for dizygotic twins unless clinical or ultrasonographic data suggest IUGR or discordance. When NSTs are discordant, additional testing may be necessary. The use of contraction stress testing is controversial and rarely used as it might precipitate preterm delivery.

  - **Amniocentesis** should be performed for both fetuses, if indicated, for prenatal diagnosis of genetic disorders or alloimmunization. One to 5 mL of indigo carmine is injected into the first sac following fluid aspiration to ensure that both sacs are sampled. To establish lung maturity, amniotic fluid evaluation from one fetal sac is adequate. For discordant twins, amniotic fluid should be obtained from the larger twin, which usually reaches pulmonary maturity later.

  - **Multifetal pregnancy reduction** may be offered to reduce risk in higher order pregnancies. Because the presence of three or more fetuses is associated with such increased maternal and perinatal mortality and morbidity, fetal reduction may be appropriately offered. The risk of subsequent pregnancy loss is 5% to 10%. **Selective termination** refers specifically to the termination of one or more specific fetuses with structural or chromosomal anomalies.

  - **Management of fetal demise** is based on gestational age and the condition of the surviving fetus. Until the surviving twin develops lung maturity, weekly fetal surveillance and maternal coagulation profile testing should be performed. Consider delivery when fetal lung maturity is demonstrated, if fetal status deteriorates, or if disseminated intravascular coagulation (DIC) develops in the mother. In TTTS, one fetal demise should prompt consideration for delivery, particularly after 28 weeks.

- The optimal **route of delivery** for twins remains controversial and should be assessed on a case-by-case basis. Decisions about delivery must consider the presentations, gestational age, maternal or fetal complications, the experience of the obstetrician, and the availability of anesthesia and neonatal intensive care support.

  - **Vertex/vertex** (43%) presentation can have a successful vaginal delivery in 70% to 80% of cases. Surveillance of twin B between deliveries is advised.

  - **Vertex/nonvertex** (38%) presentation can have a vaginal delivery if estimated fetal weights are concordant. External cephalic version or internal podalic version and breech extraction of twin B may be attempted. Vaginal delivery of twin B in nonvertex presentation may be considered for infants with an estimated weight between 1,500 and 3,500 g. Success rates are more than 96%. There is insufficient data to advocate a specific route of delivery for a second twin weighing <1,500 g.

- **Nonvertex presenting twins** (19%) are typically delivered by cesarean for both fetuses.
- **Locked twins** is a rare condition occurring with breech/vertex twins, when the body of twin A delivers, but the chin "locks" behind the chin of twin B. Hypertonicity, monoamnionic twinning, or reduced amniotic fluid may contribute to interlocking fetal heads.

## POSTTERM PREGNANCY

**Postterm pregnancy** is defined as 294 days or 42 *completed* weeks since the first day of the last menstrual period (LMP). However, there is growing evidence that perinatal morbidity and mortality significantly increase weeks before a pregnancy is designated postterm. The incidence of postterm pregnancy ranges between 7% and 12% of all pregnancies. Approximately, 4% of all pregnancies extend beyond 43 weeks. About 30% to 40% of women with a prior postterm pregnancy will have prolonged gestation in subsequent pregnancies.

- **Diagnosis** of postterm pregnancy is based on accurate estimation of gestational age. Obstetric dates should be validated by two or more of the following: certain LMP, positive urine pregnancy test within 6 weeks of LMP, fetal heart tone detected with Doppler testing at 10 to 12 weeks' gestation, fundal height at the umbilicus at 20 weeks' gestation, pelvic examination consistent with LMP before 13 weeks' gestation, and ultrasonographic dating by crown-rump length between 6 and 12 weeks' gestation or by biparietal diameter before 26 weeks' gestation. The best estimate of gestational age is confirmed by as many criteria as possible.
- The **etiology** is usually incorrect dating. Risk factors for postterm pregnancy include primiparity, previous postterm pregnancy, placental sulfatase deficiency, fetal anencephaly, family history, and fetal male sex.
- **Complications** of postterm pregnancy include:
  - **Postmaturity syndrome** exhibiting subcutaneous wasting, intrauterine growth failure, meconium staining, oligohydramnios, absent *vernix caseosa* and lanugo hair, and peeling newborn skin. Such findings are described in only 10% to 20% of true postterm newborns.
  - **Macrosomia** is more common in postterm pregnancies. Twice as many postterm fetuses weigh more than 4,000 g compared to term infants. Birth injuries caused by shoulder dystocia and delivery complications are increased postterm.
  - **Oligohydramnios** is more common in postterm pregnancies, probably due to decreasing uteroplacental function. Low AFV is associated with increased intrapartum fetal intolerance of labor and cesarean delivery.
  - **Meconium**-stained amniotic fluid and meconium aspiration syndrome increase in postterm gestation.
- **Management** of singleton pregnancy after 40 completed weeks (i.e., at 41 weeks) includes daily fetal movement assessment (kick counts), semiweekly fetal testing (NST), and AFV testing (AFI).
- A recent, large cohort study with over 3.8 million deliveries demonstrated that after 39 weeks, the risk of fetal demise is greater with expectant management than the risk of infant death with induction of labor. However, the number needed to be induced between 39 and 41 weeks to prevent one fetal death is excessive and induction before 41 weeks has not been shown to be cost-effective. Women should

be offered the option of membrane stripping commencing at 38 to 41 weeks to enhance the probability of spontaneous labor. Unless the cervix is favorable, it is common to induce at 41 weeks as the present evidence reveals a decrease in perinatal mortality without increased risk of cesarean section, although fetal surveillance until 42 weeks' gestation is acceptable.

## FETAL DEMISE IN UTERO

**FDIU**, also called intrauterine fetal demise (IUFD), is the antenatal diagnosis of a stillborn infant after 20 weeks' gestation. Approximately 50% of perinatal deaths are stillbirths. Of all fetal deaths in the United States, over two thirds occur before 32 weeks' gestation, 20% occur between 36 and 40 weeks' gestation, and approximately 10% occur beyond 41 weeks' gestation.

- FDIU is suspected with any maternal report of more than a few hours of absent fetal movement. Definitive diagnosis is by absent fetal cardiac activity on real-time ultrasonography.
- Fetal deaths can be categorized by occurrence during the antepartum period or during labor (intrapartum stillbirth). The antepartum fetal death rate in an unmonitored population is approximately 8 in 1,000 and represents 86% of fetal deaths.
- The etiology of antepartum fetal death can be divided into broad categories: chronic hypoxia of diverse origin (30%), congenital malformation or chromosomal anomaly (20%), complications of pregnancy such as Rh alloimmunization (<1%), abruptio placentae (20% to 25%), fetal infection (<5%), and idiopathic/ unexplained (25% or more).
- **Antepartum fetal assessment** may not prevent but can significantly reduce the frequency of antenatal fetal deaths. Inclusion criteria for antepartum fetal assessment are uteroplacental insufficiency, postterm pregnancy, diabetes mellitus requiring medication, hypertension requiring medication, previous stillbirth, IUGR, decreased fetal movement, and Rh disease.
- Both expectant and active **management** are acceptable after fetal demise. Spontaneous labor occurs within 2 to 3 weeks in 80% of cases. In cases of prolonged demise, induction of labor should be offered due to emotional burden and the risk of chorioamnionitis and DIC with prolonged demise. Dilation and evacuation early in the second trimester is an option. Testing to determine the cause of the loss is usually negative but can include chromosomes, infection evaluation (TORCH), maternal thyroid screening, and fetal autopsy.

## SUGGESTED READINGS

American College of Obstetricians and Gynecologists. ACOG practice bulletin no. 102: management of stillbirth. *Obstet Gynecol* 2007;113:748–761.

American College of Obstetricians and Gynecologists. Practice bulletin no. 134: fetal growth restriction. *Obstet Gynecol* 2013;121(5):1122–1133.

American College of Obstetricians and Gynecologists. Practice bulletin no. 144: multifetal gestations: twin, triplet, and higher-order multifetal pregnancies. *Obstet Gynecol* 2014;123(5):1118–1132.

American College of Obstetricians and Gynecologists. Practice Bulletin no. 146: management of late-term and postterm pregnancies. *Obstet Gynecol* 2014;124(2, pt 1):390–396.

Creasy RK, Resnik R, Iams JD, et al, eds. Intrauterine growth restriction. In *Creasy and Resnik's Maternal-Fetal Medicine: Principles and Practice*, 7th ed. Philadelphia, PA: Saunders Elsevier, 2009:743–755.

Creasy RK, Resnik R, Iams JD, et al, eds. Multiple gestation: clinical characteristics and management. In *Creasy and Resnik's Maternal-Fetal Medicine: Principles and Practice*, 7th ed. Philadelphia, PA: Saunders Elsevier, 2009:578–598.

Creasy RK, Resnik R, Iams JD, et al, eds. Multiple gestation: the biology of twinning. In *Creasy and Resnik's Maternal-Fetal Medicine: Principles and Practice*, 7th ed. Philadelphia, PA: Saunders Elsevier, 2009:53–65.

Creasy RK, Resnik R, Iams JD, et al, eds. Stillbirth. In *Creasy and Resnik's Maternal-Fetal Medicine: Principles and Practice*, 7th ed. Philadelphia, PA: Saunders Elsevier, 2009:718–731.

Nabhan AF, Abdelmoula YA. Amniotic fluid index versus single deepest vertical pocket as a screening test for preventing adverse pregnancy outcome. *Cochrane Database Syst Rev* 2008;(3):CD006593.

Robyr R, Quarello E, Ville Y. Management of fetofetal transfusion syndrome. *Prenat Diagn* 2005;25:786.

Rosenstein MG, Cheng YW, Snowden JM, et al. Risk of stillbirth and infant death stratified by gestational age. *Obstet Gynecol* 2012;120:76–82.

Silver RM, Varner MW, Reddy U, et al. Workup of stillbirth: a review of the evidence. *Am J Obstet Gynecol* 2007;196(5):433–444.

Snijders RJ, Nicolaides KH. Fetal biometry at 14–40 weeks' gestation. *Ultrasound Obstet Gynecol* 1994;4:34.

# 9

# Preterm Labor and Preterm Premature Rupture of Membranes

Julie S. Solomon and Janyne E. Althaus

## PRETERM LABOR

**Preterm labor (PTL)** is defined as:
- Regular uterine contractions with cervical change before 37 weeks' gestation
- *Extreme PTL* occurs before 28 weeks' gestation.

### Incidence and Significance
- PTL is the leading cause of neonatal morbidity in developed countries (Fig. 9-1).
- PTL accounts for 40% to 50% of preterm births. Other causes include preterm premature rupture of membranes, placental abruption, and indicated deliveries. Of the 4 million US births in 2010, 480,000 or 12% were preterm deliveries.
- Short-term neonatal morbidity includes respiratory distress syndrome (RDS), hypothermia, hypoglycemia, jaundice, intraventricular hemorrhage, necrotizing enterocolitis, bronchopulmonary dysplasia, sepsis, and patent ductus arteriosus.
- Long-term neonatal morbidity includes cerebral palsy, mental retardation, and retinopathy of prematurity.

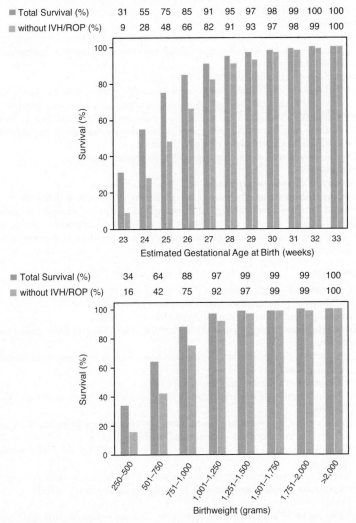

**Figure 9-1.** Outcomes for nonanomalous preterm neonates from 23 to 33 weeks (**top panel**) and from 250 to 2,000 g (**bottom panel**) are shown. Prognosis is affected by many factors other than gestational age and birthweight and is evaluated on an individual basis. Intraventricular hemorrhage (IVH) and retinopathy of prematurity (ROP) are only two possible major complications of prematurity. (Adapted from Pediatrix Medical Group. Outcomes data. Pediatrix Medical Group Web site. http://www.pediatrix.com/body_university.cfm?id=596. Accessed August 14, 2010.)

## Etiology

**Risk factors** include:
- **Previous spontaneous preterm delivery (PTD):**
  - Most significant risk factor for PTL
  - Recurrence rate is 17% to 30%.
- **Infection:**
  - Systemic or local infections including urinary tract infections, pyelonephritis, bacterial vaginosis, sexually transmitted infections, pneumonia, appendicitis, periodontal disease
  - Chorioamnionitis affects 25% of PTDs.
    - Pathogens include *Ureaplasma urealyticum, Mycoplasma hominis, Gardnerella vaginalis, Peptostreptococci,* and *Bacteroides* species.
    - Release of cytokines from endothelial cells, including interleukin-1, interleukin-6, and tumor necrosis factor-$\alpha$, stimulates a cascade of prostaglandin production that stimulates uterine contractions.
- **Uterine overdistension:** multiple gestation, polyhydramnios
- **Short cervix**
- **History of cervical manipulation**
- **Uterine malformations:** bicornuate uterus, leiomyomata, uterine didelphys
- **Second- or third-trimester vaginal bleeding:** placenta previa, placental abruption
- **Other:** anxiety, depression, stressful life events (divorce, separation, death), low level of education, low socioeconomic status, African American race, maternal age (younger than 18 or older than 40 years)

## Prevention

Any discussion on the prevention of PTD should note that the most important risk factor, history of prior spontaneous PTD, cannot be modified.
- **Educate** patients about the early signs of PTL.
- **Treat infections** promptly, especially urinary tract infections and lower genital tract infections.
  - It is notable that treatment of some infections, such as trichomoniasis, actually increase risk of PTD.
    - Treatment of infection may not remove risks.
    - The mechanism of causation may be from associated inflammation rather than infection.
  - Empiric broad-spectrum antibiotics have not been shown to reduce PTL and delivery and are associated with neonatal morbidity.
  - Chorioamnionitis is an indication for delivery, and PTD should not be avoided in this case.
    - Broad-spectrum treatment should take place while moving towards delivery.
- **Progesterone supplementation** with 17-hydroxyprogesterone (17-OHP)
  - Dose:
    - 250 mg of 17-alpha-hydroxyprogesterone caproate intramuscularly (IM) every week
    - progesterone vaginal suppositories (90 to 200 mg) every night at bedtime
  - Progesterone has been shown to prolong gestation for women with prior history of PTL.
  - Vaginal progesterone has been shown to prolong gestation for women with a short cervix <20 mm.

- Suggested therapy begins at 16 to 22 weeks of gestation and is continued until 33 to 36 weeks of gestation.
- There is no evidence to support progesterone therapy for patients with *active* PTL.
- **Cerclage**
  - There are different techniques of cerclage placement, and a variety of nonabsorbable suture material can be used (see Chapter 8).
  - Progesterone supplementation can be considered, where indicated, in addition to a cerclage if placed.
    - An additive effect has not been demonstrated in the literature.
  - Cerclage may be considered for a variety of indications:
    - Patient with both a cervix <25 mm before 24 weeks of gestation *and* a history of PTD <37 weeks
      - Meta-analyses of randomized controlled trials have demonstrated that cerclage may be beneficial in this population.
      - Patients with a cervix <25 mm and *no* history of PTD are optimally treated with vaginal progesterone without cerclage placement.
    - Cervical incompetence based on patient history
      - Generally placed around 12 to 14 weeks of gestation
      - There is limited evidence demonstrating the benefit of cerclage in this population.
    - "Rescue" cerclage placed with advanced cervical dilation in the second trimester to prevent further dilation
      - There is little evidence demonstrating the benefit of this intervention.
  - Cerclage has many limitations:
    - Cerclage is contraindicated in cases of infection, ruptured membranes, or active labor.
    - There is no evidence to support its use in multiple gestations for any indication and the suggestion that risk may outweigh benefits.
    - The wide variety of indications and patients selected for cerclage have led to limited evidence-based recommendations.
    - Cerclage, even when evidence based, may only be beneficial in one third of cases.
  - Abdominal cerclage may be considered in future pregnancies where vaginal cerclages have previously failed.

## Screening

- **History of prior spontaneous PTD is the largest risk factor.**
- **Cervical length (CL):**
  - Patients with a CL <25 mm have a high risk of PTL/PTD and are eligible for either progesterone therapy (with CL<20 mm) or with cerclage therapy (if they have a history of a prior PTD). Screening is specifically indicated in patients with known or suspected risk for PTL/PTD (including personal history).
- **Fetal fibronectin (FFN)—optional adjunct to clinical management:**
  - Should only be used as an adjunct to clinical management and is not indicated for routine screening
  - Collect from 24 to 34 weeks' gestation with signs and symptoms of PTL.
  - Should be the first test performed during exam. The sample is taken from the posterior fornix
  - Invalid with vaginal bleeding, ruptured membranes, or a history of intercourse or vaginal exam within 24 hours

- FFN has a negative predictive value of 99% for delivery within 7 days.
- The positive predictive value for delivery within 7 days is as low as 14%; a positive result provides little clinical insight.

## Evaluation

- **Establish best dating** for gestational age using last menstrual period, fundal height, ultrasound data, and prenatal records if available.
- **Obtain vital signs**
  - A temperature >38°C or fetal or maternal tachycardia may indicate an underlying infection.
  - Hypotension with fetal or maternal tachycardia may suggest placental abruption.
- **Physical exam**
  - Fundal tenderness on exam may suggest chorioamnionitis or placental abruption.
  - Costovertebral angle tenderness may suggest pyelonephritis.
  - Initiate continuous fetal heart monitoring and tocodynamometry.
    - Nonreassuring fetal heart tracing may indicate chorioamnionitis, abruption, or cord compression.
- **Sterile speculum examination (SSE)**
  - Inspect visually for bleeding, amniotic fluid pooling, advanced dilation, bulging membranes, and purulent cervical discharge.
  - Perform FFN if desired (see earlier discussion) prior to any other cervical manipulation or sampling.
  - Swab vaginal pool fluid for nitrazine and fern tests to evaluate for rupture of membranes.
  - Membrane status significantly alters management and should be determined early during evaluation.
    - Normal vaginal pH is <5.5, with amniotic fluid pH usually 7.0 to 7.5. A vaginal pH >6.5 (or blue on nitrazine paper) is consistent with rupture of membranes.
    - False-positive tests can be observed with blood, semen, trichomoniasis or other infection (such as *Proteus infection*), cervical mucus, or urine contamination.
    - The presence of ferning of vaginal fluid on a slide can indicate rupture of membranes.
      - Ferning may be falsely absent (or negative) in the presence of blood.
      - Cervical fluid can give false-positive ferning; avoid swabbing cervical mucus.
  - For pooling, have the patient cough or Valsalva to see whether apparent amniotic fluid accumulates in the vagina.
  - Obtain group B streptococci (GBS) anovaginal culture (will determine GBS need for antibiotics in labor for 4 to 5 weeks).
  - Obtain cervical cultures for *Chlamydia trachomatis* and *Neisseria gonorrhea*.
  - Evaluate wet mount for bacterial vaginosis, *Trichomonas*, and yeast.
- *After* ascertaining intact membranes, **digital examination** is performed to assess cervical dilation, effacement, and station.
- Obtain **laboratory studies** including a complete blood count, urinalysis with microscopic evaluation, and all cultures obtained in the SSE. Obtain cultures before antibiotics are given.
- Perform **ultrasound** to assess for multiple gestation, fetal presentation, estimated fetal weight (EFW), gestational age, placental location, amniotic fluid index, and fetal or uterine anomalies. CL can also be examined transvaginally where indicated.

## Management

- **Goals** of management are the following:
  - To delay delivery, if possible, where fetal and maternal status are reassuring in the absence of chorioamnionitis
  - To optimize neonatal outcomes with the administration of steroids and GBS prophylaxis per guidelines
- **Oral or intravenous hydration** can be used as an initial approach to preterm contractions due to dehydration.
  - Randomized trials have shown that hydration does not reduce the incidence of preterm birth.
  - Clinical experience will guide the initial treatment and consideration for admission.
- **Bed rest** has historically been recommended on admission to the hospital, with gradual liberalization of activity as tolerated.
  - Clinical trials have failed to demonstrate any benefit of bed rest for the prevention of PTD and there are significant potential risks including deep vein thrombosis formation.
  - Any consideration of bed rest for the prevention of PTL or delivery is in the absence of evidentiary support.
    ○ In the setting of ruptured membranes and malpresentation, bed rest might help avoid umbilical cord prolapse.
  - Thromboembolic prophylaxis should be considered and a physical therapy consultation obtained in all patients with activity limitations.
  - Limited evidence associates prolonged standing, strenuous activity, or sexual activity with PTL.
    ○ The association might be with uterine contractions or irritation rather than uterine contractions with cervical change.
- **Tocolysis**
  - No study to date shows that tocolysis beyond 48 hours improves fetal or maternal outcomes. It may be considered to permit transport to tertiary center for advanced care and to allow time for maximum efficacy of steroid treatment.
  - Contraindications: nonreassuring fetal status, chorioamnionitis, eclampsia or severe preeclampsia, fetal demise, fetal maturity, and maternal hemodynamic instability.
  - First-line tocolytics are nifedipine and, in pregnancies <32 weeks, indomethacin. (Table 9-1).
  - Use of multiple tocolytics concurrently should be avoided given the risk of pulmonary edema (excluding indomethacin).
- **GBS prophylaxis** is continued until cervical exam is stable and risk for progression to PTD is lower.
  - Antibiotic prophylaxis is not indicated outside of concern for active labor.
  - Prolonged empiric antibiotics in the case of intact membranes may increase neonatal risk of sepsis.
- **Corticosteroids** should considered between 24 and 34 weeks' gestation.
  - Give two doses of betamethasone (12 mg IM) 24 hours apart or four doses of dexamethasone (6 mg IM) 12 hours apart.
    ○ Benefit is optimized 24 hours after the second dose and remains up to 1 week after administration.
  - Corticosteroid administration reduces risk for neonatal respiratory depression, intraventricular hemorrhage, necrotizing enterocolitis, and neonatal death.

| TABLE 9-1 | Common Tocolytic Agents for Preterm Labor | | | | |
|---|---|---|---|---|---|
| Drug | Mechanism of Action | Dosing Regimen | Contraindications | Side Effects | Notes |
| Indomethacin | Prostaglandin synthetase inhibitor → prevents production of prostaglandin $F_{2\alpha}$, which normally stimulates uterine contractions. | Loading dose: 50–100 mg orally or per rectum Maintenance dose: 25–50 mg orally or per rectum q4–6hr × 72 hr | Peptic ulcer disease Renal disease Hepatic dysfunction Coagulopathy Oligohydramnios | Oligohydramnios Nausea GERD/gastritis Emesis Platelet dysfunction (rare) | First-line agent in gestations <32 wk Avoid at >32 weeks' gestation (associated with premature closure of fetal ductus arteriosus). Avoid using for >72 hr (associated with oligohydramnios). |
| Nifedipine | Calcium channel blocker → inhibits myometrial calcium entry | 10–20 mg orally q6hr | Hypotension Congestive heart failure Aortic stenosis | Hypotension Flushing Light-headedness Dizziness Nausea | First-line agent |

| | Mechanism | Dose | Contraindications | Side effects | Comments |
|---|---|---|---|---|---|
| Terbutaline | β-Sympathomimetic → causes uterine smooth muscle relaxation. | 0.25 mg SC injection every 20–30 min, as needed | Cardiac disease Hypertension Digitalis use Hyperthyroidism Poorly controlled diabetes mellitus | Tachycardia Pulmonary edema Elevated blood sugar levels Cardiac arrhythmias Myocardial ischemia Heart failure | $\beta_2$-Adrenergic agonists can reduce contractions, but no improvement in perinatal outcome or rate of preterm birth has been reported. |
| Magnesium | Competes for myometrial calcium entry, thereby decreases uterine contractility | Loading dose: 4–6 g IV or 10 g IM Maintenance: infusion of 2–4 g/hr Therapeutic levels are between 6 and 8 mg/dL. | Myasthenia gravis Heart block Renal failure | Respiratory depression Pulmonary edema Cardiac arrest Nausea/vomiting Flushing Muscle weakness Hypotension Hyporeflexia | Systematic review found no evidence that magnesium helps to prevent PTD. One gram of calcium gluconate is the antidote for $MgSO_4$ toxicity. |

GERD, gastroesophageal reflux disease; SC, subcutaneous; IV, intravenous; IM, intramuscular; PTD, preterm delivery; $MgSO_4$, magnesium sulfate.

- A single rescue course of two doses of steroid administration at 28 to 34 weeks 7 or more days after earlier administration may be considered with little additional neonatal risk and potential benefit.
  - We often redose betamethasone once at least 2 weeks after initial dose if imminent delivery is again suspected.
  - Particularly if prior dose was given at 30 weeks or earlier
- Serial courses or additional doses are not indicated and are associated with growth restriction and neonatal morbidity.
- Corticosteroids increase maternal white blood cell count and serum glucose, so exercise caution in interpreting those lab values.
  - Glucose monitoring is required if given to diabetics or suspected diabetics due to risk for hyperglycemia and morbidity.
    - This effect peaks with approximately 50% increased insulin requirements at 2 to 3 days and lasts about 5 days.
- **Magnesium** should be considered between 24 and 32 weeks of gestation for fetal neuroprotection.
  - Meta-analysis of studies evaluating intravenous magnesium have demonstrated that its administration can help decrease the combined outcome of neonatal death or cerebral palsy.
    - Studies included in the meta-analysis used different doses of magnesium infusions
      - 4 g bolus
      - 1g/hr for 24 hours
      - 2 g/hr for 12 hours
  - It is generally accepted to use any of these proposed regimens for neonatal neuro-protective effects. We generally consider a 4 gram bolus followed by magnesium at 1g/hr for 24 hours or until delivery. At 24 hours, the patient is re-evaluated and the magnesium may be continued if delivery is felt to be imminent. Additionally, magnesium infusions that are discontinued are considered to be restarted if delivery is felt to be imminent in the future, prior to 32 weeks' gestation.
- **Fetal monitoring**
  - No optimal schedule of fetal testing has been established.
    - Maintain external fetal monitoring/tocodynamometry until active PTL resolves (i.e., no cervical change and minimal contractions).
    - Once PTL resolves, there is no need for further continuous monitoring. On our inpatient unit, we check fetal doptones one to two times daily with vital signs and perform a fetal nonstress test one to three times per week.
- **Route of delivery varies by gestational age**
  - If <26 weeks or EFW <750 g, vaginal delivery for vertex or breech presentation may be considered by appropriately skilled providers.
    - There is limited data to suggest C-section improves neonatal outcomes at this early gestation.
    - A frank discussion of the risks and benefits of C-section for fetal distress or otherwise should take place, given the increased maternal morbidity and poor neonatal prognosis. The risks and future implications of classical cesarean section should be discussed. Document your discussion carefully in the chart, and revisit the issue as gestation progresses.
  - If the fetus is malpresenting and is either >26 weeks or EFW is >800 g, C-section should be considered to minimize neonatal morbidity.
    - C-section for breech presentation is performed to minimize the risk of head entrapment and associated morbidity.

- **Criteria for discharge** include acontractile, stable cervical exam (without advanced cervical dilation [>4 cm], bulging membranes, or significant effacement), no vaginal bleeding, no suspicion of ruptured membranes, reasonable hospital access with appropriate level of neonatology support, ability to comply with activity recommendations (modified bed rest and complete pelvic rest), and reassuring fetal status (we typically perform a nonstress test on the day of discharge).

## PRETERM PREMATURE RUPTURE OF MEMBRANES

**Preterm premature rupture of membranes (PPROM)** can be defined as spontaneous rupture of the amnion and chorion membranes before the onset of labor (**premature rupture of membranes [PROM]**) or PROM before 37 weeks' gestation. The latency period is the time from PROM or PPROM to onset of labor. At term, latency is 1 to 12 hours on average.

### Incidence and Significance
- Term PROM occurs in up to 19% of pregnancies.
- PPROM occurs in approximately 30% of pregnancies and accounts for 30% of PTD.
- Fifty percent of patients with PPROM before 26 weeks will labor within 1 week.
- Fifty percent of patients with PPROM between 28 and 34 weeks will labor within 24 hours; 80% to 90% will labor within 1 week.

### Etiology
- Risk factors include intrauterine infection, prior history of PPROM, trauma, amniocentesis, and polyhydramnios.

### Evaluation
- Same as for PTL (see earlier discussion). Make careful note of the circumstances, character, and timing of rupture of membranes (ROM) and the consistency of the fluid.
- Only an SSE should be performed. Avoid digital cervical exam unless delivery is imminent. Digital examination decreases the latency period and increases the risk of neonatal sepsis.
- When clinical suspicion of PROM is high despite negative ferning, nitrazine, and pooling, retest after prolonged recumbency (several hours).
  - Consider amnioinfusion of indigo carmine (1 ml in 9-ml sterile normal saline) for a "tampon test." A tampon or packing is placed in the vagina, and dye is injected into the amniotic fluid via the amniocentesis needle. After some time, the tampon is examined to see whether blue-stained fluid has leaked through the cervix.

### Management
**Management** for PPROM and PTL is similar.
- The **goals** are to screen for underlying chorioamnionitis or placental abruption and move toward delivery if these conditions are identified. Otherwise, prolonging the latent period is desired, depending on gestational age.
  - If the fetal vertex is not well applied to the cervix, **bed rest** should be maintained to avoid cord accident.
- Before 34 weeks in the absence of chorioamnionitis, initiate **latency antibiotics**, which delay the onset of PTL.
  - The standard latency regimen is intravenous ampicillin 2 g and erythromycin 250 mg every 6 hours for 48 hours.

- This is followed by oral amoxicillin 250 mg and erythromycin 330 mg every 8 hours (or 250 mg erythromycin every 6 hours) for 5 more days.
- In cases of penicillin allergy, cephalosporins can replace amoxicillin if the allergic reaction is mild, or clindamycin and gentamycin can be considered if the allergic reaction is severe (e.g., angioedema).
- The entire latency course is 7 days.
- Tocolysis is generally contraindicated in PPROM except for extreme prematurity to allow corticosteroid administration.
- If chorioamnionitis is suspected, tocolysis is contraindicated.
- Once the patient and fetus are stable, **fetal heart tones** should be evaluated every 8 hours and daily fetal testing performed.
- At <34 weeks of gestation, manage PPROM as outlined earlier with latency antibiotics and steroids.
- At ≥34 weeks, augment labor for delivery or proceed to C-section for standard obstetric indications.
- Evidence of chorioamnionitis or nonreassuring fetal status warrants prompt delivery.
- Continue inpatient management for PPROM until delivery unless membranes reseal, as documented by negative blue dye tampon test.

## SUGGESTED READINGS

American College of Obstetricians and Gynecologists Committee on Obstetric Practice; Society for Maternal-Fetal Medicine. Committee opinion no. 455: magnesium sulfate before anticipated preterm birth for neuroprotection. *Obstet Gynecol* 2010;115(3):669–671.

American College of Obstetricians and Gynecologists Committee on Practice Bulletins—Obstetrics. ACOG practice bulletin no. 80: premature rupture of membranes. Clinical management guidelines for obstetrician-gynecologists. *Obstet Gynecol* 2007;109(4):1007–1019.

American College of Obstetricians and Gynecologists Committee on Practice Bulletins—Obstetrics. ACOG practice bulletin no. 127: management of preterm labor. *Obstet Gynecol* 2012;119(6):1308–1317.

American College of Obstetricians and Gynecologists Committee on Practice Bulletins—Obstetrics. ACOG practice bulletin no. 130: prediction and prevention of preterm birth. *Obstet Gynecol* 2012;120(4):964–973.

Berghella V, Hayes E, Visintine J, et al. Fetal fibronectin testing for reducing the risk of preterm birth. *Cochrane Database Syst Rev* 2008;(4):CD006843.

Crowther CA, McKinlay CJ, Middleton P, et al. Repeat doses of prenatal corticosteroids for women at risk of preterm birth for improving neonatal health outcomes. *Cochrane Database Syst Rev* 2011;(6):CD003935.

Garite TJ, Kurtzman J, Maurel K, et al; Obstetrix Collaborative Research Network. Impact of a "rescue course" of antenatal corticosteroids: a multicenter randomized placebo-controlled trial. *Am J Obstet Gynecol* 2009;200(3):248.e1–248.e9.

Goldenberg RL, Culhane JF, Iams JD, et al. Epidemiology and causes of preterm birth. *Lancet* 2008;371(9606):75–84.

Haas DM, Imperiale TF, Kirkpatrick PR, et al. Tocolytic therapy: a meta-analysis and decision analysis. *Obstet Gynecol* 2009;113(3):585–594.

Meis PJ, Klebanoff M, Thom E, et al; National Institute of Child Health and Human Development Maternal-Fetal Medicine Units Network. Prevention of recurrent preterm delivery by 17 alpha-hydroxyprogesterone caproate. *N Engl J Med* 2003;348(24):2379–2385.

Mercer BM, Miodovnik M, Thurnau GR, et al; National Institute of Child Health and Human Development Maternal-Fetal Medicine Units Network. Antibiotic therapy for reduction of infant morbidity after preterm premature rupture of the membranes. A randomized controlled trial. *JAMA* 1997;278(12):989–995.

Roberts D, Dalziel SR. Antenatal corticosteroids for accelerating fetal lung maturation for women at risk of preterm birth. *Cochrane Database Syst Rev* 2006;(3):CD004454.

# 10

# Third-Trimester Bleeding

William Fletcher and Cynthia Holcroft Argani

**Third-trimester bleeding**, ranging from spotting to massive hemorrhage, occurs in 2% to 6% of all pregnancies. The differential diagnosis includes bloody show from labor, abruptio placentae (AP), placenta previa (PP), vasa previa (VP), cervicitis, postcoital bleeding, trauma, uterine rupture, and carcinoma. AP, PP, and VP can lead to significant maternal and fetal morbidity and mortality (see Table 10-1).

## ABRUPTIO PLACENTAE

**AP** is the premature separation of the normally implanted placenta from the uterine wall due to maternal/uterine bleeding into the *decidua basalis*.

### Epidemiology

- One third of all antepartum bleeding is due to AP, with an incidence of 1 in 75 to 1 in 225 births. The incidence increases with maternal age.
- AP recurs in 5% to 17% of pregnancies after one prior episode and up to 25% after two prior episodes.
- There is a 7% incidence of stillbirth in future pregnancies after AP leading to fetal death.

### Etiology

- Bleeding does not correlate with abruption size and may vary from scant to massive.
- AP without vaginal bleeding can result in delayed diagnosis and consumptive coagulopathy.
- Blood in the *basalis* layer stimulates forceful, classically tetanic, uterine contractions leading to ischemic abdominal pain.
- AP is associated with maternal hypertension, advanced maternal age, multiparity, cocaine use, tobacco use, chorioamnionitis, preterm premature rupture of membranes, coagulopathy, and trauma. Many cases are idiopathic.
- Patients with chronic hypertension, superimposed preeclampsia, or severe preeclampsia have fivefold increased risk of severe abruption compared to normotensive women. Antihypertensive medications do not reduce the risk.
- Cigarette smoking increases the risk of stillbirth from AP by 2.5-fold. The risk increases by 40% for each pack per day smoked.
- Rapid changes in intrauterine volume can lead to abruption, such as rupture of membranes, therapeutic amnioreduction for polyhydramnios, or during delivery of multiple gestations.
- Abruption occurs more frequently when the placenta implants on abnormal uterine surfaces as with submucosal myomas or uterine anomalies.
- Hyperhomocysteinemia, factor V Leiden, and prothrombin 20210 mutations (thrombophilias) are associated with an increased risk of abruption.

| TABLE 10-1 | Important Steps in the Diagnosis and Management of Third-Trimester Vaginal Bleeding |
|---|---|

- Assess maternal hemodynamic status through vital signs and laboratory studies. Ensure the patient has appropriate intravenous (IV) access and order fluid resuscitation when indicated. If bleeding is substantial, obtain a type and crossmatch.
- Assess fetal status through continuous external fetal monitoring.
- Obtain history from patient, including the duration/severity of bleeding, whether or not the bleeding is painful, and whether there has been any trauma. Be sure to rule out other sources of bleeding, such as rectal bleeding.
- Use ultrasound to assess the location and appearance of the placenta.
- Once previa is ruled out through imaging, a pelvic exam should be performed and the patient's cervix should be assessed.
- Formulate a plan for management and/or delivery, taking into account the patient's gestational age and hemodynamic status.
- Consider administering medications, when appropriate, including betamethasone, Rh D immunoglobulin, and/or magnesium for tocolysis.

## Complications

- Massive maternal blood loss may lead to **hemorrhagic shock** (see Chapter 3).
- Maternal **disseminated intravascular coagulation (DIC)** can occur and is found in 10% to 20% of AP with stillbirth.
- Extravasation of blood directly into the uterine muscle (Couvelaire uterus) can lead to **uterine atony** and massive postpartum hemorrhage.
- **Fetal hypoxia** may occur, leading to acute fetal distress, hypoxic-ischemic encephalopathy, premature delivery, and fetal death. Milder chronic abruption may lead to growth restriction, major malformations, or anemia.

## Diagnosis

*History and Physical Examination*

- Classically presents late in pregnancy with vaginal bleeding and acute severe abdominal pain. Even slight clinical suspicion should prompt rapid investigation and close monitoring.
- Maternal vital signs, fetal heart rate assessment, and uterine tone should be evaluated immediately.
- Mark or record the fundal height to follow expansion of concealed hemorrhage. Blood may be sequestered between the uterus and placenta when the placental margins remain adherent. Membranes or the fetus itself may obstruct the cervical os and prevent accurate assessment of blood loss.
- Defer digital cervical exam until PP and VP have been ruled out.
- Ultrasound is insensitive in diagnosing AP, but large abruptions may be seen as hypoechoic areas underlying the placenta.
- Perform a speculum exam to evaluate vaginal or cervical lacerations and the amount of bleeding.

*Laboratory Tests*

- **Complete blood cell count** with hematocrit and platelets (<100,000 plts/μL suggests severe abruption)
- Blood **type and screen** (crossmatch should be strongly considered)
- **Prothrombin/activated partial thromboplastin time**
- **Fibrinogen** (<200 mg/dL suggests severe abruption)
- **Fibrin split products**
- Consider holding a **whole blood** specimen at the bedside while lab work is pending. If a clot does not form within 6 minutes or forms and lyses within 30 minutes, DIC may be present.
- The **Apt test** can be performed to evaluate whether vaginal blood is from the mother or the fetus. The blood is collected and lysed in water to release hemoglobin. Sodium hydroxide is mixed with the supernatant. Fetal hemoglobin is resistant to the base and will remain pink, whereas maternal hemoglobin will oxidize and turn brown. In theory, this qualitative test could be used to identify bleeding from VP, but the short time to fetal distress after a ruptured umbilical vessel and the sensitivity of fetal heart monitoring make the test largely unnecessary.
- The **Kleihauer-Betke test** for fetal hemoglobin in the maternal circulation is not valuable in diagnosing AP.

## Management

- Large-bore **intravenous access** should be obtained.
- **Fluid resuscitation** should be initiated and a **Foley catheter** placed to monitor urine output (>0.5 mL/kg/hr or at least 30 mL/hr should be observed).
- Close monitoring of **maternal vital signs** and continuous **fetal monitoring** should be maintained.
- **Rh D immunoglobulin** should be administered to Rh-negative individuals.
- Further management depends on the gestational age and hemodynamic status of both mother and fetus.

*Term Gestation, Hemodynamically Stable*

- Plan for vaginal delivery via induction of labor, with cesarean section for usual indications.
- Follow serial hematocrit and coagulation studies.
- Consider fetal scalp electrode for accurate and continuous fetal monitoring and intrauterine pressure catheter to assess resting uterine tone.

*Term Gestation, Hemodynamic Instability*

- Aggressively fluid resuscitate.
- Transfuse packed red blood cells, fresh frozen plasma, and platelets as needed. Maintain fibrinogen level >150 mg/dL, hematocrit >25%, and platelets >60,000/μL.
- Once the mother is stabilized, proceed to urgent cesarean section, unless vaginal delivery is imminent.

*Preterm Gestation, Hemodynamically Stable*

- Eighty-two percent of patients with evidence of AP at <20 weeks' gestation will progress to term. Only 27% of patients who present after 20 weeks' gestation, however, will have a term delivery.
- *In the absence of labor*, preterm AP should be followed closely with serial ultrasound evaluation of fetal growth from 24 weeks and regular antepartum testing. Steroids

should be given to promote fetal lung maturity. If maternal instability or fetal distress arises, delivery should be performed as mentioned earlier. Otherwise, labor can be induced at term.

* *For preterm AP with labor,* completely stable hemodynamics, and reassuring fetal signs, tocolysis may be used in selected rare cases. Magnesium sulfate tocolysis at <32 weeks' gestation may delay delivery, giving time to administer a course of corticosteroids. Magnesium is preferred over terbutaline or nifedipine as it may be less likely to obscure signs of shock. Indomethacin is avoided because of its effect on platelet function. If maternal or fetal compromise arises, delivery should be performed after appropriate resuscitation.

*Preterm Gestation, Hemodynamic Instability*

* Delivery should be performed after appropriate resuscitation.

## PLACENTA PREVIA

**PP** is the presence of placental tissue over or near the internal cervical os. It can be classified into four types based on the location relative to the cervical os:

* **Complete** or **total previa:** The placenta covers the entire cervical os.
* **Partial previa:** The edge of the placenta covers part, but not all, of the internal os.
* **Marginal previa:** The edge of the placenta lies adjacent to the internal os.
* **Low-lying placenta:** The placenta is located near (within 2 cm) but not on the internal os.

### Epidemiology

* In general, the incidence of PP is approximately 1 in 300 pregnancies over 20 weeks' gestational age. The frequency varies with parity, however, giving an incidence of 0.2% in nulliparas and as high as 5% in grand multiparas.
* The placenta covers the cervical os in 5% of pregnancies in the second trimester. Usually, the placenta will migrate away from the cervical os as the uterus grows with gestational age and the upper third of the cervix develops into the lower uterine segment.

### Etiology

* The most important risk factor for PP is a **previous cesarean section**. PP occurs in 1% of pregnancies after a single cesarean section. The incidence after four or more cesarean sections increases to 10%, a 40-fold increased risk compared with no cesarean section. Anterior PP in these patients should be carefully evaluated for accreta.
* Other risk factors include increasing maternal age (especially after age 40 years), multiparity, smoking, residing at higher elevations, male fetus, multiple gestation, and previous uterine curettage.
* These risk factors suggest two explanations for PP development:
  * Endometrial scarring in the upper portion of the uterus promotes implantation in the lower uterine segment.
  * Reduced uteroplacental oxygen exchange favors increased placental surface area and thus previa formation.

### Complications

* Bleeding occurs with the development of the lower uterine segment in the third trimester in preparation for labor. The placenta separates and the thinned lower

segment cannot contract sufficiently to stop blood flow from the exposed uterine vessels. Cervical exams or intercourse may also cause separation of the placenta from the lower uterine segment. Bleeding can range from spotting to massive hemorrhage.

- PP increases the risk for other abnormalities of placentation:
  - **Placenta accreta:** The placenta adheres directly to the uterus without the usual intervening *decidua basalis*. The incidence in patients with previa who have not had previous uterine surgery is approximately 4%, increasing to as many as 25% of patients who have had a previous cesarean section or uterine surgery.
  - **Placenta increta:** The placenta invades the myometrium but does not cross the serosa.
  - **Placenta percreta:** The placenta penetrates the entire uterine wall, potentially growing into bladder or bowel.
- PP is associated with double the rate of fetal congenital malformations, including anomalies of the central nervous system (CNS), gastrointestinal (GI) tract, cardiovascular system, and respiratory system. No specific syndrome has been identified.
- PP is also associated with fetal malpresentation, preterm premature rupture of membranes, intrauterine growth restriction, velamentous cord insertion, and VP.

## Diagnosis

*History and Physical Exam*

- Seventy percent to 80% of PP presents with the acute onset of **painless vaginal bleeding** with bright red blood.
- The first bleeding episode is usually around 34 weeks. About one third of patients develop bleeding before 30 weeks, whereas another third present after 36 weeks and 10% go to term. The number of bleeding episodes is unrelated to the degree of PP or the prognosis for fetal survival.
- A thorough medical, obstetric, and surgical history should be obtained along with documentation of previous ultrasound examinations. Other causes of vaginal bleeding must also be ruled out, such as placental abruption.
- Maternal vital signs, abdominal exam, uterine tone, and fetal heart rate monitoring should be assessed.
- Vaginal **sonography** is the gold standard for diagnosis of previa. The placenta must be within 2 cm of the cervical os to make the diagnosis and may be missed by a transabdominal scan, especially if the placenta lies in the posterior portion of the lower uterine segment where it is poorly visualized. Having the patient empty her bladder may help in identifying anterior PP. Trendelenburg position may be useful in diagnosing posterior PP. If ultrasound findings are suspicious for accreta, magnetic resonance imaging (MRI) may be helpful in making the diagnosis, particularly with a posterior placenta.
- *If PP is present or suspected, digital examination is contraindicated.* A gentle speculum exam can be used to evaluate the presence and quantity of vaginal bleeding, but in most cases, this can be assessed adequately by inspecting the perineum and thereby avoid exacerbating the hemorrhage.

*Laboratory Studies*

- **Complete blood cell count**
- **Type and crossmatch**
- **Prothrombin time** and **activated thromboplastin time**
- **Kleihauer-Betke test** to assess for fetomaternal hemorrhage in Rh-negative unsensitized patients. Not useful for the diagnosis of PP.
- **Apt test** (as described earlier for abruption)

## Management

- In general, patients diagnosed with PP but *without* bleeding in the third trimester should have ultrasound confirmation of persistent previa. They should maintain **strict pelvic rest** (i.e., nothing in the vagina, including intercourse or pelvic exams) and avoid strenuous activity or exercise. They should receive advice about when to seek medical attention and be scheduled for fetal growth **ultrasounds** every 3 to 4 weeks.
- In general, patients with PP who *are* bleeding should be hospitalized for hemodynamic stabilization and continuous **maternal and fetal monitoring**. **Laboratory studies** should be ordered as described. **Steroids** are administered to promote lung maturity for gestations between 24 and 34 weeks, and **Rh D immunoglobulin** should be administered to Rh-negative mothers.
- Management of placenta accreta, or its variants, can be challenging. In patients with PP and a prior history of cesarean section, cesarean hysterectomy may be required. In cases where uterine preservation is highly desired and no bladder invasion has occurred, bleeding might be successfully controlled with selective arterial embolization or packing of the lower uterine segment, with removal of the pack through the vagina in 24 hours. The Bakri balloon catheter has also been used to help control bleeding from the placental bed.
- Specific management of PP is based on gestational age and assessment of the maternal and fetal status.

### *Term Gestation, Hemodynamically Stable*

- Patients with **complete previa** at term require cesarean section.
- Patients with **partial or marginal previa** at term may deliver vaginally, with thorough consent regarding risks for blood loss and need for transfusion. The staff and facilities for immediate emergent cesarean section must be available. If maternal or fetal stability is compromised at any point in labor, urgent cesarean section is performed.

### *Term Gestation, Hemodynamic Instability*

- Stabilize the mother with fluid resuscitation and blood products
- Delivery via cesarean section is indicated for nonreassuring fetal heart monitoring, life-threatening maternal hemorrhage, or bleeding after 34 weeks with documented fetal lung maturity. If the mother is stable and intrauterine fetal loss occurs or the fetus is <24 weeks' gestational age, vaginal delivery can be considered.

### *Preterm Gestation, Hemodynamically Stable*

- Patients at 24 to 37 weeks' gestation with PP *in the absence of labor can be* managed expectantly until term or until fetal lung maturity is documented.
- There is no evidence-based consensus on management of bleeding PP without hemodynamic compromise. In general, once a patient has been hospitalized for three separate episodes of bleeding, she should remain in the hospital until delivery. For each bleeding episode, the following are recommended:
  - Hospitalization on bed rest with bathroom privileges until stabilized.
  - Periodic assessment of maternal hematocrit and maintenance of an active type and screen.
  - Red blood cell transfusion as needed to maintain hematocrit above 30% for slight but continuous bleeding.
  - Corticosteroids and RhoGAM as indicated.

- Fetal testing and growth ultrasounds to assess for intrauterine growth restriction.
- Tocolysis is not warranted unless to administer a course of steroids in an otherwise stable patient.
- Amniocentesis can be used to assess fetal lung maturity.
- After initial hospital management, outpatient care may be considered if bleeding stops for >48 hours, no other complications exist, and the following criteria are met:
  - The patient can maintain bed rest at home and is adherent to medical care.
  - There is a responsible adult present at all times who can assist in an emergency.
  - The patient lives near the hospital with dependable transportation.
- For preterm gestations with PP *and contractions*, it can be difficult to diagnose labor. Cervical exams are contraindicated, and 20% of patients with PP show some uterine activity. If the patient and fetus are stable, tocolysis may be considered with magnesium sulfate. As with AP, terbutaline, nifedipine, and indomethacin should be avoided.

### Preterm Gestation, Hemodynamic Instability

- Appropriate stabilization and resuscitation are initiated with rapid delivery by cesarean section.

## VASA PREVIA

**VP** occurs when the umbilical cord inserts into the membranes instead of the central placental disc. When the vessels traverse the membranes near the internal os in advance of the fetal presenting part, they are at risk of rupture, causing fetal hemorrhage. VP can also occur when a velamentous cord insertion or vessels to an accessory lobe are located near the cervical os. Velamentous cord insertion is much more common in multiple gestations.

### Epidemiology

- The incidence of VP is estimated to be approximately 1 in 5,000 pregnancies.
- Fetal mortality may be as high as 60% with intact membranes and 75% when membranes rupture.

### Etiology

- The cause of VP is unknown. Because of the association between velamentous cord insertion, multiple gestations, and VP, one theory suggests that it develops due to trophoblastic growth and placental migration toward the more vascular uterine fundus. The initial cord insertion at the center of the placenta becomes more peripheral as one portion of the placenta actively grows and another portion does not. In vitro fertilization (IVF) may also be a risk factor.

### Complications

- Even small amounts of fetal hemorrhage can result in morbidity and possible death due to the small total fetal blood volume.
- Rupture of the membranes can result in rapid exsanguination of the fetus.

### History

- The patient usually presents with acute onset vaginal bleeding after rupture of membranes.

- The bleeding is associated with an acute change in fetal heart pattern. Typically, fetal tachycardia occurs, followed by bradycardia with intermittent accelerations. Short-term variability is often maintained. Occasionally, a sinusoidal pattern may be seen.

## Diagnosis

- **Transvaginal ultrasound**, in combination with color Doppler ultrasonography, is the most effective tool in antenatal diagnosis.
- In one study, there was a 97% survival rate in cases diagnosed antenatally compared to a 44% survival rate in those without prenatal diagnosis.

## Management

- Third-trimester bleeding caused by VP is often accompanied by acute and severe fetal distress. **Emergency cesarean section** is indicated.
- If VP is diagnosed antenatally, **planned cesarean section** should be scheduled at 36 to 38 weeks under controlled circumstances and before the onset of labor to reduce fetal mortality. Earlier delivery can be considered with documented fetal lung maturity.

## SUGGESTED READINGS

Love CD, Wallace EM. Pregnancies complicated by placenta praevia: what is appropriate management? *Br J Obstet Gynecol* 1996;103(9):864–867.

Magann EF, Cummings JE, Niederhauser A, et al. Antepartum bleeding of unknown origin in the second half of pregnancy: a review. *Obstet Gynecol Surv* 2005;60(11):741–745.

McCormack RA, Doherty DA, Magann EF, et al. Antepartum bleeding of unknown origin in the second half of pregnancy and pregnancy outcomes. *BJOG* 2008;115(11):1451–1457.

Oyelese Y, Smulian JC. Placenta previa, placenta accreta, and vasa previa. *Obstet Gynecol* 2006; 107(4):927–941.

# Perinatal Infections

Stephen Martin and Andrew J. Satin

Perinatal infections encompass a range of viruses, parasites, and bacteria that can be transmitted during pregnancy from mother to embryo or fetus. Infection can occur antepartum or intrapartum by transplacental or transcervical transmission, respectively. The acronym TORCH was originally used to characterize perinatal infections including toxoplasmosis, "other," rubella, cytomegalovirus, and herpes simplex virus. The expansive "other" has grown to include, but is not limited to, parvovirus, syphilis, group B *Streptococcus*, hepatitis, and influenza.

Asymptomatic or undiagnosed maternal disease can result in significant fetal and neonatal morbidity and mortality. For this reason, it is important to understand the clinical manifestations, diagnostic criteria, and management of these perinatal infections.

# VIRUSES

## Cytomegalovirus

*Epidemiology*

- **Cytomegalovirus (CMV)** is the most common congenital viral infection, with intrauterine infection occurring in 0.2% to 2.5% of live births. CMV is a ubiquitous DNA herpes virus, with approximately 50% of the US population having antibodies to CMV. Transmission occurs through direct contact with infected saliva, semen, cervical and vaginal secretions, urine, breast milk, or blood products. Vertical transmission can occur transplacentally, during delivery, or postpartum. An estimated 40,000 infants are born with CMV infection in the United States annually.

*Clinical Manifestations*

- **Maternal infection:** In immunocompetent adults, CMV infection is typically silent. Symptoms, however, can be flu-like, including fever, malaise, swollen glands, and rarely hepatitis. After the primary infection, the virus becomes dormant, with periodic episodes of reactivation and viral shedding.
- **Congenital (fetal) infection:** Most fetal infections are due to recurrent maternal infection and lead to congenital abnormalities in approximately 1.4% of cases. Previously acquired maternal immunity confers protection from clinically apparent disease by maternal antibodies. Mothers determined to be seronegative for CMV before conception or early in gestation have a 1% to 4% risk of acquiring the infection during pregnancy and 30% rate of fetal transmission after seroconversion.
  - Approximately 90% of infants with congenital CMV infection will be asymptomatic at birth. Ten percent to 15% of these may later develop symptoms including developmental delay, hearing loss, and visual and dental defects.
  - Unlike recurrent infection, primary maternal infection during pregnancy can often lead to serious neonatal sequelae with neonatal mortality of approximately 5% but as high as 30% in some investigations. Approximately 5% to 20% of newborns of mothers with primary CMV infection are overtly symptomatic at birth. Infection in the first trimester leads to higher risk of sequelae than in the third trimester.
  - The most common clinical findings at birth include the presence of petechiae, hepatosplenomegaly or jaundice, and chorioretinitis. These symptoms constitute fulminant cytomegalic inclusion disease. Infants show signs of respiratory distress, lethargy, and seizures. Long-term sequelae include mental retardation, motor disabilities, and hearing and visual loss.

*Diagnosis*

- **Maternal** CMV screening is not routine. Women at high risk, such as day care workers and health care providers, should be offered testing with both immunoglobulin G and M (IgG and IgM). Screening may also be indicated as part of the workup for mononucleosis-like symptoms. Presence of CMV IgM is not helpful for timing the onset of infection because it is present in only 75% to 90% of women with acute infection, can remain positive following acute infection, and may represent reactivation or reinfection with a different strain. High anti-CMV IgG avidity suggests that the primary infection occurred more than 6 months in the past, while low avidity suggest the primary infection was more recent.
- **Fetal** ultrasound may demonstrate microcephaly, ventriculomegaly, intracranial calcifications, oligohydramnios, and intrauterine growth restriction. Amniocentesis

and cordocentesis for polymerase chain reaction (PCR) DNA testing have also been used to diagnose intrauterine infection.

## Management

- There is no effective in utero therapy for CMV. Because it is difficult to predict the severity of sequelae, counseling patients appropriately about pregnancy termination is problematic. Limited studies have suggested a role for hyperimmunoglobulin therapy, while use is limited to a case-by-case base until further research confirm that benefits outweigh risks. Use of antiviral drugs in immunocompetent individuals is not indicated. The majority of infected fetuses do not suffer serious sequelae. The benefits of breast-feeding outweigh the risk of infection transmission by breast-feeding and may be encouraged.

## Prevention

- CMV transmission requires close personal contact or contact with contaminated bodily fluids. Preventive measures include transfusing only CMV-negative blood products, safe sex practices, and frequent hand washing.

## Varicella Zoster Virus

### Epidemiology

- **Primary varicella infection** is estimated to affect only 1 to 5 of every 10,000 pregnancies. Less than 2% of cases occur in adults, but this group represents 25% of mortality from **varicella zoster virus (VZV). Herpes zoster** is also uncommon in women of childbearing age.
- The major mode of transmission is respiratory, although direct contact with vesicular or pustular lesions may also result in disease. In the past, nearly all persons were infected before adulthood, 90% before age 14 years. Since the advent of varicella vaccine, most people in the United States have vaccine-induced immunity.
- Varicella outbreaks occur most frequently during the winter and spring. The incubation period is 10 to 21 days. Infectivity is greatest 24 to 48 hours before the onset of rash and lasts 3 to 4 days into the rash. The virus is rarely isolated after the lesions have crusted over.

### Clinical Manifestations

- **Maternal:** The characteristic pruritic rash starts as macules, evolves into papules, and then vesicles. Primary varicella infection tends to be more severe in adults than in children and can be especially severe in pregnancy. A particularly morbid complication of VZV in pregnancy is **varicella pneumonia**. Maternal mortality with varicella pneumonia may reach 40% in the absence of antiviral therapy (3% to 14% with antiviral therapy). In contrast, herpes zoster infection (reactivation of varicella) is more common in older and immunocompromised patients and poses little risk to the fetus.
- **Congenital:** Fetal infection with varicella zoster can occur in utero, intrapartum, or postpartum. Intrauterine infection infrequently causes congenital abnormalities including cutaneous scars, limb reduction anomalies, malformed digits, muscle atrophy, growth restriction, cataracts, chorioretinitis, microphthalmia, cortical atrophy, microcephaly, and psychomotor retardation.
  - The risk of congenital malformation after fetal exposure to primary maternal varicella before 20 weeks' gestation is estimated to be <2% and is <0.4% before 12 weeks.
  - Infection after 20 weeks' gestation may lead to postnatal disease, with symptoms ranging from typical varicella with a benign course to fatal disseminated infection

or shingles appearing months to years after birth. If maternal infection occurs within 5 days of delivery, hematogenous transplacental viral transfer may cause significant infant morbidity and neonatal mortality rates as high as 25%. Sufficient transplacental antibody transfer to confer fetal immunity requires at least 5 days after the onset of the maternal rash. Women who develop chickenpox, especially near term, should be observed. Delay in delivery may offer the fetus the benefit of passive immunity. Neonatal therapy with immunoglobulin is also important when a mother develops signs of chickenpox within 3 days postpartum. Herpes zoster infection during pregnancy is not associated with fetal sequelae due to maternal antibody transfer.

## Diagnosis

- **Clinical:** The diagnosis of acute varicella zoster in the mother usually can be established by the characteristic cutaneous manifestations described as chickenpox. The generalized vesicular rash usually appears on the head and ears and then spreads to the face, trunk, and extremities. Mucous membrane involvement is common. Vesicles and pustules evolve into crusted lesions, which then heal and may scar. Herpes zoster, or shingles, demonstrates a unilateral vesicular eruption in a dermatomal distribution.
- **Laboratory:** Confirmation of the diagnosis may be obtained by examining scrapings of vesicular lesions that will reveal multinucleated giant cells. For rapid diagnosis, varicella zoster antigen may be demonstrated in exfoliated cells from lesions by immunofluorescent antibody staining.
- **Ultrasonography:** Detailed ultrasonographic examination is the best means for assessing a fetus for major limb abnormalities or growth disturbances associated with varicella infection. Ultrasound findings in combination with PCR testing of amniotic fluid can estimate the risk of intrauterine infection and the congenital syndrome.

## Management

- **Varicella exposure during pregnancy:** An IgG titer should be obtained within 24 to 48 hours of exposure to a person with noncrusted lesions. The presence of IgG reflects prior immunity, whereas absence of varicella IgG indicates susceptibility.
- **Varicella zoster immune globulin (VZIG)** may be administered to susceptible women (i.e., women without detectable varicella IgG) within 72 hours of exposure to reduce the severity of maternal infection. VZIG is administered intramuscularly (IM) at a dose of 125 U/10 kg to a maximum of 625 U. Maternal administration of VZIG, however, does not ameliorate or prevent fetal infection.
- Usually, the disease course is similar in pregnant and nonpregnant patients. Supportive care with fluids and analgesics should be administered. In addition, oral acyclovir, when started within 72 hours of symptom onset, has been shown to be associated with faster healing of lesions, shorter fever times, and less progression to pneumonia. It has low rates of teratogenicity, and its use is recommended by the American College of Obstetricians and Gynecologists (ACOG).
- Varicella pneumonia is a medical emergency with significant risk for mortality. Patients should be admitted to the hospital for treatment with intravenous (IV) acyclovir. Acyclovir administered to pregnant women with varicella pneumonia during the second or third trimester decreases maternal morbidity and mortality. The dosage of acyclovir is 10 to 15 mg/kg IV every 8 hours for 7 days, or 800 mg by mouth (PO) five times per day. Tocolytics are generally avoided in women with varicella pneumonia. Delivery should be performed for obstetric indications.

*Prevention*

- Preconception counseling plays an important role in prevention of VZV. An **attenuated live vaccine** was approved by the U.S. Food and Drug Administration (FDA) in 1995. One dose is recommended for all children between ages 1 and 12 years. Two doses, given 4 to 8 weeks apart, are recommended for adolescents and adults without history of varicella infection. The seroconversion rate after vaccination is approximately 82% in adults and 91% for children. Use of the vaccine during pregnancy is not recommended, but it is appropriate for breast-feeding mothers.

## Parvovirus B19

*Epidemiology*

- Parvovirus B19 is a single-stranded DNA virus passed primarily by respiratory secretions. Also known as *erythema infectiosum* or *fifth disease*, it commonly occurs in school-aged children. By adulthood, 30% to 60% of women have acquired immunity (IgG) to the virus. Outbreaks usually occur in the midwinter to spring months. Prevalence in pregnancy is approximately 3.3% and is highest among teachers, day care workers, and homemakers.

*Clinical Manifestations*

- **Maternal:** Adults may present with typical clinical features: a red, macular rash and facial erythroderma, which gives a characteristic "slapped cheek" appearance. The rash may also cover the trunk and extremities. Infected adults often have acute joint swelling, usually with symmetric involvement of peripheral joints. The arthritis may be severe and chronic. Cases may also present with constitutional symptoms of fever, malaise, myalgia, and headaches. Some adults have a completely asymptomatic infection. Parvovirus B19 preferentially affects rapidly dividing cells and is cytotoxic to erythroid progenitor cells. It may cause aplastic crisis in patients with chronic anemia (e.g., sickle cell disease or thalassemia).
- **Congenital:** Approximately one third of maternal infections are associated with fetal infection via transplacental transfer of the virus. Infection of fetal red blood cell precursors can result in fetal anemia, which, if severe, leads to nonimmune hydrops fetalis. Hydrops can lead to rapid fetal death or can resolve spontaneously. In cases of mild to moderate hydrops, approximately one third resolves; this number decreases in cases of severe hydrops. The likelihood of severe fetal disease is increased if maternal infection occurs during the first 18 weeks of pregnancy, but the risk of hydrops fetalis persists even when infection occurs in the late third trimester. Fetal IgM production after 18 weeks' gestation probably contributes to the resolution of infection in fetuses who survive. The overall risk of fetal death after maternal infection before 20 weeks is 6% to 11% and after 20 weeks' gestation is <1%. Parvovirus B19 infection has not been directly associated with specific congenital abnormalities.

*Diagnosis*

- The illness may be suspected if a regional outbreak is ongoing or if family members are affected. Children are the most common vectors for parvovirus B19 transmission.
- A pregnant woman who has been exposed to fifth disease and presents with clinical symptoms or who has a known history of chronic hemolytic anemia and presents

with an aplastic crisis should be evaluated with parvovirus B19 immunoglobulin titers. Parvovirus B19 IgM appears 3 days after the onset of illness, peaks in 30 to 60 days, and may persist for 3 to 4 months. Parvovirus B19 IgG is usually detected by the seventh day of illness and persists for years. PCR of amniotic fluid can be used to detect fetal infection in a woman who was recently exposed or has ultrasound findings of fetal hydrops.

*Management*
- No specific antiviral therapy exists for parvovirus B19 infection. IV gamma globulin may be administered on an empiric basis to immunocompromised patients with known exposure to parvovirus B19 and should be used for treatment of women in aplastic crisis with viremia.
- Parvovirus B19 can infect the fetal bone marrow, which may lead to severe fetal anemia. Therefore, when maternal infection is confirmed, serial screening sonograms should be performed to assess for fetal signs such as hydrops. Hydrops fetalis usually develops within 6 weeks but can develop as late as 10 weeks after maternal infection. Fetal middle cerebral artery (MCA) Doppler evaluation can be used to predict fetal anemia. Weekly or biweekly ultrasonographic scans can be useful.
- If severe anemia is suspected based on ultrasound findings, then fetal hemoglobin levels may be determined with percutaneous umbilical vein sampling. Intrauterine blood transfusion can be used to correct fetal anemia and hydrops. Single or serial intrauterine transfusions may be undertaken.

*Prevention*
- Conscientious hand washing and avoiding known infected contacts are advised.

## Rubella Virus
*Epidemiology*
- Despite widespread immunization programs in the United States, the Centers for Disease Control and Prevention (CDC) reports 10% to 20% of adults remain susceptible to rubella. The annual number of reported cases in the United States, however, remains extremely low, with fewer than 10 cases of congenital rubella occurring annually. The disease remains endemic in many areas of the world, and positive rubella antibodies in individuals from these areas can represent active infection.

*Clinical Manifestations*
The disease is communicable for 1 week before and for 4 days after the onset of the rash, with the most contagious period occurring a few days before the onset of the maculopapular rash. The incubation period ranges from 14 to 21 days. Transmission results from direct contact with the nasopharyngeal secretions of an infected person.
- **Maternal:** Rubella usually presents as a maculopapular rash that persists for 3 days; generalized lymphadenopathy (especially postauricular and occipital), which may precede the rash; transient arthritis; malaise; and headache. Rubella typically follows the same mild course in pregnancy and may be asymptomatic. The majority of women with affected infants report no history of a rash during their pregnancies.

- **Congenital:** Maternal viremia leads to fetal infection in 25% to 90% of cases. Fetal sequelae are dependent on gestational age, with 90% of first-trimester exposures resulting in clinical signs, 54% at 13 to 14 weeks, and 25% by the end of the second trimester. Congenital rubella syndrome involves multiple organs. The most common manifestations are sensorineural hearing loss, developmental delay, growth retardation, and cardiac and ophthalmic defects.
- As many as one third of asymptomatic exposed infants may develop late manifestations, including diabetes mellitus, thyroid disorders, and precocious puberty. The extended rubella syndrome (progressive panencephalitis and type 1 diabetes mellitus) may develop as late as the second or third decade of life.

*Diagnosis*

- Infection is confirmed by serology. Specimens should be obtained as soon as possible after exposure, 2 weeks later, and, if necessary, 4 weeks after exposure. Serum specimens from both acute and convalescent phases should be tested; a fourfold or greater increase in titer or seroconversion indicates acute infection. If the patient is IgG-seropositive on the first titer, no risk to the fetus is apparent. Primary rubella confers lifelong immunity. Reinfection with rubella is usually subclinical, rarely associated with viremia, and infrequently results in a congenitally infected infant.
- Prenatal diagnosis is made by identification of rubella-specific IgM antibody in fetal blood samples obtained at 22 weeks' gestation or later. IgM does not cross the placenta, and therefore, its presence indicates fetal infection.

*Management*

- If a pregnant woman is exposed to rubella, serologic evaluation is recommended. If primary rubella is diagnosed, the mother should be informed about the implications of the infection for the fetus including the high rate of fetal infection and the option for termination discussed. Women electing to continue the pregnancy may be given immune globulin, which may modify clinical rubella in the mother. Immune globulin, however, does not prevent infection or viremia and affords no protection to the fetus.

*Prevention*

- Pregnant women should undergo rubella serum evaluation as part of routine prenatal care. A clinical history of rubella is unreliable. If the patient is nonimmune, she should receive rubella vaccine after delivery. The rubella vaccine is a live attenuated virus, so it should be avoided in pregnancy due to the theoretic risk of teratogenicity. The CDC maintains a registry to monitor fetal effects of vaccination, and there have been no reported cases of congenital rubella syndrome after vaccination. Nonetheless, the CDC recommends contraception for 28 days after vaccination.

## Influenza

*Epidemiology*

In recent years, the number of cases of influenza has increased in the general population. The pattern of outbreaks is determined by the changing antigenic properties of the virus and their effect on the transmissibility and infectivity of the virus. During pregnancy, physiologic changes make women more likely to become infected with influenza and more likely to have severe infection with significant morbidity and mortality.

### Clinical Manifestations

- **Maternal:** Clinical manifestations of influenza in pregnancy are similar to the general population. The symptoms include fever, cough, rhinorrhea, sore throat, myalgia, and headaches. During the pandemics of 1918, 1957, and 2009, pregnant women were noted to have a disproportionate risk of mortality compared to the general population.
- **Fetal:** There is some evidence that pandemic influenza infection may increase the risk of spontaneous abortion, preterm delivery, and low-birth-weight fetuses. However, this is not well studied.

### Management/Prevention

Antiviral therapies have not been well studied but can be used for postexposure chemoprophylaxis and treatment of influenza. Oseltamivir 75 mg daily for 10 days and zanamivir 10 mg daily are currently used. The CDC maintains a website with up-to-date treatment recommendations: http://www.cdc.gov/flu/antivirals/index .htm. Treatment is otherwise supportive with antipyretics and fluids. The CDC and ACOG recommend use of the trivalent inactivated influenza vaccine at any point during pregnancy.

## Hepatitis A Virus

### Epidemiology

- An estimated 200,000 cases of **hepatitis A virus (HAV)** infection occur annually in the United States, and HAV affects approximately 1 in 1,000 pregnancies. HAV is transmitted primarily through fecal–oral contamination and typically is not excreted in urine or other bodily fluids. Obstetric patients at highest risk of developing HAV infection are those who have emigrated from or traveled to countries where the virus is endemic (e.g., Southeast Asia, Africa, Central America, Mexico, and the Middle East).

### Clinical Manifestations

- **Maternal:** Symptoms of HAV infection include malaise, fatigue, anorexia, nausea, and abdominal pain, typically right upper quadrant or epigastric. Physical findings include jaundice, upper abdominal tenderness, and hepatomegaly.
- **Congenital:** Perinatal transmission of HAV has not been documented.

### Diagnosis

- A complete travel history suggests the diagnosis in a jaundiced patient. Laboratory studies may reveal transaminitis (elevated alanine aminotransferase [ALT] and aspartate aminotransferase [AST]) and hyperbilirubinemia. Abnormal coagulation studies and hyperammonemia may suggest more significant liver injury. The presence of IgM antibody to HAV confirms the diagnosis. IgG antibody will persist in patients with a history of exposure.

### Management

- Individuals with close personal or sexual contact with an affected individual may receive HAV immune globulin in a single IM dose.

- Treatment of HAV is supportive. There is no antiviral therapy. Activity level should be decreased, and upper abdominal trauma should be avoided. Patients with hepatitis-induced encephalopathy or coagulopathy and debilitated patients should be hospitalized.

*Prevention*

- The HAV vaccine, an inactivated vaccine, may be used in pregnancy. The vaccine is recommended for individuals traveling to endemic areas and is administered in two injections 4 to 6 months apart.

## Hepatitis B Virus

*Epidemiology*

- In North America, **hepatitis B virus (HBV)** transmission occurs most commonly via parenteral exposure or sexual contact. Approximately 43,000 persons in the United States are newly diagnosed each year, with an estimated 2.2 million chronic carriers. Acute HBV occurs in 1 to 2 per 1,000 pregnancies and chronic HBV in 5 to 15 per 1,000. Mother-to-child transmission (MTCT) is an important cause of chronic HBV infection worldwide. Transmission can occur prenatally, during delivery, or postpartum and is highest in women who are HBV envelope antigen (HBeAg)-positive. The vertical transmission rate in these women is as high as 90% in the puerperium if prophylaxis is not given to their neonates.

- **Natural history:** HBV contains three principal antigens: HBV surface antigen (HBsAg), HBV core antigen (HBcAg), and HBeAg. HBsAg is detectable in serum during acute and chronic infection. HBcAg compromises the central nucleocapsid of the virus; it is found only in hepatocytes during active viral replication and is not detected in serum. HBeAg is a secretory product that is processed from the precore protein; it is a marker of active HBV replication and increased infectivity. The presence of HBeAg is usually associated with high levels of HBV DNA in serum and higher rates of HBV transmission. Circulating antibodies against these viral antigens develop in response to infection.

*Clinical Manifestations*

- **Maternal:** The clinical manifestations of HBV during pregnancy are similar to those for the nonpregnant patient. HBV infection presents with nonhepatic prodromal symptoms, including rash, arthralgia, myalgia, and occasionally frank arthritis. Jaundice occurs in a minority of patients. In adults, between 95% and 99% of acute infections resolve completely, and the patient develops protective levels of antibody. The remaining 1% to 5% of patients become chronically infected. These patients are clinically asymptomatic and usually have normal liver function tests. They nonetheless have detectable levels of HBsAg. The incidence of cirrhosis in a chronic HBV carrier is 8% to 20% over 5 years. Acute hepatitis B carries a 1% risk of maternal mortality. Physiologic changes in immunity, metabolism, and hemodynamics during pregnancy may unmask underlying liver disease in otherwise asymptomatic patients.

- **Fetal infection:** Maternal–fetal transmission can occur at any time during pregnancy but most commonly occurs at the time of delivery. In women who are seropositive for both HBsAg and HBeAg (indicating active replication), the vertical transmission rate approaches 90%. However, in a woman who is HBsAg-positive and anti-HBV surface antibody–positive with an undetectable hepatitis B viral load (carrier state), the risk of transmission drops to 10% to 30%. The frequency of vertical transmission is also affected by the timing of maternal infection. When maternal infection occurs in the first trimester, 10% of neonates are seropositive; when it occurs in the third trimester, 80% to 90% of neonates are infected. Whether infection occurs in utero or intrapartum, the presence of HBeAg in the neonates carries an 85% to 90% likelihood of progression to chronic HBV infection and the associated hepatic sequelae. Prophylactic administration of hepatitis B immunoglobulin to infants after birth reduces transmission from 5% to 10%. Fetal malformation, intrauterine growth restriction, spontaneous abortion, or stillbirth is not associated with HBV infection.

### Diagnosis

- Diagnosis is confirmed by serology.
- HBsAg appears in the serum 1 to 10 weeks after an acute exposure prior to the onset of clinical symptoms then becomes undetectable after 4 to 6 months in patients who eventually recover. Persistence of HBsAg for >6 months implies chronic infection.
- The disappearance of HBsAg is followed by the appearance of anti-HBs. In most patients, anti-HBs persist for life, conferring long-term immunity.
- HBeAg is detected during active viral replication. The disappearance of HBeAg and the appearance of anti-HBeAg IgG signal a decrease in infectivity. The presence of anti-HBsAg IgG indicates immunity or recovery.
- If a patient is tested during the period in which results for HBsAg are negative, HBV can be identified by the presence of anti-HBsAg IgM.

### Management

- Patients with acute hepatitis B infection may require hospitalization and supportive care. The disease is generally self-limited, and symptoms resolve within 1 to 2 weeks. Therapeutic options for HBV include antiviral nucleoside analogues and pegylated interferon. These therapies have the theoretical risk of teratogenicity but have been shown to be safe.
- Current CDC recommendations include universal screening of all pregnant women for HBV at the first prenatal visit. Serum transaminase levels should be measured in seropositive patients to assess active chronic hepatitis.
- Women exposed to HBV should receive passive immunization with HBV immune globulin (HBIG) and receive recombinant HBV vaccine, preferably in the contralateral arm. HBIG is 75% effective in preventing maternal HBV infection.
- HBIG should be administered to the neonate of an infected mother within the first 12 hours of life. HBIG is followed immediately by the standard three-dose HBV immunization series. The combination of HBIG and HBV vaccine prevents vertical transmission in 85% to 90% of cases.
- Invasive intrapartum fetal monitoring (fetal scalp electrodes or fetal scalp blood sampling) should be avoided if maternal infection is known to help minimize vertical transmission risk.

### Prevention

- Vaccination for hepatitis B is recommended for all women of reproductive age, preferably during preconception or routine gynecologic care but is also safe to use during pregnancy.

## Hepatitis C Virus

*Epidemiology*

- Transmission of the **hepatitis C virus (HCV)** is similar to that of HBV but occurs via percutaneous blood contamination and rarely through sexual contact. An increased incidence of HCV is noted among IV drug abusers and recipients of blood products. Mass screening of the blood supply for HCV has markedly decreased the risk of HCV infection to <1 per 1,000,000 screened units of blood.

*Clinical Manifestations*

- **Maternal:** Acute HCV infection presents after an incubation period of 30 to 60 days. Asymptomatic infection occurs in 75% of patients, and at least 50% of infected individuals progress to chronic infection, regardless of the mode of acquisition or severity of initial infection. Of these patients, approximately 20% subsequently develop chronic active hepatitis or cirrhosis. Concomitant infection with HIV may accelerate the progression and severity of hepatic injury. Unlike HBV antibodies, antibodies to HCV are not protective. HCV causes acute hepatitis in pregnancy but may go undetected if liver function tests and HCV antibody tests are not performed.
- **Congenital:** Vertical transmission is proportional to the maternal serum HCV viral RNA titer. Transmission is approximately 2% in women with HCV viremia and is approximately 19% in the setting of maternal coinfection with HIV. Higher HCV RNA levels in pregnancy are associated with vertical transmission. Currently, there is no method or technique to prevent prenatal transmission. If transmission occurs transplacentally, the neonate is at increased risk of acute hepatitis and of probable chronic hepatitis or carrier status. To date, no teratogenic syndromes associated with HCV have been described.

*Diagnosis*

- Anti-HCV antibody is detected in serum but may take up to 1 year from exposure to test positive. HCV viral RNA can be detected by PCR assay of serum soon after infection and in chronic disease and can be used to quantify active viral replication (see Table 11-1).

*Management*

- Because there is no prophylaxis for transmission, primary prevention of maternal infection is the mainstay of management. Treatment with interferon alpha in pregnant women has not been well studied and is generally considered contraindicated. During labor, invasive procedures such as a fetal scalp electrode or fetal scalp blood sampling should be avoided. Prolonged rupture of membranes has been shown to increase transmission in several studies. According to CDC guidelines, maternal infection with hepatitis C is not an absolute contraindication to breast-feeding.

## Herpes Simplex Virus

*Epidemiology*

- Type 1 **herpes simplex virus (HSV)** is responsible for most nongenital herpetic infections and up to 50% of genital lesions. Type 2 HSV is usually recovered from the genital tract. Approximately 1 in 7,500 live-born infants contract HSV perinatally. Whether pregnancy alters the rate of recurrence or frequency of cervical

| TABLE 11-1 | Interpretation of Hepatitis Serology Results |

| Significance | Anti-HAV IgM | HBsAg | HBeAg | Anti-HBcAg IgG | Anti-HBcAg IgM | Anti-HBsAg IgG | Anti-HCV IgG/IgM |
|---|---|---|---|---|---|---|---|
| Acute HAV infection | + | − | − | − | − | − | − |
| Acute HBV infection | − | + | + | − | + | − | − |
| Chronic HBV infection, active replication | − | + | + | + | − | − | − |
| Chronic HBV infection, quiescent | − | + | − | + | − | − | − |
| HBV infection, resolved | − | − | − | − | − | + | − |
| Post-HBV vaccine | − | − | − | − | − | + | − |
| Acute or chronic HCV infection | − | − | − | − | − | − | + |

+, present; −, absent; HAV, hepatitis A virus; IgM, immunoglobulin M; HBsAg, hepatitis B surface antigen; HBeAg, hepatitis B envelope antigen; HBcAg, hepatitis B core antigen; IgG, immunoglobulin G; HCV, hepatitis C virus; HBV, hepatitis B virus.

shedding of virus is debated. The incidence of asymptomatic shedding in pregnancy is 10% after a first episode and 0.5% after a recurrent episode.
- Primary maternal infection with HSV results from direct contact with mucous membranes or skin infected with the virus, commonly through sexual contact.
- Fetal infection with HSV can occur transplacentally, as an ascending infection from the cervix, or most commonly through direct contact with infectious maternal genital lesions during delivery.

*Clinical Manifestations*
- **Maternal:** Primary infections range from mild or asymptomatic to severe. Vesicles appear on the cervix, vagina, or vulva from 2 to 10 days after exposure. Swelling, erythema, pain, and regional lymphadenopathy are common. The lesions persist for 1 to 3 weeks with concomitant viral shedding. Reactivation occurs in 50% of patients within 6 months of the initial outbreak and subsequently at irregular intervals. Symptoms of recurrent outbreaks are generally milder, with viral shedding lasting less than a week. In pregnancy, primary outbreaks are not associated with spontaneous abortion but may increase the incidence of preterm labor in the latter half of pregnancy.

• **Fetal** infection is usually the result of primary maternal infection. Transmission from a recurrent maternal infection is rare, accounting for <1% of fetal infections. The most common form of transmission is direct contact with vaginal secretions during delivery. Viral shedding during labor is the strongest predictor of transmission, with 5% of neonates becoming infected. Overall, congenital infections are very rare, and few are asymptomatic. The majority ultimately produce disseminated or central nervous system (CNS) disease. Localized infection is usually associated with a good outcome, but infants with disseminated infection have a mortality rate of 60%, even with treatment. At least half of infants surviving disseminated infection develop serious neurologic and ophthalmic sequelae.

*Diagnosis*
• When HSV is suspected, a swab specimen may be obtained from the lesion for culture and immunofluorescent or PCR studies. Seven to 10 days must be allowed for isolation of the virus via tissue culture, but the sensitivity is 95% and specificity is also high. Serology is of limited value in diagnosis because a single antibody titer is not predictive of viral shedding and IgG will be positive indefinitely after the primary outbreak. Smears of scrapings from the bases of vesicles may be stained using the Tzanck or Papanicolaou technique. PCR for HSV DNA is sensitive and rapid.

*Management*
• Patients with a history of genital herpes should undergo a careful perineal examination at the time of delivery. Vaginal delivery is permitted if no signs or symptoms of HSV are present. Active genital HSV in patients in labor or with ruptured membranes at or near term is an indication for cesarean section, regardless of the duration of rupture. Evidence shows that HSV recurrences in the regions of the buttocks, thighs, and anus are associated with low rates of cervical virus shedding. Lesions in these areas should not preclude a vaginal delivery; however, it is recommended that the lesion(s) be covered for delivery. Acyclovir may be used to treat HSV infection in pregnancy; however, valacyclovir hydrochloride (Valtrex) is more easily tolerated due to a twice-daily dosing schedule. Third-trimester suppression with valacyclovir, 500 mg PO daily or twice daily, should be considered in women with frequent outbreaks during their pregnancies.

*Prevention*
• Barrier contraception can be recommended to avoid primary maternal infection as part of routine safe sex counseling.

## PROTOZOA

### Toxoplasma
*Epidemiology*
• In the United States, the incidence of acute **toxoplasmosis** infection in pregnancy is estimated at 0.2% to 1.0%. Congenital toxoplasmosis occurs in 1 to 8 per 1,000 live births. The infective agent is the oocyst, shed by the alimentary tract of cats. Transmission occurs primarily by eating undercooked or raw meat containing cysts, ingesting food or water contaminated by the oocyst of an infected cat,

inhaling aerosolized oocysts from cat litter, or handling material contaminated by the feces of an infected cat. Approximately one third of American women carry antibodies to *Toxoplasma gondii*.

## Clinical Manifestations

- **Maternal:** Up to 90% of acute toxoplasmosis infections are asymptomatic. A mononucleosis-like syndrome, including fatigue, malaise, cervical lymphadenopathy, sore throat, and atypical lymphocytosis, may occur. Placental infection and subsequent fetal infection occur during the spreading phase of the parasitemia.
- **Congenital:** The rate of fetal transmission is approximately 15% in the first trimester, 30% in the second trimester, and 70% in the third trimester. Fetal morbidity and mortality rates are higher after early transmission, with 11% risk of perinatal death from infection in the first trimester, 4% in the second trimester, and minimal to zero in the third trimester. Infected neonates often exhibit low birth weight, hepatosplenomegaly, icterus, and anemia. Sequelae such as vision loss and psychomotor and mental retardation are common. Hearing loss is demonstrated in 10% to 30% and developmental delay in 20% to 75%. Up to 90% of infants with congenital toxoplasmosis are asymptomatic at birth.

## Diagnosis

- Screening for toxoplasmosis is not routine in the United States. Because most women with acute toxoplasmosis are asymptomatic, the diagnosis is not suspected until an affected infant is born. For women who do present with symptoms of acute infection, both IgM and IgG titers should be measured as soon as possible (Table 11-2).
- Negative IgM excludes acute or recent infection, unless the serum has been tested so early that an immune response has not yet been mounted. A positive test is more difficult to interpret because IgM may be elevated for more than a year after infection. Seroconversion of IgG on repeat testing can be useful as well.
- PCR testing for toxoplasma DNA can be performed on amniotic fluid. This is the best method for confirming congenital infection.
- Sonographic findings include bilateral dilated cerebral ventricles, intracranial and intrahepatic lesions, and placental hyperdensities. Occasionally, pericardial and pleural effusions are observed.

| **TABLE 11-2** | Interpretation of *Toxoplasma* Serology Results | |
|---|---|---|
| **IgM**[a] | **IgG** | **Interpretation** |
| + | − | Possible acute infection; IgG titers should be reassessed in several weeks |
| + | + | Possible acute infection |
| − | + | Remote infection |
| − | − | Susceptible; uninfected |

[a]IgM titers may remain elevated for up to 1 year. IgM, immunoglobulin M; IgG, immunoglobulin G; +, positive; −, negative.

*Management*

- For women who elect to continue their pregnancies after a diagnosis of toxoplasmosis, therapy should be started immediately and continued in the infant for 1 year or more to decrease risk for developmental sequelae. There is debate concerning the effectiveness of antibiotics, but the mainstay of treatment is spiramycin, pyrimethamine, and sulfadiazine.
- **Spiramycin** reduces the incidence but not necessarily the severity of fetal infection. It is recommended for the treatment of acute maternal infections diagnosed before the third trimester and should then be continued for the duration of the pregnancy. If amniotic fluid PCR results for *Toxoplasma* are negative, spiramycin is used as a single agent; if results are positive, pyrimethamine and sulfadiazine should be added. Spiramycin dosing is 500 mg PO five times daily, or 3 g/day in divided doses.
- **Pyrimethamine and sulfadiazine:** Patients with documented *T gondii* infection of the fetus may be offered treatment with pyrimethamine 25 mg PO daily and sulfadiazine PO 1 g four times daily for 28 days. Folinic acid, 6 mg IM or PO, is administered three times per week to prevent toxicity. During the first trimester, pyrimethamine is not recommended due to teratogenic risk. Sulfadiazine is omitted from the regimen at term.

*Prevention*

- Pregnant women should eat only fully cooked meats, wash their hands after preparing meat for cooking, wash fruits and vegetables well, and avoid contact with cat litter boxes.

## BACTERIA

### Group B *Streptococcus*

*Epidemiology*

- **Group B *Streptococcus* (GBS)** (*Streptococcus agalactiae*), a Gram-positive bacteria, can be isolated from the vagina and/or rectum in 5% to 40% of pregnant women in the United States. Neonatal colonization may occur as a result of ascending infection from the maternal genital tract or during passage of the fetus through the birth canal during a vaginal delivery. The vertical transmission rate may be as high as 72%, but invasive disease in term neonates is rare. In preterm infants, however, invasive disease is more common and is accompanied by significant morbidity and mortality.

*Clinical Manifestations*

- **Maternal:** GBS is a common urinary pathogen in pregnant women. GBS is isolated in 5% to 29% of cases of asymptomatic bacteriuria and in 1% to 5% of cases of acute cystitis during pregnancy. When inadequately treated, both asymptomatic bacteriuria and acute cystitis can progress to pyelonephritis, necessitating hospitalization. Maternal GBS infection has also been associated with premature rupture of membranes, preterm labor, chorioamnionitis, bacteremia, puerperal endometritis, and postoperative wound infections after cesarean section.
- **Congenital:** Neonatal colonization with GBS results from contamination from the mother's genital tract in 75% of cases. One percent to 2% of colonized infants will develop early-onset GBS infection (infection occurring within the first 7 days of life), with a case fatality of 11% to 50%. Preterm and/or low-birth-weight

infants are at higher risk than term neonates. Maternal risk factors that predispose a neonate to early-onset GBS infection include preterm delivery, prolonged rupture of membranes (>18 hours), intrapartum temperature of at least 38°C or 100.4°F, or a prior infant who had GBS infection.

- Late-onset GBS infection, which occurs 7 days or more after birth, affects 0.5 to 1.8 per 1,000 live births. It may result from maternal–neonatal transmission, nosocomial, or community contacts. Mortality for late-onset disease is approximately 10%.
- Meningitis occurs in 85% of all colonized neonates, but infants may also present with bacteremia without localizing symptoms. Other clinical syndromes include pneumonia, osteomyelitis, cellulitis, and sepsis. Neurologic sequelae develop in 15% to 30% of meningitis survivors.

*Diagnosis*

- GBS colonization can be detected by culture or rapid DNA-based testing. Anorectovaginal culture remains the gold standard and can be performed in a single swab of the areas. Samples must be inoculated immediately into Todd-Hewitt broth or onto selective blood agar to inhibit the growth of competing organisms. The predominant limitation of culture is time. Results are not available for 24 to 48 hours, making management difficult if delivery is imminent. Rapid diagnostic tests are available that detect specific polysaccharide antigens. They are easy to perform, generally less expensive than a culture, and produce results within a short period of time (usually 1 hour). The tests are highly sensitive in patients who are heavily colonized with GBS; however, their lower sensitivity and higher false-negative rate compared with those of cultures prevent their widespread clinical application in obstetrics. Rapid DNA-based testing is also available with excellent sensitivity.

*Management*

- Treatment of uncomplicated GBS lower urinary tract infection is with amoxicillin or penicillin. Hospitalization is required for cases of pyelonephritis, and patients should be treated with an appropriate regimen until afebrile and asymptomatic for 24 to 48 hours. She may then be discharged to complete a total of 10 days of antibiotics.
- ACOG recommends universal screening for GBS at 35 to 37 weeks' gestation with a swab of the lower vagina and rectum. Women with a positive screen, a previous infant with GBS infection, urine colonization (>10,000 colony-forming units (CFUs)/mL) or infection with GBS during the current pregnancy, labor before 37 weeks with unknown GBS status, rupture of membranes >18 hours at term with unknown GBS status, or signs of chorioamnionitis should receive intrapartum antibiotics. Treatment is typically with penicillin 5-million-U IV loading dose followed by 2.5 million U IV every 4 hours. Prophylaxis is most effective if started at least 4 hours before delivery. For patients with a penicillin allergy, cephalosporins can be used if the allergy is mild as with a rash but should be avoided for more severe allergies that may lead to anaphylaxis. Genital culture results should be evaluated for sensitivity to clindamycin and erythromycin, where resistance to either precludes effectiveness of clindamycin. If culture results demonstrate resistance or sensitivities are unknown and the patient has a severe penicillin allergy, vancomycin should be administered.

## SEQUELAE OF PERINATAL INFECTIONS

Table 11-3 summarizes the **sequelae of the perinatal infections** discussed earlier.

| TABLE 11-3 | Maternal and Fetal Manifestations of Perinatal Infections | | |
|---|---|---|---|
| Infection | Maternal Disease | Fetal Sonographic Findings | Congenital Disease |
| Toxoplasmosis | Usually asymptomatic; may include mononucleosis-like syndrome | Nonspecific but may include intracranial calcification or ventricular dilatation | Usually asymptomatic at birth. Triad of congenital toxoplasmosis: chorioretinitis, hydrocephalus, and intracranial calcifications |
| Rubella | Maculopapular rash, generalized lymphadenopathy, low-grade fever, malaise | Increased risk of spontaneous abortion, stillbirth, and intrauterine growth restriction. No specific sonographic findings | Sensorineural deafness, cataracts, glaucoma, patent ductus arteriosus, peripheral pulmonary artery stenosis, mental retardation, growth restriction. Classic purpuric skin lesions at birth called "blueberry muffin" lesions |
| CMV | May be asymptomatic or may include fever, malaise, and lymphadenopathy. Rarely includes hepatitis | May present with microcephaly, hepatosplenomegaly, and intracranial calcification. Normal ultrasound does not exclude infection. | Up to 90% are asymptomatic at birth. Symptomatic infection includes petechiae, hepatosplenomegaly, jaundice, chorioretinitis, and seizures. |
| HSV | Usually localized vesicular lesions on cervix, vagina, or vulva. Disseminated disease is uncommon. | None | Most neonates appear normal at birth. Disease subsequently develops in one of three patterns: localized lesions on skin, eyes, and mouth; localized CNS disease; and disseminated multiorgan disease. |

| | | | |
|---|---|---|---|
| Varicella | Prodromal symptoms include fever, malaise, and myalgia followed by "chickenpox" vesicular rash. Risk of varicella pneumonia increased in pregnancy. | May include hypoplastic limbs, malformed digits, clubbed feet, microcephaly, intrauterine growth restriction | Dermatomal scarring, cataracts, chorioretinitis, Horner syndrome, microphthalmos, nystagmus, low birth weight, cortical atrophy, mental retardation, and hypoplastic limbs |
| Parvovirus B19 | Facial macular rash with "slapped cheek" appearance, arthritis, and rarely, aplastic anemia | Fetal anemia, which may lead to nonimmune hydrops fetalis. May also cause fetal hydrocephaly, cleft lip and palate, cardiomyopathy, and ocular defects when infection present in first trimester. | No specific congenital syndrome |
| GBS | Usually asymptomatic but may cause urinary tract infection | None | Early-onset disease may present as generalized sepsis, pneumonia, or meningitis. Late-onset disease most often presents as bacteremia without a focus. |

CMV, cytomegalovirus; HSV, herpes simplex virus; CNS, central nervous system; GBS, group B *Streptococcus*

## SUGGESTED READINGS

American College of Obstetricians and Gynecologists. ACOG practice bulletin. Perinatal viral and parasitic infections. Number 20, September 2000. (Replaces educational bulletin number 177, February 1993). *Int J Gynaecol Obstet* 2002;76(1):95–107.

Centers for Disease Control and Prevention. Perinatal group B streptococcal disease after universal screening recommendations—United States, 2003–2005. *MMWR Morb Mortal Wkly Rep* 2007;56(28):701–705.

Corey L, Wald A. Maternal and neonatal herpes simplex virus infections. *N Engl J Med* 2009;361(14):1376–1385.

Lin K, Vickery J. Screening for hepatitis B virus infection in pregnant women: evidence for the U.S. Preventive Services Task Force reaffirmation recommendation statement. *Ann Intern Med* 2009;150(12):874–876.

Malm G, Engman ML. Congenital cytomegalovirus infections. *Semin Fetal Neonatal Med* 2007;12(3):154–159.

Sharma D, Spearman P. The impact of cesarean delivery on transmission of infectious agents to the neonate. *Clin Perinatol* 2008;35(2):407–420.

Winn HN. Group B streptococcus infection in pregnancy. *Clin Perinatol* 2007;34(3):387–392.

# Congenital Anomalies

Jill Berkin and Melissa L. Russo

**Congenital anomalies** are among the most common causes of neonatal morbidity and mortality. According to the Centers for Disease Control and Prevention, they occur in 3% of live births and account for 25% of all pediatric hospital admissions. Birth defects can involve an isolated organ system or multiple organ systems; multiple anomalies may encompass a syndrome. The causes of congenital anomalies are genetic, environmental, or unknown etiology. There are multiple risk factors that have been associated with increased risk of congenital anomalies.

## ETIOLOGY

- Causes of congenital anomalies may be chromosomal, familial, multifactorial, or idiopathic; hence, obtaining a thorough family history and screening of low-risk populations are important.
- **Genetic etiologies** include the following: chromosomal disorders such as trisomy (e.g., Down syndrome), deletion (e.g., DiGeorge syndrome), or monosomy (e.g., Turner syndrome); monogenic disorders such as Noonan syndrome and Smith-Lemli-Opitz syndrome; and multifactorial disorders such as isolated congenital heart disease, cleft lip and palate, and arthrogryposis which result from interactions of several genes and environmental factors.
- **Nongenetic/environmental etiologies** include the following teratogens: ethanol, certain medications such as tretinoin (Retin-A) and warfarin (Coumadin), illicit

| TABLE 12-1 | Factors Associated with Increased Risk for Congenital Abnormalities |
|---|---|

Advanced maternal age (maternal age ≥35 years at time of delivery)
Pregestational diabetes
Exposure to a known teratogen
History of having a child with birth defect
Personal or family history of a known genetic abnormality (e.g., balanced translocation, mutation, or aneuploidy)
Abnormal serum screening
Multiple gestation
Assisted reproductive technology

drugs, maternal nutritional deficiencies, and maternal medical conditions such as diabetes and maternal infections such as toxoplasmosis or syphilis (see Chapter 11).
• Ninety percent of infants with congenital anomalies are born to women with no risk factors (Table 12-1).

## SCREENING AND MANAGEMENT

• Given the significant morbidity and mortality of congenital defects, all patients should be offered screening for fetal chromosomal abnormalities preferably during the first trimester and a level II anatomy ultrasound at 18 to 22 weeks. Detailed ultrasonography by an experienced technician can detect up to 80% of fetal anomalies, allowing the full range of management options: expectant management, in utero therapy, further workup (e.g., karyotyping, microarray and/or viral studies), and pregnancy termination.
• Management should include counseling that takes into consideration the fetus, the mother, and the family. Treatment options and prognosis should be discussed. With a fetal congenital anomaly, multidisciplinary approach facilitates a unified plan of care. The obstetrician or maternal fetal medicine (MFM) specialist can coordinate care with genetic counselors, neonatologists, and other pediatric specialists such as surgeons, cardiologists, urologists, and neurosurgeons. Social work and bereavement counseling can also be part of the care plan if indicated. The care plan must be timely, unbiased, and sensitive to the concerns and values of the patient and her family.
• **Ultrasonography** can be used to diagnose many major anomalies. The other clinical uses for ultrasound entail confirmation of gestational age, definition of placental location, determination of amniotic fluid volume, and evaluation of fetal growth.
• Optimal timing for the anatomic survey is between 18 and 20 weeks' gestation. At this gestational age, organogenesis is complete, bony ossification in the skull does not yet obscure sonography, and structures are large enough for accurate assessment but still small enough to visualize within a single ultrasound window. With a detected anomaly, a patient can pursue a genetic workup and has a full set of options available to her at the time the anomaly is discovered.

- The structures that are assessed in the level II anatomy screen include the following:
  - **Head:** The biparietal diameter and head circumference are measured, both in the same view at the level of the thalamus and cavum septum pellucidum. The intracranial contents, ventricular structures, cerebellar diameter, and cisterna magna are evaluated.
  - **Spine:** Sagittal, transverse, or coronal views are obtained at all levels to screen for neural tube defects.
  - **Heart:** Four-chamber view and visualization of left and right outflow tracts are required. If an abnormality is suspected, fetal echocardiography should be performed.
  - **Abdomen:** The stomach and umbilical vein should be visualized in the same plane for the abdominal circumference measurement. Abdominal wall defects are ruled out by verifying normal cord insertion and the absence of bowel loops in the amniotic fluid. The kidneys, renal pelvises, and bladder are evaluated for location, structure, and evidence of obstruction.
  - **Limbs:** The four limbs should be imaged to their distal ends and the humerus and femur measured. The hands should be seen to open and close and the feet examined for normal positioning and appearance.
- Several sonographic "soft markers" occur more frequently in fetuses with aneuploidy, specifically trisomy 21. These markers include increased nuchal translucency, renal pelvis dilation, echogenic intracardiac focus (small bright spot within the fetal heart on ultrasound), echogenic bowel, and short long bones. Aneuploidy risk increases with an increased number of markers identified; previous studies have reported likelihood ratios for the individual markers.

## CHROMOSOMAL ABNORMALITIES WITH ASSOCIATED CONGENITAL ANOMALIES

In many specific chromosomal syndromes, there are characteristic findings prenatally that assist in prenatal diagnosis. Common aneuploidies will be discussed with their associated findings (Table 12-2A,B).

### Trisomy 21 (Down syndrome)

- Down syndrome is the most common aneuploidy where the fetus survives, with a frequency of 1:660 to 1:800 births. With trisomy 21, there is an extra copy of chromosome 21. The frequency of nondisjunction increases with increasing maternal age.
- Down syndrome can be complete trisomy 21 in which all cells have three copies of chromosome 21 (94% of cases) or mosaic trisomy 21 in which only some cells in the body have an abnormal number of chromosome 21 (2% to 3%). A third etiology of Down syndrome results from a mother who has a balanced translocation, in which an extra piece of chromosome 21 is attached to another chromosome and is given to the fetus.
- The finding of an echogenic intracardiac focus is not an indication for a fetal echocardiogram, as this is not a structural defect, but should prompt a search for other markers of Down syndrome and a discussion of a potential increased risk in the pregnancy. If Down syndrome is suspected, a fetal echocardiogram is recommended, as these fetuses have a higher incidence of congenital heart defects.
- Children with Down syndrome have some degree of intellectual disability, and in prenatal counseling, it is important to discuss that there is a spectrum of disease and the severity of disease cannot be predicted prenatally or by genetic testing.

| TABLE 12-2A | Common Aneuploidies with Associated Findings | |
| --- | --- | --- |
| **Chromosomal Defect** | **Prenatal Ultrasound Findings** | **Neonatal Clinical Features** |
| Trisomy 21 (Down syndrome) | • Short femur/humerus<br>• Clinodactyly<br>• Sandal gap between first and second toes<br>• Echogenic intracardiac focus<br>• Echogenic bowel<br>• Renal pyelectasis | • Hypotonia<br>• Flat facial profile<br>• Upslanting palpebral fissures<br>• Small ears<br>• Excess dorsal nuchal skin<br>• Single palmar crease<br>• Hypoplasia of fifth finger middle phalanx |
| Monosomy X (Turner syndrome) | • Cystic hygroma<br>• Edema of hands/feet | • Low hairline<br>• Webbed neck<br>• Short stature<br>• Shield chest<br>• Wide-spaced hypoplastic nipples<br>• Gonadal dysgenesis<br>• Coarctation of the aorta |
| Triploidy | • Severe IUGR<br>• Cystic placenta<br>• Ventriculomegaly<br>• Syndactyly<br>• Cardiac defects<br>• Renal anomalies | |

IUGR, intrauterine growth restriction.

| TABLE 12-2B | Common Aneuploidies with Associated Findings |
| --- | --- |
| **Chromosomal Defect** | **Neonatal Findings** |
| Trisomy 13 (Patau syndrome) | Holoprosencephaly; cardiac defects; hypotelorism; abnormalities of orbits, nose, and palate; abnormal ears, omphalocele, polycystic kidneys, radial bone aplasia, skin aplasia, polydactyly |
| Trisomy 18 (Edwards syndrome) | IUGR; cardiac defects; prominent occiput; rotated and malformed ears; short palpebral fissures; small mouth; clenched hands with second and fifth fingers overlapping third and fourth fingers; horseshoe kidney; radial bone aplasia; hemivertebrae; imperforate anus |

IUGR, intrauterine growth restriction.

## Trisomy 13 and 18

- **Trisomy 13** (Patau syndrome) is usually due to meiotic primary nondisjunction giving rise to a 47 +13, XX or XY genotype. Trisomy 13 is invariably fatal; approximately 50% of newborns die in the first month of life and 90% die by 1 year. Of those that survive, they have multiple anomalies and severe intellectual disability.
- **Trisomy 18** (Edwards syndrome) is most commonly due to meiotic primary nondisjunction giving rise to a 47 +18, XX or XY genotype. Life expectancy for these infants is usually very limited.

## Turner Syndrome

- **Turner syndrome** (monosomy X) is usually 45, X genotype. Some individuals are mosaic, with both 45, X and 46, XX cell lines, with resultant variable characteristics. These individuals can have some degree of learning disability.

## Triploidy

- **Triploidy** has one extra haploid set of chromosomes (i.e., 69 chromosomes). Most cases are 69, XXY (60%) or 69, XXX (37%). Only 3% of cases are 69, XYY. Triploidy is uniformly fatal within the first few months of life.

# COMMON SPECIFIC CONGENITAL ANOMALIES

## Congenital Heart Abnormalities

**Congenital heart abnormalities** are among the most common birth defects (Table 12-3). There are some known etiologies for congenital heart disease (CHD), namely maternal diabetes, teratogen exposure, and certain genetic causes such as 22q11 microdeletion (i.e., DiGeorge syndrome). There is a long-established association between congenital heart defects and aneuploidy. The frequency of chromosomal abnormalities with a congenital heart defect has been estimated to be 16% to 45% prenatally and 5% to 10% postnatally; the discrepancy in these rates is secondary to antenatal death occurring in fetuses with chromosomal abnormalities. The likelihood of a cardiac defect exceeds 50% for Down syndrome and is 90% for trisomies 13 and 18.

- **Prenatal diagnosis** of CHD has increased secondary to advances in ultrasound resolution and fetal echocardiography. A fetal echocardiogram is recommended for any abnormality detected in the standard heart views and for any fetus at high risk of a congenital heart defect (e.g., diabetic mother, exposure to a teratogen in the first trimester, previous child with CHD). Some CHDs need a higher level of surveillance during the pregnancy to watch for signs of fetal heart failure in utero. Hydrops in utero is a poor prognostic sign.
- The functional consequences of cardiac anomalies are usually not evident until conversion from fetal to neonatal circulation after birth. Some common defects, such as ventriculoseptal defects and coarctation of the aorta, can be missed on prenatal ultrasounds and fetal echocardiograms.
- **Management** depends on the specific type of cardiac defect. Prenatal management entails offering genetic counseling secondary to the association of a chromosomal or genetic etiology for the CHD, the option of prenatal diagnosis with amniocentesis, appropriate pediatric cardiology, and pediatric cardiac surgery consultation. Most cardiac defects can be corrected surgically, although multiple procedures are usually required. Secondary to the complex nature of these cases, delivery at a tertiary care center is recommended.

| TABLE 12-3 | Most Common Congenital Cardiac Defects |
|---|---|

| Name | Percentage of Cardiac Defects[a] | Findings |
|---|---|---|
| Hypoplastic left heart syndrome (HLHS) | 2%–4% | Small left ventricle, aortic atresia, hypoplastic mitral valve |
| Endocardial cushion defect/atrioventricular septal defect (AVSD) | 2%–7% | Missing "crux" of the heart in four-chamber view |
| Ventricular septal defect (VSD) | 20%–40% | Abnormal communication between left and right ventricles, causing shunt |
| Persistent truncus arteriosus | 1%–2% | Single overriding arterial trunk |
| Transposition of great arteries (TGA) | 2.5%–5% | Aorta arises from right ventricle and pulmonary artery from left. |
| Double outlet right ventricle (DORV) | 1%–2% | Both great arteries arise from right ventricle. |
| Tetralogy of Fallot (TOF) | 3%–7% | VSD, overriding aorta, pulmonary artery stenosis, right ventricular hypertrophy |

[a]Does not add to 100%; minor cardiac defects are not listed. Adapted from Woodward PJ, Kennedy A, Roya S, et al, eds. *Diagnostic Imaging: Obstetrics*, 1st ed. Salt Lake City, UT: Amirsys/Elsevier, 2005.

## Neural Tube Defects

**Neural tube defects (NTDs)** are congenital structural abnormalities of the brain and spine and are the second most common form of structural congenital anomalies. NTDs result from failure of neuropore closure during the third and fourth weeks of gestation. They occur in 1 to 2 per 1,000 births. The main forms of NTD are anencephaly and spina bifida (Table 12-4). Spina bifida can be closed or open and there are different types. NTD risk factors include family history of NTD, poorly controlled diabetes, seizure medications, and poor nutritional status or low folate stores.

- **Prevention** with preconception folate supplementation (0.4 mg/day) significantly lowers the incidence of NTDs. For women with a previously affected pregnancy, a higher dose of 4.0 mg of daily folate is recommended.
- **Prenatal screening** with maternal serum alpha-fetoprotein (MSAFP) should be offered to all pregnant women in the second trimester. The alpha-fetoprotein (AFP) is elevated in 89% to 100% of pregnancies complicated by NTDs and an abnormal value is defined as more than 2.5 times the normal.
- **Prenatal diagnosis** can be made by ultrasound with confirmation by amniocentesis for AFP and acetylcholinesterase levels. The prenatal ultrasound shows splaying of dorsal vertebral elements and a meningeal sac. Other intracranial findings are the "lemon sign" from scalloping of the frontal bones and the "banana sign" of the compressed cerebellum. Ventriculomegaly is also common along with Arnold-Chiari II abnormalities.

| TABLE 12-4 | Types of Neural Tube Defects | |
|---|---|---|
| | **Anencephaly** | **Spina Bifida** |
| **Ultrasound findings** | • Absent cranial vault<br>• Absent telencephalon and encephalon<br>• Polyhydramnios | • Vertebral splaying +/− overlying soft tissue<br>• Lemon sign<br>• Banana sign |
| **Associations** | | • Arnold-Chiari type II malformation<br>• Ventriculomegaly |
| **Outcomes** | Fatal | Severity depends on level of the lesion→ worse with higher level defects<br>With lumbar/sacral: possible bowel, bladder, mobility, and neurologic dysfunction |

- **Management** of NTDs entails delivery at a tertiary care center where neonatology and neurosurgery are available. Delivery at term is preferred. The mode of delivery is determined on an individual basis; however, there have been no improved outcomes with C-section for these fetuses. In terms of when to repair this defect, the Management of Myelomeningocele Study trial recently compared prenatal versus postnatal closure and found that the children who had prenatal surgery had some improved outcomes but with an increased risk of preterm delivery and uterine dehiscence at delivery.

## Hydrocephalus and Ventriculomegaly

**Hydrocephalus** is a pathologic increase in intracranial cerebrospinal fluid (CSF) volume; hydrocephalus results from fluid production that exceeds absorption or primary atrophy of brain parenchyma. The majority of cases are secondary to an obstruction at some level.

**Ventriculomegaly** is a descriptive term of enlarged ventricles and this finding can be secondary to various causes. Some of these include obstruction, inability to resorb CSF, maldevelopment of a ventricle or agenesis of a structure in the brain, ex vacuo destructive phenomenon from cerebral atrophy, fetal aneuploidy, genetic such as X-linked hydrocephalus, or infections such as cytomegalovirus or toxoplasmosis. A less common cause of ventriculomegaly is cerebral hemorrhage. If this diagnosis is being considered, a workup for neonatal alloimmune thrombocytopenia (NAIT) should be offered (see Chapter 20).

- **Prenatal diagnosis** of enlarged ventricles on ultrasound is the definitive finding. The fetal biparietal diameter may or may not be increased with the finding of enlarged ventricles. The method for assessing ventricular size is the atrial diameter measured in a transverse view. If the mean diameter is greater than 10 mm, this indicates the presence of ventriculomegaly. The incidence of associated anomalies with enlarged ventricles varies from 54% to 84%; thus, it is important to have targeted sonographic exam to ensure there are no other abnormalities. **Management** of the pregnancy with enlarged ventricles includes a determination of the cause. The diagnostic studies include amniocentesis for karyotype, DNA analysis for L1CAM mutations, and viral studies. A multidisciplinary team that includes perinatologists, genetic counselors, pediatric neurosurgery, and neonatology should be involved in the care of this pregnancy. Pregnancy termination may be considered in some cases. Fetuses with ventriculomegaly should be delivered at a tertiary care center where a pediatric neurosurgery team is available. The **mode of delivery** is individualized, and if there is no significant head enlargement, a vaginal delivery is reasonable. Significant head enlargement may preclude vaginal delivery and may be an indication for early delivery.

- **Prognosis** for ventriculomegaly depends on etiology, severity of ventriculomegaly, and the presence of associated abnormalities. The degree of ventricular dilation does not appear to be associated with poor long-term outcome.

## Congenital Diaphragmatic Hernia

**Congenital diaphragmatic hernia** (CDH) is a failure of the diaphragm to fuse properly during embryologic development, resulting in abdominal contents occupying the thoracic cavity. This creates a mass effect that prevents normal lung development and leads to pulmonary hypoplasia and persistent pulmonary hypertension, with significant morbidity and mortality in the newborn. Approximately 1 in 2,000 to 3,000 newborns have CDH. Hernias are more often unilateral, posterior, and left sided.

- **Prenatal diagnosis** of CDH is accomplished in 60% to 90% of cases by ultrasonography or fetal magnetic resonance imaging. On ultrasound, abdominal contents (stomach, bowel, and/or liver) are seen in the thoracic cavity. Other signs seen on ultrasound are mediastinal shift, polyhydramnios, and abnormal cardiac axis. Associated structure anomalies are found in approximately 40% of cases, and the most common anomalies are congenital heart defect, renal anomalies, central nervous system anomalies, and gastrointestinal anomalies.

- **Management** of the pregnancy includes a detailed ultrasound, to ensure there are no other associated abnormalities, and a fetal echocardiogram. Secondary to an association with chromosomal anomalies and some genetic syndromes, amniocentesis should be offered for karyotype and array. The option of termination of pregnancy should be discussed in some cases depending on gestational age and parental choice. A multidisciplinary team that involves neonatology, pediatric surgery, MFM, and genetic counselors can help the patient and her family determine a treatment plan. Delivery should be performed at a tertiary center where pediatric extracorporeal membrane oxygenation (ECMO) is available.

- **Prognosis** has significantly improved in recent years due to advances in techniques of ventilation and ECMO. Overall survival now exceeds 80%.

## Congenital Cystic Adenomatoid Malformation and Bronchopulmonary Sequestration

**Congenital cystic adenomatoid malformation (CCAM)** and **bronchopulmonary sequestration (BPS)** are two common congenital lung malformations in the differential for a fetal chest mass. CCAM is a cystic malformation of pulmonary tissue and BPS is a mass of nonfunctioning lung tissue that does not communicate with the bronchial tree. These two abnormalities can exist in isolation or as a hybrid of the two lesions. The distinguishing feature is that CCAM typically has a pulmonary blood supply, whereas BPS has blood supply from anomalous systemic vessels.

- **Prenatal diagnosis** is possible for both lesions. In CCAM, prenatal ultrasound shows a lung tumor that may be cystic or solid and there is an absence of systemic vascular flow. In BPS, an echodense triangular area of tissue is seen, with a systemic feeding vessel on color Doppler sonography. Additional ultrasound findings with BPS are pleural effusion, mediastinal shift, hydrops, and polyhydramnios.

- **Management** of pregnancy with either of these lesions entails a detailed ultrasound examination to ensure there are no other anomalies. With both of these lesions, fetal echocardiography should be performed because of an increased incidence in congenital heart defects. In CCAM, the association with chromosomal abnormalities is uncertain; however, amniocentesis is offered to exclude these abnormalities. In BPS, amniocentesis should be offered for fetal karyotype, as chromosomal anomalies have been described with this anomaly. These fetuses should be delivered at tertiary care centers, and prenatal consultation with MFM, pediatric surgery, and neonatology is recommended. These pregnancies need to be serially monitored by an MFM specialist with ultrasound to watch for signs of progression or regression or an associated fetal complication such as hydrops. In the postnatal period, if these lesions persist, surgical excision is usually recommended.
- **Prognosis** is generally good for fetuses with CCAM and BPS. The long-term outcome of infants with CCAM following resection is excellent. The long-term outcome from BPS depends on the location of the lesion (intrathoracic vs. extrathoracic) and the degree of pulmonary hypoplasia.

## Gastroschisis and Omphalocele

**Gastroschisis** and **omphalocele** are the two classic diagnoses for abdominal wall defects that are detected in utero. Gastroschisis is an isolated abdominal wall defect where the herniated abdominal contents have no covering membrane. Omphalocele is a defect in the abdominal wall in which a membrane of peritoneum and amnion covers the herniated abdominal contents. Differences between these two abdominal wall defects are reviewed in Table 12-5.

- **Prenatal screening** is accomplished by measuring AFP in the second trimester; both of these defects are associated with an elevated MSAFP.
- **Prenatal diagnosis** is usually made by ultrasound. Gastroschisis is not associated with an increased risk for aneuploidy. Omphalocele has a high incidence of

| TABLE 12-5 | Omphalocele and Gastroschisis | |
|---|---|---|
| | Omphalocele | Gastroschisis |
| **Umbilical cord location** | Umbilical cord enters into the center of the sac. | Umbilical cord inserts to left of the defect. |
| **Physical findings** | • Covered by membrane <br> • Varies in size <br> • Contains bowel loops +/− liver | • No covering <br> • Varies in size <br> • Small bowel +/− liver |
| **Additional anomalies** | Common (up to 45%) | Usually isolated <br> Increased risk for IUGR <br> Intestinal atresia in 10%–15% |
| **Associated chromosomal abnormality** | Up to 30% with chromosomal abnormality <br> Association with Beckwith-Wiedemann and other syndromes | No association with chromosomal problem |

IUGR, intrauterine growth restriction.

associated malformations and chromosomal abnormalities. The option of amniocentesis for fetal karyotype and genetic testing should be offered in the case of omphalocele. Additionally, there is an increased incidence of congenital heart defects in cases of omphalocele, and fetal echocardiography is recommended.

- **Management** in pregnancy entails serial ultrasound assessments to follow the amount and type of abdominal contents that are herniated. A multidisciplinary team should be involved including MFM, genetic counselors, neonatology, and pediatric surgery. Delivery at a tertiary care center enables optimal care of the newborn. The mode of delivery can be vaginal in most cases, if other standard obstetric indications are met.
- **Prognosis** of infants with abdominal wall defects depends on whether this is an isolated anomaly, other anomalies, or an underlying chromosomal anomaly.

## Renal Anomalies

**Congenital renal anomalies** can be diagnosed in the prenatal period, including renal agenesis, multicystic dysplastic kidney disease, infantile polycystic kidney disease, and hydronephrosis secondary to ureteropelvic junction obstruction and outlet obstruction.

- **Renal agenesis** can be unilateral or bilateral. Unilateral renal agenesis has a normal prognosis and there is usually compensatory hypertrophy of the contralateral side. A portion of patients with unilateral renal agenesis have contralateral vesicoureteral reflux. Bilateral renal agenesis is diagnosed after 18 weeks' gestation, as the fetal kidneys do not contribute to the majority of amniotic fluid until after this gestation. On prenatal ultrasound of these fetuses, the kidneys and bladder are not visualized. This condition causes severe oligohydramnios or anhydramnios and is lethal secondary to severe pulmonary hypoplasia.
- **Multicystic dysplastic kidney disease** (MCKD) is a severe renal abnormality characterized by increased renal size and numerous large noncommunicating cysts alternating with areas of increased echogenicity on ultrasound. Because of the size of the kidney and the numerous cysts, this is usually detected by prenatal ultrasound. MCKD is usually unilateral. In almost half of cases, the contralateral kidney has other malformations, the severity of which determines the overall prognosis. There is also an association with other nongenitourinary anomalies and some genetic syndromes. Amniocentesis should be offered during a prenatal consultation. With unilateral MCKD, prenatal pediatric urology consultation is recommended. Bilateral multicystic dysplasia is associated with severe oligohydramnios and is fatal secondary to pulmonary hypoplasia.
- **Polycystic kidney disease** encompasses two inherited disorders with diffuse involvement of both kidneys. The so-called infantile polycystic kidney disease (**autosomal recessive polycystic kidney disease** [**ARPKD**]) is inherited in an autosomal recessive fashion. From the perspective of prenatal diagnosis and neonatal presentation, the recessive polycystic kidney disease is much more common. This disease is characterized by bilateral, enlarged, echogenic kidneys. Oligohydramnios can be present. **Autosomal dominant polycystic kidney disease (ADPKD)** rarely presents in the prenatal period; this disease usually has clinical findings in the third or fourth decade of life. Sonogram reveals enlarged kidneys with multiple cysts. Individuals with this form of polycystic kidney disease also have liver cysts, pancreatic cysts, and intracranial aneurysms. Renal ultrasound is recommended in both parents to evaluate for ADPKD. The main cause of perinatal morbidity and mortality is pulmonary hypoplasia. Aggressive neonatal management has lead to 1-year survival rates of 82% to 85% in ARPKD. If infants survive the first month of life, they are predicted to live for many years.

- **Ureteropelvic junction (UPJ) obstruction** is the most common cause of significant neonatal hydronephrosis. UPJ obstruction prevents urinary flow from the renal pelvis to the ureter. Most cases are unilateral; bilateral cases have a worse prognosis. Pregnancy management is generally unchanged in unilateral cases, but with bilateral UPJ obstruction, a fetal intervention of urinary shunting may be necessary. There is an overall increased incidence of chromosomal abnormalities with obstructive uropathy; thus, the option of amniocentesis for prenatal karyotype should be offered. A consultation with a pediatric surgeon or pediatric urologist should be offered to the patient as well. With isolated UPJ obstruction, the prognosis is usually favorable.
- Bladder outlet obstructions have the potential to affect the entire urinary and pulmonary system. In males, the most common cause of bladder outlet obstruction is **posterior urethral valves** (PUVs). In females, the most common cause is **urethral atresia**. The characteristic prenatal finding on ultrasound is a dilated bladder (megacystis) and bilateral hydroureteronephrosis. With PUVs, the bladder wall is thickened and the urethra may have a characteristic keyhole appearance. There is an association with chromosomal abnormalities; thus, amniocentesis and fetal karyotype should be offered in cases of bladder outlet obstruction. In utero interventions may be helpful in some cases, but there is often severe irreversible renal impairment. Pediatric urology consultation should be offered prenatally. Prognosis is determined

| **TABLE 12-6** | Skeletal Dysplasias | |
|---|---|---|
| **Type of Dysplasia and Gene Mutation** | **Description** | **Outcome** |
| Achondroplasia FGFR3 | • Rhizomelic shortening of limbs<br>• Frontal bossing<br>• "Collar hoop" sign: rounded metaphyseal epiphyseal interface at the femur | Normal intelligence comorbidities:<br>• Joint problems<br>• Craniocervical junction problems<br>• Obstructive sleep apnea<br>• Middle ear dysfunction<br>• Kyphosis |
| Thanatophoric dysplasia FGFR3 | • Very short extremities<br>• Platyspondyly-flattened vertebral ossification centers<br>• Small chest<br>• Telephone receiver femur—type I<br>• Cloverleaf skull—type II | Usually lethal |
| Osteogenesis imperfecta (OI) COL1A1 COL1A2 CRTAP/LEPRE1 | • Bone fractures<br>• Irregularity and angulation to long bones<br>• Decreased skull ossification<br>• Irregular shape of ribs | Type II perinatal lethal Severity and features are variable based on the type of OI |

by evaluation of amniotic fluid volume. The degree of oligohydramnios determines the extent of pulmonary hypoplasia and the ultimate outcome for the fetus.

## Collagen and Bone Disorders

**Collagen/bone disorders** can be diagnosed prenatally. The most common skeletal dysplasia disorders that are diagnosed prenatally are **achondroplasia**, **thanatophoric dysplasia**, and **osteogenesis imperfecta** (Table 12-6). Ultrasound findings include shortened limbs, 3 to 4 standard deviations below the mean for gestational age, as well as abnormalities in the skull, spine, and thorax. Options for further management of the pregnancy may depend on these ultrasound findings, as type II osteogenesis imperfecta and thanatophoric dysplasia are lethal.

## SUGGESTED READINGS

Adzick NS, Thom EA, Spong CY, et al. A randomized trial of prenatal versus postnatal repair of myelomeningocele. *NEJM* 2011;364(11):993–1004.

Allen LD, Sharland GK, Chita SK, et al. Chromosomal anomalies in fetal congenital heart disease. *Ultrasound Obstet Gynecol* 1991;1:8–11.

American College of Obstetricians and Gynecologists Committee on Practice Bulletins. ACOG practice bulletin no. 77: screening for chromosomal abnormalities. *Obstet Gynecol* 2007;109(1):217–227.

Barboza JM, Dajani NK. Prenatal diagnosis of congenital cardiac anomalies: a practical approach using two basic views. *Radiographics* 2002;22:1125–1138.

Centers for Disease Control and Prevention. National Center on Birth Defects and Developmental Disabilities. Centers for Disease Control and Prevention Web site. http://www.cdc.gov/ncbddd/index.html. Accessed November 13, 2014.

Copel JA, Cullen M, Green JJ, et al. The frequency of aneuploidy in prenatally diagnosed congenital heart disease: an indication for fetal karyotyping. *Am J Obstet Gynecol* 1988; 158:409–413.

Cuckle HS, Malone FD, Wright D, et al. Contingent screening for Down syndrome—results from the FaSTER trial. *Prenat Diagn* 2008;28(2):89–94.

Cunningham FG, Leveno K, Bloom SL, et al. Fetal imaging. In Cunningham FG, Leveno K, Bloom SL, et al, eds. *Williams Obstetrics*, 23rd ed. New York, NY: McGraw-Hill, 2010:349–373.

Cunningham FG, Leveno K, Bloom SL, et al. Prenatal diagnosis and fetal therapy. In Cunningham FG, Leveno K, Bloom SL, et al, eds. *Williams Obstetrics*, 23rd ed. New York, NY: McGraw-Hill, 2010:287–311.

Gabbe SG, Niebyl JR, Simpson JL, et al. Prenatal genetic diagnosis. In Gabbe SG, Niebyl JR, Simpson JL, et al, eds. *Obstetrics: Normal and Problem Pregnancies*, 6th ed. Philadelphia, PA: Saunders, 2012:210–236.

Laurence KM, James N, Miller MH, et al. Double blind randomized controlled trial of folate treatment before conception to prevent recurrence of neural tube defects. *JAMA* 1988; 260:3141–3145.

Leschot NJ, Verjaal M, Treffers PE. Risks of midtrimester amniocentesis: assessment in 3000 pregnancies. *Br J Obstet Gynaecol* 1985;92:804–807.

Malone FD, Canick JA, Ball RH, et al; First- and Second-Trimester Evaluation of Risk Research Consortium. First-trimester or second-trimester screening, or both, for Down's syndrome. *N Engl J Med* 2005;353:2001–2011.

Nyberg DA, Souter VL, El-Bastawissi A, et al. Isolated sonographic markers for detection of fetal Down syndrome in the second trimester. *J Ultrasound Med* 2001;20:1053–1063.

Rhoads GG, Jackson LG, Schlesselman SE, et al. The safety and efficacy of chorionic villus sampling for early prenatal diagnosis of cytogenetic abnormalities. *N Engl J Med* 1989; 320:609–617.

Taipale P, Hiilesmaa V, Salonen R, et al. Increased nuchal translucency as a marker for fetal chromosomal defects. *N Engl J Med* 1997;337:1654–1658.

# 13 Endocrine Disorders of Pregnancy

Clark T. Johnson and Lorraine A. Milio

## DIABETES MELLITUS

**Diabetes mellitus (DM)** is the most common medical complication of pregnancy in the United States, affecting nearly 7% of all pregnancies. As the incidence of type 2 DM increases nationwide, cases of gestational diabetes mellitus (GDM) have grown also. In 90% of diabetic pregnancies, the cause is GDM.

- Diabetes in pregnancy is categorized as pregestational diabetes (diagnosed prior to pregnancy) or GDM (diagnosed during pregnancy). Pregestational diabetes is further classified as type 1 or type 2 (Table 13-1). One half percent to 1% of pregnancies are complicated by pregestational DM.
- Carbohydrate metabolism changes during pregnancy to provide adequate nutrition for both the mother and the fetus.
  - In the fasting state, maternal serum glucose is lower in pregnancy than in the nonpregnant state (55 to 65 mg/dL), whereas free fatty acid, triglyceride, and plasma ketone concentrations are increased. A state of relative maternal starvation exists in pregnancy, during which glucose is spared for fetal consumption and alternate fuels are used by the mother.
  - GDM is similar to type 2 DM, in which increased pancreatic secretion cannot overcome decreased insulin sensitivity of maternal target tissues. Increased metabolism in pregnancy also increases insulin clearance. These changes are due to the effects of estrogen, progesterone, cortisol, prolactin, and human placental lactogen. The net result is hyperglycemia.

### Diagnosis and Screening

- Diagnosis of type 1 and 2 DM before pregnancy is by standard criteria: two abnormal fasting glucose levels ≥126 mg/dL or a random glucose level of ≥200 mg/dL (Table 13-2). Classic symptoms are polydipsia, polyuria, and polyphagia. Clinical signs include weight loss, hyperglycemia, persistent glucosuria, and ketoacidosis.
- Universal screening for GDM is standard in the United States, whether by patient history, clinical risk factors, or laboratory testing. Testing is typically performed at 24 to 28 weeks, but if strong risk factors such as obesity, family history, or a personal history of GDM are present, blood glucose screening may be performed at the first prenatal visit. Not all patients require screening via blood glucose testing (Table 13-3).
- Screening for GDM has undergone much scrutiny in recent years as a result of the Hyperglycemia and Adverse Pregnancy Outcome (HAPO) study in which progressive hyperglycemia was linked to adverse perinatal outcomes. For many years, a two-step screening/diagnostic protocol has been widely used. In this screening, a 50-g oral glucose challenge is consumed, followed by serum glucose measurement at

| TABLE 13-1 | Comparison of Type 1 and Type 2 Diabetes Mellitus |
|---|---|

| Type 1 | Type 2 |
|---|---|
| Pathophysiology is absolute insulin deficiency. | Pathophysiology is tissue resistance to insulin. |
| Patients are at risk for severe hypoglycemia and DKA. | Patients may develop hyperosmolar non-ketotic coma (HONK). DKA is rare. |
| DKA can be encountered at relatively low blood sugars (<200 mg/dL). | HONK usually encountered at higher blood sugars (>500mg/dL). |
| Increased risk for chronic micro-vascular disease at an early age | Lower incidence of microvascular disease during reproductive age range |

DKA, diabetic ketoacidosis.

1 hour. No fasting or dietary preparation is required. A serum glucose ≥140 mg/dL identifies 80% of GDM, whereas decreasing the cutoff to ≥130 mg/dL identifies over 90% of GDM but with more "false positives." A serum glucose ≥200 mg/dL diagnoses GDM without additional testing.

• If the screening test is positive, then a diagnostic 3-hour glucose tolerance test (GTT) should be performed with 100-g oral glucose after at least 8 hours of fasting (Table 13-4). With abnormal fasting or any other two abnormal values, the diagnosis of DM is confirmed. In patients at high risk for GDM with a normal GTT, a follow-up GTT can be performed at 32 to 34 weeks to identify late-onset diabetes.

| TABLE 13-2 | Diabetic Screening in the Nonpregnant Patient |
|---|---|

1. A1C ≥6.5%. The test should be performed in a laboratory using a method that is NGSP certified and standardized to the DCCT assay.[a]

OR

2. FPG ≥126 mg/dL (7.0 mmol/L). Fasting is defined as no caloric intake for at least 8 hr.[a]

OR

3. Two-hour plasma glucose ≥200 mg/dL (11.1 mmol/L) during an OGTT. The test should be performed as described by the World Health Organization using a glucose load containing the equivalent of 75-g anhydrous glucose dissolved in water.[a]

OR

4. In a patient with classic symptoms of hyperglycemia or hyperglycemic crisis, a random plasma glucose ≥200 mg/dL (11.1 mmol/L).

[a]Diagnoses based on 1, 2, or 3 should undergo repeat testing to confirm findings.
NGSP, National Glycohemoglobin Standardization Program; DCCT, Diabetes Control and Complications Trial; FPG, fasting plasma glucose; OGTT, oral glucose tolerance test.
From American Diabetes Association. Standards of medical care in diabetes 2011. *Diabetes Care* 2011;34(suppl 1):S11–S61.

| TABLE 13-3 | Gestational Diabetes Risk Assessment |

**Low risk**

Age younger than 25 years

Not a member of an ethnic group with increased risk for type 2 DM (Hispanic, African, Native American, South or East Asian, or Pacific Islander ancestry)

BMI <25; normal weight at birth

No history of abnormal glucose tolerance

No history of poor obstetric outcomes

No first-degree relatives with DM

**High risk**

Severe obesity

Strong family history of type 2 diabetes

Previous history of GDM, impaired glucose metabolism, or glucosuria

Patients who meet all low-risk criteria and have no high-risk factors may forgo oral glucose challenge testing if appropriate.

DM, diabetes mellitus; BMI, body mass index; GDM, gestational diabetes mellitus.

Adapted from Metzger BE, Buchanan TA, Coustan DR, et al. Summary and recommendations of the Fifth International Workshop-Conference on gestational diabetes mellitus. *Diabetes Care* 2007;30(suppl 2):S251–S260.

- Based on the HAPO study, the International Association of Diabetes and Pregnancy Study group, in 2010, recommended that a universal 75-g, 2-hour GTT be used in a single-step screening/diagnosis of GDM. In this schemata, the diagnosis of GDM would be made when any single threshold value was reached or exceeded (fasting value = 92 mg/dL, 1-hour value = 180 mg/dL, and 2-hour value = 153 mg/dL).
- This protocol was endorsed by the American Diabetes Association. However, there has been concern that using this criterion for diagnosis of GDM would result in 17% to 18% of pregnancies diagnosed with GDM and would improved

| TABLE 13-4 | Criteria for Diagnosis of Gestational Diabetes from Oral Glucose Tolerance Testing |

| Time Since 100-g Glucose Load (hr) | Modified O'Sullivan Scale | Carpenter and Coustan Scale |
|---|---|---|
| Fasting | ≥105 | ≥95 |
| 1 | ≥190 | ≥180 |
| 2 | ≥165 | ≥155 |
| 3 | ≥145 | ≥140 |

Values are plasma glucose levels in milligrams per deciliter.

Adapted from O'Sullivan JB, Mahan CM. Criteria for the oral glucose tolerance test in pregnancy. *Diabetes* 1964;13:278–285; Carpenter MW, Coustan DR. Criteria for screening tests for gestational diabetes. *Am J Obstet Gynecol* 1982;144:768–773.

perinatal outcomes justify the increased burden of managing such a surge in diagnosed patients. In 2013, a National Institute of Child Health and Human Development consensus panel concluded that there was not enough evidence to date to warrant recommendation of this protocol for universal diagnosis of GDM.

* Classification of GDM depends on the management required to control blood glucose levels. Type A1 achieves euglycemia by dietary changes alone. Type A2 requires additional (i.e., medical) therapy.

## Fetal Complications of Diabetes Mellitus

* Fetal and neonatal complications of DM in pregnancy are increased with both gestational and pregestational DM, but the incidence is much higher in pregestational DM and with poor glycemic control. Fetal glucose levels are similar to maternal blood glucose levels, and both fetal hyperglycemia and hypoglycemia have important effects.

* Spontaneous abortion ranges between 6% and 29% with pregestational DM and correlates with poor glucose control and an elevated hemoglobin A1C (HbA1C) around the time of conception. Type 1 and type 2 DM carry the same risk of pregnancy loss, but the main causes of fetal loss for type 1 DM are congenital anomalies and complications of prematurity, whereas for type 2 DM, they are in utero fetal demise, fetal hypoxia, and chorioamnionitis. There is no increased incidence of spontaneous abortion in diabetics with excellent preconception glucose control (i.e., HbA1C <6%).

* Congenital malformations are the most common cause of perinatal mortality in pregestational diabetic pregnancies and correlate with elevated HbA1C. Congenital anomalies account for 30% to 50% of perinatal mortality from diabetes. Maternal hyperglycemia is considered to be the principal factor causing congenital malformations. Six percent to 10% of infants of diabetic mothers have a major congenital anomaly (see Chapter 12). Again, there is no increase in congenital malformations when euglycemia and a normal HbA1C is present from conception through the first trimester.

    * The most common congenital malformations in diabetic pregnancies are in the cardiovascular system. Defects include transposition of the great vessels, ventricular and atrial septal defects, hypoplastic left ventricle, situs inversus, aortic anomalies, and complex cardiac anomalies. The rate of cardiac malformations is fivefold higher in diabetics.

    * Sacral agenesis/caudal regression is highly suggestive of diabetic fetopathy. It is a rare malformation but diagnosed up to 400 times more frequently in diabetic pregnancies and is nearly pathognomonic.

    * There is a 10-fold increase in the incidence of central nervous system malformations in infants of diabetic mothers, including anencephaly, holoprosencephaly, open spina bifida, microcephaly, encephalocele, and meningomyelocele.

    * Gastrointestinal (GI) system malformations, including tracheoesophageal fistula, bowel atresia, and imperforate anus, are also increased in diabetic gestations.

    * Genitourinary system anomalies including absent kidneys (leading to Potter syndrome), polycystic kidneys, and double ureter are more common in pregnancies complicated by diabetes.

* Polyhydramnios occurs in 3% to 32% of diabetic pregnancies, 30 times the rate for nondiabetic gestations. Diabetes alone is the leading known cause of polyhydramnios. Furthermore, diabetes-associated congenital anomalies of the central nervous and GI systems can also lead to polyhydramnios. Mechanisms of polyhydramnios include increased fetal glycemic load resulting in polyuria, decreased fetal swallowing, and fetal GI obstructions. Higher perinatal morbidity and mortality rates are

associated with polyhydramnios, attributed in part to the higher incidence of both congenital anomalies and preterm delivery.

- Macrosomia is defined as an estimated fetal weight more than 4,000 to 4,500 g or more than the 90th percentile at any gestational age, depending on the authority. It occurs in 25% to 42% of hyperglycemic versus 8% to 14% of euglycemic pregnancies, and maternal diabetes is the most significant single risk factor. Diabetic macrosomia is characterized specifically by a large fetal abdominal circumference and decreased head to abdominal circumference ratio because fetal hyperinsulinemia leads to abnormal fat distribution. Macrosomic fetuses have an increased mortality rate and higher risk for hypertrophic cardiomyopathy, vascular thrombosis, neonatal hypoglycemia, and birth trauma. They are more likely to be delivered by cesarean section and are at increased risk for shoulder dystocia during birth, which may result in fractured clavicles, facial paralysis, Erb palsy, Klumpke palsy, phrenic nerve injury, and intracranial hemorrhage.

- Intrauterine growth restriction (IUGR) may complicate pregnancy for pregestational diabetic women with microvascular disease. Placentae of diabetic pregnancies can be compromised and may exhibit pathohistologic changes, including fibrinoid necrosis, abnormal villus maturation, and proliferative endarteritis of fetal stem arteries. There is wide variation, but these observations occur even with good glucose control, suggesting that irreversible placental abnormalities occur very early in gestation.

- Poorly controlled diabetes increases risk for fetal demise in utero during the third trimester. Cord thrombosis and accelerated placental aging may be the cause.

- Shoulder dystocia is increased threefold in diabetic gestations at any estimated fetal weight and is of even greater concern when macrosomia is also present. If shoulder dystocia occurs, infants of diabetic mothers are more likely to have brachial plexus injury than infants of women without DM. In macrosomic infants of diabetic mothers, vaginal delivery carries a 2% to 5% risk of brachial plexus injury.

- Twenty-five percent to 40% of infants of diabetic mothers develop neonatal hypoglycemia. The serum glucose nadirs at about 24 hours of life. Poor maternal glycemic control during late pregnancy and at delivery increases the risk. The pathogenesis is in utero stimulation of the fetal pancreas by maternal hyperglycemia leading to fetal islet cell hypertrophy and beta cell hyperplasia. When the maternal glucose source is eliminated, the continued overproduction of insulin leads to newborn hypoglycemia with cyanosis, convulsions, tremor, apathy, diaphoresis, and a weak or high-pitched cry, if untreated. Severe or prolonged hypoglycemia is associated with neurologic sequelae and death. Standard of care includes testing neonatal blood glucose value within 1 hour of birth. Treatment should be instituted when the infant's blood glucose drops below 40 mg/dL.

- Neonatal hypocalcemia and hypomagnesemia are common in infants of diabetic mothers and correlate with the degree of glycemic control.

- Thirty-three percent of infants born to diabetic mothers have polycythemia (hematocrit higher than 65%). Chronic intrauterine hypoxia increases erythropoietin production, resulting in vigorous hematopoiesis. Alternatively, elevated glucose may lead to early increased red blood cell destruction, followed by increased erythrocyte production.

- Neonatal hyperbilirubinemia and neonatal jaundice occur more commonly in infants of diabetic mothers than in infants of nondiabetic patients of comparable gestational age because poor glycemic control delays fetal liver maturation.

- Neonatal respiratory distress syndrome (RDS) may occur more frequently in diabetic pregnancies as a result of delayed fetal lung maturation. Fetal hyperinsulinemia may suppress production and secretion of surfactant required for normal lung function at birth.

- The risk of fetal cardiac septal hypertrophy and hypertrophic cardiomyopathy is increased in diabetic pregnancies (up to 10% have hypertrophic changes). There is a strong correlation between cardiomyopathy and poor maternal glycemic control. As an isolated finding, cardiac septal hypertrophy is a benign neonatal condition. However, it increases the risk of morbidity and mortality in neonates with sepsis or congenital structural heart disease.

## Maternal Complications of Diabetes Mellitus

- Maternal complications are increased with diabetes.
- Diabetic ketoacidosis (DKA) is a potentially life-threatening metabolic emergency for both mother and fetus. In pregnant patients, DKA can occur at lower blood glucose levels (i.e., <200 mg/dL) and more rapidly than in nonpregnant diabetics. Although maternal death is rare with proper treatment, fetal mortality rates from 10% to 30% are reported. About half of DKA cases are due to medical illness, usually infection; another 20% result from dietary or insulin noncompliance. In 30% of cases, no precipitating cause is identified. Antenatal steroids for fetal lung maturity and beta-adrenergic tocolytics can precipitate or exacerbate hyperglycemia and DKA in pregestational diabetics.
- The pathophysiology of DKA is relative or absolute insulin deficiency. The resulting hyperglycemia and glucosuria lead to osmotic diuresis, promoting urinary potassium, sodium, and fluid loss. Insulin deficiency also increases lipolysis and hepatic oxidation of fatty acids, producing ketones and eventually causing metabolic acidosis.
- Diagnosis is by objective documentation of maternal hyperglycemia, acidemia, and serum ketosis. Signs and symptoms include abdominal pain, nausea and vomiting, polydipsia, polyuria, hypotension, rapid deep respiration, and impaired mental status (ranging from mild drowsiness to profound lethargy). Acidosis can be defined as a plasma bicarbonate level <15 mEq/L or arterial pH <7.3. In the presence of hyperglycemia, ketosis is presumed and can be verified by serum testing. Because pregnancy is a state of physiologic respiratory alkalosis, profound DKA may occur at a higher pH.
- Initial management consists of vigorous intravenous (IV) hydration followed by IV insulin drip and frequent blood sugar checks to titrate dosing. Potassium and bicarbonate supplementation may be necessary. Insulin cannot be given if potassium is less than 3.0 mEq/L because insulin drives potassium into the cells and can cause profound hypokalemia with resultant cardiac arrhythmias. Check electrolytes every 4 hours and blood sugar hourly until DKA is resolved (Fig. 13-1). Evaluating for the underlying cause and pursuing treatment (e.g., antibiotics for a urinary tract infection) is part of the management.
- Severe hypoglycemia, requiring hospitalization, may occur in up to 45% of mothers with type 1 DM. Patients with poorer glycemic control can have blunted autonomic responses and milder symptoms so they may present with more severe or prolonged episodes. Vomiting in early pregnancy also predisposes diabetics to low blood sugars. Severe hypoglycemia may be teratogenic in early gestation, but the effects on the developing fetus are not fully understood.
  - Symptoms include nausea, headache, diaphoresis, tremors, blurred or double vision, weakness, hunger, confusion, paresthesia, and stupor. Diagnosis is by careful history and review of symptoms and confirmed with a blood glucose measurement <60 mg/dL.

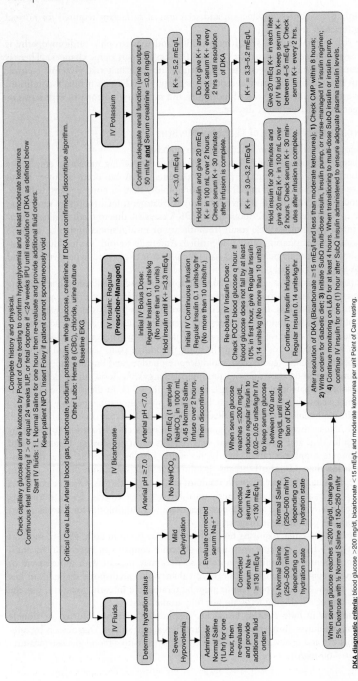

**Figure 13-1.** Prescriber guidelines for management of obstetric patient with diabetic ketoacidosis.

**DKA diagnostic criteria:** blood glucose >200 mg/dl, bicarbonate <15 mEq/l, and moderate ketonurea per unit Point of Care testing.

* Serum Na should be corrected for hyperglycemia (for each 100 mg/dl above normal value, add 1.6 mEq to sodium value for corrected serum sodium value).

Adapted from Kitachci, A.E. et al (July 2009). **Hyperglycemic Crises in Adult Patients With Diabetes.** Diabetes Care, Vol. 32, No. 7, pp: 1335–1343; doi:10.2337/dc09-9032.

- Treatment starts with 4 oz of juice or a glucose tablet. Assess serum glucose after 15 to 20 minutes, and repeat feeding until blood sugar is >70 mg/dL, followed with complex carbohydrates or a scheduled meal or snack. If the patient is unable to tolerate food and drink, a subcutaneous injection of glucagon is appropriate or an ampule of dextrose 10% can be given IV push followed by IV fluids containing 5% dextrose.

- The Somogyi effect is rebound hyperglycemia after hypoglycemia secondary to counterregulatory hormone release. It usually occurs in the middle of the night but can happen after any hypoglycemic episode, manifesting as wide variations in blood glucose levels over a short period of time (e.g., between 2:00 and 6:00 A.M.). Diagnosis is by checking additional blood sugars (i.e., 3:00 A.M.) to identify unrecognized hypoglycemia. Treatment involves adding or modifying a nighttime snack or decreasing the overnight insulin dose in order to better match insulin needs with dietary intake.

- The dawn phenomenon is also an early morning increase in plasma glucose, possibly due to normal nighttime production of growth hormone (GH), catecholamines, and cortisol. It is also diagnosed by checking early morning (i.e., 3:00 A.M.) blood sugar level. If the patient is euglycemic overnight, she may require increased bedtime insulin dosing to cover the effect of normal morning hormones. Differentiating between the Somogyi effect and the dawn phenomenon helps tailor the insulin regimen and achieve optimal glucose control.

- Rapid progression of microvascular and atherosclerotic disease can occur in pregnant diabetics. Any evidence of ischemic heart disease, heart failure, peripheral vascular disease, or cerebral ischemia should be evaluated carefully. A pregestational diabetic older than age 30 years should have a baseline electrocardiogram (ECG). Maternal echocardiogram and cardiology consultation may be warranted. Preconception counseling is useful for these patients. For the most severe maternal disease, termination in early pregnancy may be considered and offered.

- Nephropathy complicates 5% to 10% of diabetic pregnancies. In renal failure, with creatinine >1.5 mg/dL, there may be worsening failure with advancing pregnancy, but it is unclear if pregnancy actually hastens progression to end-stage disease. Diabetic nephropathy increases the risk for maternal hypertensive complications, preeclampsia, preterm birth, fetal growth restriction, and perinatal death. A new diagnosis of diabetic nephropathy is made in pregnancy if persistent proteinuria >300 mg/day in the absence of urinary tract infection is detected prior to 20 weeks' gestation. Creatinine clearance <50 mL/min is associated with increased incidence of severe preeclampsia and fetal loss. Treatment with an angiotensin-converting enzyme inhibitor (ACE-I) before pregnancy has a prolonged maternal renal protective effect and improves outcomes; however, ACE-I is teratogenic especially in the second half of pregnancy. Intensive maternal and fetal surveillance throughout gestation is required with renal disease but can result in fetal survival rates >90% (see Chapter 16).

- Diabetic retinopathy is the most common vascular manifestation of diabetes and a principal cause of adult-onset blindness in the United States. Proliferative retinopathy is believed to be a consequence of persistent hyperglycemia and is directly related to the duration of disease. Pregnancy does not change the long-term prognosis, but an ophthalmologic evaluation is recommended in preconception counseling or at the time of the pregnancy diagnosis. Progressive disease may be treated with laser treatment during pregnancy.

- The incidence of chronic hypertension is increased in patients with pregestational DM, especially those with nephropathy (see Chapter 14).

- Preeclampsia is two to four times more common in pregestational diabetics. The risk is increased with longer duration of disease, nephropathy or retinopathy, and chronic hypertension. Up to a third of women with long-standing diabetes (>20 years) will develop preeclampsia. Even in GDM, the risk of preeclampsia is 13% to 18%. The threshold for preeclampsia workup in these women should be very low (see Chapter 14).

- Preterm labor and delivery may be three to four times higher in patients with DM. Worsening maternal medical status, poor glycemic control, noncompliance with diabetic management, and nonreassuring fetal status result in many iatrogenic preterm deliveries.
  - Corticosteroids should be administered as indicated when there is an increased risk for preterm delivery before 34 weeks. Additional insulin or oral agents may be required for 5 to 7 days after steroid administration.
- Diabetics also have increased maternal risk for adverse obstetric outcomes including third- and fourth-degree perineal lacerations and wound infection. Additionally, they are at increased risk for intrauterine fetal demise, particularly after 40 weeks' gestation.

## Management of Diabetes in Pregnancy

- Ideally, diabetic women desiring pregnancy should seek preconception consultation and maintain euglycemia before conception. The initial prenatal visit should include a detailed history and physical examination, an ophthalmologic examination, an ECG (for women older than age 30 years, smokers, or hypertensives), and 24-hour urine collection for protein and creatinine clearance. Echocardiography and cardiology consultation should be obtained for known or suspected cardiovascular disease. HbA1C is helpful in evaluating recent (8 to 12 weeks) glycemic control and in assessing risk for fetal malformations. HbA1C ≥9.5% carries >20% risk of major fetal malformation. Strict glucose control (i.e., HbA1C ≤6%) during organogenesis dramatically reduces embryopathy to nondiabetic levels. Early nutrition consult and counseling may be beneficial.
- Blood glucose goals in pregnancy are given in Table 13-5.
  - Patients should start or continue intensive glucose monitoring early in pregnancy using a home glucometer. They should record fasting and 1-hour (or 2-hour) postprandial blood sugar levels for each meal.
  - Postprandial glycemic control correlates most strongly with risk for neonatal hypoglycemia, macrosomia, fetal death, and neonatal complications. Home monitoring records are reviewed every 1 to 2 weeks and therapy is optimized.

| TABLE 13-5 | Goals for Glycemic Control in Pregnancy |
| --- | --- |
| | **Goal Blood Sugar Values** |
| Fasting | 60–90 mg/dL |
| Premeal | <100 mg/dL |
| 1 hr postprandial | <140 mg/dL |
| 2 hr postprandial | <120 mg/dL |
| Bedtime | <120 mg/dL |
| 2:00–6:00 A.M. | 60–90 mg/dL |

From Metzger BE, Buchanan TA, Coustan DR, et al. Summary and recommendations of the Fifth International Workshop-Conference on Gestational Diabetes Mellitus. *Diabetes Care* 2007;30(suppl 2): S251–S260.

*Gestational Diabetes Mellitus Management*

- Management for GDM initially consists of diet and exercise. If good glucose control is not achieved, oral hypoglycemic agents or insulin are then prescribed.
  - Women with newly diagnosed GDM are started on a carbohydrate-controlled diet with three meals and three snacks daily.
  - Moderate exercise can improve glycemic control in GDM. Patients are encouraged to maintain a consistent level of activity throughout pregnancy provided there are no contraindications (e.g., preterm labor).
  - Oral hypoglycemic agents are acceptable in GDM management when dietary efforts fail to achieve euglycemia. One agent frequently used in pregnancy, glyburide, works by increasing tissue insulin sensitivity and has minimal placental transfer. The starting dose is usually 2.5 mg orally (PO) at bedtime or 2.5 mg PO twice daily, titrated to a maximum dose of 20 mg daily. Glyburide side effects include hypoglycemia, nausea, heartburn, and allergic skin reactions. Metformin is also safe and effective. Four percent to 20% of patients will need additional therapy with insulin, particularly if fasting blood sugars are high.
  - Insulin therapy can improve glycemic control for GDM. Different types of insulin are combined to maintain euglycemia throughout the day and night (Fig. 13-2).
  - Neutral protamine Hagedorn (NPH) insulin is an intermediate-acting insulin given in the morning and at night, with peak activity at 5 to 12 hours.
  - Rapid-acting insulin (e.g., Humalog or NovoLog) is administered with meals because its onset is 5 to 15 minutes and peak activity occurs at 2 to 4 hours.
  - Fetal monitoring is not required for GDM-A1 diabetics. They are not at increased risk for fetal demise before 40 weeks' gestation. Women with GDM-A2 require antenatal testing similar to that recommended for pregestational DM (twice weekly nonstress tests or biophysical profile from 32 to 34 weeks until delivery). Delivery by 40 weeks' gestation is recommended due to increased risk of intrauterine demise after that time.

*Pregestational Diabetes Mellitus Management*

- Management of pregestational DM
  - The recommended diet for pregnant diabetic women is 1,800 to 2,400 kcal daily, made up of 20% protein, 60% carbohydrates, and 20% fat. Carbohydrate

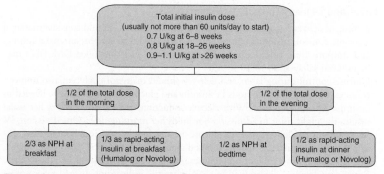

**Figure 13-2.** Calculation and dose distribution for initial insulin management in pregnancy. (Adapted from Gabbe SG. Management of diabetes mellitus complicating pregnancy. *Obstet Gynecol* 2003;102[4]:857.)

counting, with 180 to 210 g of daily carbohydrates, is becoming more common and replacing caloric guidelines. Three meals and three snacks are recommended for all diabetics in pregnancy. Nutrition consult should be part of preconception or early pregnancy planning.

- Patients are usually continued on their normal prepregnancy insulin regimen while initial blood sugar monitoring is performed. Monitoring and goals are the same for GDM and pregestational DM (see Table 13-5).

  o The American Diabetes Association recommends insulin for pregnant women with DM and for women with DM considering pregnancy. Patients taking oral hypoglycemic agents (except glyburide or metformin) or a 70/30 (NPH/regular) mixed insulin regimen are switched to NPH and a rapid-acting insulin analog. Patients with type 1 DM usually require 50% to 100% increased insulin doses in the second half of pregnancy. Type 2 DM insulin dosing is frequently more than doubled in pregnancy.

  o Insulin pumps provide a continuous subcutaneous infusion of insulin. Pump dosing must be managed carefully because the risk of severe hypoglycemia causing seizures and death is increased in pregnancy. Patients must be carefully selected; however, diabetic control may be improved in the correct patient population.

- Fetal assessment and monitoring for pregestational diabetes varies according to gestational age.

  - First trimester: Obtain an early dating sonogram to confirm gestational age and document fetal viability.

  - Second trimester: Offer maternal serum alpha-fetoprotein screening for neural tube defects (either alone or as part of aneuploidy screening if desired by the patient; see Chapter 12). Ultrasonography at 18 to 20 weeks is recommended for complete anatomy evaluation. Fetal echocardiography is also recommended at 19 to 22 weeks for pregestational diabetics.

  - Third trimester: Twice-weekly antenatal testing should be initiated for all diabetic pregnancies starting at 32 to 34 weeks' gestation. Patients with comorbidities or very poor glycemic control may start assessment as early as 28 weeks. Serial ultrasonographic exams for fetal growth should be considered at 28 to 30 weeks and again at 34 to 36 weeks. Monthly fetal growth ultrasounds with umbilical artery Doppler velocimetry may be required to assess for IUGR in patients with microvascular disease (see Chapter 6).

## Labor and Delivery in Diabetic Pregnancies

- Timing of delivery in an insulin-requiring diabetic patient should consider maternal glycemic control, maternal comorbidities, estimated fetal weight, antenatal testing, and amniotic fluid volume. In many patients with well-controlled DM, labor may be induced safely at 39 to 40 weeks.

- Glucose control during labor and delivery should maintain euglycemia to improve neonatal outcomes. Continuous IV insulin and glucose infusions may be needed to optimize glycemic control. With elective induction, the patient receives her usual insulin the night prior to admission but holds her morning dose. On admission, IV fluids are started along with serial glucose monitoring (every 1 to 2 hours). The infusion fluids are adjusted to maintain blood glucose levels between 70 and 110 mg/dL (Table 13-6). Short-acting insulin boluses may be required in addition to the IV drip.

- Route of delivery is determined by usual obstetric indications. If fetal macrosomia >4,500 g is suspected, cesarean section is considered to avoid the risk of a shoulder dystocia. Otherwise, induction of labor is warranted.

| TABLE 13-6 | Low-Dose Continuous Insulin Infusion for Labor and Delivery |
|---|---|

| Blood Glucose (mg/dL) | Insulin Dosage (U/hr)[a] | Fluids (125 mL/hr) |
|---|---|---|
| <60 | 0 | One ampule D50 or D5NS by severity |
| 60–100 | 0[a] | D5NS |
| 101–140 | 1.0[b] | D5NS |
| 141–180 | 1.5[b,c] | D5NS |
| 181–220 | 2.0[b,c] | D5NS |
| >220 | 2.5[b,c] | Normal saline |

[a]Type 1 diabetic patients need baseline insulin when blood glucose is >60 mg/dL; 0.5 U/hr is reasonable to start.
[b]Increase as needed.
[c]Boluses of insulin may be required in addition to an increase in the insulin drip.
D5NS, 5% dextrose in normal saline.
Adapted from Rosenberg V, Eglinton GS, Rauch ER, et al. Intrapartum glycemic control in women with insulin requiring diabetes: a randomized clinical trial of rotating fluids versus insulin drip. *Am J Obstet Gynecol* 2006;195(5):1095–1099.

## Postpartum Care for Diabetics

• Postpartum management of diabetic mothers depends on the severity and type of DM.
• For GDM, no immediate postpartum testing is required. Most gestational DM diagnosed in the third trimester resolves rapidly after delivery. Glucose tolerance testing is strongly recommended for these patients at their postpartum visit, with a 2-hour fasting GTT, because some women with GDM will persist as type 2 diabetics after delivery (Table 13-7). GDM will recur in 30% to 50% of subsequent pregnancies. Because women with a history of GDM have a sevenfold increased risk of developing type 2 diabetes, they should be advised postpartum on weight control, a healthy diet, exercise, and yearly evaluation for diabetes.

| TABLE 13-7 | Postpartum Glucose Tolerance Test |
|---|---|

| | No DM | Impaired Glucose Tolerance | Overt DM |
|---|---|---|---|
| 8-hr fasting | <100 | 100–125 | ≥126 |
| 2 hr after 75-g glucose load | <140 | 140–199 | ≥200 |

Values are plasma glucose levels in milligrams per deciliter.
Adapted from Metzger BE, Buchanan TA, Coustan DR, et al. Summary and recommendations of the Fifth International Workshop-Conference on Gestational Diabetes Mellitus. *Diabetes Care* 2007;30(suppl 2):S251–S260; American Diabetes Association. Standards of medical care in diabetes—2010. *Diabetes Care* 2010;33:S11–S61.

• For pregestational diabetics, blood sugar can be monitored with nonpregnant regimen. The insulin dose is typically one half of the dose at the end of pregnancy, and oral hyperglycemics are significantly decreased. Blood sugar testing every 4 to 6 hours for 24 hours after cesarean section, with sliding scale insulin dosing, may be helpful until the patient can resume her normal routine. Keeping blood sugar <180 mg/dL can help prevent wound breakdown, although strict glucose leading to hypoglycemia should be avoided.

## THYROID DISORDERS

Thyroid disorders are common in women of reproductive age and are present in 3% to 4% of pregnancies. However, only 10% exhibit symptomatic disease.

### Thyroid Hormones in Pregnancy

• Thyroid hormone levels are altered in pregnancy (Table 13-8).
• Total T3 and T4 increase due to human chorionic gonadotropin (hCG) stimulation of thyroid-stimulating hormone (TSH) receptors. In the first trimester, total serum T4 can increase two- to threefold and TSH may decrease, but hyperthyroid disease is not present because estrogen stimulates the liver to increase thyroxine-binding globulin (TBG), maintaining a constant proportion of active free T3 (fT3) and free T4 (fT4). Therefore, serum fT4 may offer better specificity for thyroid testing

| TABLE 13-8 | Thyroid Function Test Results in Pregnancy Compared with Hyperthyroid and Hypothyroid Conditions | | |
|---|---|---|---|
| Test | Normal Pregnancy | Hyperthyroidism | Hypothyroidism |
| Thyroid-stimulating hormone (TSH) | No change | Decreased | Increased |
| Thyroxine-binding globulin (TBG) | Increased | No change | No change |
| Total T4 (T4) | Increased | Increased | Decreased |
| Free T4 (fT4) or free T4 index (FTI) | No change | Increased | Decreased |
| Total triiodothyronine (T3) | Increased | Increased or no change | Decreased or no change |
| Free T3 (fT3) | No change | Increased or no change | Decreased or no change |
| T3 resin uptake (T3RU) | Decreased | Increased | Decreased |
| Iodine uptake | Increased | Increased or no change | Decreased or no change |

Adapted from American College of Obstetricians and Gynecologists. ACOG practice bulletin. Clinical management guidelines for obstetrician-gynecologists. Number 37, August 2002. (Replaces practice bulletin number 32, November 2001). Thyroid disease in pregnancy. *Obstet Gynecol* 2002;100:387–396; Rashid M, Rashid MH. Obstetric management of thyroid disease. *Obstet Gynecol Surv* 2007;62(10):680–688.

| TABLE 13-9 | Indications for Thyroid Function Testing in Pregnancy |
| --- | --- |

Patient on thyroid therapy
Large goiter or thyroid nodularity
History of hyperthyroidism or hypothyroidism
History of neck irradiation
Previous infant born with thyroid dysfunction
Type 1 diabetes mellitus
Family history of autoimmune thyroid disease
Fetal demise in utero

Adapted from Mestman JH. Thyroid diseases in pregnancy other than Graves' disease and postpartum thyroid dysfunction. *Endocrinologist* 1999;9:294–307.

during pregnancy. The free T4 index (FTI) can be used as an indirect estimation of free T4, but direct fT4 measurement is preferred.

- The serum TSH level is more useful for diagnosing primary hypothyroidism than hyperthyroidism in pregnancy. TSH is not protein bound and does not cross the placenta. Normal TSH with low free T4 may suggest secondary hypothyroidism from a central hypothalamic pituitary defect.
- The thyroid gland itself is moderately enlarged in normal pregnancy, although nodularity or frank thyromegaly should provoke thorough evaluation.
- There are few strong indications for thyroid testing during pregnancy (Table 13-9). Universal screening is not necessary or recommended.
  - Figure 13-3 outlines a thyroid testing algorithm.
  - Testing for anti-TSH receptor antibodies is indicated in only certain circumstances (Table 13-10). IgG antibodies cross the placenta and can affect the fetal thyroid function. TSH-stimulating immunoglobulin (TSI) will stimulate,

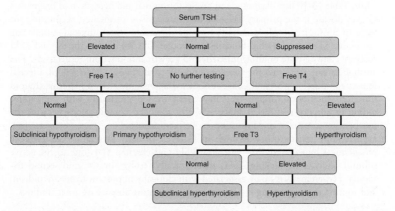

**Figure 13-3.** Thyroid testing algorithm. (Adapted from Mestman JH. Thyroid and parathyroid diseases in pregnancy. In Gabbe SM, Niebyl JR, Simpson JL, et al, eds *Obstetrics: Normal and Problem Pregnancies*. Philadelphia, PA: Churchill Livingstone, 2007:1011–1037.)

| TABLE 13-10 | Indications for Thyroid-stimulating Hormone Receptor Antibody Testing in Pregnancy |
|---|---|

Graves disease (TSI)
    Fetal or neonatal hyperthyroidism in previous pregnancy
    Euthyroid, postablation, in the presence of
        Fetal tachycardia
        IUGR
        Incidental fetal goiter on ultrasound
Incidental fetal goiter on ultrasound (TRAb)
Infant born with congenital hypothyroidism (TRAb)

---

TSI, TSH receptor–stimulating immunoglobulin; IUGR, intrauterine growth retardation; TRAb, TSH receptor–blocking antibodies.
Adapted from Mestman JH. Hyperthyroidism in pregnancy. *Best Pract Res Clin Endocrinol Metab* 2004;18(2):267–288.

whereas TSH receptor–blocking antibodies (TRAb) will inhibit fetal thyroid function. The presence of these antibodies in high titers can produce fetal or neonatal hyperthyroidism or hypothyroidism.

## Hyperthyroid Conditions

- Specific hyperthyroid conditions include Graves disease, hyperemesis gravidarum, gestational trophoblastic disease, struma ovarii, toxic adenoma, toxic multinodular goiter, subacute thyroiditis, TSH-producing pituitary tumor, metastatic follicular cell carcinoma, and painless lymphocytic thyroiditis. Thyrotoxicosis occurs in up to 1 in 500 pregnancies and increases risk for complications such as preeclampsia, thyroid storm, congestive heart failure, IUGR, preterm delivery, and stillbirth.
  - Clinical signs of thyrotoxicosis include tachycardia, exophthalmos, thyromegaly, onycholysis, heat intolerance, pretibial myxedema, menstrual irregularities, and weight loss. Table 13-10 lists diagnostic test results for normal and hyperthyroid pregnancy.
- Graves disease is the primary cause of thyrotoxicosis in pregnancy, accounting for 90% to 95% of cases. It is an autoimmune disease in which thyroid-stimulating antibodies (TSAs) or thyroid-blocking antibodies (TRAb) bind to the thyroid TSH receptors and activate or antagonize thyroid growth and function, respectively. The antibodies can also cross the placenta and affect the fetus. Up to 5% of affected fetuses can develop neonatal Graves disease, which is unrelated to maternal thyroid function. Infants of women who have been treated previously with radioactive iodine or surgery may be at higher risk for neonatal complications because the mothers are not maintained on suppressive medications.
- Hyperemesis gravidarum with high hCG levels in early pregnancy can produce biochemical hyperthyroidism with low TSH and elevated fT4 (due to the active subunit of hCG mimicking TSH) that typically resolves by the mid second trimester. Hyperemesis is rarely associated with clinically important hyperthyroidism, and routine thyroid testing is not recommended in the absence of other findings.

### *Hyperthyroid Management*

- Medical management is with propylthiouracil (PTU) or methimazole. Both cross the placenta and can potentially cause fetal hypothyroidism and goiter.

Maintaining high normal range thyroid hormone levels with a minimum drug dosage is the goal.

- PTU blocks iodide organification in the thyroid and reduces the peripheral conversion of T4 to T3. It is traditionally preferred to methimazole, although placental transfer of the two drugs is nearly equivalent. Both drugs have <0.5% risk of agranulocytosis and <1% risk of thrombocytopenia, hepatitis, and vasculitis. Breast-feeding is allowed for mothers taking PTU because only a small fraction of PTU passes into milk.
  - Initial dose of PTU is 300 to 400 mg daily (divided into an 8-hour dosing schedule). fT4 should be checked regularly (every 2 to 4 weeks) and the PTU dose adjusted to a maximum of 1,200 mg daily to maintain fT4 levels in the normal range.
- Methimazole can also be used in pregnancy. The dose is 15 to 100 mg daily (divided into three times daily). The association of methimazole with fetal aplasia cutis has largely been refuted.
- Beta-blockers are used for symptom management in thyrotoxicosis until thyroid hormone levels are normalized with suppressive therapy. Propranolol hydrochloride is the most widely used. Adverse side effects include decreased ventricular function resulting in pulmonary edema. The dose of propranolol is 20 to 80 mg PO every 4 to 6 hours to maintain heart rate below 100 beats per minute.
- Iodine 131 thyroid ablation is contraindicated in pregnancy.
- Surgical management is reserved for severe cases that are unresponsive to medical therapy. Subtotal thyroidectomy may be performed at any time during pregnancy if required.
- Thyroid storm is a medical emergency occurring in <1% of pregnant patients with hyperthyroidism. Heart failure due to the long-term effects of increased T4 is more frequent and can be exacerbated during pregnancy by preeclampsia, anemia, or infection. Clinical signs include fever higher than 103°F, severe tachycardia, widened pulse pressure, and changes in mentation. Thyroid blood testing is sent, but treatment should be initiated immediately.
- Treatment by a standard series of medications is initiated immediately for thyroid storm. Blood work for fT3, fT4, and TSH is sent to confirm the diagnosis, but testing should not delay therapy. Oxygen, cooling blankets, antipyretics, and IV hydration are initiated. Fetal monitoring is performed when appropriate.
  - PTU 600 to 800 mg PO once then 150 to 200 mg PO every 4 to 6 hours blocks hormone synthesis and conversion.
  - Saturated potassium iodide solution two to five drops every 8 hours blocks thyroid hormone release.
  - Dexamethasone 2 mg IV or intramuscular every 6 hours for 24 hours decreases hormone release and peripheral conversion.
  - Propranolol is given as mentioned earlier for tachycardia.
  - Phenobarbital 30 to 60 mg every 6 to 8 hours can relieve extreme restlessness.

## Hypothyroid Conditions

- Hypothyroidism in pregnancy is uncommon because untreated hypothyroidism is associated with infertility. Common causes include Hashimoto thyroiditis, subacute thyroiditis, prior radioablative treatment, and iodine deficiency.
- Type 1 diabetes is associated with 5% incidence of hypothyroidism during pregnancy and has up to a 25% incidence of postpartum thyroid dysfunction.
- Complications of hypothyroidism in pregnancy include preeclampsia, abruptio placentae, anemia, and postpartum hemorrhage. Fetal complications include IUGR,

congenital cretinism (growth failure and neuropsychological deficits), and stillbirth. Infants of optimally treated hypothyroid mothers usually have no evidence of thyroid dysfunction.

- The most common etiology of hypothyroidism in the United States is Hashimoto chronic autoimmune thyroiditis, resulting from thyroid antimicrosomal and anti-thyroglobulin antibodies. Worldwide, the most common cause of hypothyroidism is iodine deficiency.
- Presentation may be asymptomatic or include disproportionate weight gain, lethargy, weakness, constipation, carpal tunnel syndrome, cold sensitivity, hair loss, dry skin, and, eventually, myxedema. Table 13-10 lists test results for hypothyroid pregnancy.
- Treatment is initiated if thyroid function testing is consistent with hypothyroidism, regardless of symptoms. Thyroxine replacement is based on the patient's clinical history and laboratory test values and adjusted until TSH remains normal and stable.
  - The starting dose for levothyroxine is 50 to 100 μg daily. It may be several weeks before the full effect is obtained. TSH can be checked every 4 to 6 weeks initially. The dose may need to be increased in pregnancy. Stable patients can be tested every trimester.

## Nodular Thyroid

- Nodular thyroid disease should be evaluated when detected during pregnancy. Thyroid cancer occurs in 1 in 1,000 pregnancies, and up to 40% of nodules will be malignant. Ultrasonography, fine-needle aspiration, or tissue biopsy can be performed in pregnancy. Surgical excision is the definitive treatment and should not be postponed because of pregnancy, whereas radiation treatment is deferred until after delivery.

## PARATHYROID DISORDERS

Parathyroid disorders and calcium dysregulation are uncommon in pregnancy. Calcium requirements do increase during pregnancy, however, so 1,000 to 1,300 mg calcium and 200 IU vitamin D supplementation are recommended. Fetal calcium uptake, increased plasma volume, renal loss from increased glomerular filtration rate (GFR), and hypoalbuminemia lead to lower total maternal serum calcium levels, but ionized calcium remains fairly constant.

- Serum calcium levels are regulated by several hormones:
  - Parathyroid hormone (PTH) increases calcium mobilization from bone, calcium recovery in the kidney, and calcium absorption in the intestine (indirectly via activation of vitamin D). PTH increases throughout pregnancy until term, possibly to counteract the inhibitory effects of estrogen on bone.
  - Parathyroid hormone–related peptide (PTHrP) is produced by the placenta and fetal parathyroid to activate active placental calcium transport and, like PTH, mobilize maternal calcium stores.
  - Calcitonin is produced in the parafollicular cells of the thyroid and acts to decrease serum calcium levels.

## Hyperparathyroidism

- Hyperparathyroidism produces hypercalcemia. Clinical manifestations include hyperemesis, weakness, constipation, polyuria, polydipsia, nephrolithiasis, mental status changes, arrhythmias, and occasionally pancreatitis. Obstetric and fetal complications include preeclampsia, stillbirth, premature delivery, neonatal tetany, and neonatal death. Poor control of maternal hyperparathyroidism is associated with significant neonatal morbidity and mortality.

- The differential diagnosis of hypercalcemia includes thyrotoxicosis, hypervitaminosis A and D, familial hypocalciuric hypercalcemia, granulomatous disease, and malignancy.
- Laboratory findings include elevated free serum calcium and decreased phosphorus levels. Disproportionately high PTH relative to serum calcium may also be found. ECG abnormalities, including arrhythmias, may be present. Ultrasonography is recommended for localization. If radiation exposure is necessary to identify local disease, it should be kept to a minimum.
- Surgical treatment (e.g., excision) of a parathyroid adenoma is considered in any patient with symptomatic hyperparathyroidism following medical stabilization. Hypercalcemic crisis is corrected with IV hydration, furosemide, electrolyte correction, and calcitonin. Oral phosphates can be used as treatment for mild cases or in preparation for surgery.

## Hypoparathyroidism

- Hypoparathyroidism is rare and usually occurs iatrogenically after neck surgery. It is the most common cause of hypocalcemia. Patients exhibit cramps, paresthesias, bone pain, hyperacute deep tendon reflexes, tetany, prolonged QT interval, arrhythmias, and laryngospasm. Trousseau sign (carpopedal spasm after blood pressure cuff inflation above systolic pressure for several minutes) or Chvostek sign (upper lip twitching after tapping of the facial nerve) may be present. Fetal skeletal demineralization, subperiosteal resorption, osteitis fibrosa cystica, growth restriction, and neonatal hyperparathyroidism can develop.
- The differential diagnosis of hypocalcemia includes prior parathyroidectomy or thyroid surgery, prior radioactive iodine or radiation treatment, vitamin D deficiency, hypomagnesemia or hypermagnesemia, autoimmune disorders (e.g., Addison disease, chronic lymphocytic thyroiditis), eating disorders, renal failure, DiGeorge syndrome, and pseudohypoparathyroidism (i.e., PTH resistance).
- Laboratory evaluation shows low serum calcium, low PTH, and elevated serum phosphate levels. 1,25-Dihydroxy vitamin D levels are decreased, and ECG changes include prolongation of the QT interval.
- Treatment is with vitamin D (50,000 to 150,000 IU/day) and calcium (1,000 to 1,500 mg/day) supplementation and low-phosphate diet. Doses may need to be increased during pregnancy and reduced postpartum. Maternal repletion with calcium gluconate during labor and delivery may prevent neonatal tetany. Acute symptomatic hypocalcemia is treated with IV calcium gluconate infusion.

# PITUITARY DISORDERS

Pituitary disorders are not common in pregnancy; pituitary dysfunction is commonly associated with anovulatory infertility.

- Pituitary hormone release is under hypothalamic control. The anterior pituitary (adenohypophysis) releases adrenocorticotropin (ACTH), TSH, prolactin, GH, follicle-stimulating hormone (FSH), luteinizing hormone (LH), and endorphins. The posterior pituitary (neurohypophysis) contains the nerve terminals projecting from the hypothalamus that release oxytocin and antidiuretic hormone (ADH; also called arginine vasopressin [AVP]).
- During normal pregnancy, the pituitary gland may more than double in size. Lactotroph growth in response to estrogen leads to increased serum prolactin levels,

whereas ACTH release increases in response to placental corticotropin-releasing hormone (CRH). LH and FSH secretion are decreased in pregnancy. Pituitary GH and TSH decrease as placental GH and hCG rise, respectively. ADH secretion may be increased in pregnancy, but placental vasopressinase increases degradation, leading to a lowered plasma osmolality setpoint (i.e., 5 to 8 mOsm/kg decrease).

- The differential diagnosis of pituitary dysfunction includes tumor, infarction, autoimmune/inflammatory disease, infection, infiltrative processes, head trauma, sporadic or familial genetic mutations, prior surgery or radiotherapy, hypothalamic lesions, and empty sella syndrome.

## Prolactinoma

- Prolactinoma is the most common pituitary tumor of reproductive age women. Elevated prolactin can cause amenorrhea, anovulation, infertility, and galactorrhea. With increasing size and mass effect, prolactinoma can cause headaches, visual changes, and diabetes insipidus.
- Pituitary adenomas are classified as **microadenomas**, which are ≤10 mm in size and rarely (<2%) progress to **macroadenomas**, which are >10 mm in diameter, during pregnancy. Up to one third of previously untreated macroadenomas, however, may become symptomatic during pregnancy.
- Initial diagnosis is by history, physical exam, and computed tomography (CT) or magnetic resonance imaging (MRI) of the head. Serum prolactin may not be useful during pregnancy due to normal pregnancy-induced elevations. Patients with microadenomas can be monitored for symptoms at each prenatal visit, with visual field testing and MRI if visual symptoms develop. Patients with macroadenomas should have baseline visual field testing early in pregnancy and referral for endocrinology and ophthalmology consults can be considered.
- Treatment of symptomatic prolactinoma is with dopamine agonists, which mimic the prolactin-inhibiting factor activity of hypothalamic dopamine. Bromocriptine (drug of choice; 2.5 to 5 mg daily) or cabergoline (0.5 to 3 mg weekly) can shrink the adenoma and decrease serum prolactin levels. Patients taking these medications should stop them during pregnancy unless they have a symptomatic or large tumor. Transsphenoidal surgical resection of the macroadenoma is indicated for macroadenomas or high prolactin levels that are not controlled with medication. Radiotherapy can also be used to treat persistent disease. Radiologic evaluation and serum prolactin testing should be followed after treatment.

## Acromegaly

- Acromegaly is caused by a GH-secreting pituitary adenoma. Symptoms include coarsened facial features, prominent chin, large feet, spade-like hands, irregular menses, headaches, visual changes, hyperhidrosis, arthralgias, and carpal tunnel syndrome. Usually, these women are infertile, with hyperprolactinemia and anovulation. In the rare patient with acromegaly who becomes pregnant, there are no deleterious or teratogenic effects for the fetus. Carbohydrate intolerance, hypertension, and cardiac abnormalities may complicate pregnancy, however. Laboratory testing shows elevated serum insulin-like growth factor 1 (IGF-1) levels and nonsuppressed GH during glucose tolerance testing (100-g glucose load normally suppresses GH release). Diagnosis during pregnancy is complicated by placental GH secretion. Head CT or MRI can localize the tumor. Treatment is with surgical excision; radioablation; or medical treatment with bromocriptine, somatostatin analogues (e.g., octreotide or lanreotide), or the newer GH receptor antagonist pegvisomant.

## Diabetes Insipidus

- Diabetes insipidus (DI) results from abnormal water homeostasis. Central DI results from decreased ADH/vasopressin release due to pituitary tumor, metastases, granuloma, infection, trauma, or global pituitary failure. Nephrogenic DI due to renal resistance to ADH hormone is rare and primarily found in males. Psychogenic DI is due to massive free water consumption. Subclinical DI may be identified during pregnancy when ADH/vasopressin metabolism is increased. Viral hepatitis, preeclampsia, HELLP syndrome, and acute fatty liver of pregnancy (AFLP) can also exacerbate or promote DI. Polyuria (>3 L/day) and polydipsia are the clinical hallmarks of DI.
- Diagnosis is by the water deprivation test, showing low urine osmolality and high plasma osmolality with fluid restriction. L-Deamino-I-D-arginine vasopressin (DDAVP) injection corrects central DI and can be helpful in confirming the diagnosis. Head CT or MRI may be used to identify pituitary lesions.
- Treatment is with synthetic ADH/vasopressin (i.e., DDAVP) at 10 to 25 µg/day intranasally. Higher doses may be required during pregnancy.

## Other Pituitary Disorders

- Sheehan syndrome results from pituitary necrosis following massive blood loss. Clinical findings include tachycardia, postural hypotension, hypoglycemia, galactorrhea, anorexia, nausea, lethargy, weakness, weight loss, decreased pigmentation, periorbital edema, normocytic anemia, and DI. Approximately 4% of patients with obstetric hemorrhage may have mild pituitary dysfunction, but frank Sheehan syndrome can present up to 20 years later. Diagnosis requires laboratory testing for stimulated pituitary hormone secretion (i.e., after injecting hypothalamic-releasing hormones). Random blood hormone levels are not useful.
- Lymphocytic hypophysitis is caused by autoimmune lymphocyte and plasma cell infiltration with destruction of the pituitary gland, similar to Sheehan syndrome. Pituitary dysfunction can vary widely, and mass effect may cause headache with visual changes. Head CT or MRI may be helpful in diagnosis. Surgery is reserved for severe symptoms from mass effect.

## ADRENAL DISORDERS

Adrenal disorders are not pregnancy induced but do persist during pregnancy, causing significant morbidity without prompt diagnosis. The adrenal gland is profoundly affected by pregnancy and its physiologic changes. CRH is secreted by the placenta, stimulating ACTH release from the pituitary that increases cortisol production in maternal adrenal glands. Cortisol clearance is also decreased, leading to more than twofold increase in total and free serum cortisol levels by the third trimester. Aldosterone production is stimulated by elevated renin/angiotensin II levels in pregnancy; renin activity peaks by the second trimester. Androgen levels are increased five- to eightfold, whereas dehydroepiandrosterone sulfate (DHEA-S) is decreased in pregnancy.

## Cushing Syndrome

- Cushing syndrome results from long-term exposure to glucocorticoids, either from exogenous steroid use (as in treatment of lupus erythematosus, sarcoidosis, or severe asthma) or from increased endogenous hormone production (from excessive pituitary ACTH production, adrenal hyperplasia, or adrenal neoplasia). Adrenal hyperplasia is the most common cause of Cushing syndrome in pregnancy (up to 50%), with a relative decrease in other etiologies.

- Signs and symptoms include moon facies, buffalo hump, truncal obesity, striae, fatigue, weakness, hirsutism, easy bruising, nephrolithiasis, mental status changes, and hypertension.
- Diagnosis is by laboratory testing, showing increased plasma cortisol levels or increased 24-hour urine free cortisol. It can be difficult to identify mild cases due to the normal pregnancy-induced changes in cortisol levels. The dexamethasone suppression test can be used to differentiate a pituitary cause (i.e., Cushing syndrome) from adrenal or exogenous sources of the increased cortisol. Head or abdominal CT or MRI is recommended to localize tumors in the pituitary or adrenal gland.
- Treatment of Cushing syndrome entails medical management of blood pressure and subsequent surgical excision of pituitary or adrenal adenoma. Medical management of the pregnant patient until delivery is usually preferred, although maternal morbidity may be higher with adrenal adenomas, prompting earlier surgical treatment. Metyrapone has been used to block cortisol secretion with adrenal hyperplasia, although it crosses the placenta, may affect fetal adrenal function, and has been associated with preeclampsia. Ketoconazole has been associated with IUGR and may have potential antiandrogen activity; mifepristone is contraindicated in pregnancy.
- Prognosis is improved with early detection and close management, although these patients are at increased risk for maternal complications including hypertension, DM, preeclampsia, cardiac problems, and death. There is increased risk for perinatal complications including IUGR, preterm delivery (up to 50%), stillbirth, and neonatal death.

## Hyperaldosteronism

- Hyperaldosteronism can result from adrenal aldosteronoma or carcinoma (about 75%) and bilateral adrenal hyperplasia (about 25%). Symptoms include hypertension, hypokalemia, and weakness. Laboratory testing shows increased serum or urine aldosterone and low plasma renin levels. MRI can be used to identify and localize an adrenal tumor. Definitive treatment is tumor resection, which can be performed laparoscopically in the second trimester. Medical management is potassium supplementation and treatment of hypertension. Calcium channel blockers or beta-blockers are preferred agents for blood pressure control, with spironolactone contraindicated in pregnancy.

## Pheochromocytoma

- Pheochromocytoma is a rare catecholamine-secreting tumor of chromaffin cells. Ninety percent arise in the adrenal medulla and 10% in sympathetic ganglia. Ten percent of tumors are bilateral. Ten percent are malignant. It is associated with medullary thyroid cancer and hyperparathyroidism in multiple endocrine neoplasia (MEN) type 2 syndromes.
- When diagnosed during pregnancy, pheochromocytoma increases maternal mortality to approximately 10%. Fetal mortality increases to nearly 50%, even though the catecholamines do not cross the placenta or directly affect the fetus. IUGR is common, but there is no increased neonatal mortality after delivery. When the diagnosis is not made before delivery, postpartum maternal mortality increases to about 50%.
- Signs and symptoms of pheochromocytoma include paroxysmal or sustained hypertension, headaches, anxiety, chest pain, visual changes, palpitations, diaphoresis, nausea and vomiting, pallor or flushing, abdominal pain, and seizures. The differential diagnosis should include preeclampsia and other hypertensive diseases.
- Diagnosis is by laboratory testing showing elevated catecholamines, metanephrines, and vanillylmandelic acid in a 24-hour urine specimen. Methyldopa should be discontinued before this test, as it will give a false-positive result. Abdominal CT or MRI can be used for localizing the tumor in pregnancy; myocardial perfusion scan can identify extra-adrenal sites.

- Definitive treatment is adrenalectomy, although timing of surgical intervention is controversial: generally, it is recommended either <24 weeks' gestation or following delivery. Medical therapy is primarily with alpha-adrenergic blockers: phenoxybenzamine (10 to 30 mg PO two to four times daily) or phentolamine (for acute treatment IV). Beta-adrenergic blockers are useful to treat tachycardia (e.g., propranolol 20 to 80 mg PO four times daily). Cesarean delivery is recommended to avoid the catecholamine surges of labor and delivery, which may increase mortality.

## Adrenal Insufficiency

- Adrenal insufficiency may be primary (Addison disease) or secondary to pituitary failure (Sheehan syndrome) or adrenal suppression following exogenous steroids. Destruction of more than 90% of the gland is required to significantly deplete all steroid hormones and cause symptomatic primary failure. When treated, adrenal insufficiency is not associated with adverse fetal or neonatal outcomes.
- Signs and symptoms include hypotension, weakness, fatigue, anorexia, nausea and vomiting, weight loss, and hyperpigmentation of the skin. Pregnancy can exacerbate adrenal insufficiency resulting from Addison disease.
- The differential diagnosis includes idiopathic autoimmune adrenalitis, tuberculosis, histoplasmosis, hemorrhagic necrosis, and infiltrative neoplasms. Other autoimmune disease may also be present, such as Hashimoto thyroiditis, premature ovarian failure, type 1 DM, and Graves disease.
- Diagnosis of primary adrenal insufficiency is by laboratory testing showing low plasma cortisol levels and an abnormal ACTH stimulation test (injection of 0.25 mg ACTH without plasma cortisol response at 1 hour).
- Treatment includes maintenance replacement of corticosteroids with hydrocortisone (20 mg PO each morning and 10 mg PO each evening) or prednisone (5 mg each morning and 2.5 mg each evening). Fludrocortisone (0.05 to 0.1 mg PO daily) is given for mineralocorticoid replacement. Patients should continue their usual regimen during pregnancy, with careful follow-up. Stress-dose steroids (e.g., hydrocortisone 100 mg IV every 8 hours with taper following stress) should be administered during labor and delivery, at the time of major surgical procedures, for severe infection, or other significant stresses.

## SUGGESTED READINGS

American College of Obstetricians and Gynecologists Committee on Practice Bulletins. ACOG practice bulletin no. 30: clinical management guidelines for obstetrician-gynecologists: gestational diabetes. *Obstet Gynecol* 2001;98:525–538.

American College of Obstetricians and Gynecologists Committee on Practice Bulletins. ACOG practice bulletin no. 32: clinical management guidelines for obstetrician-gynecologists: thyroid disease in pregnancy. *Obstet Gynecol* 2001;98(5, pt 1):879–888.

American College of Obstetricians and Gynecologists Committee on Practice Bulletins. ACOG practice bulletin no. 60: clinical management guidelines for obstetrician-gynecologists: pregestational diabetes mellitus. *Obstet Gynecol* 2005;105:675–685.

Cooper MS. Disorders of calcium metabolism and parathyroid disease. *Best Pract Res Clin Endocrinol Metab* 2011;25(6):975–983.

De Groot L, Abalovich M, Alexander EK, et al. Management of thyroid dysfunction during pregnancy and postpartum: an Endocrine Society clinical practice guideline. *J Clin Endocrinol Metab* 2012;97(8):2543–2565.

de Valk HW, Visser GH. Insulin during pregnancy, labour and delivery. *Best Pract Res Clin Obstet Gynaecol* 2011;25(1):65–76.

Dhulkotia JS, Ola B, Fraser R, et al. Oral hypoglycemic agents vs insulin in management of gestational diabetes: a systematic review and metaanalysis. *Am J Obstet Gynecol* 2010;203(5): 457.e1–457.e9.

HAPO Study Cooperative Research Group. Hyperglycemia and adverse pregnancy outcomes. *NEJM* 2008;358:1991.

HAPO Study Cooperative Research Group. Hyperglycemia and Adverse Pregnancy Outcome (HAPO) study: associations of maternal A1C and glucose with pregnancy outcomes. *Diabetes Care* 2012;35(3):574–580.

Karaca Z, Kelestimur F. Pregnancy and other pituitary disorders (including GH deficiency). *Best Pract Res Clin Endocrinol Metab* 2011;25(6):897–910.

Lekarev O, New MI. Adrenal disease in pregnancy. *Best Pract Res Clin Endocrinol Metab* 2011; 25(6):959–973.

Metzger BF, Gabbe SG, Persson B, et al. International Association of Diabetes and Pregnancy Study Groups recommendations on the diagnosis and classification of hyperglycemia in pregnancy. *Diabetes Care* 2010;33:676–682

Nicholson W, Baptiste-Roberts K. Oral hypoglycaemic agents during pregnancy: the evidence for effectiveness and safety. *Best Pract Res Clin Obstet Gynaecol* 2011;25(1):51–63.

Schnatz PF, Thaxton S. Parathyroidectomy in the third trimester of pregnancy. *Obstet Gynecol Surv* 2005;60(10):672–682.

# 14 Hypertensive Disorders of Pregnancy

Veena Choubey and Frank R. Witter

## DEFINITIONS OF HYPERTENSIVE DISORDERS

**Hypertensive disorders** affect 5% to 10% of all pregnancies.

- **Hypertension** is defined as systolic blood pressure (BP) ≥140 mm Hg or diastolic BP ≥90 mm Hg on two separate occasions at least 6 hours but not more than 7 days apart.
- **Chronic hypertension** is high BP diagnosed before pregnancy or before 20 weeks' gestation or first recognized during pregnancy but persisting longer than 12 weeks postpartum.
- **Gestational hypertension**, formerly known as pregnancy-induced or transient hypertension, is defined as BP ≥140/90 mm Hg during pregnancy or within the first 24 hours postpartum without a history of chronic hypertension and without the signs and symptoms of preeclampsia. If the BP is ≥160/110 for more than 6 hours, the diagnosis is severe gestational hypertension.
- **Preeclampsia** is diagnosed by elevated BP and proteinuria after 20 weeks' gestation in a patient known to be previously normotensive. Trophoblastic disease or multiple gestation can present with preeclampsia before 20 weeks' gestation.
  - **Mild preeclampsia** is defined by the following criteria:
    ○ **BP** ≥140/90 mm Hg confirmed on two measures at least 6 hours but not more than 7 days apart, *and*

- **Proteinuria** ≥300 mg on a 24-hour urine collection or two random urine dipstick results of at least 30 mg/dL ("1+"). Spot urine protein: Creatinine ratios are used by some investigators instead of 24-hour urine collection and show good predictive value in the lower and higher ranges.
  - Preeclamptic patients often have wide variation in urine protein values over time, possibly from renal vasospasm. Discrepancies between the random urine dipstick and 24-hour urine collection measurements have been well described. The 24-hour urine collection, therefore, remains the preferred measure for diagnosing preeclampsia.
- **Severe preeclampsia** is classified by the following criteria:
  - **BP** during bed rest of ≥160 mm Hg systolic or ≥110 mm Hg diastolic; *or*
  - **Proteinuria** ≥5 g on a 24-hour urine collection even if BP is in the mild range. Persistent urine dipstick ≥3+ also qualifies; *or*
  - **Signs, symptoms, or lab values** of severe preeclampsia with any elevated BP.
- **Symptoms** of preeclampsia may include the following: cerebral or visual disturbances (e.g., persistent headache, blurred vision, scotomata, and blindness from retinal detachment); epigastric, right upper quadrant, or constant low abdominal pain from liver dysfunction or from abruptio placentae; nausea and vomiting; dyspnea from pulmonary edema; decreased urine output, hematuria, or rapid weight gain >5 pounds in 1 week; and absent or decreased fetal movement.
- **Physical findings** of preeclampsia may include the following:
  - Elevated BP measured in the sitting or semireclined position with the arm positioned roughly at heart level
  - Nondependent or generalized edema
  - **Pulmonary edema**, with rales or crackles on lung examination
  - **Epigastric** or **right upper quadrant tenderness** without a known cause, likely secondary to hepatic edema
  - Uterine tenderness or tetany secondary to placental abruption
  - **Oliguria** with 24-hour urine output <500 mL
- **Laboratory findings** of preeclampsia may include the following:
  - Diagnostic proteinuria (described earlier)
  - Decreased hematocrit secondary to severe hemolysis in HELLP (hemolysis, elevated liver enzymes, and low platelets) syndrome
  - **Microangiopathic hemolytic anemia** with abnormal findings on peripheral smear, increased serum bilirubin, elevated serum lactate dehydrogenase (LDH), or decreased serum haptoglobin
  - Elevated hematocrit resulting from decreased intravascular volume secondary to third spacing of fluid
  - Elevated serum uric acid level of 5 mg/dL or greater
  - Elevated serum creatinine of 1.2 mg/dL or greater. Creatinine normally decreases in pregnancy, thus even slight increases warrant further investigation.
  - Elevated serum transaminases (aspartate aminotransferase >70 IU/L)
  - **Thrombocytopenia** with platelet count of 100,000/L or less
  - Prolonged prothrombin and partial thromboplastin times that may be due to primary coagulopathy, hepatic synthesis dysfunction, or abruptio placentae leading to disseminated intravascular coagulation
  - Decreased fibrinogen, increased fibrin degradation products, or both, as a result of coagulopathy or abruptio placentae
- **Fetal findings** of preeclampsia may include **intrauterine growth restriction (IUGR)**, **oligohydramnios**, and other signs of **uteroplacental insufficiency**.

- **Preeclampsia superimposed on chronic hypertension** occurs in patients with preexisting high BP. Differentiating chronic hypertension with superimposed preeclampsia from a gestational exacerbation of chronic hypertension can be difficult, especially if there is baseline proteinuria. In general, diagnosis requires a significant change from baseline proteinuria and worsening hypertension or the development of symptoms.
- **HELLP syndrome** is a variant of preeclampsia defined by the following criteria:
  - **Hemolysis** identified by burr cells and schistocytes on an abnormal peripheral smear, an elevated serum bilirubin (>1.2 mg/dL) or LDH level (>600 IU/L), or a low serum haptoglobin
  - **Thrombocytopenia** with platelets ≤100,000/μL is the most consistent finding in HELLP syndrome.
  - **Elevated liver function tests** (i.e., transaminases) greater than two times the upper limit of normal
  - Note that hypertension may be absent (12% to 18% of cases), mild (15% to 50%), or severe (50%). Proteinuria may be absent as well (13%).
- **Eclampsia** is seizure or unexplained coma in a patient with preeclampsia. Eclampsia can present without hypertension (16%) or proteinuria (14%).

## CHRONIC HYPERTENSION

**Chronic hypertension** carries increased risk for superimposed preeclampsia, preterm delivery, abruptio placentae, and IUGR. See Chapter 1 for general classification and treatment of hypertension.
- The **differential diagnosis** of chronic hypertension in pregnancy includes the following:
  - Essential hypertension, which accounts for 90% of hypertension outside of pregnancy
  - Kidney disease, adrenal disorders (e.g., primary aldosteronism, congenital adrenal hyperplasia, Cushing syndrome, pheochromocytoma), hyperthyroidism, new-onset collagen vascular disease, systemic lupus erythematosus, aortic coarctation, chronic obstructive sleep apnea, and cocaine use
  - Worsening chronic hypertension is difficult to distinguish from superimposed preeclampsia. If seizures, thrombocytopenia, pulmonary edema, unexplained hemolysis, or elevation in liver enzyme levels develop, superimposed preeclampsia should be diagnosed. Monitoring trends in BP and urine protein may also be helpful.
    - A 24-hour urine calcium measurement may be useful. Urine calcium with preeclampsia is lower than in patients with hypertension alone.
    - A value <195 mg total urine calcium in 24 hours predicts preeclampsia with a sensitivity of 86% and specificity of 84%.
- Obtain **baseline information** early in pregnancy for chronic hypertension, including:
  - History of first diagnosis, etiology, duration, and current and prior treatments
  - Complete medical history including cardiovascular risk factors (e.g., smoking, increased plasma lipid levels, obesity, and diabetes mellitus) and complicating medical factors (e.g., headaches, history of chest pain, myocardial infarction, stroke, renal disease)
  - Complete medication list including vasoactive over-the-counter drugs (e.g., sympathomimetic amines, nasal decongestants, diet pills)

- Baseline complete blood count (CBC) and serum creatinine, urea nitrogen, uric acid, and calcium levels
- Baseline electrocardiogram (ECG) if not documented within the prior 6 months. Echocardiogram may be indicated if evidence of left ventricular hypertrophy is present.
- Baseline 24-hour urine protein
- **Treatment** is tailored to the severity of illness and presence of comorbidities.
- Mild hypertension often responds to conservative management.
  - Sodium restriction of ≤2.4 g/day. Dietary modifications with increased fruits and vegetables and decreased total and saturated fats can be encouraged.
  - Smoking and alcohol cessation
  - Mild activity restrictions, due to concern for decreased uteroplacental blood flow increasing risk of preeclampsia
  - Serial fetal growth ultrasounds every 4 to 6 weeks starting after the anatomy scan at 18 to 20 weeks' gestation. More severe or worsening hypertension may require **drug therapy** and requires closer monitoring of fetal well-being. Patients receiving antihypertensive agents should undergo antepartum fetal surveillance with nonstress test (NST) or biophysical profile (BPP) and a BP check one or two times per week starting at 28 weeks' gestation (earlier if severe hypertension or suspected IUGR).
- Treatment for chronic hypertension or persistently elevated BPs can include the following during pregnancy:
  - **Labetalol**—an $\alpha_1$ and nonselective β-adrenergic antagonist that can be used as monotherapy or combined with hydralazine or a diuretic. The initial dose is 100 mg twice daily and may be increased in increments of 100 mg twice daily every 2 to 3 days to a maximum of 2,400 mg daily. It is contraindicated in patients with greater than first-degree heart block. Chronic beta-blocker use in pregnancy has a mild association with IUGR.
  - **Nifedipine**—a calcium channel blocker used commonly in pregnancy that allows convenient daily dosing with the sustained release formulation. A multicenter prospective study of first-trimester drug exposure to calcium antagonists found no increased teratogenicity. The initial dose of nifedipine is 30 mg daily. The dose can be increased to 60 mg daily if adequate response is not seen in 7 days. The maximum daily dose is 90 mg. There is a theoretical risk of neuromuscular blockade when magnesium and nifedipine are administered together, although this was not supported in retrospective studies.
  - **Methyldopa** (Aldomet)—a centrally acting sympathetic outflow inhibitor that decreases systemic vascular resistance and is safe in pregnancy. Side effects include hepatic damage; therefore, liver function tests should be monitored at least once per trimester. Starting dose is 250 mg orally three times daily with a maximum dose of 3 g/day. The dose may be adjusted at increased in intervals of not less than every 2 days.
  - **Hydralazine**—a direct peripheral vasodilator that can be combined with methyldopa or a beta-blocker. It can cause a lupus-like syndrome but usually only at doses higher than 200 mg/day for an extended time. The starting oral dose is 10 mg four times a day and may be increased to a maximum of 200 mg/day.
  - **Thiazide diuretics**—inhibit renal sodium and chloride reabsorption. A large meta-analysis found no adverse outcomes in pregnancy; however, decreased plasma volume from diuresis carries a theoretic risk of placental insufficiency,

which deters its use as a first-line agent. The initial dose of hydrochlorothiazide (HCTZ) is 12.5 to 25 mg daily, titrated every 2 to 3 weeks to a maximum daily dose of 50 mg daily. Diuretics are not recommended in the setting of pre-eclampsia, uteroplacental insufficiency, or IUGR. Serum uric acid increases with thiazide diuretics, limiting diagnostic options for preeclampsia.

○ **Angiotensin-converting enzyme (ACE) inhibitors**—inhibit angiotensin I conversion to the vasoconstrictor angiotensin II. ACE inhibitors are *contraindicated* in pregnancy due to the risk of fetal death in the second and third trimesters and neonatal renal failure and pulmonary failure. There is also an unconfirmed report of first-trimester teratogenicity. Angiotensin antagonists are also contraindicated due to their similar effects on the angiotensin-renal system.

• **Severe range BPs:** Elevated sustained BPs ≥160 systolic or ≥105 to 110 diastolic warrant immediate therapy with intravenous (IV) antihypertensives, including labetalol or hydralazine for the prevention of acute morbidity from hypertensive urgency. See discussion later under "Preeclampsia" and antihypertensive therapy.

• **Delivery:** Timing of delivery should be tailored to the individual patient. In general, those who do not require antihypertensive medications should be delivered at 38 0/7 to 39 6/7 weeks. Those controlled with antihypertensive medication should be delivered at 37 0/7 to 39 6/7 weeks, and those with difficult to control hypertension at 36 0/7 to 37 6/7 weeks.

## GESTATIONAL HYPERTENSION

**Gestational hypertension** is the most common etiology of hypertension in pregnancy, affecting 6% to 7% of nulliparous and 2% to 4% of parous women. The incidence increases with a history of preeclampsia and in multiple gestations. Earlier diagnosis of gestational hypertension increases the risk of preeclampsia; up to 50% of those with hypertension before 30 weeks will progress to preeclampsia.

• **Prognosis and management** depend on timing and severity.
• **Mild gestational hypertension** after 37 weeks has a similar outcome to normotensive patients but an increased rate of labor induction and cesarean section.
  ○ If <37 weeks, monitor closely for progression to severe hypertension, preeclampsia, and fetal growth restriction.
  ○ If >37 weeks (full term), deliver if the cervix is favorable; otherwise, close follow-up may be permitted with delivery achieved between 37 0/7 and 38 6/7 weeks.
• **Severe gestational hypertension**, especially in early pregnancy, increases fetal and maternal morbidity even more than mild preeclampsia. Risks include placental abruption, preterm delivery, and small-for-gestational-age infants.
  ○ When BP is 160/110 or greater, antihypertensive therapy is indicated, as mentioned earlier. The goal is to maintain uteroplacental perfusion but gently reduce systolic and diastolic BP to the mild hypertensive range.
  ○ If the response to medical therapy is inadequate, the patient must be admitted to the antepartum service for close monitoring.

## PREECLAMPSIA

**Preeclampsia** occurs in 2% to 7% of healthy nulliparous women and 1% to 5% of parous women. The incidence is higher in twin pregnancies (14%) and for women with a history of preeclampsia (18%). It is the third leading cause of maternal mortality, responsible for over 17% of maternal deaths, and a major cause of neonatal morbidity and mortality.

- **Risk factors** for preeclampsia include:
  - Nulliparity
  - Multiple gestation
  - Obesity
  - Chronic hypertension (15% to 50% of cases)
  - Systemic lupus erythematosus
  - Thrombophilia
  - Pregestational diabetes (10% to 36% of cases)
  - Kidney disease
  - History of preeclampsia or eclampsia
  - Poor outcome in a previous pregnancy
  - Family history of preeclampsia, eclampsia, or cardiovascular disease
  - Molar pregnancy
  - Conception via assisted reproductive technologies
  - Abnormal uterine Doppler studies at 18 and 24 weeks
- The **pathophysiology** of preeclampsia requires the presence of trophoblastic tissue but not necessarily a fetus (e.g., molar pregnancy). Proposed mechanisms include impaired trophoblastic differentiation and invasion, immunologic response to pregnancy, and placental or endothelial abnormalities. The temporal sequence and relative importance of these alterations are under investigation.
- The best **preventive** measures for preeclampsia are early evaluation, risk reduction, and optimizing maternal health. Women with preeclampsia in the second trimester have a recurrence rate as high as 65%. In patients at high risk for development of preeclampsia (history of early onset or severe growth restriction), low-dose aspirin therapy has been shown to reduce the risk of preeclampsia, perinatal mortality, preterm birth, and small-for-gestational-age infants. Supplementation with fish oil, calcium, or vitamins C and E and early antihypertensive therapy are ineffective.
- **Diagnosis** of preeclampsia is by symptoms and signs, including elevated BP and abnormal laboratory findings (described earlier).
- Definitive **management** for gestational hypertension, preeclampsia, and eclampsia is delivery.
  - In general, **mild preeclampsia** (see definitions earlier) at term is treated by delivery.
    - Optimal treatment prior to 37 weeks is usually expectant management. The benefits of bed rest, antihypertensive medications, and hospitalization are not clearly established. There are no large, randomized trials on the management of mild preeclampsia.
    - Close maternal and fetal observation is essential, but there is no standard protocol for testing or frequency.
    - Fetal monitoring can include growth ultrasound and amniotic fluid assessment every 3 to 4 weeks; umbilical artery Doppler velocimetry, and once or twice weekly NST or BPP.
    - Maternal monitoring can include weekly or semiweekly BP check and evaluation and periodic lab testing such as 24-hour urine protein, serum creatinine, platelet count, and serum transaminases to detect progression to severe preeclampsia.
    - A gestational age of >34 weeks with progressive labor, uncontrolled hypertension, abnormal fetal testing, or growth restriction should prompt delivery.

- The first priority in treating **severe preeclampsia** is to assess and stabilize the mother.
  - **At ≥34 weeks**, delivery is indicated, although immediate cesarean section is not usually warranted.
    - Patients in labor, or with a favorable cervix, can deliver vaginally. Careful monitoring, at least hourly assessments, and strict intake/output recordings should be maintained.
  - **Between 24 and 34 weeks**, expectant management is acceptable if BP is adequately controlled with antihypertensive agents, fetal testing is reassuring, and there is no evidence of IUGR.
    - Magnesium sulfate and IV antihypertensives may be given initially while betamethasone is administered for fetal lung maturity.
    - Fluid status should be monitored.
    - CBC, platelets, and liver function tests should be checked daily.
    - Fetal surveillance with NST or BPP should be performed at least weekly and patients should be instructed regarding maternal assessment of fetal movement.
    - Delivery is indicated by the following: IUGR, nonreassuring fetal tracing, eclampsia, neurologic deficits, pulmonary edema, right upper quadrant/epigastric pain, oliguria <500 mL in 24 hours or creatinine >1.5, disseminated intravascular coagulation, HELLP, placental abruption, or uncontrolled severe BP.
  - **At 24 weeks' gestation and earlier**, expectant management is associated with high maternal morbidity and limited perinatal benefit.
  - Expectant management of severe preeclampsia with IUGR has been associated with increased risk of fetal death (rate of perinatal death is 5.4%).
- **Seizure prophylaxis** during labor and for 24 hours postpartum is recommended for patients with preeclampsia. Some patients with severe persistent preeclampsia need seizure prophylaxis for longer periods *before and after* delivery.
  - **Magnesium sulfate (MgSO$_4$)** is the agent of choice for eclamptic seizure prophylaxis. MgSO$_4$ has been shown to decrease the risk of eclampsia by more than 50%.
    - For prophylaxis, we administer a loading dose of 4 g MgSO$_4$ IV over 15 to 20 minutes.
    - Maintenance dose is 2 g/hr IV (dose should be titrated down if the patient has poor urine output, poor kidney function, or an elevated serum creatinine).
    - If there is no IV access, the loading dose is 5 g MgSO$_4$ (50% solution) administered intramuscularly in each buttock (10 g total), with a maintenance dose of 5 g in alternating buttocks every 4 hours.
    - The therapeutic serum magnesium level for seizure prophylaxis depends on the laboratory. In general, the therapeutic range is 4 to 6 mEq/L. However, it is our practice to follow magnesium levels only for those patients in whom we are unusually concerned for developing supratherapeutic levels. For such patients, check serum magnesium level 4 hours after the loading dose, then every 6 hours as needed or if symptoms suggest magnesium toxicity.
    - Diuresis is a useful criterion for early cessation of seizure prophylaxis. Urine output equal to or exceeding 100 mL/hr for 2 hours suggests resolving preeclampsia with no or rare complications.
    - Patients are monitored hourly for signs and symptoms of magnesium toxicity:
      - Loss of patellar reflexes at 8 to 10 mEq/L
      - Respiratory depression or arrest at 12 mEq/L

- Mental status changes at >12 mEq/L followed by ECG changes and arrhythmias
- If magnesium toxicity develops, check the patient's vital signs, stop magnesium and check plasma levels, administer 1 g calcium gluconate IV over 3 minutes, and consider diuretics (e.g., furosemide, mannitol).

o **Phenytoin (Dilantin)** is a secondary agent for eclamptic seizure prophylaxis. Magnesium was clearly superior in a large randomized clinical trial and is preferred. It may, however, be contraindicated as in patients with myasthenia gravis.

o The loading dose is maternal weight based. For <50 kg, load 1,000 mg; for 50 to 70 kg, load 1,250 mg; and for >70 kg, load with 1,500 mg phenytoin.

o The first 750 mg of the loading dose should be given at 25 mg/min and the rest at 12.5 mg/min. If the patient maintains normal cardiac rhythm and has no history of heart disease, ECG monitoring is not necessary at this infusion rate.

o Check the serum phenytoin level at 30 to 60 minutes after infusion.

o A therapeutic level is >12 μg/mL; recheck level in 12 hours.

o If the level is <10 μg/mL, reload with 500 mg and check again in 30 to 60 minutes.

o If the level is 10 to 12 μg/mL, reload with 250 mg and check again in 30 to 60 minutes.

- **Antihypertensive therapy** is indicated for patients with a systolic BP of 160 mm Hg or greater or diastolic BP of 105 mm Hg or greater. Acute treatment aims to reduce BP in a controlled manner without compromising uteroplacental perfusion.

o It is reasonable to reduce the patient's systolic BP to 140 to 155 mm Hg and the diastolic BP to 90 to 100 mm Hg. It is more important to decrease the diastolic pressure.

o Useful antihypertensive agents for acute management include the following:

o **Hydralazine hydrochloride** has an onset of action within 10 to 20 minutes. The duration of action is 4 to 6 hours.

- Begin with a 5 mg IV bolus, and repeat every 20 minutes to a maximum of 20 mg as needed.

o **Labetalol hydrochloride** has an onset of action within 5 to 10 minutes and lasts for 3 to 6 hours. It is contraindicated in greater than first-degree maternal heart block.

- Begin with a 20 mg IV loading dose, then continuous infusion or an escalating bolus protocol.
- The escalating bolus protocol uses labetalol doses of 20, 40, 80, 80, and 80 mg given at 10-minute intervals to a maximum of 300 mg/24 hours.
- The continuous infusion protocol starts at 0.5 mg/kg/hr and increases every 30 minutes by 0.5 mg/kg/hr to a maximum dose of 3 mg/kg/hr.

- **Fluid management:** Patients with preeclampsia are frequently hypovolemic due to third spacing from low serum oncotic pressure and increased capillary permeability. These same abnormalities also increase risk for pulmonary edema. Diuretics may be used to treat pulmonary edema but should not be used otherwise in preeclamptic patients.

o Oliguria is defined as urine output of <100 mL in 4 hours. It is treated with 500-mL crystalloid bolus if the lungs are clear. If there is no response, another

500-mL bolus can be administered. If there is no response after 1 L, central hemodynamic monitoring can be considered (see Chapter 3).

- o Central venous pressure monitoring does not correlate well with pulmonary capillary wedge pressure. A Swan-Ganz catheter may be required to help guide fluid management and prevent flash pulmonary edema.

- o Patients usually begin to effectively diurese about 12 to 24 hours after delivery. In cases of severe renal compromise, it may take 72 hours or more for adequate diuresis to resume.

- **Maternal complications** of severe preeclampsia require a high index of clinical suspicion and include renal failure (acute tubular necrosis), acute cardiac failure, pulmonary edema, thrombocytopenia, disseminated intravascular coagulopathy, and cerebrovascular accidents.

- **Perinatal outcome:** There is a high perinatal morbidity and mortality in pregnancies complicated by severe preeclampsia. Fetal mortality rates range from 5% to more than 70%.

## HELLP SYNDROME

**HELLP syndrome** often presents with nonspecific complaints such as malaise, abdominal pain, vomiting, shortness of breath, or bleeding.

- The **differential diagnosis** for HELLP syndrome includes:
  - Acute fatty liver of pregnancy (AFLP)
  - Thrombotic thrombocytopenic purpura (TTP)
  - Hemolytic uremic syndrome (HUS)
  - Immune thrombocytopenic purpura (ITP)
  - Systemic lupus erythematosus flare
  - Antiphospholipid antibody syndrome
  - Cholecystitis
  - Fulminant hepatitis (of any cause)
  - Acute pancreatitis
  - Disseminated herpes zoster

- **Management** is the same as for severe preeclampsia. Platelet transfusion may be required immediately prior to delivery depending on severity of thrombocytopenia. Short-term expectant management in order to allow for administration of betamethasone for fetal lung maturity *may* be possible in a very select group of patients with HELLP prior to 34 weeks; however, there are no data suggesting improved perinatal outcomes with this approach.

## ECLAMPSIA

**Eclampsia** should be the presumed diagnosis in obstetric patients with seizures and/or coma without a known history of epilepsy. The incidence of eclampsia is between 1 in 2,000 and 1 in 3,500 pregnancies in developed countries. Eclampsia occurs in about 1% of patients with preeclampsia. Virtually all eclampsia is preceded by preeclampsia.

- The **pathophysiology** of eclamptic seizures is unknown but may occur when mean arterial pressure exceeds the capacity of cerebral autoregulation, leading to cerebral edema and increased intracranial pressure.

- Eclampsia can occur antepartum, peripartum, or postpartum and has been reported as late as 3 to 4 weeks postpartum. Patients may have associated hypertension and proteinuria; a small percentage has neither.

- **Management** of eclampsia is an obstetric emergency that requires immediate treatment, including:
  - Appropriate management of ABCs (airway, breathing, and circulation) with measures taken to avoid aspiration
  - Seizure control with 4 to 6 g MgSO$_4$ IV bolus. If the patient has a seizure during or after the loading dose, an additional 2 g IV bolus of MgSO$_4$ can be given.
  - Treatment of seizures refractory to MgSO$_4$ with IV phenytoin or a benzodiazepine (e.g., lorazepam)
  - Treatment of *status epilepticus* with lorazepam 0.1 mg/kg IV at a rate ≥2 mg/min. Patients with *status epilepticus* may require intubation to correct hypoxia and acidosis and to maintain a secure airway.
  - Prevention of maternal injury with padded bedrails and appropriate positioning
  - Control of severe hypertension (see medications mentioned earlier)
  - Delivery after maternal stabilization
    - During acute eclamptic episodes, fetal bradycardia is common. It usually resolves in 3 to 5 minutes. Allowing the fetus to recover in utero from the maternal seizure, hypoxia, and hypercarbia before delivery is optimal. However, if fetal bradycardia persists beyond 10 minutes, abruptio placentae should be suspected.
    - Emergency cesarean section should always be anticipated in case of rapid maternal or fetal deterioration.
- **Outcomes** depend on the severity of disease. Perinatal mortality in the United States ranges from 5.6% to 11.8%, mainly due to extreme prematurity, placental abruption, and IUGR. The maternal mortality rate is from <1.8% in the developed world to 14% in underresourced countries. Maternal complications include aspiration pneumonitis, hemorrhage, cardiac failure, intracranial hemorrhage, and transient or permanent retinal blindness.
- Long-term neurologic sequelae of eclampsia are rare. Central nervous system (CNS) imaging with computed tomography (CT) or magnetic resonance imaging (MRI) should be performed if seizures are of late onset (longer than 48 hours after delivery) or if neurologic deficits are clinically evident. The signs and symptoms of preeclampsia usually resolve within 1 to 2 weeks postpartum. Approximately 25% of eclamptic patients develop preeclampsia in subsequent pregnancies, with recurrence of eclampsia in 2% of cases.

## SUGGESTED READINGS

American College of Obstetricians and Gynecologists. ACOG practice bulletin no. 125: chronic hypertension in pregnancy. *Obstet Gynecol* 2012;119(2, pt 1):396–407.

American College of Obstetricians and Gynecologists Committee on Practice Bulletins—Obstetrics. ACOG practice bulletin no. 33: diagnosis and management of preeclampsia and eclampsia. *Obstet Gynecol* 2002;99:159–167.

Haddad B, Kayem G, Deis S, et al. Are perinatal and maternal outcomes different during expectant management of severe preeclampsia in the presence of IUGR? *Am J Obstet Gynecol* 2007;196:237.e1–237.e5.

National High Blood Pressure Education Program. Working Group report on high blood pressure in pregnancy. *Am J Obstet Gynecol* 2000;183(suppl 1):S1–S51.

Sibai B. Diagnosis, prevention and management of eclampsia. *Obstet Gynecol* 2005;105:402–410.

Sibai B. Expectant management of severe preeclampsia remote from term: patient selection, treatment and delivery indications. *Am J Obstet Gynecol* 2007;196:514.

Spong CY, Mercer BM, D'alton M, et al. Timing of indicated late-preterm and early-term birth. *Obstet Gynecol* 2011;118(2, pt 1):323–333.

# Cardiopulmonary Disorders of Pregnancy

Stephen Martin and Ernest M. Graham

## CARDIAC DISORDERS

**Cardiac diseases** complicate 1% to 4% of pregnancies in women without preexisting cardiac abnormalities. Pregnancy is associated with major alterations in circulatory physiology, and cardiovascular disease remains a major cause of nonobstetric maternal morbidity in the United States.

### Hemodynamic Changes During Pregnancy

- Profound **hemodynamic alterations** occur during pregnancy, labor, delivery, and the postpartum period. These changes begin during the first 5 to 8 weeks of pregnancy and peak in the late second trimester. Normal pregnancy is associated with fatigue, dyspnea, decreased exercise capacity, peripheral edema, and jugular venous distention. Most pregnant women have audible physiologic systolic murmurs created by augmented blood flow and a physiologic third heart sound (S3) that reflects the volume-expanded state. The enormous changes in the cardiovascular system during pregnancy carry many implications for management of pregnant patients with cardiac disease.

- **Blood volume** increases 40% to 50% during normal pregnancy, in part due to estrogen-mediated activation of the renin-aldosterone axis leading to sodium and water retention. The rise in blood volume is greater than the increase in red blood cell mass (20% to 30%), contributing to the fall in hemoglobin concentration causing physiologic anemia in pregnancy. Peak dilution occurs at 24 to 26 weeks.

- **Cardiac output** increases 30% to 50% above baseline by 20 to 26 weeks' gestation, peaks at the end of the second trimester, and then plateaus until delivery. The change in cardiac output is mediated by the following: (a) increased preload due to the rise in blood volume, (b) reduced afterload due to a fall in systemic vascular resistance, and (c) a rise in maternal heart rate of 10 to 15 beats per minute. Stroke volume increases during the first and second trimesters but declines in the third trimester due to caval compression by the gravid uterus. Cardiac output in twin pregnancies is 20% above that of singleton pregnancies. Blood pressure typically falls slightly during the first two trimesters of pregnancy because of reduction in peripheral vascular resistance related to increased progesterone production.

- **Labor and delivery:** During labor and delivery, hemodynamic fluctuations can be profound. Each uterine contraction results in the displacement of 300 to 500 mL of blood into the general circulation. Stroke volume increases, causing a rise in cardiac output of an additional 50% with each contraction. Mean systemic pressure also rises due to maternal pain and anxiety. Blood loss during delivery can further alter the hemodynamic state.

- **Postpartum:** Immediately postpartum, uterine involution leads to autotransfusion, which increases cardiac output dramatically. In addition, there is a relief of vena caval compression after delivery. Increased venous return augments cardiac output and prompts brisk diuresis. The cardiovascular system returns to the prepregnant baseline within 3 to 4 weeks postpartum.

## Cardiac Disease in Pregnancy

- **Signs and symptoms** of cardiac disease overlap common symptoms and findings in pregnancy including fatigue, shortness of breath, orthopnea, palpitations, edema, systolic flow murmur, and a third heart sound.
- **Evaluation** of cardiac disease includes a thorough history and physical examination. Noninvasive testing includes an electrocardiogram (ECG), chest radiograph, and an echocardiogram. The ECG may reveal a leftward shift of the electrical axis, especially during the third trimester when the diaphragm is pushed upward by the uterus. Ventricular extrasystoles are a common finding. Routine chest radiographs are used to assess cardiomegaly and pulmonary vascular prominence. Echocardiographic evaluation of ventricular function and structural anomalies is invaluable for diagnosis of cardiac disease in pregnancy. Many changes including mild valvular regurgitation and chamber enlargement are normal findings on echocardiogram during pregnancy.

### Management of Patients with Known Cardiac Disease

- **Before conception:** Whenever possible, women with preexisting cardiac lesions should receive preconception counseling regarding maternal and fetal risks during pregnancy and long-term maternal morbidity and mortality. The New York Heart Association (NYHA) functional class (Table 15-1) is used as a predictor of outcome. Women with NYHA class III and IV face a mortality rate of 7% and morbidity over 30%. These women should be strongly cautioned against pregnancy. A risk index using four risk factors has been shown to accurately predict a woman's chance of having adverse cardiac or neonatal complications: (a) a prior cardiac event, (b) cyanosis or poor functional class, (c) left heart obstruction, and (d) systemic ventricular dysfunction. With two or more risk factors, the chance of cardiac event approaches 75%.

| TABLE 15-1 | New York Heart Association (NYHA) Functional Classification |
|---|---|

| NYHA Class | Symptoms |
|---|---|
| I | No symptoms and no limitation in ordinary physical activity such as shortness of breath when walking or climbing stairs. |
| II | Mild symptoms (mild shortness of breath and/or angina) and slight limitation during ordinary activity. |
| III | Marked limitation in activity due to symptoms, even during less-than-ordinary activity such as walking short distances (20–100 m). Comfortable only at rest. |
| IV | Severe limitations. Experiences symptoms even while at rest. Mostly bedbound. |

Criteria Committee of the New York Heart Association. *Nomenclature and Criteria for Diagnosis of Diseases of the Heart and Great Vessels*, 8th ed. Boston, MA: Little Brown, 1979.

- **After conception:** Pregnant patients with significant history require cardiac assessment as early as possible. If the pregnancy poses a serious threat to maternal health, the patient should be counseled about the option of pregnancy termination. Patients need close monitoring and follow-up by both a perinatologist and cardiologist, with attention to signs or symptoms of worsening congestive heart failure (CHF) throughout the pregnancy. Each visit should include the following: (a) cardiac examination and cardiac review of systems; (b) documentation of weight, blood pressure, and pulse; and (c) evaluation of peripheral edema.
- **During pregnancy:** The most common cardiac complications of pregnancy include arrhythmia and CHF. If symptoms worsen, hospitalization, bed rest, diuresis, or correction of an underlying arrhythmia may be required. Sometimes, surgical correction during pregnancy becomes necessary. When possible, procedures should be performed during the early second trimester to avoid the period of fetal organogenesis and before more significant hemodynamic changes of pregnancy occur. Pregnancy is also a time of hypercoagulability, and anticoagulation should be started if appropriately indicated.

### Antibiotic Prophylaxis for Endocarditis

- American College of Obstetricians and Gynecologists (ACOG) has endorsed the 2007 American Heart Association (AHA) guidelines for prevention of infective endocarditis (IE) which represent a marked change from prior AHA guidelines. Antibiotic prophylaxis is no longer recommended, as IE is more likely to result from frequent random bacteremia with daily activities than from bacteremia caused by specific dental, gastrointestinal (GI), or genitourinary (GU) procedures. Prophylaxis is now based on the risk of adverse outcome with the procedure, and it is not recommended for GU procedures, except in high-risk patients with GU infections, to prevent wound infection and sepsis. Antibiotic prophylaxis for IE is not recommended for vaginal delivery or hysterectomy (see Chapter 27).

## Specific Cardiac Conditions

### Cardiomyopathy

- **Cardiomyopathy** can be genetic, idiopathic, or caused by myocarditis or toxins and manifests during pregnancy with signs and symptoms of CHF. These include chest pain, dyspnea, paroxysmal nocturnal dyspnea, and cough. Echocardiography demonstrates chamber enlargement and reduced ventricular function. The heart becomes uniformly dilated, filling pressures increase, and cardiac output decreases. Eventually, heart failure develops and is often refractory to treatment. The 5-year survival rate is approximately 50%; therefore, careful preconception counseling is important, even if the patient is asymptomatic.
  - **Hypertrophic cardiomyopathy** with or without left ventricular outflow tract obstruction is an autosomal dominant disorder with a variable phenotype and incidence of 0.1% to 0.5% in pregnancy. Most women with hypertrophic cardiomyopathy do well in pregnancy, and complications are uncommon with prior prepregnancy risk stratification via NYHA functional class and multidisciplinary specialist management. Risk is increased in patients that are symptomatic or if there is significant left ventricular outflow obstruction. The potential exists for poor tolerance of the circulatory overload of pregnancy. Major complications include pulmonary edema secondary to diastolic dysfunction, dysrhythmias secondary to myofibrillar disarray, functional class decline, obstetric complications, and poor fetal outcomes. During pregnancy, beta-blockers should be continued and the judicious use of diuretics may be required to treat symptoms of dyspnea.

- **Peripartum cardiomyopathy** is an idiopathic dilated cardiomyopathy that typically develops in the last month of pregnancy or within 5 months of delivery and is characterized by left ventricular systolic dysfunction with ejection fraction (EF) <45%. Incidence is 1 in 1,300 to 1 in 15,000. Risk factors include advanced maternal age; multiparity; multiple gestations; black race; obesity; malnutrition; gestational hypertension (HTN); preeclampsia; poor antenatal care; breast-feeding; cesarean section; low socioeconomic status; family history; and abuse of tobacco, alcohol, or cocaine. The most common clinical complaints are dyspnea, cough, orthopnea, paroxysmal nocturnal dyspnea, and hemoptysis. Workup and diagnosis are completed with ECG, echocardiography, and lab studies such as brain natriuretic peptide.

  ○ Of the patients who survive, approximately 50% recover normal left heart function. The mortality rate is 25% to 50%; half of those die within the first month of presentation, and the majority dies within 3 months postpartum. Prognosis is related to left ventricular dysfunction at presentation. Death results from progressive CHF, thromboembolic events, and arrhythmias.

  ○ Medical management includes fluid and salt restriction, digoxin, diuretics, vasodilators, and anticoagulants; bed rest can predispose to thromboembolism. Cardiac transplantation may be required in advanced unresolving disease. For patients diagnosed antenatally, invasive cardiac monitoring should be considered during labor and until at least 24 hours postpartum. Supplemental oxygen and regional analgesia for pain control should be administered and a passive second stage of labor facilitated by operative vaginal delivery. Cesarean section is reserved for obstetric indications. Intensive care unit monitoring should continue immediately postpartum, including detection and management of possible autotransfusion-induced pulmonary edema.

## Valvular Disease

- **Mitral valve prolapse (MVP)** is the most common congenital heart defect in women. It rarely has implications for maternal or fetal outcomes. It is the most common cause of mitral regurgitation (MR) in women.
- **MR** is usually well tolerated during pregnancy. The fall in systemic vasoresistance improves cardiac output in pregnancy. Medical management includes diuretics in the rare event of pulmonary congestion or vasodilators for systemic HTN. Acute, severe worsening of MR can result from ruptured chordae and must be repaired surgically. Women with severe MR before pregnancy should undergo operative repair before conception. Patients with advanced disease may require central monitoring during labor.
- **Aortic regurgitation (AR):** AR may be encountered in women with rheumatic heart disease, a congenitally bicuspid or deformed aortic valve, IE, or connective tissue disease. AR is generally well tolerated during pregnancy. Medical management includes diuretics and vasodilators. Ideally, women with severe AR should undergo operative repair before conception; as in MR, surgery during pregnancy should be considered only for control of refractory NYHA functional class III or IV symptoms.
- **Aortic stenosis (AS):** The most common etiology of AS in pregnant women is a congenitally bicuspid valve. Mild AS with normal left ventricular function is usually well tolerated during pregnancy. Asymptomatic severe stenosis can be managed conservatively with bed rest, oxygen, and beta-blockade. Moderate to severe AS markedly increases the medical risk of pregnancy; patients are advised to delay conception until correction is performed. Symptoms, such as dyspnea, angina pectoris, or syncope, usually become apparent late in the second trimester or early

in the third trimester. Women with bicuspid aortic valves are also at increased risk for aortic dissection and should be followed carefully. Aortic root enlargement >40 mm or an increase in aortic root size during pregnancy are risk factors for dissection. Beta-blockers may be indicated in these patients.

- Severe symptomatic AS can be managed by percutaneous aortic balloon valvuloplasty prior to labor and delivery but not without significant risk to both mother and fetus. If presenting early in pregnancy, termination should be discussed before surgical correction of severe AS (EF <40%). Spinal and epidural anesthesia are discouraged because of their vasodilatory effects. This disorder is characterized by a fixed afterload, thus adequate end-diastolic volume, and therefore adequate filling pressure, are necessary to maintain cardiac output. Consequently, great care must be taken to prevent hypotension, tachycardia, and hypoperfusion caused by blood loss, regional anesthesia, or other medications. Patients should be hydrated adequately and placed in the left lateral position to maximize venous return. As with mitral stenosis, hemodynamic monitoring with a pulmonary arterial catheter should be considered during labor and delivery.
- **Pulmonic stenosis (PS)** frequently accompanies other congenital cardiac anomalies, but as an isolated lesion, PS rarely complicates pregnancy. Patients with cyanotic congenital cardiac disease tolerate pregnancy less well than those with acyanotic lesions. Echocardiogram-guided percutaneous valvotomy is a potential treatment option.
- **Mitral stenosis (MS)** in women of childbearing age is usually due to rheumatic fever. Patients with moderate to severe MS often experience hemodynamic deterioration during the third trimester and/or during labor and delivery. Increased blood volumes and heart rate lead to an elevation of left atrial pressure, resulting in pulmonary edema. Additional displacement of blood volume into the systemic circulation during contractions makes labor particularly hazardous. Mild to moderate MS can be managed with judicious diuresis and beta-blockade, although aggressive diuresis should be avoided so as to preserve uteroplacental perfusion. Cardioselective beta-blockers such as metoprolol and atenolol are used to treat or prevent tachycardia, optimizing diastolic filling while preventing deleterious effects of epinephrine blockade on myometrial activity. These patients should be comanaged with a cardiologist. Patients with severe MS who develop NYHA functional class III to IV symptoms during pregnancy should undergo percutaneous balloon valvotomy.
  - Atrial fibrillation in pregnant patients with MS may result in rapid decompensation. Digoxin and beta-blockers can reduce heart rate, and diuretics may be used to reduce blood volume and left atrial pressure. With atrial fibrillation and hemodynamic deterioration, electrocardioversion can be performed safely and promptly. Atrial fibrillation also increases the risk of stroke and necessitates anticoagulation.
  - Most patients with MS can undergo vaginal delivery. However, patients with symptoms of CHF or moderate to severe MS should undergo hemodynamic monitoring with a Swan-Ganz catheter during labor, delivery, and for several hours postpartum. Epidural anesthesia is usually better tolerated hemodynamically than general anesthesia.

### Congenital Heart Disease

- During pregnancy, women with **congenital heart disease** are at increased risk of cardiac events including pulmonary edema and symptomatic sustained arrhythmias (supraventricular tachycardia [SVT] and ventricular tachycardia [VT]). Risk factors include prior history of heart failure, NYHA class III, decreased subpulmonary ventricular EF, severe pulmonary regurgitation, and smoking. These women also face increased risks of adverse neonatal outcomes including preterm delivery and infants with growth restriction, respiratory distress syndrome, and intraventricular hemorrhage. The risk of intrauterine or neonatal death is approximately 12% and 4%, respectively. Additionally, there is an increased incidence of congenital heart disease in children of women with a congenital abnormality ranging from approximately 3% overall to 50% in women carrying single-gene defects with autosomal dominant inheritance (e.g., Marfan syndrome). Because of the heterogeneity of congenital heart lesions, each patient needs individual assessment for ability to tolerate the hemodynamic changes of pregnancy.

- **Minimal risk lesions** include small ventricular septal defects (VSDs), atrial septal defects (ASDs), and bicuspid aortic valves without stenosis, insufficiency, or aortic enlargement. These patients have near-normal physiology with only minimally increased risk during pregnancy and can receive routine care.
- **Moderate risk lesions** include repaired tetralogy of Fallot without significant pulmonary insufficiency or stenosis, complex congenital heart disease with anatomic right ventricle serving as systemic ventricle, and mild left side valve stenosis.
- **High-risk lesions** for which patients should be counseled against pregnancy due to the risk of maternal cardiac decompensation and death include Eisenmenger syndrome, severe pulmonary HTN, severe AS or left ventricular outflow tract obstruction, Marfan syndrome with aortic dilation >45 mm, or symptomatic ventricular dysfunction with EF <40%. Moderate- and high-risk patients should be followed at tertiary care centers with perinatologists and cardiologists experienced in managing pregnant patients with congenital heart disease.
  - **Tetralogy of Fallot**, characterized by right ventricular outflow tract obstruction, VSD, right ventricular hypertrophy, and overriding aorta, is associated with right-to-left shunting and cyanosis. If the defect goes uncorrected, the affected patient rarely lives beyond childhood. In developed countries, almost all patients have had surgical correction with good survival rates (85% to 86% at 32 to 36 years) and good quality of life. Pregnancy is generally well tolerated in patients who have had surgical repair, although these women are at increased risk of right-sided heart failure and arrhythmia.
  - **Coarctation of the aorta:** Severe cases of coarctation of the aorta are usually corrected in infancy. Surgical correction during pregnancy is recommended only if dissection occurs. Some studies suggest that patients with a history of coarctation have increased rates of preeclampsia, gestational HTN, and preterm labor. Coarctation of the aorta is associated with other cardiac lesions such as berry aneurysms. Two percent of infants of mothers with coarctation of the aorta may have other cardiac lesions. Coarctation of the aorta is characterized by a fixed cardiac output. Therefore, the patient's heart cannot increase its rate to meet the increased cardiac demands of pregnancy, and extreme care must be taken to prevent hypotension, as with AS.
  - **Septal defects:** Young women with uncomplicated secundum-type ASD or isolated VSD usually tolerate pregnancy well. ASD is the most common congenital heart lesion in adults. ASDs are usually very well tolerated unless they are associated with pulmonary HTN. Complications, such as atrial arrhythmias, pulmonary HTN, and heart failure, usually do not arise until the fifth decade of

life and are therefore uncommon in pregnancy. VSDs usually close spontaneously or are closed surgically if the lesion is large. For this reason, significant VSDs are rarely seen in pregnancy. Rarely, uncorrected lesions lead to significant left-to-right shunts with pulmonary HTN, right ventricular failure, arrhythmias, and reversal of the shunt. The incidence of VSD in the offspring of affected parents is 4%; however, small VSDs are often difficult to detect antenatally.

- **Patent ductus arteriosus (PDA):** PDA is not associated with additional maternal risk for cardiac complications if the shunt is small to moderate and if pulmonary artery pressures are normal. Moderate to large PDA may be associated with increased volume, left heart failure, and pulmonary HTN or other pulmonary abnormalities. Therefore, pregnancy is not recommended for patients with large PDA and associated complications.

- **Eisenmenger syndrome** occurs when an initial left-to-right shunt results in pulmonary arterial obliteration and pulmonary HTN, eventually leading to a right-to-left shunt. This serious condition carries a maternal mortality rate of 50% and a fetal mortality rate of more than 50% if cyanosis is present. In addition, 30% of fetuses exhibit intrauterine growth restriction. Because of increased maternal mortality, pregnancy is generally contraindicated, and termination of the pregnancy should be discussed. If the pregnancy is continued, special precautions must be taken during the peripartum period. Women with Eisenmenger syndrome tolerate hypotension poorly. The patient should be monitored with a Swan-Ganz catheter, and care should be taken to avoid hypovolemia. Postpartum death most often occurs within 1 week after delivery; however, delayed deaths up to 4 to 6 weeks after delivery have been reported.

- **Marfan syndrome** is an autosomal dominant disorder of the fibrillin gene characterized by connective tissue fragility. Cardiovascular manifestations include aortic root dilation and dissection, MVP, and aneurysms. Genetic counseling is recommended. According to the 2010 American College of Cardiology (ACC)/AHA/American Association of Thoracic Surgeons guidelines, patients with a dilated aortic root >40 mm are considered high-risk. If cardiovascular involvement is minor and the aortic root diameter is smaller than 40 mm, the risk in pregnancy is less than 1%. If cardiovascular involvement is more extensive or the aortic root is larger than 40 mm, complications during pregnancy and aortic dissection are increased significantly. Patients should be monitored with serial physical exams as well as echocardiography. HTN should be avoided. Beta-blockade is recommended for patients with Marfan syndrome from the second trimester onward, particularly if the aortic root is dilated. Regional anesthesia during labor is considered safe. Women should labor in the left lateral decubitus position with the second stage shortened by operative vaginal delivery. Cesarean section should be reserved for obstetric indications.

- **Idiopathic hypertrophic subaortic stenosis** is an autosomal dominant disorder that manifests as left ventricular outflow tract obstruction secondary to a hypertrophic interventricular septum. Genetic counseling is advised for affected patients. Patients' conditions improve when left ventricular end-diastolic volume is maximized. Pregnant patients fare quite well initially because of an increase in circulating blood volume. There is less progression of disease in those patients who are asymptomatic before pregnancy. Later in pregnancy, however, decreased systemic vascular resistance and decreased venous return may worsen the obstruction. This may cause left ventricular failure as well as supraventricular arrhythmias from left atrial distention. The following labor management points should be kept in mind: (a) Inotropic agents may exacerbate obstruction, (b) medications that decrease systemic vascular resistance should be avoided or limited, (c) cardiac rhythm should be monitored and tachycardia treated promptly, and (d) the patient should undergo labor in the left lateral decubitus position with the second stage of labor shortened by operative vaginal delivery.

• **Transposition of the great arteries (TGA)** is characterized by correct atrioventricular connections and inappropriate ventriculoarterial connections; the aorta arises anteriorly from the right ventricle, and the pulmonary artery arises posteriorly from the left ventricle. The Senning operation (using atrial and septal tissues) and Mustard operation (using extrinsic material such as pericardium) redirect atrial blood via baffles to deliver oxygenated pulmonary venous blood to the systemic right ventricle and deoxygenated systemic venous blood to the pulmonary left ventricle. Long-term follow-up demonstrates an 80% survival at 28 years with the majority of survivors in NYHA class I. Pregnancy in women after Senning or Mustard repair is associated with arrhythmias (VT, SVT, atrial flutter), heart failure, and NYHA functional class deterioration as well as a high incidence of serious obstetric complications (65%) and offspring mortality (11.7%).

• **Congenital atrioventricular block:** Although affected patients may need a pacemaker, they usually fare well and do not require special treatment during pregnancy.

## Arrhythmias

• **Premature atrial and/or ventricular complexes** are not associated with adverse maternal or fetal outcomes and do not require antiarrhythmic therapy. **Atrial fibrillation** and **atrial flutter** are rare during pregnancy. Rate control can be safely achieved with digoxin or beta-blockers. Electrical cardioversion can be performed safely during any stage of pregnancy. Other arrhythmias should be managed with the assistance of a cardiologist. Nonsustained arrhythmias in the absence of organic cardiac disease are best left untreated or managed with lifestyle and dietary modifications (e.g., decreasing smoking, caffeine, and stress). Serious, life-threatening arrhythmias associated with an aberrant reentrant pathway should be treated before pregnancy by ablation. If medical therapy is necessary during pregnancy, established drugs such as beta-blockers should be used. Artificial pacing, electrical defibrillation, and cardioversion should have no effect on the fetus.

## Ischemic Heart Disease

• **Ischemic heart disease** is an uncommon but potentially devastating event in pregnancy. Risk factors include HTN, thrombophilia, diabetes, smoking, transfusion, postpartum infection, obesity, and age >35 years. Anterior wall myocardial infarctions (MIs) are most common. Diagnosis and evaluation of acute cardiac events is similar as in nonpregnant patients. Approximately 67% of MI during pregnancy occurs during the third trimester. If it occurs before 24 weeks' gestation, the option of pregnancy termination should be discussed due to the high incidence of maternal mortality. If delivery takes place within 2 weeks of the acute event, the mortality rate reaches 50%; survival is much improved if delivery takes place more than 2 weeks after the acute event.

- Coronary angioplasty is the preferred reperfusion therapy in cases of ST-elevated MI. Medical therapy for acute MI should be modified in the pregnant patient. Thrombolytic agents increase the risk of maternal hemorrhage to 8% for women who receive thrombolytic therapy shortly after delivery. Low-dose aspirin and nitrates are considered safe. Beta-blockers are safe, although some have been linked to a slight decrease in fetal growth. Short-term heparin administration has not been associated with increased maternal or fetal adverse effects. Angiotensin-converting enzyme (ACE) inhibitors and statins are contraindicated during pregnancy. Hydralazine and nitrates may be used as substitutes for ACE inhibitors.

## Cardiovascular Drugs in Pregnancy

- The most commonly used cardiovascular drugs and their potential adverse effects during pregnancy are shown in Table 15-2.
- **Anticoagulation:** Several conditions require the initiation or maintenance of anticoagulation during pregnancy. Anticoagulation choice depends on patient and physician preferences after consideration of the maternal and fetal risks. The three most common agents considered during pregnancy are warfarin, unfractionated heparin (UFH), and low-molecular-weight heparin (LMWH).
  - **UFH** does not cross the placenta and is safe for the fetus. Its use, however, has been associated with maternal osteoporosis, hemorrhage at the uteroplacental junction, thrombocytopenia (heparin-induced thrombocytopenia [HIT]), thrombosis, and a high incidence (12% to 24%) of thromboembolic events with older generation mechanical valves. High doses of UFH are often required to achieve the desired activated partial thromboplastin time (aPTT) due to the hypercoagulable state associated with pregnancy. Parenteral infusions should be stopped at least 4 hours before cesarean sections. UFH can be reversed with protamine sulfate.
  - **LMWH**, in comparison to UFH, produces a more predictable anticoagulant response, is less likely to cause HIT, is easier to administer and monitor, and has lower risk of osteoporosis and bleeding complications. LMWH does not cross the placenta and is safe for the fetus. Antifactor-Xa levels can be checked 4 hours after the morning dose and the dose adjusted to attain antifactor-Xa levels of 0.7 to 1.2 U/mL. Although data support the use of LMWH for DVT treatment in pregnant women, there are no data to guide its use in pregnant patients with mechanical valve prostheses and several small studies have shown increased rates of serious complications.
  - **Warfarin**, a vitamin K antagonist, freely crosses the placenta and can harm the fetus. The incidence of warfarin embryopathy (abnormalities of fetal bone and cartilage formation) has been estimated at 4% to 10%; the risk is highest when warfarin is administered during the 6th through 12th weeks' gestation. Clinically important embryopathy may be lower if the warfarin dose is <5 mg/day. Fetal central nervous system (CNS) abnormalities can occur after exposure during any trimester. Warfarin must be discontinued and switched to a heparin compound several weeks before delivery to avoid risk of fetal hemorrhage. Specifically, in the setting of mechanical prosthetic heart valves, warfarin has been associated with a lower risk of maternal thromboembolic complications compared to heparin (by ~2% to 4%). Treatment of this high-risk population must balance potentially improved thrombotic prophylaxis against risks of embryopathy; some

**TABLE 15-2  Cardiovascular Drugs in Pregnancy**

| Drug | Use | Side Effects | Pregnancy Risk Category | Safe during Breast-Feeding |
|------|-----|-------------|------------------------|---------------------------|
| Adenosine | Arrhythmia | None reported | C | No data |
| Amiodarone | Arrhythmia | IUGR, prematurity, hypothyroidism, neonatal prolonged QT | C/D | Not recommended |
| ACE inhibitors | HTN | Oligohydramnios, IUGR, PDA, prematurity, renal failure, neonatal hypotension, anemia musculoskeletal abnormalities | C (first trimester), D (second, third) | Not recommended |
| Beta-blockers (labetalol, metoprolol, propranolol) | HTN, MI, MS, HCM, arrhythmias, hyperthyroidism, Marfan syndrome | Fetal bradycardia, LBW, hypoglycemia, respiratory depression | C/D | Compatible |
| Digoxin | Arrhythmia, CHF | LBW, prematurity | C | Compatible |
| Diltiazem | Myocardial ischemia, tocolysis | Limited data | C | Compatible |
| Disopyramide | Arrhythmias | Limited data | C | Compatible |
| Diuretics | HTN, CHF | Uteroplacental hypoperfusion, fetal hypoglycemia, thrombocytopenia, hyponatremia, hypokalemia | C | Compatible |
| Flecainide | Arrhythmia | Limited data | C | Compatible |
| Heparin (UFH) | Anticoagulation | Maternal osteoporosis, hemorrhage, thrombocytopenia | C | Compatible |
| Hydralazine | HTN | None reported | C | Compatible |

*(Continued)*

**TABLE 15-2** Cardiovascular Drugs in Pregnancy *(Continued)*

| Drug | Use | Side Effects | Pregnancy Risk Category | Safe During Breast-Feeding |
|------|-----|--------------|-------------------------|----------------------------|
| Lidocaine | Arrhythmia, anesthesia | Neonatal CNS depression | B/C | Compatible |
| LMWH | Anticoagulation | Hemorrhage | B | Limited data |
| Nifedipine | HTN, tocolysis | Fetal distress with maternal hypotension | C | Compatible |
| Nitrates | HTN, MI, pulmonary edema | Limited data | C | No data |
| Procainamide | Arrhythmia | Limited data | C | Compatible |
| Propafenone | Arrhythmias | Limited data | C | No data |
| Quinidine | Arrhythmias | Premature labor, abortion, (minimal oxytocic effect) | C | Compatible |
| Sodium nitroprusside | HTN, aortic dissection | Fetal thiocyanate toxicity | C | No data |
| Sotalol | Arrhythmia, HTN | Limited data | B | Compatible |
| Verapamil | Arrhythmia, HTN, tocolysis | Limited data | C | Compatible |
| Warfarin | Anticoagulation | Warfarin embryopathy, fetal CNS abnormalities, fetal hemorrhage | D/X[a] | Compatible |

[a]Warfarin is listed as a category D drug by the U.S. Food and Drug Administration (FDA) but category X by its manufacturer. IUGR, intrauterine growth restriction; ACE, angiotensin-converting enzyme; HTN, hypertension; PDA, patent ductus arteriosus; MI, myocardial infarction; MS, mitral stenosis; HCM, hypertrophic cardiomyopathy; LBW, low birth weight; CHF, congestive heart failure; UFH, unfractionated heparin; CNS, central nervous system; LMWH, low-molecular-weight heparin. Adapted from Elkayam U. Pregnancy and cardiovascular disease. In Braunwald E, ed. *Heart Disease. A Textbook of Cardiovascular Medicine*, 6th ed. Philadelphia, PA: WB Saunders, 2001:2172–2191, with permission.

groups recommend prophylaxis in patients with mechanical heart valves using heparin agents in the first trimester, with consideration to transitioning to Coumadin until the last weeks of pregnancy, when the patient is transitioned back to heparin.

## RESPIRATORY DISORDERS

### Pulmonary Changes during Pregnancy

- Pregnancy causes mechanical and biochemical changes that affect maternal respiratory function and gas exchange. The most prominent factors are the mechanical effect of the gravid uterus on the diaphragm and the effect of increased circulating progesterone on ventilation. Progesterone is thought to increase the sensitivity of the respiratory center to carbon dioxide.
- Elevation of the diaphragm in the second half of pregnancy decreases functional residual capacity (FRC), the resting volume of the lungs at the end of a normal expiration. Despite the alteration in resting diaphragm position, excursion is unaffected and therefore vital capacity is maintained. Airway function is normal during pregnancy, as FEV1 (forced expiratory volume in the first second) and FEV1/FVC (forced vital capacity) are normal. Resting minute ventilation increases by 50% due to increased tidal volume of 40%. Both FEV and peak expiratory flow remain unchanged. As a result of increased minute ventilation, arterial $PCO_2$ decreases, which is offset by renal bicarbonate excretion, and arterial $PO_2$ levels are slightly increased. Oxygen consumption increases by 15% to 20% throughout pregnancy, which is compensated by the increased cardiac output. Arterial pH rises slightly from the decrease in $PCO_2$, resulting in a mild maternal respiratory alkalosis.

### Specific Respiratory Disorders

*Asthma*

- **Asthma** is the most common chronic condition in pregnancy and affects 3% to 12% of gestations. This condition is more likely to worsen in women with prepregnancy severe asthma. Exacerbations are most frequent between 24 and 36 weeks' gestation and are most commonly precipitated by viral respiratory infections and noncompliance with inhaled corticosteroid regimens. For women with severe asthma, a pulmonary examination, peak flow measurement, and review of symptoms should be performed at each visit. Smoking cessation must be encouraged. In addition, patients may monitor their peak flow at home and begin treatment before they become dangerously symptomatic. Influenza vaccination is recommended for all healthy pregnant patients and pregnant women with high-risk medical conditions. Low birth weight (LBW) is more common in infants born to mothers reporting daily symptoms of moderate asthma.
  - Because asthma exacerbations can be severe, they should be treated aggressively in pregnancy. Pregnant women tend to decrease use of asthma medications because of fear of fetal malformations. Physicians should provide reassurance that it is safer to take asthma medications in pregnancy than to risk adverse perinatal outcomes from a severe exacerbation.
  - **Inhaled corticosteroids** including beclomethasone, fluticasone, budesonide, flunisolide, and triamcinolone are the cornerstone of treatment for persistent asthma of all severities. They remain active locally with little systemic absorption

and effectively prevent exacerbations. Patients must be reassured that side effect profile is not the same for inhaled corticosteroids as for systemic/oral glucocorticoids to ensure compliance.

- **Oral steroids** are indicated for acute exacerbations when patients do not respond adequately to other measures. In acute settings, hydrocortisone 100 mg intravenous (IV) every 8 hours or methylprednisolone 125 mg IV every 6 hours may be used, followed by a tapered dose of oral prednisone.
- **Beta-sympathomimetic** drugs help control asthma via bronchial smooth muscle relaxation and can be used for symptomatic relief in conjunction with inhaled corticosteroids. Short-acting preparations are safe in pregnancy. Few data are available on long-acting preparations.
- **Anticholinergics**, such as aerosolized ipratropium bromide or glycopyrrolate, can also be used to treat severe symptoms. Side effects include tachycardia.
- **Cromolyn and leukotriene antagonists** are useful alternatives for mild persistent asthma or additional treatment for more severe exacerbations.
- **Theophylline**, a phosphodiesterase inhibitor, is a last treatment option in moderate or severe asthma, although it is rarely used. Blood levels are required during the third trimester as clearance increases during this period.
- **Acute asthma exacerbations** that require hospital observation or admission are treated with 40% humidified oxygen and beta-agonists initially. Chest radiograph should be obtained. Anticholinergics and inhaled or systemic steroids can be added as needed. Intubation should be considered if the $PCO_2$ is >40 mm Hg or hypoxia develops.
- **Exacerbations during labor** are rare, perhaps because of the increase in endogenous cortisol. Patients who received steroids throughout their pregnancies may require stress-dose steroids during labor and delivery. General endotracheal anesthesia should be avoided, if possible, because of the increased incidence of bronchospasm and atelectasis.

### Cystic Fibrosis

- **Cystic fibrosis (CF)** is an autosomal recessive disorder occurring in approximately 1 in 2,500 live births and is characterized by abnormal epithelial cell chloride transport and thickened glandular secretions. Diagnosis is confirmed by elevated sweat chloride concentration with pilocarpine iontophoresis or by mutation analysis of the cystic fibrosis transmembrane conductance regulator (CFTR) gene. Due to improved treatment modalities, women with CF are living longer—the median survival age for women is now 29 years—and they are more frequently reaching childbearing age.
  - Pregnancy does not compromise long-term survival in CF nor does it affect overall severity or maternal survival. Poor prognostic factors include a vital capacity of <50% of predicted value, cor pulmonale, and pulmonary HTN. Affected patients may have pancreatic insufficiency manifested as diabetes, malabsorption, or liver cirrhosis. Early diabetes screening in pregnancy is indicated.
  - Genetic counseling and screening should be offered. Pulmonary function tests should be performed monthly throughout pregnancy and pulmonary infection should be managed aggressively. During labor, fluid and electrolytes should be followed closely. The increased sodium content of sweat in affected patients may make them prone to hypovolemia during labor. Overall, 70% to 80% of pregnant mothers with CF have successful deliveries of healthy infants.

- Breast milk should be evaluated for sodium content before the infant is allowed to breast-feed; in the event of significant sodium elevation, breast-feeding is contraindicated.

## Tuberculosis

- **Tuberculosis (TB)** is a worldwide public health issue and highly prevalent in many urban areas.
  - Screening is by subcutaneous injection of purified protein derivative (PPD). Only 80% of results are positive in the setting of reactivation of disease, however, and if a patient previously received the bacille Calmette-Guérin (BCG) vaccine, the PPD result may remain positive for life. If the PPD test is positive or TB is suspected, chest radiography with abdominal shielding should be performed, preferably after 20 weeks' gestation. Alternative methods of screening are being developed but have yet to be widely accepted to replace PPD screening.
  - A definitive diagnosis of TB can be made with culture of *Mycobacterium tuberculosis* or acid-fast stain. Sputum samples may be induced using aerosolized saline; the first morning sputum should be collected for 3 consecutive days. If sputum is positive for acid-fast bacilli, antibiotic therapy should be initiated while final culture and sensitivity results are pending.
  - Standard treatment in pregnancy consists of isoniazid (INH) with pyridoxine supplementation, ethambutol, and pyrazinamide. Streptomycin sulfate should be avoided because of the risk of fetal cranial nerve VIII damage. Rifampin should also be avoided during pregnancy unless INH and ethambutol cannot be used. INH prophylaxis for 6 to 9 months is recommended for asymptomatic patients younger than age 35 years with positive PPD results and negative findings on chest radiograph.
  - If the patient has converted to positive PPD results within the last 2 years, INH therapy should be initiated during the pregnancy after the first trimester. If the time since conversion is unknown or longer than 2 years, INH is started during the postpartum period. INH prophylaxis is not recommended for patients older than age 35 years due to its hepatotoxicity. If treated, TB should not affect the pregnancy, and pregnancy should not alter the course of the disease.

## SUGGESTED READINGS

Cunningham FG, Leveno KJ, Bloom SL, et al., eds. Cardiovascular disease. In *Williams Obstetrics*, 23rd ed. New York, NY: McGraw-Hill, 2010.

Cunningham FG, Leveno KJ, Bloom SL, et al., eds. Pulmonary disorders. In *Williams Obstetrics*, 23rd ed. New York, NY: McGraw-Hill, 2010.

Easterling TR, Stout K. Heart disease. In Gabbe SG, Niebyl JR, Simpson JL, eds. *Obstetrics: Normal and Problem Pregnancies*, 5th ed. Philadelphia, PA: Elsevier, 2007.

Whitty JE, Dombrowski MP. Respiratory diseases in pregnancy. In Gabbe SG, Niebyl JR, Simpson JL, eds. *Obstetrics: Normal and Problem Pregnancies*, 5th ed. Philadelphia, PA: Elsevier, 2007.

Wilson W, Taubert KA, Gewitz M, et al. Prevention of infective endocarditis: guidelines from the American Heart Association. *J Am Dent Assoc* 2007;138:739–760.

# 16 Genitourinary Assessment and Renal Disease in Pregnancy

Katherine Ikard Stewart and Robert M. Ehsanipoor

## KIDNEY AND URINARY TRACT DISORDERS

### Renal Physiology in Pregnancy

- The renal system undergoes many physiologic changes during a normal pregnancy. In addition, as the gravid uterus increases in size, it produces a mass effect on the renal system.
- **Structural changes:** During pregnancy, the kidneys increase 1 to 1.5 cm in length and 30% in volume. The collecting system expands more than 80%, with greater dilation on the right side.
  - Mild right-sided physiologic hydronephrosis is seen as early as 6 weeks of gestation. Renal volume returns to normal within the first week postpartum, but hydronephrosis and hydroureter may not normalize until 3 to 4 months after delivery. Elective pyelography should, therefore, be deferred until at least 12 weeks postpartum.
  - These structural changes increase the risk of pyelonephritis in the setting of asymptomatic bacteriuria or urinary tract infections.
- **Renal filtration:** Blood volume expansion during pregnancy increases renal plasma flow by 50% to 80%, which in turn results in an increased glomerular filtration rate (GFR). Increased GFR can be seen within 1 month after conception, peaking at 40% to 50% above prepregnancy levels by the end of the first trimester.
  - Elevated GFR increases creatinine clearance, so formulas for GFR based on age, height, and weight do not apply; creatinine clearance must be calculated with a 24-hour urine collection in pregnancy.
  - Increased GFR results in lower mean serum blood urea nitrogen (BUN) and serum creatinine during pregnancy (8.5 and 0.46 mg/dL, respectively). A serum creatinine which may be considered normal outside of pregnancy may suggest renal insufficiency in pregnancy.
- **Renal tubular function:** Decreased tubular resorption in pregnancy increases urinary excretion of electrolytes, glucose, amino acids, and protein.
  - Increased calcium clearance is balanced by increased gastrointestinal (GI) tract absorption. Ionized calcium remains stable despite decreased total serum calcium because of the lower serum albumin concentration.
  - Physiologic hyponatremia occurs, with plasma sodium concentration falling by 5 mEq/L during pregnancy. Sodium levels return to baseline by 1 to 2 months postpartum.
  - Urinary excretion of glucose increases 10- to 100-fold, and glucosuria is observed routinely in normal pregnancy. Increased urinary glucose increases the risk of bacteriuria and urinary tract infections.

- Renal resorption of bicarbonate decreases to compensate for the respiratory alkalosis of pregnancy, lowering serum bicarbonate by about 5 mEq/L in pregnancy.
- **Routine assessment of renal function:** Proteinuria should be assessed at every prenatal visit. A urine dipstick value $>1+$ should prompt further evaluation by clean-catch urine sample for culture and microscopy. If proteinuria persists despite negative culture, further evaluation is warranted and may include either a 24-hour urine protein collection or a random protein to creatinine ratio. A 24-hour total urine protein exceeding 150 mg is abnormal.
- Patients with chronic hypertension, diabetes, preexisting renal disease, or other diseases may have abnormal levels of proteinuria prior to pregnancy and should undergo a baseline 24-hour urine protein collection early in pregnancy.
- Serum creatinine persistently $>0.9$ mg/dL should prompt investigation for intrinsic renal disease. The presence of comorbidities should be assessed and further evaluation should be considered. Renal biopsy during pregnancy should be considered when the results will change management before delivery.

## Urinary Tract Disorders in Pregnancy
### *Urinary Tract Infection*

- **Urinary tract infections (UTIs)** are common in pregnancy. Urinary stasis secondary to hydroureter and hydronephrosis, bladder trauma due to compression or edema, vesicoureteral reflux, and increased glucosuria may all contribute to the increased risk of infection. Women with two or more UTIs or a diagnosis of pyelonephritis during pregnancy should be considered for daily suppressive antibiotic therapy until delivery.
- **Asymptomatic bacteriuria (ASB)** is the presence of bacteria within the urinary tract, excluding the distal urethra, without signs or symptoms of infection. ASB is associated with low-birth-weight infants and preterm delivery, and its treatment in pregnancy is indicated. The prevalence of ASB during pregnancy ranges from 2% to 7%. If left untreated, 20% to 30% of ASB in pregnant women progresses to pyelonephritis; treatment reduces this to 3%. Screening for bacteriuria with a urine culture is recommended at the first prenatal visit. Women with sickle cell trait have a twofold increased risk of ASB and can be screened every trimester.
  - A clean-catch urine culture with $>100,000$ colonies/mL or catheterized urine culture with $>100$ colonies/mL warrants treatment.
  - *Escherichia coli* accounts for 75% to 90% of infections. *Klebsiella, Proteus, Pseudomonas, Enterobacter*, and coagulase-negative *Staphylococcus* are other common pathogens.
  - Initial therapy is usually empiric and may be altered based on urine culture sensitivities. Repeat urine culture is obtained 1 to 2 weeks after treatment and again each trimester. If bacteriuria persists after two or more treatment courses, suppressive therapy should be considered for the remainder of the pregnancy.
- **Acute cystitis** occurs in approximately 1% to 3% of pregnant women. Symptoms include urinary frequency, urgency, dysuria, hematuria, and/or suprapubic discomfort. Empiric treatment regimens are the same as for ASB. If possible, a urine culture should be sent prior to initiating antibiotic therapy.
- **Urethritis** is usually caused by *Chlamydia trachomatis*, and it should be suspected in patients with symptoms of acute cystitis and a negative urine culture. Mucopurulent cervicitis may also be present. The treatment of choice is azithromycin 1 g as a single oral dose for both the patient and her partner. A test of cure should be sent 3 to 4 weeks after treatment.

*Pyelonephritis*

- **Acute pyelonephritis** occurs in approximately 1% to 2% of all pregnancies and is the leading cause of septic shock in pregnancy. Complications include preterm labor, preterm premature rupture of membranes (PPROM), bacteremia, sepsis, acute respiratory distress syndrome, and hemolytic anemia. Prompt diagnosis and treatment of pyelonephritis in pregnancy are crucial.
  - Symptoms include fever, chills, flank pain, nausea, and vomiting. Frequency, urgency, and dysuria are variably present.
  - Pyelonephritis is a clinical diagnosis. Urine culture, complete blood count (CBC), serum creatinine, and electrolytes should be obtained at admission. Blood cultures need not be routinely performed in pyelonephritis and can be reserved for severely ill patients.
  - Treatment includes administration of intravenous (IV) broad-spectrum antibiotics, hydration, and antipyretics. Cefazolin or ceftriaxone are commonly used and are equivalent to ampicillin plus gentamicin. For penicillin allergy, clindamycin plus gentamicin is appropriate. Fluoroquinolones are generally avoided during pregnancy.
  - Pregnant women with pyelonephritis are at significant risk for developing acute respiratory distress syndrome. They should be closely monitored for evidence of respiratory symptomatology with provision of respiratory support as needed.
  - Transition to an oral regimen is appropriate after an afebrile period of greater than 48 hours. Antibiotic regimen should be chosen based on urine culture sensitivities. Oral therapy is continued to complete a 14-day antibiotic course. Daily suppressive therapy (Table 16-1) is then initiated for the remainder of pregnancy due to the recurrence risk of approximately 20%.

| TABLE 16-1 | Antimicrobial Agents for Treatment of Urinary Tract Infection and Asymptomatic Bacteriuria |
|---|---|

**Single dose**
Amoxicillin, 3 g
Ampicillin, 2 g
Cephalexin, 2 g
Nitrofurantoin, 200 mg
Sulfisoxazole, 2 g
Trimethoprim-sulfamethoxazole, 320/1,600 mg

**Short course (3–7 days)**
Amoxicillin, 250–500 mg tid
Ampicillin, 250 mg qid
Cephalexin, 250–500 mg qid
Nitrofurantoin, 100 mg bid
Sulfisoxazole, 1 g then 500 mg qid
Trimethoprim-sulfamethoxazole, 320/1,600 mg bid

**Suppression therapy**
Nitrofurantoin, 100 mg qhs
Ampicillin, 250 mg po qd
Trimethoprim-sulfamethoxazole, 160/800 mg qd

tid, three times a day; qid, four times a day; bid, twice a day; qhs, at bedtime; po, by mouth; qd, every day.

- If there is no response to antibiotic treatment within 48 hours, review antibiotic dosing and sensitivities, send repeat urine culture, and obtain renal ultrasonography to evaluate for anatomic anomalies, nephrolithiasis, and intrarenal or perinephric abscess.

## Nephrolithiasis

- **Nephrolithiasis** should be considered in a pregnant patient with acute onset of abdominal or flank pain. The incidence is between 0.3 and 4.0 per 1,000 pregnancies. Increased urinary excretion of calcium, urinary stasis, and dehydration are risk factors associated with development of renal stones in pregnancy.
  - Diagnosis is primarily clinical. Classic symptoms include acute onset of colicky flank pain, hematuria, and pyuria. In more than 50% of cases, the stone passes spontaneously after hydration and may be observed directly by filtering the patient's urine. Renal ultrasonography should be performed to rule out obstruction, but pathologic obstruction from a renal stone must be differentiated from physiologic hydronephrosis of pregnancy. If the diagnosis remains uncertain and there is a negative ultrasound, magnetic resonance (MR) urography or noncontrast computed tomography (CT) scan can be considered.
  - Initial treatment is administration of IV hydration and analgesia, with the patient lying on her side with the symptomatic side up. This helps reduce the pressure from the gravid uterus on the affected side. Approximately 75% of stones will pass spontaneously. Associated infections must be treated aggressively. Indications for surgical intervention include impairment of renal function, obstruction, protracted severe pain, or signs of sepsis. Extracorporeal shock wave lithotripsy is contraindicated in pregnancy.

## Glomerular Disease

- **Glomerular disease** is caused by a wide spectrum of diseases, and its clinical presentation can vary from asymptomatic to renal failure. Clinical syndromes are defined to differentiate these patients, with nephritic and nephrotic syndrome being the most common. Definitive diagnosis ultimately requires a renal biopsy. However, with potential risks, renal biopsy should only be pursued in pregnancy if results will change management.
- **Acute nephritic syndrome**
  - Usually presents with hypertension, hematuria, urinary red cell casts, pyuria and mild to moderate proteinuria.
  - Causes include poststreptococcal glomerulonephritis, lupus nephritis, immunoglobulin A (IgA) nephropathy, membranoproliferative glomerulonephritis, endocarditis-associated glomerulonephritis, antiglomerular basement membrane disease, Goodpasture syndrome, Wegener syndrome, and Churg-Strauss syndrome.
  - Goodpasture, Wegener, Churg-Straus, Henoch-Schönlein purpura, or cryoglobulinemia can also present as a pulmonary renal syndrome with significant hemoptysis along with glomerulonephritis.
- **Nephrotic syndrome**
  - Usually presents with severe proteinuria (>3.5 g/day), hypertension, edema, hyperlipidemia, and minimal hematuria. Minimal cells or casts are present in urine other than fatty casts.
  - Causes include minimal change disease, focal segmental glomerulosclerosis often secondary to HIV, membranous glomerulonephritis, diabetic nephropathy, hepatitis C, systemic lupus erythematosus (SLE), and amyloidosis.

- Complications of glomerular disease in pregnancy include preterm delivery, intrauterine growth restriction (IUGR), stillbirth, maternal hypertension, preeclampsia, and impaired renal function.

### Chronic Kidney Disease

- **Chronic kidney disease** is present in less than 0.2% of all pregnancies. It is defined as impaired renal function or damage for 3 or more months. The most common causes are diabetes, hypertension, glomerulonephritis, and polycystic kidney disease.
- The degree of renal impairment is the major determinant of pregnancy outcome and can be categorized as *mild* (serum creatinine <1.5 mg/dL), *moderate* (serum creatinine 1.5 to 3.0 mg/dL), or *severe* (serum creatinine >3.0 mg/dL). In general, patients with mild renal dysfunction experience little disease progression during pregnancy, whereas patients with moderate to severe renal insufficiency are at high risk for potentially irreversible loss of renal function. Chronic renal disease in the setting of poorly controlled hypertension markedly increases both maternal and fetal risks. Thus, it is very important to optimize blood pressure in addition to other comorbidities such as diabetes or connective tissue disorders that may worsen renal disease.
- **Pregnancy complications** with chronic renal disease include fetal demise, fetal growth restriction, preeclampsia, eclampsia, and preterm delivery. Maternal and fetal outcomes correlate with severity of baseline renal function and presence of comorbidities.
- **Antepartum management** includes the following:
  - Early pregnancy diagnosis and dating.
  - Preconception planning and counseling are encouraged.
  - Baseline laboratory studies including serum creatinine, electrolytes, BUN, 24-hour urine protein and creatinine clearance, urinalysis, and urine culture. Serial monitoring of maternal renal function, as clinically indicated.
  - Consider increased frequency of prenatal visits, depending on disease severity.
  - Consider serial ultrasonographic fetal growth examinations.
  - Consider antepartum fetal testing in the third trimester.

### Renal Dialysis

- Conception occurs in approximately 1% per year of reproductive aged women on dialysis. Between 40% and 75% of these pregnancies result in delivery of a surviving infant. There is a high rate of spontaneous abortion and pregnancy complications. Most infants are born premature usually secondary to severe maternal hypertension or preeclampsia. These patients are also at increased risk of IUGR, polyhydramnios, PPROM, nonreassuring fetal testing, and placental abruption. With significant maternal risks of pregnancies being maintained on dialysis, including severe hypertension, cardiac events, and death, delaying pregnancy until after renal transplantation may be advantageous.
  - Neonatal outcomes are improved with maintenance of the BUN <50 mg/dL on dialysis. This is typically achieved by increasing frequency of dialysis to 5 to 7 days per week.
  - Blood pressure must be controlled, especially during dialysis, to avoid fetal compromise.
  - Electrolytes should be monitored and appropriately corrected. Bicarbonate concentrations, for example, must be managed carefully to avoid dialysis-induced alkalemia. Ultrafiltration goals may be difficult to estimate and should consider

fetal and placental growth as well as the plasma volume expansion associated with pregnancy.

- Continuous fetal monitoring during dialysis after 24 weeks' gestation should be considered to assess fetal tolerance to hemodynamic changes.
- Anemia is common due to the combined effects of renal failure and pregnancy. Pregnant women may require higher doses of erythropoietin and/or blood transfusions to maintain a hemoglobin of 10 to 11 g/dL.

Renal Transplant

- Approximately 5% to 12% of renal transplant patients who are of reproductive age will become pregnant. The hormonal aberrations associated with end-stage renal disease are usually reversed after kidney transplant, and women often rapidly resume cyclic ovulation and regular menstruation. Pregnancy complications for these patients include increased infections secondary to chronic immunosuppression, hypertension, preeclampsia, preterm labor, PPROM, and IUGR.
- Transplant patients are generally advised to wait at least 1 year after a living related donor transplant and 2 years after a deceased donor transplant before attempting to become pregnant.
- Factors associate with favorable outcomes include serum creatinine <1.5 mg/dL, well-controlled blood pressure, proteinuria <500 mg/day, no recent episodes of acute rejection, maintenance level of immunosuppression, and normal appearance of transplanted kidney on ultrasound.
- Cyclosporine and tacrolimus are commonly used immunosuppressant medications that have favorable safety profiles in pregnancy. Frequent monitoring of drug levels and renal function is imperative to avoid potential toxicity.
- Mycophenolate mofetil and sirolimus are preferably avoided in pregnancy and have been associated with adverse fetal effects. Patients trying to conceive should be switched from these medications to either tacrolimus or cyclosporine where possible.
- Mode of delivery is based on obstetric indications. The pelvic allograft does not usually obstruct the birth canal, and vaginal delivery is preferred. When cesarean section is indicated, prophylactic antibiotics and careful attention to wound closure are recommended to minimize infectious complications. In addition, knowledge of allograft placement is essential in order to avoid operative injury, although the transplanted kidney is not usually positioned in an area that is vulnerable when using standard approaches to cesarean section.

## SUGGESTED READINGS

American College of Obstetrics and Gynecologists Task Force Report on Hypertension in Pregnancy. *Hypertension in Pregnancy*. Washington, DC: American College of Obstetrics and Gynecologists, 2013.

Cunningham FG, Cox SM, Harstad TW, et al. Chronic renal disease and pregnancy outcome. *Am J Obstet Gynecol* 1990;163:453–459.

Macejko AM, Schaeffer AJ. Asymptomatic bacteriuria and symptomatic urinary tract infections during pregnancy. *Urol Clin North Am* 2007;34(1):35–42.

Nevis IF, Reitsma A, Dominic A, et al. Pregnancy outcomes in women with chronic kidney disease: a systematic review. *Clin J Am Soc Nephrol* 2011;6(11):2587–2598.

Vidaeff AC, Yeomans ER, Ramin SM. Pregnancy in women with renal disease. Part I: general principles. *Am J Perinatol* 2008;25(7):385–397.

Vidaeff AC, Yeomans ER, Ramin SM. Pregnancy in women with renal disease. Part II: specific underlying renal conditions. *Am J Perinatol* 2008;25(7):399–405.

# Gastrointestinal Disease in Pregnancy

Christopher C. DeStephano and
Abimbola Aina-Mumuney

## GASTROINTESTINAL PHYSIOLOGY AND ANATOMY IN PREGNANCY

During pregnancy, anatomic and physiologic changes undergone by the gastrointestinal tract can influence the diagnosis of gastrointestinal disorders. The displacement of the gastrointestinal organs by the gravid uterus changes the location, character, and intensity of gastrointestinal symptoms. This chapter summarizes the normal changes in pregnancy in contrast to pathologic conditions.

### Liver Disorders

*Hepatic Physiology in Pregnancy*

- As the gravid uterus expands into the upper abdomen, the liver is displaced posteriorly and to the right, decreasing its estimated size on physical examination. A palpable liver in pregnancy is abnormal and a workup is indicated. Table 17-1 summarizes the normal changes in liver function tests during pregnancy, some of which are considered abnormal in nonpregnant patients.

*Hepatic Disorders Unique to Pregnancy*

Cholestasis of Pregnancy

- **Intrahepatic cholestasis of pregnancy (ICP)** occurs in about 1 in 1,000 pregnancies in the United States but has significant genetic and geographic variations. Risk factors include a personal or family history of ICP, multiple gestations, and chronic hepatitis C infection. The cause is postulated to be secondary to incomplete bile acid clearance. Complications include preterm labor, meconium ileus, and intrauterine fetal demise. These risks increase progressively with duration, regardless of symptoms. The cause of fetal demise is unknown and rarely happens before term.
  - Initial **diagnosis** is clinical, with confirmation by laboratory testing. The cardinal symptom is pruritus, especially of the palms and soles that worsens at night. Anorexia, malaise, steatorrhea, and dark urine are also common complaints. Jaundice develops in 15% of patients but resolves quickly after delivery. Fever, abdominal pain, hepatosplenomegaly, and stigmata of chronic liver disease are usually absent. Onset is typically late in pregnancy (80% after 30 weeks) but occasionally occurs in the second trimester.
  - **Differential diagnosis** includes preeclampsia, viral hepatitis, and gallbladder disease.
  - **Laboratory findings** include elevated total bilirubin, aminotransferases, and fasting serum total bile acids (>10 to 14 μmol/L). Cholic acid is raised more than chenodeoxycholic acid, which results in an elevation of the cholic/chenodeoxycholic

| TABLE 17-1 | Liver Function Test Changes during Normal Pregnancy |
|---|---|
| Alkaline phosphatase | ↑ |
| Aminotransferases | ↔ |
| Bilirubin | ↔ |
| Albumin | ↓ |
| Hormone-binding proteins | ↑ |
| Lipids | ↑ |
| Fibrinogen | ↑ |
| PT/aPTT | ↔ |

↑, increased or elevated; ↓, decreased; ↔, unchanged. PT, prothrombin time; aPTT, activated partial thromboplastin time.

acid ratio compared to pregnant women without ICP. Lab abnormalities arise a mean of 3 weeks after the development of pruritus. Serum alkaline phosphatase and transaminase levels are modestly elevated. Serum gamma glutamyl transpeptidase, albumin, and prothrombin time remain normal.

- **Treatment** is mainly for symptomatic relief until delivery, which is the definitive therapy. Diphenhydramine, topical emollients, and dexamethasone (12 mg/day for 7 days) can relieve pruritus. Ursodeoxycholic acid (8 to 10 mg/kg/day) is the most effective treatment and works by increasing bile flow, thereby decreasing serum bile acid levels and decreasing pruritus. Cholestyramine (8 to 16 g, two to four times per day) decreases intestinal absorption of bile salts and is effective for mild to moderate symptoms but does not improve lab values. Fat-soluble vitamins (A, D, E, and K) and prothrombin time should be checked periodically for patients taking cholestyramine for extended treatment. If the prothrombin time is elevated, 10 mg/day of oral vitamin K should be administered until the coagulation profile normalizes.
- ICP at term is associated with 3% risk of fetal demise. Antepartum fetal testing is recommended, although intrauterine demise may occur despite reassuring testing. Delivery should be performed no later than 38 weeks' gestation. When cholestasis is severe, delivery at 36 weeks with or without fetal lung maturity may be considered.
- Recurrence risk in subsequent pregnancies is approximately 70% and is usually more severe. Estrogen-containing oral contraceptives can cause cholestasis in these patients.

Acute Fatty Liver of Pregnancy

- **Acute fatty liver of pregnancy (AFLP)** is uncommon, occurring in 1 in 10,000 pregnancies. It typically occurs in primigravid women in the third trimester and is associated with multiple gestations, male fetuses, and with a fetal mitochondrial gene mutation causing long chain 3-hydroxyacyl-CoA-dehydrogenase deficiency. Patients present with nausea, vomiting, epigastric pain, anorexia, jaundice, and malaise. Intra-abdominal bleeding or altered mental status may indicate disease progression to disseminated intravascular coagulation (DIC) or hepatic failure. Laboratory tests may reveal hypoglycemia, elevated aminotransferases to 1,000 IU/L, leukocytosis, thrombocytopenia, coagulopathy, markedly reduced antithrombin III, metabolic acidosis, hyperuricemia, and renal failure. Treatment includes maternal stabilization with intensive supportive care and prompt delivery, either with induction of labor with close maternal and fetal surveillance or cesarean delivery. Liver function usually normalizes within 1 week postpartum, and recurrence in subsequent pregnancy is uncommon.

*Hepatic Disorders Not Directly Related to Pregnancy*

Hepatitis

• **Acute and chronic hepatitis**—See Chapter 11.

Cirrhosis

• **Hepatic cirrhosis** leads to metabolic and hormonal derangements that usually induce anovulation, amenorrhea, and infertility. Cirrhosis is associated with 30% to 40% risk of spontaneous abortion, 25% risk of preterm delivery, and up to 18% risk of neonatal mortality. Maternal mortality is estimated at 10% but may be up to 50% in patients with portal hypertension who develop gastrointestinal bleeding during pregnancy. Outcomes are generally poor, but hepatic dysfunction before pregnancy and the presence of portal hypertension correlate with worse maternal/fetal prognosis.
  • Esophageal variceal bleeding is the most common complication, occurring in 18% to 32% of pregnant women with cirrhosis. To reduce portal pressure and the risk of acute bleeding, beta-blockers such as propranolol should be considered. As in nonpregnant patients, endoscopic variceal ligation is the mainstay of therapy for acute episodes of hemorrhage. Portal decompression shunt placement is required when hemorrhage cannot be controlled by endoscopy. If endoscopy is unavailable, balloon tamponade can be employed to control severe bleeding. Other complications include ascites and bacterial peritonitis, splenic artery aneurysm, portal vein thrombosis, portal vein hypertension, hepatic encephalopathy or coma, postpartum uterine hemorrhage, and death.
  • Vaginal delivery is preferred over cesarean delivery due to the high rate of intraoperative and postoperative complications. In patients with portal hypertension, however, repetitive Valsalva in the second stage of labor can increase the risk of significant variceal bleeding. A passive second stage with forceps-assisted delivery may be beneficial.

Budd-Chiari Syndrome

• **Budd-Chiari syndrome** is a veno-occlusive disease of the hepatic vein that increases hepatic sinusoidal pressure and can result in portal hypertension or hepatic necrosis. The disease presents with abdominal pain and the abrupt onset of ascites and hepatomegaly. Cases are often caused by congenital vascular anomalies, myeloproliferative disorders, and thrombophilic disorders. In obstetrics, the disease typically occurs postpartum. Diagnosis is by hepatic Doppler ultrasonography to identify venous occlusion and evaluate the direction and amplitude of blood flow. Acute therapy includes selective thrombolytics and a surgical shunt or transjugular intrahepatic portosystemic shunt (TIPS) for portal hypertension. Chronic Budd-Chiari syndrome is treated with anticoagulation therapy.

Choledochal Cyst

• **Choledochal cysts** are rare, occurring in 1 in 100,000 people. They generally produce abdominal pain, jaundice, and a palpable abdominal mass. Compression by the gravid uterus may lead to cyst rupture, potentially resulting in cholangitis. Surgical management is generally recommended.

## Gallbladder Disorders

### Cholelithiasis

- **Cholelithiasis** occurs in up to 10% of pregnancies and is often clinically silent. Biliary stasis from progesterone-induced smooth muscle relaxation and the pro-lithogenic effect of elevated estrogen levels in pregnancy may predispose to gallstone formation. Symptomatic patients typically complain of vague intermittent right upper quadrant discomfort that occurs with meals. Asymptomatic cholelithiasis requires no treatment during pregnancy.
- **Symptomatic cholelithiasis** and **acute cholecystitis**—See Chapter 22.

## Other Gastrointestinal Disorders

### Hyperemesis Gravidarum

- **Hyperemesis gravidarum** is a severe form of nausea and vomiting in pregnancy, characterized by intractable vomiting, dehydration, alkalosis, hypokalemia, and weight loss usually exceeding 5% of prepregnant body weight. It affects 0.3% to 2% of pregnancies and peaks between the 8th and 12th weeks of pregnancy. The etiology may be multifactorial, involving hormonal, neurologic, metabolic, toxic, and psychosocial factors.
  - Nausea (with or without vomiting) occurs in up to 90% of pregnancies at any time of day, despite the general term "morning sickness." Mean onset of symptoms is 5 to 6 weeks' gestation. Although symptoms typically abate by 16 to 18 weeks of gestation, they continue into the third trimester in 15% to 20% of pregnant women and until delivery in 5%.
  - With true hyperemesis gravidarum, persistent vomiting leads to plasma volume depletion and elevated hematocrit and metabolic derangements that include increased blood urea nitrogen, hyponatremia, hypokalemia, hypochloremia, and metabolic alkalosis. A complete workup includes pelvic sonogram to identify multiple gestation or molar pregnancy and thyroid function tests to evaluate for hyperthyroidism. Some patients with hyperemesis gravidarum have transient benign hyperthyroidism most likely due to thyroid stimulation by the human chorionic gonadotropin (hCG) molecule, which is structurally similar to thyroid-stimulating hormone (TSH) and has been shown in animal studies to be a weak thyrotropin. This usually resolves spontaneously as pregnancy continues.
- **Treatment** depends on the severity of symptoms. Usually, intravenous (IV) hydration and antiemetic therapy are sufficient. Patients may require hospitalization for intractable emesis, electrolyte abnormalities, and severe hypovolemia. Thiamine supplementation (100 mg daily intramuscularly [IM] or IV) is given prior to administration of glucose to prevent Wernicke encephalopathy. Oral feeding with a bland diet should be introduced slowly as tolerated. If symptoms are refractory to medical and supportive care, a psychiatry consultation may be considered.
  - There are no drugs approved specifically for the treatment of nausea and vomiting in pregnancy; however, the following medications have been clinically effective:
    - Pyridoxine (vitamin $B_6$) 10 to 25 mg PO three times daily
    - Doxylamine succinate 12.5 mg PO three times daily taken with pyridoxine 10 to 50 mg. A recent formulation of delayed release tablets of 10 mg of

doxylamine and 10 mg of pyridoxine has recently become available in the United States, which may be taken as needed up to two tablets in the morning and one in the afternoon and evening.

- ○ Metoclopramide hydrochloride (Reglan) 5 to 10 mg PO or IV three times daily
- ○ Promethazine hydrochloride (Phenergan) 12.5 to 25 mg PO or IV four times daily
- ○ Prochlorperazine (Compazine) 10 to 50 mg PO, IV, or IM three or four times daily
- ○ Ondansetron hydrochloride (Zofran) 4 to 8 mg PO or IV three times daily
- ○ Methylprednisolone (Medrol) 16 mg PO or IV every 8 hours for 3 days may be used for refractory cases after 10 weeks' gestation. There is a theoretical risk of cleft lip and palate when administered in the early to mid-first trimester.

- ○ In severe cases requiring prolonged IV hydration, enteral feeds via gastric tube or parenteral nutrition may be initiated. Complications from parenteral nutrition are common and severe. Peripherally inserted catheters (PICC) appear to have a lower complication than centrally inserted catheters, although the complication rate of both is near 50%. Potential complications include pneumothorax, hemothorax, brachial plexus injury, thromboembolism, and catheter sepsis. Risk of line infection can be as common as one in three, with resulting bacteremia or fungemia that can significantly complicate a pregnancy. Vitamin K should be supplemented in addition to the standard parenteral nutrition formula secondary to the risk of fetal intracranial hemorrhage secondary to maternal vitamin K deficiency. Due to these risks, initiation of enteral feeding is strongly recommended preferentially prior to proceeding with parenteral nutrition.

*Acid Reflux*

- **Gastroesophageal reflux disease (GERD)** and the resulting symptom of pyrosis ("heartburn") are common during pregnancy secondary to the altered position of the stomach, decreased lower esophageal sphincter tone (due to elevated progesterone levels), and lower intraesophageal pressures. The incidence is 30% to 50% but may approach 80% in selected populations. Symptoms begin late in the first trimester and become more frequent and severe with increasing gestational age. Risk factors include multiparity and history of GERD before pregnancy.
  - **Treatment** is medical and aimed at neutralizing or decreasing reflux. Lifestyle modification is key in treating mild diseases. Elevating the head of the bed at night, avoiding meals within 3 hours of bedtime, and consuming smaller but more frequent meals can help. Dietary modification is recommended, including reduced consumption of fatty foods, chocolate, and caffeine. Cigarette smoking and alcohol consumption can exacerbate GERD and are discouraged in all patients.
  - More persistent symptoms can be treated with over-the-counter antacids (e.g., calcium carbonate) or sucralfate 1 g orally thrice daily. An $H_2$ blocker, such as ranitidine 150 mg orally twice daily, may be considered. Proton pump inhibitors (e.g., omeprazole) and promotility agents (e.g., metoclopramide) are generally effective and may be used if necessary. Endoscopy is considered if therapeutic measures are unsuccessful and symptoms are severe.

*Peptic Ulcer Disease*

- **Peptic ulcer disease(PUD)** is not common in pregnancy, and the hormonal changes of pregnancy usually decrease PUD severity and symptoms.
  - **Treatment** during pregnancy is similar to treatment for GERD and consists of diet modification, avoiding nonsteroidal anti-inflammatory drugs (NSAIDs), and starting $H_2$ blockers or proton pump inhibitors. Avoid indomethacin for tocolysis of patients with PUD. Diagnosis of *Helicobacter pylori* infection is usually reserved for those with active ulcers; treatment regimens for *H. pylori* without tetracycline are selected.

*Inflammatory Bowel Disease*

- **Inflammatory bowel disease (IBD)**, including **ulcerative colitis** and **Crohn disease**, often presents in reproductive age women. IBD increases the risk for preterm birth, low birth weight, and intrauterine growth restriction. There is no evidence that pregnancy influences disease activity; however, patients with active disease around the time of conception often fail to achieve remission during the pregnancy.
  - **Treatment** is largely pharmacologic, usually with sulfasalazine and corticosteroids. Because sulfasalazine may interfere with folate absorption, supplemental folate should be prescribed. Immunosuppressive agents, such as azathioprine, 6-mercaptopurine, cyclosporine, or infliximab, are used for more severe disease. Limited experience shows that all these medications are safe during pregnancy. Methotrexate and mycophenolate are not used in pregnancy. Antibiotics, particularly metronidazole and cephalosporins, are used for perirectal abscesses/fistulae. There is limited data regarding the safety of antidiarrheal medications such as Kaopectate, Lomotil, and Imodium in pregnancy, but significant teratogenicity is unlikely. Surgical intervention is indicated only for severe complications of IBD.
  - The **mode of delivery** may be affected by IBD depending on disease activity and past surgical history. Vaginal delivery can usually be attempted unless there is severe perineal disease or previous colorectal surgery. In such cases, a colorectal surgery consultation should be obtained. Operative vaginal delivery or episiotomy may be avoided to prevent excessive perineal trauma as possible. Cesarean section should be considered in patients with active perianal disease due to the risk of wound complications and fistulae formation.

*Pancreatitis*

- **Pancreatitis** is an uncommon cause of abdominal pain in pregnancy, with an incidence of 1 in 1,000 to 1 in 3,800 pregnancies.
  - The **presentation** is usually midepigastric or left upper quadrant pain with radiation to the back, nausea, vomiting, ileus, and low-grade fever. Cholelithiasis is the most common cause of pancreatitis during pregnancy. Ultrasound is of limited use for acute pancreatitis in pregnancy because of the enlarged uterus and overlying bowel gas.
  - **Management** consists of IV hydration, analgesics, and bowel rest. Most cases of gallstone pancreatitis can be managed medically. See Chapter 22 for surgical management.

*Appendicitis*

- **Appendicitis** can be a challenging diagnosis in the gravid patient due to the changes of pregnancy. See Chapter 22.

## SUGGESTED READINGS

Bacq Y, Sentilhes L, Reyes HB, et al. Efficacy of ursodeoxycholic acid in treating intrahepatic cholestasis of pregnancy: a meta-analysis. *Gastroenterology* 2012;143(6):1492–1501.

Brites D, Rodrigues CM, Oliveira N, et al. Correction of maternal serum bile acid profile during ursodeoxycholic acid therapy in cholestasis of pregnancy. *J Hepatol* 1998;28(1):91–98.

Holmgren C, Aagaard-Tillery KM, Silver RM, et al. Hyperemesis in pregnancy: an evaluation of treatment strategies with maternal and neonatal outcomes. *Am J Obstet Gynecol* 2008;198(1):56.e1–e4.

Kenyon AP, Piercy CN, Girling J, et al. Obstetric cholestasis, outcome with active management: a series of 70 cases. *Br J Obstet Gynaecol* 2002;109(3):282–288.

Ogura JM, Francois KE, Perlow JH, et al. Complications associated with peripherally inserted central catheter use during pregnancy. *Am J Obstet Gynecol* 2003;188(5):1223–1225.

Russo-Stieglitz KE, Levine AB, Wagner BA, et al. Pregnancy outcome in patients requiring parenteral nutrition. *J Matern Fetal Med* 1999;8(4):164–167.

# 18 Autoimmune Disease in Pregnancy

Katherine Latimer and Donna Neale

Autoimmune disease is characterized by the production of antibodies against self-antigens. One of many medical mysteries is how the fetus, that is genetically partially foreign to the mother, implants and survives a pregnancy. This chapter aims to review common autoimmune diseases encountered during pregnancy, including their management concerns and medical therapies.

## PATHOPHYSIOLOGY

### Cytokine Milieu during and after Pregnancy

During pregnancy, the immune system undergoes several changes to allow the mother to carry the fetus. Traditional teaching suggests that pregnancy reflects a switch from the normal predominant proinflammatory (T helper 1 [$T_H1$]) state to an anti-inflammatory (T helper 2 [$T_H2$]) state. It is this switch that is thought to protect the antigen-distinct fetus from being rejected by its mother. More recent study suggests that the immune changes in pregnancy are not so simplistic but represent a constant interplay between the proinflammatory and anti-inflammatory systems. Because of these changes in the maternal immune profile, autoimmune diseases can present and behave very differently during various times of the pregnancy than in the nonpregnant state. Furthermore, the switch back to the predominant proinflammatory state in the postpartum period can affect disease activity during this time. Clinical applications of these changes help explain exacerbations in $T_H2$-driven diseases such as systemic lupus erythematous and improvement in $T_H1$-driven diseases such as rheumatoid arthritis, multiple sclerosis, and autoimmune thyroiditis during pregnancy with increased "flaring" in the postpartum period.

## Autoantibodies in Pregnancy

Maternal immunoglobulin G (IgG) crosses the placenta, not immunoglobulin M (IgM) or immunoglobulin A (IgA). Notably, even in the presence of transplacental transfer of antibodies, fetal sequelae vary widely from no harm to permanent disability due to patient-dependent differences in antibody titer, specificity, and avidity as well as fetal factors such as antigen distribution, blocking, or inhibiting factors. Following delivery, the newborn's titers of maternal autoantibodies drop quickly over a period of 1 to 3 weeks; therefore, neonatal disease is often limited.

## COMMON MANAGEMENT CONCERNS

- Care should be taken at the **initial prenatal visit** to outline baseline function/disability, recent history, and symptoms of flares. Ideally, patients should have stable disease or remission prior to embarking on pregnancy. Whenever there is a concern for the presence of anti-Ro, anti-La, or antiphospholipid antibodies, titers should be checked. C3/C4 levels may also be helpful. Patients should be asked about flare symptoms at each visit. Generally, patients exhibiting one autoimmune disease should be carefully evaluated for others because these frequently coexists.
  - **Anti-Ro and anti-La antibodies** are found frequently in patients with systemic lupus erythematosus and Sjögren disease and occasionally seen in scleroderma and mixed connective tissue disorder (MCTD). If present, fetal echocardiography should be performed at 22 weeks' gestation. M-mode with PR interval measurements should start at 16 to 18 weeks' gestation and repeated weekly to assess for possible fetal heart block. If it is found, maternal dexamethasone administration may be helpful to protect the fetal cardiac tissue from further damage.
  - **Baseline renal function** should be determined because many autoimmune diseases affect the kidney. For instance, systemic lupus erythematosus, scleroderma, MCTD, and vasculitis can cause renal insufficiency. Renal crises during pregnancy carry high morbidity and mortality. Patients at risk should be carefully evaluated early in pregnancy with 24-hour urine protein and creatinine for baseline function. Patients with significant, known renal disease (serum creatinine, SCr > 2.5 mg/dL) are generally advised against becoming pregnant.

## Pregnancy Complications

- Several autoimmune diseases put patients at increased risk for **intrauterine growth restriction (IUGR)** including systemic lupus erythematosus, scleroderma, MCTD, dermatosytis/polymyositis, antiphospholipid syndrome, and autoimmune bullous disease. An ultrasound should be performed every 4 weeks following the anatomy ultrasound. In the presence of IUGR, serial fetal Doppler ultrasonographic studies should be performed.
- **Increased risk of preeclampsia:** These patients should have baseline 24-hour urine collection for total protein and creatinine clearance, even in the absence of known renal disease. Serial samples should be collected at least in every trimester in high-risk patients.
- **Increased risk of stillbirth:** Antenatal testing is normally initiated at 32 weeks of gestation, unless there is evidence of maternal/fetal compromise prior to this time.

- **Increased risk of premature birth:** Betamethasone/dexamethasone should be administered to patients with poor fetal testing results or worsening maternal disease before 34 weeks.

## MEDICATION CONSIDERATIONS DURING PREGNANCY

Generally, immunosuppressive medications are the cornerstone therapy for autoimmune disease. The need for medications in pregnancy must be balanced against fetal affects. **Breast-feeding** may be contraindicated based on the immunosuppressant medications mothers resume postpartum.

- **Glucocorticoids** such as prednisone and methylprednisolone are often first-line therapies. They are generally considered safe in pregnancy.
- **Nonsteroidal anti-inflammatory drugs (NSAIDs)** are typically limited during pregnancy after the first trimester up to 32 weeks given the concern for fetal renal agenesis, premature closure of the fetal ductus arteriosus, and oligohydramnios. If used during pregnancy, consider short pulse courses.
- **Low-dose aspirin** (81 mg) can be used safely in pregnancy. In most cases, it is discontinued at 36 weeks; however, in high-risk pregnancies such as symptomatic antiphospholipid antibody syndrome, it can be continued throughout the entire pregnancy.
- Immunosuppressant **azathioprine** and antimalarial **hydroxychloroquine** are used for a variety of autoimmune conditions and are generally considered relevantly safe.
- The monoclonal antibody **rituximab** and immunosuppressant **mycophenolate** are less commonly used due to limited safety data.
- **Cyclophosphamide** is an alkylating agent used to treat severe vasculitis and other autoimmune disorders. It should be avoided in the first trimester due to risk of congenital anomalies.
- **Methotrexate** should not be used during pregnancy. It is an antimetabolite/antifolate drug associated with spontaneous neural tube defects, abortion, and other significant congenital anomalies. Patients on methotrexate prior to conceiving should begin folate supplementation prior to becoming pregnant.
- **Antihypertensives:** When autoimmune disease is associated with hypertension, the need for medications should be reevaluated in the context of pregnancy. If possible, patients on angiotensin-converting enzyme (ACE) inhibitors, which have fetal renal effects, should be transitioned to alternatives such as labetalol, nifedipine, hydralazine, or methyldopa.

## DISORDERS COMMONLY ENCOUNTERED IN PREGNANCY

- **Systemic lupus erythematosus (SLE)** is a multisystem, chronic autoimmune disease that commonly affects women in their 20s and 30s. Symptoms can include arthritis, photosensitive rash, alopecia, mucocutaneous lesions, renal insufficiency, Raynaud phenomenon, pulmonary involvement, gastrointestinal (GI) disease, neurologic symptoms, pericarditis, and hematologic effects. Autoantibodies involved include antinuclear antibodies (ANAs), anti-Ro, anti-La, anti-Sm, anti-dsDNA, and antiphospholipid antibodies.
  - Lupus is associated with poor obstetric outcomes including IUGR, prematurity, stillbirth, and spontaneous abortion. Active lupus nephritis poses the greatest maternal risk.
  - Disease should be inactive for at least 6 months prior to pregnancy.

- One third of patients experience **flares** during pregnancy, which should be treated with hydroxychloroquine, low-dose prednisone, pulse intravenous (IV) methylprednisolone, or azathioprine. High-dose prednisone and cyclophosphamide should only be used in severe flares when necessary.
- Distinction between a flare versus **preeclampsia** (PEC) may be difficult, as both can result in proteinuria, thrombocytopenia, hypertension, or hyperuricemia. Transaminitis supports PEC. Generally, during a lupus flare, complement levels will be decreased. Red blood cell casts may be present on urinalysis.
- **Neonatal lupus syndrome** is rare, characterized by skin, hematologic, and other systemic lupus lesions and sometimes by congenital heart block appearing up to a month after birth. Subsequent pregnancies carry up to 25% recurrence risk.
- **Antiphospholipid syndrome**
  - Antiphospholipid (APL) antibodies interfere with coagulation, thrombus formation, and complement pathways.
  - **Diagnosis** requires the presence of at least one of the clinical criteria in Table 18-1 and testing positive for lupus anticoagulant, anticardiolipin antibodies (IgG and IgM), or anti-$\beta$2-glycoprotein I antibodies (IgG and IgM) on two separate occasions at least 12 weeks apart. Notably, 1% to 5% of healthy individuals may test positive for APL antibodies.
  - Gravidas are at increased risk for venous or arterial thrombosis, IUGR, fetal loss, preeclampsia, and pregnancy-induced hypertension.
  - American College of Obstetricians and Gynecologists expert's opinion on pharmacologic management differs by patient history. During the antepartum period and 6 weeks postpartum, women with:
    - **History of thrombosis** should receive prophylactic heparin
    - **No history of thrombosis** should receive clinical surveillance or prophylactic heparin

| TABLE 18-1 | Clinical Criteria for Diagnosis of Antiphospholipid Syndrome |
| --- | --- |
| Vascular thrombosis | One or more clinical episodes of arterial, venous, or small vessel thrombosis in any tissue or organ |
| Pregnancy morbidity | One or more unexplained deaths of a morphologically normal fetus at or beyond the 10th week of gestation, with normal fetal morphology documented by ultrasound or by direct examination of the fetus |
| | One or more premature births of a morphologically normal neonate before the 34th week of gestation because of eclampsia or severe preeclampsia or features consistent with placental insufficiency |
| | Three or more unexplained consecutive spontaneous pregnancy losses before the 10th week of pregnancy, with maternal anatomic or hormonal abnormalities and paternal and maternal chromosomal causes excluded |

Adapted from American College of Obstetricians and Gynecologists. Practice bulletin no. 132: antiphospholipid syndrome. American College of Obstetricians and Gynecologists. *Obstet Gynecol* 2012;120(6):1514–1521.

○ **Recurrent pregnancy loss** should receive prophylactic heparin and low-dose aspirin

- **Neonatal thrombosis** attributable to APL antibodies is rare. Fetal factors such as thrombophilia or prematurity often contribute to risk in affected infants.
- **Autoimmune thyroid disease**
  - *Graves disease* involves thyroid-stimulating antibodies that bind the thyroid-stimulating hormone (TSH) receptor, causing hyperfunctioning and potential thyrotoxicosis.
  - *Hashimoto thyroiditis* involves destruction of the thyroid by autoantibodies, such as antithyroid peroxidase antibodies. Despite transplacental transfer of autoantibodies and rare reports of effects on fetal thyroid function, most maternal autoantibodies do not result in fetal thyroid dysfunction. Untreated maternal disease can have significant consequences (see Chapter 13.)
- **Type 1 diabetes**—See Chapter 13.
- **Rheumatoid arthritis** is a chronic polyarthritis of unclear etiology characterized by morning stiffness and decreased range of motion in affected joints. Diagnosis is based on symptoms and lab findings such as rheumatoid factor, anti-cyclic citrullinated peptides (anti-CCP), or elevated erythrocyte sedimentation rate (ESR). During pregnancy, symptoms improve in 50% to 90% of patients; however, up to 90% will experience flares postpartum, particularly in the first 3 months. No obvious adverse fetal effects are known. Need-based treatment includes NSAIDs, low-dose acetylsalicylic acid (ASA), glucocorticoids, and potentially hydroxychloroquine.
- **Sjögren syndrome** is a chronic inflammatory disorder with diminished lacrimal and salivary gland function and potential extraglandular symptoms. Autoantibodies involved commonly include Ro, La, ANA, rheumatoid factor (RF) and potentially Sm, ribonucleoprotein (RNP), anticardiolipin, and lupus anticoagulant. Treatment of dry mouth involves diet modifications, regular hydration, and regular dental care. Artificial tears can be given for dry eyes. Extraglandular symptoms may require immunosuppressive therapy.
- **Scleroderma (Sc)** is a chronic, inflammatory disorder with nearly universal dermatologic involvement including skin hardening or sclerosis. Patients have varying degrees of pulmonary fibrosis and hypertension, renal insufficiency, GI dysmotility, cardiac, and musculoskeletal effects.
  - Pregnancy has no clear impact on flares. However, morbidity is high when renal crises occur. There is an increased risk of hypertension and IUGR.
  - Pregnancy exacerbates GI dysmotility. Proton pump inhibitor (PPI) may be helpful.
  - When present, perineal/cervical involvement impacts vaginal delivery and may increase risk of shoulder dystocia.
  - Skin symptoms are managed with antihistamines and lotion.
- **Dermatomyositis/polymyositis:** Myositis-specific autoantibodies are believed to contribute these inflammatory myopathies. Diagnosis is aided by elevated muscle enzymes, electromyelogram, and confirmed by biopsy. Treatment involves glucocorticoids and/or azathioprine. Dermatomyositis (DM) has characteristic skin changes, of which 15% are associated with a malignant tumor. There is an increased risk of IUGR and perinatal death. Active disease is associated with worse outcome.
- **Mixed connective tissue disease** is an autoimmune disease associated with anti-U1 ribonucleoprotein (RNP) that is characterized by a combination of symptoms of SLE, Sc, rheumatoid arthritis, and myositis. Other autoantibodies sometimes associated with the condition include anti-dsDNA, Sm, and Ro. Presentation is

highly variable with patients with predominant Sc or myositis-like features generally having a worse prognosis. Treatment is tailored to features of illness, including autoantibody management as mentioned earlier. SLE features are typically steroid-responsive, whereas Sc-like features are not.

- **Myasthenia gravis** is characterized by IgG-mediated damage to acetylcholine receptors or muscle-specific tyrosine kinase at the neuromuscular junction resulting in contractile muscle weakness of the face, oropharynx, eyes, limbs, and respiratory muscles.
  - **Crisis** can be life-threatening, particularly with oropharyngeal or respiratory involvement, and is more likely in the first trimester and postpartum period.
  - Suspected infections should be treated promptly to decrease risk of crisis.
  - The gravid uterus increases baseline fatigue and difficulty breathing.
  - **Labor** is possible because smooth muscle is unaffected. Fatigue with expulsive efforts in the second stage may necessitate operative delivery.
  - **Magnesium sulfate can precipitate a crisis**, and phenytoin worsens weakness. Seizure prophylaxis typically involves levetiracetam or valproic acid.
  - Pyridostigmine, an anticholinesterase, is used in **treatment**, as well as glucocorticoids and azathioprine. Plasmapheresis or intravenous immunoglobulin (IVIG) may be needed for crisis.
  - Both treatment and maternal antibodies can pass transplacentally. In rare instances where fetal movement is inhibited, the contracture syndrome **arthrogryposis multiplex congenital** develops. **Transient neonatal symptoms** are noted in 10% to 20% of infants following delivery.
- **Multiple sclerosis** is an autoimmune disease of the central nervous system characterized by demyelination, inflammation, and axon degeneration. Various cell types including $T_H17$ and inflammatory T and B cells have been implicated. The disease exists in relapsing-remitting and progressive forms. Neurologic symptoms such as weakness and visual and sensory loss vary depending on the tissues involved.
  - The Pregnancy in Multiple Sclerosis (PRIMS) study suggests that patients have fewer relapses during pregnancy and tend to flare postpartum.
  - Women with bladder involvement may be more prone to urinary tract infections (UTIs).
  - Methylprednisolone intravenously can be used for treatment of acute attacks. Limited data suggest that continuing use of natalizumab and glatiramer acetate during pregnancy is safe. Similarly, patients taking interferon beta have a slightly lower birth weight and increased incidence of preterm birth without increased risk of anomalies.
- **Immune thrombocytopenic purpura**—See Chapter 20.
- **Autoimmune hemolytic anemia**
  - *Cold agglutinin disease* is caused by IgM (rarely IgA or IgG) antibodies against polysaccharide components of the red blood cell. Symptoms are prominent in cold temperatures. Rapid hemoglobin drops may result in miscarriage or stillbirth. Fetal effects are rare because the antibody is normally IgM, which does not cross the placenta. Treatment is supportive, including warm clothing. In severe cases, rituximab is used. Plasmapheresis is rarely necessary. If transfusion is necessary, fluids should be warmed.
  - *Warm agglutinin disease* is due to IgG antibodies and may be associated with SLE, viral infection, connective tissue disease, or immune deficiency. When IgG antibodies cross the placenta, fetal effects are usually mild. Maternal treatment options

include glucocorticoids and azathioprine. Splenectomy can lead to remission, and IVIG is used for refractory cases. Neonates will transiently be Coombs-positive and rarely require transfusion or plasmapheresis.

- **Autoimmune neutropenia** is characterized by granulocyte-specific antibodies and an absolute neutrophil count (ANC) less than 1,500 cells/μL. It is commonly developed in childhood with remission in adulthood. Transplacental passage of antibodies from affected gravidas has been documented. The transient effect on neonates is mild; however, severe infections may occur.
- **Vasculitic syndrome** involves damage to blood vessels, often through immune complexes. Relatively rare in pregnancy, information is limited to small cases series and reports.
  - *Polyarteritis nodosa* (PAN) is a necrotizing vasculitis involving small- and medium-sized arteries that is characterized by neuropathy, hypertension, GI disorders, and renal failure. Treatment consists of glucocorticoids, cyclophosphamide, and ACE inhibitors. During pregnancy, this regime must be reevaluated (see medications discussed earlier). Thirty percent of cases are associated with hepatitis B and require antiviral treatment. Although rare, PAN can be devastating when identified in pregnancy, with morality rates greater than 50%.
  - *Wegener granulomatosis* is a necrotizing granulomatous vasculitis with pulmonary, ear/nose/throat, and renal involvement. Treatment includes corticosteroids, cyclophosphamide, rituximab, or azathioprine.
  - *Takayasu arteritis* is a vasculitis that affects large vessels including the upper aorta and its branches. Surgery prior to pregnancy may improve survival. Most case series report good fetal outcomes; however, the incidence of maternal adverse events varies widely. Baseline function, abdominal aorta involvement, and prenatal care may explain these differences. Hypertension poses significant risk and should be managed aggressively. Invasive monitoring may be necessary.
  - *Henoch-Schönlein purpura* is a small vessel vasculitis characterized by abdominal pain, hematuria, purpura, and arthritis that is more common in childhood. Treatment is supportive, and pregnancy outcomes are generally favorable.
  - *Behçet disease* is a systemic vasculitis characterized by uveitis and oral and genital ulcers. Disease is usually stable during pregnancy; early miscarriage rates are higher.
- **Autoimmune bullous disease**
  - In *pemphigus vulgaris*, IgG antibodies against desmoglein result in intraepidermal bullae on the skin and mucous membranes. Its milder variant, *pemphigus foliaceus*, does not have mucous membrane involvement. Therapy includes systemic glucocorticoids and occasionally azathioprine. Refractory cases are treated with rituximab and IVIG.
  - In *bullous pemphigoid* (BP), IgG antibodies against hemidesmosomes in the basement membrane result in subepidermal bullae. When onset occurs during pregnancy, the condition is called *pemphigoid gestationis* or *herpes gestationis*. Exacerbations can occur postpartum and in subsequent pregnancies. Maternal treatment includes topical corticosteroids and antihistamines. Systemic therapy is used for refractory cases.
  - Fetal deaths have been reported in women with high antibody titers. Therefore, rising titers should prompt aggressive maternal treatment.
  - Due to risk of stillbirth, prematurity, and IUGR, antenatal testing may be indicated.
  - **Neonatal bullous disease** occurs in 3% to 40% of infants. Treatment is supportive because lesions resolve as maternal antibodies degrade.
- **Autoimmune hepatitis** has a heterogeneous presentation ranging from asymptomatic to liver failure. Autoantibodies present include antinuclear (ANA), antiactin

(AAA), and anti-smooth muscle (ASMA) in type 1 and anti-liver/kidney microsomes (ALKM-1) and anti-liver cytosol (ALC-1) in type 2. Healthy pregnancy outcome is possible, although there is an increased risk of prematurity, low birth weight, and stillbirth. Common treatment options include glucocorticoids and azathioprine.

## SUGGESTED READINGS

American College of Obstetricians and Gynecologists. Practice bulletin no. 132: antiphospho-lipid syndrome. *Obstet Gynecol* 2012;120(6):1514–1521.

Baer AN, Witter FR, Petri M. Lupus and pregnancy. *Obstet Gynecol Surv* 2011;66(10):639–653.

Chaouat G. The Th1/Th2 paradigm: still important in pregnancy? *Semin Immunopathol* 2007;29(2):95–113.

Cunningham FG, Leveno KJ, Bloom SL, et al., eds. Connective-tissue disorders. In *Williams Obstetrics*, 23rd ed. New York, NY: McGraw-Hill, 2010.

Cunningham FG, Leveno KJ, Bloom SL, et al., eds. Neurological and psychiatric disorders. In *Williams Obstetrics*, 23rd ed. New York, NY: McGraw-Hill, 2010.

Hoftman AC, Hernandez MI, Lee KW, et al. Newborn illnesses caused by transplacental anti-bodies. *Adv Pediatr* 2008;55:271–304.

Seo P. Pregnancy and vasculitis. *Rheum Dis Clin North Am* 2007;33(2):299–317.

# 19 Neurologic Diseases in Pregnancy

Sarahn M. Wheeler and Irina Burd

A wide range of neurologic disorders can complicate pregnancy. The obstetric care provider is often challenged with managing these symptoms with a limited spectrum of medications known to be safe in pregnancy and a desire to minimize radiographic studies during parturition. Additionally, women with complex preexisting neuro-logic conditions often achieve pregnancy, necessitating the obstetric provider to be well versed in the treatment of these conditions and the unique implications of these diseases in the setting of pregnancy. This section will review common neurologic com-plaints and preexisting neurologic conditions and their management during pregnancy.

## HEADACHE

- Headache is a common complaint in pregnancy.
- Although most of these headaches are due to benign causes, it is imperative that obstetric providers perform a thorough history and physical examination to identify those headaches that warrant further workup (Table 19-1).
- In the presence of concerning signs or symptoms, neurologic consultation and diagnostic workup should be performed.

| TABLE 19-1 | History and Physical Exam Findings that Should Prompt Further Headache Workup |
| --- | --- |

| History | Physical Exam |
| --- | --- |
| • Sudden or rapid onset<br>• Prior or coexisting infection<br>• Onset during exertion<br>• Immunosuppression<br>• Environmental exposure<br>• No relief from pain medication | • Toxic appearance<br>• Fever<br>• Decreased mental status<br>• Papilledema<br>• Any localizing or lateralizing signs<br>• Meningismus |

Adapted from Contag SA, Bushnell C. Contemporary management of migrainous disorders in pregnancy. *Curr Opin Obstet Gynecol* 2010;22:437.

## Imaging/Diagnosis

• Lumbar puncture (LP), magnetic resonance imaging (MRI), and head computed tomography (CT) can be considered for headache with concerning features.
  • MRI poses no radiation exposure risks to the fetus and is the imaging of choice for pregnant patients. However, MRI is expensive and often not readily available.
  • Head CT is the imaging of choice for nonpregnant patients, as it is less expensive and more readily available in most settings. Although head CT does expose the fetus to some radiation, it is approximately 0.05 rad. A fetus must be exposed to 5 rad prior to significantly increased fetal risks, including fetal anomalies or pregnancy loss (Fig. 19-1). As such, the diagnostic benefit of a head CT, as with any clinical test, should be weighed against its risks.
• LP is not contraindicated in pregnancy and should be used if clinically indicated.

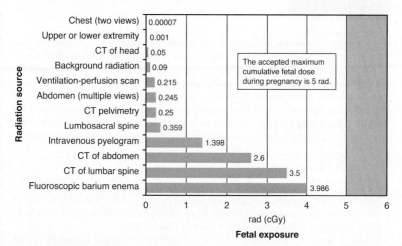

**Figure 19-1.** Fetal exposure to radiation with varying imaging studies. (From Toppenburg KS, Hill DA, Miller DP. Safety of radiographic imaging during pregnancy. *Am Fam Physician* 1999;59:1813–1818, 1820.)

## Common Obstetric Causes of Headache

- Any headache beyond 20 weeks' gestation and up to 12 weeks' postpartum should be included on the differential diagnosis **preeclampsia**, and the patient should have a blood pressure check and evaluation for proteinuria. If suspicion for preeclampsia is high, further workup including 24-hour urine collection and laboratory evaluation may be indicated (see Chapter 14).
- Post-epidural headache should be considered in postpartum patients particularly in postural headaches. Although acetaminophen, nonsteroidal anti-inflammatory drugs (NSAIDs), and caffeine are often sufficient treatment, anesthesia consultation for blood patching should be considered in patients who are refractory to conservative treatments.

### Migraine

- Although many chronic migraine sufferers report improved symptoms during pregnancy, it remains a common cause of headache in pregnancy.
- Approximately 2% of women have their first migraine while pregnant.
- **Typical migraine symptoms** include unilateral headache with a throbbing quality, nausea, vomiting, and sensitivity to light and sound. Some patients also describe precipitating symptoms such as visual changes or weakness, known as an aura.
- **Treatment of migraines in pregnancy**: Many of the same pharmacologic and nonpharmacologic treatments that are useful outside of pregnancy are also used intrapartum.
  - **Acute symptom management:** Treatment of acute migraines can involve a variety of medications (Table 19-2).
  - **Chronic symptom management:** Preventive therapy for frequent migraines with beta-blockade and calcium channel blockers can be used in pregnancy. Patients should be aware that prolonged use of beta-blockers may be associated with mild intrauterine growth restriction, transient bradycardia of the neonate, or hyperbilirubinemia.
  - **Refractory symptom management:** Selective serotonin reuptake inhibitors (SSRI), serotonin norepinephrine reuptake inhibitors (SNRI), and tricyclic antidepressants may be useful, particularly for patients with comorbid depression.
- Although most of the medications used for migraine treatment are safe in pregnancy, there are some notable exceptions. Ergotamine is contraindicated in pregnancy due to its association with hypertonic uterine contractions. Isometheptene is generally avoided due to concern for compromising uterine blood flow.

### Tension Headaches

- These are the most common type of headache.
- Patients describe tightness or tension in their head often with radiation to the neck.
- The frequency of tension headaches typically not altered by pregnancy
- Treatment: Nonpharmacologic treatments such as heat, massage, rest, and stress management are often helpful. Acetaminophen is the first-line pharmacologic therapy. NSAIDs can be used in the second trimester. Muscle relaxants can often be a useful adjunct. Opioids should be reserved for rare circumstances and for a limited course.

### Cluster Headaches

- These are recurrent, unilateral headaches that are accompanied by autonomic symptoms such as nasal stuffiness, tearing, facial swelling, or eyelid edema.

| TABLE 19-2 | Treatment Options for Acute Migraine Headache in Pregnancy |
|---|---|

**First-Line Therapies**

| Acetaminophen | • Extensive evidence of its safety in pregnancy<br>• Inexpensive<br>• May be used in combination with other drugs<br>• Maximum of 4 g daily to avoid liver toxicity |
|---|---|
| Caffeine | • Up to 200 mg daily considered safe in pregnancy<br>• Can be used in combination with acetaminophen |
| Metoclopramide | • Often helpful with headache reduction and alleviates associated nausea<br>• Can cause dystonic reaction |

**Second-Line Therapies**

| NSAIDs/aspirin | • Not used in first trimester due to possible teratogenicity<br>• Safe in second trimester<br>• Use in third trimester should be limited to 48 hr or less due to possible premature ductal closure, platelet dysfunction, and oligohydramnios |
|---|---|

**Third-Line Therapies**

| Opioids | • Should be used for short duration, as dependence can develop in the mother or fetus with high doses over long duration<br>• Can cause constipation and worsen nausea/vomiting associated with migraines<br>• No teratogenic effects associated with opioids |
|---|---|

**Severe Symptoms**

| Triptans | • Studies show no association with triptans and birth defects<br>• Use in third trimester associated with slight increased risk of uterine atony and increased blood loss at delivery |
|---|---|

NSAIDs, nonsteroidal anti-inflammatory drugs.

- Recurrent headaches are more common in males.
- Treatment: Oxygen therapy is first line for both pregnant and nonpregnant patients. Intranasal lidocaine and triptans can also be useful adjunct therapies.

## CARPAL TUNNEL SYNDROME

- Diagnosed clinically. Symptoms include pain and numbness in the median nerve distribution.

- Pregnant patients at increased risk due to swelling of carpal tunnels leading to compression of median nerves.
- Symptoms most often present in the third trimester and can remain for up to a year after delivery.
- Treatment with conservative measures such as a wrist brace is usually effective. In rare cases, corticosteroid injections or surgery is indicated.

## CHRONIC NEUROLOGIC DISEASES

### Multiple Sclerosis

- Multiple sclerosis (MS) is an autoimmune demyelinating disease characterized by relapsing and remitting neurologic deficits.
- Common symptoms during a flare include optic neuritis, asymmetric numbness, weakness, or ataxia.
- There are no current recommendations regarding whether women should become pregnant in the setting of MS.
- MS can have a variable course in pregnancy.
  - The intrapartum period is associated with **decreased** MS flare risk, whereas postpartum patients have an **increased** risk.
  - Taken together, pregnancy overall has not been shown to alter the long-term disease course.
  - Many of the common treatment options for MS are teratogenic. Patients are often advised to discontinue disease-modifying drugs due to teratogenic concerns and decreased risk of flare intrapartum.
  - Acute flares in pregnancy are typically managed with glucocorticoids.
- Classically, MS was considered a contraindication for spinal anesthesia. More recently, data has supported individualizing the plan of anesthetic care and spinal anesthesia.

### Epilepsy

- Many of the drugs used to control epilepsy are teratogenic; therefore, patients should be weaned to the lowest dose possible prior to pregnancy or weaned off of the medications entirely.
- Valproate, carbamazepine, phenobarbital, and lamotrigine are commonly used antiepileptics and are all associated with an increased risk of neural tube defects. Recent data suggests that when used as single agents, these medications cause less frequent severe congenital defects than previously thought (Fig. 19-2).
- Women with epilepsy who are pregnant or planning a pregnancy should be supplemented with **4 mg of folic acid** daily to help prevent neural tube defects.
- Pregnancy does not typically affect the frequency of seizures. However, a confounding factor is that pregnant mothers are often noncompliant with medications for fear of teratogenicity.
- Seizure during pregnancy can cause fetal hypoxia. Fetal monitoring may reflect fetal hypoxia for up to 30 minutes after the seizure. Emergent delivery is not indicated based on this tracing alone.
- Preeclampsia must be considered in the differential in the setting of seizures, particularly in the third trimester (see Chapter 14).

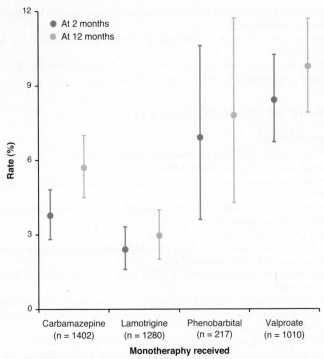

**Figure 19-2.** The rates of major anomalies associated with *in utero* exposure to various antiepileptic medications and 2 and 12 months of life. (From Tomson T, Battino D. Teratogenic effects of antiepileptic drugs. *Lancet Neurol* 2012;11[9]:803–813.)

## Spinal Cord Injury

Complications of pregnancy in patients with prior spinal cord injuries are often related to the level of the spinal cord lesion.

- Patients with lower lesions (T11 and below) will likely perceive labor pain. Most complications in their pregnancies are related to recurrent urinary tract infections and decubitus ulcers.
- Patients with mid lesions (T5 to T10) often have painless deliveries. These patients must be counseled carefully and monitored closely to avoid undetected labor and delivery. Patients can use home uterine monitors or be taught uterine palpation. Weekly cervical examinations should be considered near term.
- Higher lesions (above T5 to T6) are associated with **autonomic dysreflexia** leading to potentially life-threatening sympathetic hyperactivity. This is manifested by severe hypertension, loss of consciousness, headache, nasal congestion, facial erythema, sweating, piloerection, bradycardia, tachycardia, or arrhythmia. It can be very challenging to distinguish this condition from preeclampsia. Epidural anesthesia up to T10 is critical in patients with high spinal cord lesions to prevent this complication. In the setting of acute autonomic dysreflexia, labetalol or nifedipine can be used to control blood pressure. Magnesium sulfate has been

shown to have some benefit in the setting of autonomic dysreflexia (although it is not first line) and should be considered if preeclampsia cannot be definitively excluded.

## Myasthenia Gravis

- Myasthenia gravis (MG) is an autoimmune disease marked by muscle fatigue due to antibodies against acetylcholine receptors.
- There are two types of MG:
  - **Ocular MG** involves only the eyelids and extraocular muscles
  - **Generalized MG** involves ocular, bulbar, limb, and respiratory muscles affected
- Exacerbation in pregnancy noted in approximately 40% of patients. Flares are particularly likely in the first trimester and immediately postpartum.
- Treatment:
  - Acetylcholinesterase inhibitors are first-line therapy for pregnant and nonpregnant patients.
  - Glucocorticoids, azathioprine, and cyclosporine are second-line options and are safe in pregnancy.
- Medication interactions:
  - Patients with MG are often challenging to manage because a wide variety of medications can exacerbate symptoms. These medications range from anesthetics to antibiotics, even oxytocin and magnesium sulfate.
  - **Magnesium sulfate is contraindicated** for these patients. In the setting of preeclampsia, levetiracetam or valproic acid can be used for seizure prophylaxis.
- Concerns during labor:
  - First stage of labor is not affected by MG, as this stage is mediated by smooth muscles. MG only affects skeletal muscle.
  - Second stage of labor can be affected and patients can become fatigued with pushing. "Laboring down" or operative delivery can be used to minimize fatigue.
- Fetal concerns:
  - Immunoglobulin G anti–acetylcholine receptor antibodies can cross the placenta leading to fetal manifestations of MG.
  - Polyhydramnios due to impaired swallowing, decreased fetal movement, and decreased fetal breathing can be observed in fetuses of MG patients.
  - Nonstress test is often not reliable because fetal movement and therefore accelerations can be impaired by MG. Contraction stress testing can be useful.
  - Up to 20% of neonates develop transient MG postpartum, lasting for up to 3 months.
  - Most studies do not show an increased long-term risk of MG in fetuses born to MG patients, although data are limited.

## POSTPARTUM COMPRESSION NERVE INJURIES

- Risk factors include fetal macrosomia, epidural anesthesia, prolonged second stage, and poor positioning in stirrups.
- Prolonged pushing and "over"-aggressive McRoberts during second stage of labor can be associated with postpartum neuropathies. This is particularly true in patients who have an epidural during the second stage of labor.
- See Table 19-3 for common nerve palsies and the associated mechanism of injury.
- Most patients make a complete recovery. Physical therapy can be helpful.

| TABLE 19-3 | Common Postpartum Nerve Palsies and Mechanisms of Injury | |
|---|---|---|
| **Nerve Damaged** | **Common Mechanism of Injury** | **Deficit** |
| Peroneal nerve | • Prolonged knee flexion during labor<br>• Pressure of fibular head from stirrups<br>• Palmar pressure during pushing | • Inability to dorsiflex the foot, i.e., foot drop |
| Femoral nerve | • Prolonged hip flexion with McRoberts | • Weak quadriceps leading to inability to flex hip<br>• Sensory loss over anterior and medial thigh |
| Lateral femoral cutaneous | • Prolonged compression | • Purely sensory defect, often paresthesias on outer thigh |

## SUGGESTED READINGS

Boonmak P, Boonmak S. Epidural blood patching for preventing and treating post-dural puncture headache. *Cochrane Database Syst Rev* 2010;(1):CD001791.

Contag SA, Bushnell C. Contemporary management of migrainous disorders in pregnancy. *Curr Opin Obstet Gynecol* 2010;22:437.

Coyle, PK. Pregnancy and multiple sclerosis. *Neurol Clin* 2012;30(3):877–888.

Estresvag JM, Zwart JA, Helde G, et al. Headache and transient focal neurologic symptoms during pregnancy, a prospective cohort. *Acta Neurol Scand* 2005;111:233.

Ferrero S, Esposito F, Biamonti M, et al. Myasthenia gravis during pregnancy. *Expert Rev Neurother* 2008;8(6):979–988.

Osterman M, Ilyas AM, Matzon JL. Carpel tunnel syndrome in pregnancy. *Othop Clin North Am* 2012;43(4):515–520.

Pasto L, Portaccio E, Ghezzi A, et al. Epidural analgesia and cesarean delivery in multiple sclerosis post-partum relapses: the Italian cohort study. *BMC Neurol* 2012;12:165.

Pearce CF, Hansen WF. Headache and neurological diseases in pregnancy. *Clin Obstet Gynecol* 2012;55(3):810–828.

Signore C, Spong CY, Krotoski D, et al. Pregnancy in women with physical disabilities. *Obstet Gynecol* 2011;117(4):935–947.

Tomson T, Battino D. Teratogenic effects of antiepileptic drugs. *Lancet Neurol* 2012;11(9):803–813.

Toppenburg KS, Hill DA, Miller DP, et al. Safety of radiographic imaging during pregnancy. *Am Fam Physician* 1999;59:1813–1818.

Wong CA, Scavone BM, Dugan S, et al. Incidence of postpartum lumbosacral spine and lower extremity nerve injuries. *Obstet Gynecol* 2003;101:279.

# Hematologic Disorders of Pregnancy

Nina Resetkova and Linda M. Szymanski

## ANEMIA

- The Centers for Disease Control and Prevention's **definition of anemia in pregnancy** is hemoglobin (Hgb) or hematocrit (Hct) value less than the fifth percentile in a healthy reference population at the same stage of pregnancy.
- Typical values include Hgb <11.0 g/dL in the first and third trimesters and <10.5 in the second trimester (Fig. 20-1).
- Racial differences have been noted, with lower Hgb and Hct levels seen in African American women compared with white women. The Institute of Medicine suggests lowering the normal value for Hgb by 0.8 g/dL and Hct by 2% in African Americans.

### Common Types of Anemia

- Anemia is commonly classified by mean corpuscular volume (MCV) as normocytic, microcytic, and macrocytic (Table 20-1).

*Physiologic Anemia of Pregnancy*

- **Physiologic anemia of pregnancy** occurs because plasma volume increases more (25% to 50%) than red blood cell mass (10% to 25%), causing hemodilution and reduction in Hct of 3% to 5%. These changes begin at approximately 6 weeks' gestation and normalize by 6 weeks postpartum.

*Iron Deficiency Anemia*

- **Iron deficiency anemia** is the most common anemia diagnosed during pregnancy, accounting for nearly 50% to 75% of all cases.
  - **Diagnosis** is based on insidious symptom onset, such as weakness and lethargy, and in severe cases, glossitis, stomatitis, koilonychia (in which the outer surfaces of the nails are concave), pica, impaired thermogenesis, and gastritis.
  - **Laboratory findings:** If a microcytic anemia is present, iron studies are indicated (Table 20-2). Measurement of serum ferritin levels has the greatest sensitivity and specificity for the diagnosis of iron deficiency. Serum ferritin levels <10 to 15 ng/mL (or µg/L) generally indicate iron deficiency anemia. A typical diagnostic cut-off is <12 ng/mL.
  - **Treatment:** Although it is important for pregnant women to maintain healthy iron levels, insufficient data exist regarding the benefits of iron supplementation for anemia prophylaxis and treatment during pregnancy. The Centers for Disease Control and Prevention currently recommends daily elemental iron supplementation (30 mg) for prophylaxis and 60 to 120 mg of daily elemental iron if iron deficiency anemia has been diagnosed. A 325-mg tablet of ferrous sulfate contains 65-mg elemental iron; a 300-mg tablet of ferrous gluconate contains 34-mg elemental iron. The American College of Obstetricians and Gynecologists (ACOG)

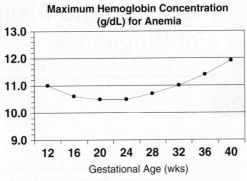

**Figure 20-1.** Cutoff values for anemia, defined as a hemoglobin level below the fifth percentile based on values from pregnant women with adequate iron supplementation. (Data adapted from Centers for Disease Control and Prevention. Recommendations to prevent and control iron deficiency in the United States. *MMWR Recomm Rep* 1998;47[RR-3]:1–29.)

guidelines recommend supplemental iron for women with iron deficiency anemia. For patients who do not respond to or cannot tolerate oral therapy, or for those with severe anemia, intravenous (IV) iron is an alternative. In women with Hgb <6 g/dL, fetal well-being may be compromised secondary to abnormal fetal oxygenation, and maternal transfusion may be indicated.

*Hemoglobinopathies*

- **Hemoglobinopathies** are genetic abnormalities in the globin portion of the hemoglobin molecule (HbA) that can either be qualitative, resulting in structural abnormalities

| TABLE 20-1 | Classification of Anemia by Mean Corpuscular Volume | |
|---|---|---|
| **Microcytic (MCV <80 fL)** | **Normocytic (MCV 80–100 fL)** | **Macrocytic (MCV >100 fL)** |
| Iron deficiency | Early iron deficiency | Vitamin $B_{12}$ deficiency |
| Thalassemias | Acute blood loss | Folic acid deficiency |
| Anemia of chronic disease (late) | Sickle cell disease | Drug induced (zidovudine) |
| Sideroblastic anemia | Anemia of chronic disease | Ethanol abuse |
| Lead poisoning | Infection (osteomyelitis, HIV, mycoplasma, EBV) | Liver disease |
| Copper deficiency | Bone marrow disease | Myelodysplastic syndromes |
| | Chronic renal insufficiency | |
| | Hypothyroidism | |
| | Autoimmune hemolytic anemia | |

MCV, mean corpuscular volume; EBV, Epstein-Barr virus.
Adapted from American College of Obstetricians and Gynecologists. ACOG practice bulletin no. 95: anemia in pregnancy. *Obstet Gynecol* 2008;112:201–207.

| TABLE 20-2 | Laboratory Studies in Various Anemias | | |
|---|---|---|---|
| Type of Anemia | Serum Iron | Serum Ferritin | Total Iron-Binding Capacity (TIBC) |
| Iron deficiency anemia | ↓ | ↓ | ↑ |
| Anemia of chronic disease | ↓ | ↑ | ↓ |
| Sideroblastic anemia | ↑ | ↑ | ↓ |
| Thalassemia | ↔ | ↔ | ↔ |

↓, decreased; ↑, increased; ↔, no change.
Adapted from American College of Obstetricians and Gynecologists. ACOG practice bulletin no. 95: anemia in pregnancy. *Obstet Gynecol* 2008;112:201–207.

like sickle cell anemia, or quantitative, resulting in a decreased number of normal globin chains as in the thalassemias. Normal Hgb is composed of 96% to 97% HbA, 2% to 3% hemoglobin alpha 2 (HbA2), and <1% fetal hemoglobin (HbF).

Sickle Cell Disease

- **Sickle cell disease (SCD)** describes a group of hemoglobinopathies that involve sickle hemoglobin (HbS), including SCD (often called "sickle cell anemia"), sickle cell hemoglobin C (HbSC), and sickle-thalassemia hemoglobin (HbS-Thal). Homozygosity for HbS (HbSS) is the most common phenotype, occurring primarily among people from sub-Saharan Africa, South and Central America, Saudi Arabia, India, and Mediterranean countries. Approximately 1 in every 500 to 600 African American newborns has SCD, an autosomal recessive disorder. Affected patients may experience hemolytic anemia, recurrent pain crises, infection, and infarction of more than one organ system. HbS results from a single substitution of valine for glutamic acid at the sixth position of the beta (β)-globin chain. When deoxygenated, HbS is less soluble and tends to polymerize into rigid aggregates and distort the red blood cell into a sickle shape. These cells undergo extravascular hemolysis, leading to a severe chronic anemia, and may become trapped in the microvasculature, causing vascular obstruction, ischemia, and infarction. This cascade results in a vaso-occlusive crisis, which can be associated with severe pain, fever, organ dysfunction, and tissue necrosis. Vaso-occlusive crises may be triggered by infection, hypoxia, acidosis, dehydration, or psychological stress. A serious complication is acute chest syndrome, one of the leading causes of hospitalization and death in patients with SCD. Acute chest syndrome is characterized by a combination of respiratory symptoms, new lung infiltrates, and fever.
- **Diagnosis:** The anemia is normocytic, normochromic with an Hgb concentration of 6 to 10 g/dL and Hct of 18% to 30%. The reticulocyte count is increased to 3% to 15%. Lactate dehydrogenase is elevated, and haptoglobin is decreased. The peripheral blood smear may show sickle cells, target cells, and Howell-Jolly bodies. Diagnosis is confirmed by Hgb electrophoresis, which typically shows 85% to 100% HbS, absent HbA, normal HbA2, and moderately elevated HbF (usually <15%). Jaundice may result from red blood cell destruction, leading to unconjugated hyperbilirubinemia.
- **Treatment:** Hydroxyurea may be used to reduce intracellular sickling but is not recommended in pregnancy because it is teratogenic in animal studies. Infections are treated aggressively with antibiotics. Severe anemia is treated with blood transfusion. Pain crises are managed with oxygen, hydration, and analgesia. Controversy surrounds prophylactic exchange transfusion and is reserved for the most severe cases. Additionally,

the risks involved with transfusions must be taken into account. Advantages of transfusion are an increase in HbA level, which improves oxygen-carrying capacity and a decrease in HbS-carrying erythrocytes. If a transfusion is given, leukocyte-depleted packed red cells, phenotyped for major and minor antigens, should be used.

- **Pregnancy considerations:** Patients with SCD are at increased risk for sickling during pregnancy because of increased metabolic requirements, vascular stasis, and a relative hypercoagulable state. Complications during pregnancy in women with SCD include an increased risk of spontaneous abortion, intrauterine growth restriction (IUGR), fetal death in utero, low birth weight, preeclampsia, and premature birth. Women with SCD also experience greater risk of urinary tract infection (UTI), bacteriuria, pulmonary infections and infarction, and, possibly, more painful crises. Due to elevated risk of UTI, a urine culture should be evaluated at minimum in every trimester and treated correspondingly. Women with SCD should receive the pneumococcal vaccine before pregnancy and folate supplementation of 1 to 4 mg/day. Iron supplements should be prescribed only if iron is deficient. The intensity of fetal surveillance varies according to the clinical severity of the disease. In severe cases, twice weekly assessment of fetal well-being should begin at 32 weeks' gestation, and monthly sonography should be performed to evaluate fetal growth. All African American patients should undergo an Hgb electrophoresis to assess carrier status. If both the patient and the father of the baby are found to be hemoglobinopathy carriers, genetic counseling is indicated. Amniocentesis or chorionic villus sampling (CVS) may be offered for prenatal diagnosis. After delivery, patients should practice early ambulation and wear thromboembolic deterrent stockings to prevent thromboembolism.

- Regarding contraception, the levonorgestrel-containing intrauterine device (IUD) and progestin-only implants are considered excellent contraceptive options for patients with SCD. No well-controlled studies have evaluated oral contraceptives in SCD; however, low-dose combined contraceptives appear to be a good choice in some women with SCD. The benefits of copper-containing IUDs are debated due to a potential for increased blood loss but copper-containing IUDs are generally considered a safe and effective method of contraception for women with SCD. Progestin-only pills, depot medroxyprogesterone, and barrier devices are also safe for contraception. Medroxyprogesterone acetate (Depo Provera) injections may decrease the number of pain crises.

## Sickle Trait

- **Sickle cell trait (HbAS)** is common in African Americans (1 in 12, or 8%) and is also prevalent in persons of Mediterranean, Middle Eastern, Indian, Caribbean, and Central and South American descents. Women with sickle cell trait have approximately twice the frequency of UTIs compared to the general population, especially during pregnancy, and should be screened each trimester. No direct fetal compromise exists from maternal sickle cell trait. Partners should be screened because the risk of having a child with SCD becomes one in four if the father is also a carrier.

## Thalassemias

- The term **thalassemia** encompasses a group of inherited blood disorders that can cause severe microcytic hypochromic anemia. Alpha ($\alpha$)-thalassemia and beta ($\beta$)-thalassemia result from absent or decreased production of structurally normal $\alpha$- and $\beta$-globulin chains, respectively, generating an abnormal ratio of $\alpha$ to non-$\alpha$ chains (see Table 20-3). The excess chains form aggregates that lead to ineffective erythropoiesis and/or hemolysis. A broad spectrum of syndromes is possible, ranging from no symptoms to transfusion-dependent anemia and death. Both diseases are transmitted as autosomal recessive traits.

**TABLE 20-3** Findings in Thalassemia

| | Genotype[a] | Lab/Clinical Findings | Specifics |
|---|---|---|---|
| **Alpha-thalassemias** | | | |
| Silent carrier | $-\alpha/\alpha\,\alpha$ | Normal or slight microcytosis. | Asymptomatic. 25%–30% of African Americans. |
| α-Thalassemia trait | $-\,-/\alpha\,\alpha$ (Asian) $-\,\alpha/-\,\alpha$ (African) | Mild microcytic, hypochromic. Normal Hgb electrophoresis. | Asymptomatic anemia not treatable with iron. Both genotypes identical clinically; position of deleted genes determines severity in offspring ($-\,-/\alpha\,\alpha$ at risk of fetus with HbH or hydrops). |
| HbH disease | $-\,-/-\,\alpha$ | Moderate to severe microcytic, hypochromic anemia (Hgb 8–10 g/dL). ↑ reticulocytes (5%–10%). HbH = 2%–40%; ↓ HbA2, HbF normal. Normal serum iron. Heinz bodies on peripheral smear. Splenomegaly, bony abnormalities. | Anemia worsens during pregnancy, infection, and with oxidant drugs. Treat with long-term transfusion, splenectomy, and iron chelation. May have cholelithiasis. |
| Hydrops fetalis "Hb Bart disease" | $-\,-/-\,-$ | Marked anemia (Hgb 3–10), ↑ nucleated erythrocytes, 80%–90% Hgb Bart; 10%–20% HbH. No HbA. Hydrops, heart failure, pulmonary edema, transverse limb reduction defects, hypospadias. | Diagnosis often made in pregnancy by sonogram noting hydropic fetus. Usually results in death. Survival possible with intrauterine transfusion. |

*(Continued)*

| TABLE 20-3 | Findings in Thalassemia *(Continued)* | | |
|---|---|---|---|
| | Genotype[a] | Lab/Clinical Findings | Specifics |
| **Beta-thalassemias** | | | |
| β-Thalassemia minor | $\beta^0/\beta$ | Asymptomatic or mild microcytic anemia (Hgb 8–10 g/dL). ↑ HbA2, ↑ HbF, ↓ HbA. | Heterozygous. Confers resistance to falciparum malaria. Often misdiagnosed as iron deficient. |
| "β-Thalassemia trait" | $\beta^+/\beta$ | Mild or no anemia. Basophilic stippling. ↔ ↑ erythrocytes. No splenomegaly, MCV 60 to normal. | |
| β-Thalassemia intermedia | Varies, 2 β mutations (at least 1 mild) | Mild to moderate anemia. Prominent splenomegaly, bony deformities, growth retardation, iron overload. | Clinical diagnosis. May be asymptomatic to severely symptomatic. Present with symptoms later in life. Chronic transfusions not required. |
| Thalassemia major "Cooley anemia" | $\beta^0/\beta^0$ $\beta^+/\beta^+$ | Hgb as low as 2–3 g/dL. MCV <67 fL. ↓ reticulocytes. ↑↑ HbF, variable HbA2, no HbA ↑ HbF, ↓ HbA, variable HbA2 Splenomegaly; bone changes (increased hematopoiesis), severe iron overload. | Homozygous. Severity depends on amount of globin produced ($\beta^0/\beta^0$ more severe—no globin.) Manifests at age 6–9 mo when HbF changes to HbA. With transfusions and chelation, may survive into third to fifth decade. Die young from infectious or cardiac complications. |

[a]Genotype: β and δ—single gene per chromosome. α Gene is duplicated producing two genes per haploid and four per diploid.

Hgb, hemoglobin; HbH, hemoglobin H; HbA, hemoglobin A; HbA2, hemoglobin alpha 2; HbF, fetal hemoglobin; MCV, mean corpuscular volume.

Adapted from American College of Obstetricians and Gynecologists. ACOG practice bulletin no. 78: hemoglobinopathies in pregnancy. *Obstet Gynecol* 2007;109:229–237.

- **Alpha-thalassemia** is associated with Southeast Asian, African, Caribbean, and Mediterranean origin and results from a deletion of one to all $\alpha$ genes, located on chromosome 16. Excess $\beta$ globins then form $\beta$-globin tetramers called HbH. A fetus would be affected because fetal Hgb also requires $\alpha$ chains.
- **Beta-thalassemia** is associated with Mediterranean, Asian, Middle Eastern, Caribbean, and Hispanic origin. More than 200 alterations (mostly point mutations) in $\beta$-globin genes, located on chromosome 11, have been reported. The two consequences of these gene defects are the following: $\beta^0$, which is the complete absence of the $\beta$ chain, and $\beta^+$, which is decreased synthesis of the $\beta$ chain.
  - **Diagnosis:** Thalassemia is usually microcytic and hypochromic with an MCV of $<80$ fL similar to iron deficiency anemia but with important differences in clinical presentation and laboratory testing.
  - **Laboratory findings:** In general, thalassemias, especially the traits, are often misdiagnosed as iron deficiency anemia. However, the anemia is not corrected with iron repletion. A microcytic anemia in the absence of iron deficiency suggests thalassemia and additional testing including electrophoresis and iron studies are warranted. Suspicion for the presence of $\alpha$-thalassemia is raised by the finding of microcytosis and a normal red cell distribution width with minimal or no anemia in the absence of iron deficiency or $\beta$-thalassemia. Pedigree studies are often helpful during workup of patients with $\alpha$-thalassemia. Molecular genetic testing, such as quantitative polymerase chain reaction (PCR), is needed for diagnosis. Quantitative Hgb electrophoresis is required for the diagnosis of $\beta$-thalassemia and should be suspected in cases of elevated HbA2 ($>3.5\%$).
- **Pregnancy and thalassemia**
  - Women with trait status for either thalassemia require no special care.
  - Women diagnosed with or at high risk for thalassemia should be offered preconception counseling and information about the availability of prenatal diagnosis. First-trimester, DNA-based prenatal testing (CVS) is available if both members of the couple are carriers. Preimplantation genetic diagnosis may also be an option for affected parents.
  - Women with HbH may have successful pregnancies, with maternal outcome related to the severity of anemia.
  - Pregnancy may exacerbate the anemia, necessitating transfusions, and place women at an increased risk for preeclampsia, congestive heart failure, and premature delivery.
  - Information on pregnancy in women with $\beta$-thalassemia major or intermedia is more limited, although successful pregnancies have been reported. These women require close medical evaluation and follow-up.
  - If asplenic, vaccinations for pneumococcus, *Haemophilus influenzae*, and meningococcus need to be up-to-date.
  - Thalassemia may confer an increased risk of neural tube defects secondary to folic acid deficiency, so up to 4 mg/day periconceptional folic acid supplementation is recommended. Iron supplements should be prescribed only if iron deficiency is present; otherwise, iron overload can result.
- **Antepartum fetal testing** should be undertaken in anemic thalassemia patients.
  - Periodic fetal sonography to assess fetal growth as well as nonstress testing to evaluate fetal well-being is recommended.
  - Ultrasonography is also useful to detect hydrops fetalis but usually at a later gestational age. Options for affected fetuses include intrauterine blood transfusions, which have shown good success in fetuses with hydrops fetalis.

*Megaloblastic Anemia*

- **Megaloblastic anemia** is the result of impaired DNA synthesis, leading to ineffective erythropoiesis.
  - Megaloblastic anemia is a much greater problem in underdeveloped countries and is primarily the result of dietary folic acid deficiency. Folic acid requirements increase from 50 µg/day in the nonpregnant state to up to 800 µg/day during pregnancy. Phenytoin, nitrofurantoin, trimethoprim, and alcohol decrease absorption of folic acid.
  - A less common cause of megaloblastic anemia is vitamin $B_{12}$ deficiency, often from a long-term vegan diet or decreased intestinal absorption due to tropical sprue, regional enteritis, gastrointestinal resection for bariatric surgery, or chronic giardiasis.
  - Megaloblastic anemia in pregnancy may lead to poor outcomes. Animal studies suggest that it may be related to abruptio placentae, preeclampsia, IUGR, and prematurity. Folic acid deficiency is also linked to open neural tube defects.
- **Diagnosis:** Megaloblastic anemia is often slowly progressive and tends to occur in the third trimester. Weight loss and anorexia may occur in addition to the usual symptoms of anemia, roughness of the skin, and glossitis. It can also manifest as bleeding due to thrombocytopenia or as an infection resulting from leukopenia.
- **Laboratory findings:**
  - Macrocytic, normochromic anemia involving erythrocytes, leukocytes, and platelets
  - Peripheral blood smear shows hypersegmented neutrophils, oval macrocytes, and Howell-Jolly bodies.
  - To diagnose folate deficiency, consider the erythrocyte folate level, as it is a better indicator of whole body stores than the serum level, which can vary widely.
- **Treatment:** Determining which deficiency exists is important before commencing treatment.
  - Folate deficiency is generally treated with daily folic acid supplementation of 1 mg/day. Within 7 to 10 days, the white blood cell and platelet counts should normalize. Hgb gradually increases to normal levels after several weeks of therapy.
  - If the anemia is due to vitamin $B_{12}$ deficiency, folate supplementation may ameliorate the anemia, masking the $B_{12}$ deficiency; it may also precipitate neurologic deficits. Vitamin $B_{12}$ deficiency is treated with intramuscular cobalamin. Affected patients may require monthly (1 mg) injections for life.

## THROMBOCYTOPENIA

**Thrombocytopenia** is defined as a platelet count <150,000/µL and occurs in about 10% of pregnancies. Clinical signs, such as petechiae, easy bruising, epistaxis, gingival bleeding, and hematuria, are usually not seen until platelets are <50,000/µL. Counts below 50,000/µL may also increase surgical bleeding. The risk of spontaneous bleeding increases only when platelet counts fall below 20,000/µL, and significant bleeding may occur with platelet counts <10,000/µL. Thrombocytopenia, depending on the severity and etiology, may or may not be associated with serious maternal and/or fetal morbidity and mortality. Many conditions can cause thrombocytopenia during pregnancy.

## Gestational Thrombocytopenia

- **Gestational thrombocytopenia**, also referred to as incidental thrombocytopenia of pregnancy or essential thrombocytopenia, affects up to 8% of pregnancies and represents the most common diagnosis in over 75% of cases of mild thrombocytopenia during pregnancy. It generally occurs late in gestation and is not associated with fetal thrombocytopenia. The decreased platelet count is likely due to hemodilution and increased physiologic platelet turnover. Platelet counts usually return to normal within 2 to 12 weeks after delivery. Gestational thrombocytopenia can recur in subsequent pregnancies, although the recurrence rate is unknown.
- **Diagnosis:** Gestational thrombocytopenia is a diagnosis of exclusion; therefore, the first step is to take a careful history to rule out other causes. Platelet counts obtained before pregnancy and any laboratory data available from prior pregnancies should be reviewed.
  - Three criteria should be present: (a) mild thrombocytopenia (70,000 to 150,000/μL); (b) no previous history of thrombocytopenia, except during pregnancy; and (c) no bleeding symptoms.
  - There are no specific diagnostic tests to distinguish gestational thrombocytopenia from mild idiopathic thrombocytopenic purpura (ITP). In fact, many women with gestational thrombocytopenia have platelet-associated immunoglobulin G (IgG) and serum antiplatelet IgG, making it difficult to distinguish from ITP using platelet antibody testing.
- **Management:** In gestational thrombocytopenia, no intervention is necessary. Women with gestational thrombocytopenia are not at risk for maternal or fetal hemorrhage or bleeding complications.
  - Monitor platelets closely to detect decreases below 50,000.
  - Document normal neonatal platelet count. Approximately 2% of the offspring of mothers with gestational thrombocytopenia have mild thrombocytopenia (<50,000/μL). However, infants generally do not suffer from severe platelet deficiency.
  - Reevaluate platelet count in the postpartum period to ensure it returns to normal. If thrombocytopenia persists, consider referring patient for evaluation by a hematologist.

## HELLP Syndrome

- **Hemolysis, elevated liver enzymes, and low platelet (HELLP) syndrome** is the most common pathologic cause of maternal thrombocytopenia. It occurs in approximately 10% to 20% of women who have severe preeclampsia and is often an early finding in preeclampsia. Platelets usually nadir at 24 to 48 hours after delivery but typically do not drop below 20,000/μL. In women who remain severely thrombocytopenic after delivery, plasma exchange and/or corticosteroids may be considered. In addition to improving neonatal outcome before 34 weeks' gestation, corticosteroids may also improve maternal outcomes. When given in the antepartum period, transient improvements are seen in maternal platelet counts. Small placebo-controlled trials have not shown decreased morbidity when steroids are continued postpartum.

## Idiopathic Thrombocytopenic Purpura

- **ITP** occurs in 1 to 2 per 1,000 pregnancies and accounts for 5% of pregnancy-associated thrombocytopenia. ITP is the most common cause of thrombocytopenia in the first trimester. Antiplatelet antibodies are directed at platelet surface glycoproteins, leading to increased destruction of platelets by the reticuloendothelial system (primarily the spleen) that exceeds the rate of platelet synthesis by the bone marrow. The course of ITP is not typically affected by pregnancy.

- **Diagnosis:** Diagnosis is based on the history, physical exam, complete blood count, and peripheral smear. Women with ITP may report symptoms of easy bruising, petechiae, epistaxis, or gingival bleeding predating pregnancy. ITP is a diagnosis of exclusion, and there is no diagnostic test. If thrombocytopenia is mild, it is difficult to distinguish ITP from gestational thrombocytopenia. Detection of platelet-associated antibodies is consistent with, but not diagnostic of, ITP because they may also be present in women with gestational thrombocytopenia and preeclampsia. Platelet antibody testing has a fairly low sensitivity (49% to 66%). However, the absence of platelet-associated IgG makes the diagnosis of ITP less likely. ITP is more likely if the platelet count is $<50,000/\mu L$ or in the presence of an underlying autoimmune disease or history of previous thrombocytopenia. In contrast to gestational thrombocytopenia, ITP-associated thrombocytopenia is typically evident early in pregnancy. Findings include the following:
  - Persistent thrombocytopenia (platelet count $<100,000/\mu L$ with or without accompanying megathrombocytes on the peripheral smear)
  - Normal or increased megakaryocytes determined from bone marrow
  - Secondary causes of maternal thrombocytopenia should be excluded (e.g., preeclampsia, HIV infection, systemic lupus erythematosus, drugs).
  - Absence of splenomegaly
- **Antenatal management:** According to the American Society of Hematology, any adult with a new diagnosis of ITP requires testing for HIV and hepatitis C. Pregnant women with platelet counts over $50,000/\mu L$ at any time during the pregnancy and those with counts of 30,000 to $50,000/\mu L$ in the first or second trimester do not routinely require treatment. If the platelet count is $<10,000/\mu L$ at any point in pregnancy, between 10,000 and $30,000/\mu L$ in the second or third trimester, or if the patient demonstrates bleeding symptoms, treatment is required. Two treatments are available: glucocorticoids and IV gamma globulin (IVIG).
  - Glucocorticoids suppress antibody production, inhibit sequestration of antibody-coated platelets, and interfere with the interaction between platelets and antibodies.
    - Oral prednisone is started at 1 to 2 mg/kg/day and is tapered to the lowest dose supporting an acceptable platelet count (usually over $50,000/\mu L$) and tolerable side effect profile. Patients usually respond within 3 to 7 days and approximately 75% respond within 3 weeks. One fourth of patients may achieve complete remission.
    - High-dose glucocorticoids, such as methylprednisolone, may be administered at 1 to 1.5 mg/kg IV in divided doses. Very little crosses the placenta. Response is usually seen in 2 to 10 days.
    - Side effects of glucocorticoids include increased rates of gestational hypertension and diabetes.
  - High-dose IVIG (400 mg/kg/day for 5 days or 1 g/kg/day for 2 days) is another therapeutic option. The proposed mechanism of action of IVIG is prolongation of the clearance time of IgG-coated platelets by the maternal reticuloendothelial system. Eighty percent of patients treated with IVIG respond within days, and remission lasts 3 weeks. The main drawbacks are cost and inconvenience to the patient.

- Splenectomy is an option in the second trimester in women who fail glucocorticoid and IVIG therapy and are experiencing bleeding associated with platelet counts <10,000/μL. With splenectomy, remission occurs in 75% of women; however, data in pregnancy are limited. Individuals with splenectomies should be immunized against pneumococcus, *H. influenzae*, and meningococcus.
- Immunosuppressive therapy is controversial and usually not pursued because, although its efficacy is well established in nonpregnant patients, it is potentially harmful to the developing fetus. The therapeutic regimens have side effects, and the goal of therapy is to raise the platelet count to a safe level (over 20,000 to 30,000/μL), with the least amount of intervention possible, keeping in mind that a safe platelet count is not necessarily a normal platelet count.
- Pregnant women with ITP should be instructed to avoid nonsteroidal anti-inflammatory agents, salicylates, and trauma.
- **Intrapartum management:** As pregnancy approaches term, more aggressive measures to increase maternal platelet counts may be indicated to allow for adequate hemostasis during delivery and epidural anesthesia. Platelet counts over 50,000/μL are usually adequate for either vaginal or cesarean delivery and are usually also adequate for regional anesthesia, although some recommend a platelet count over 100,000/μL to avoid epidural hematomas. Prophylactic platelet transfusion may be appropriate with a maternal platelet count <10,000 to 20,000/μL before vaginal delivery or <50,000/μL before a cesarean section or if bleeding is present. For cesarean section, the transfusion should begin at the time of incision. One "pack" of platelets will increase the platelet count by 5,000 to 10,000/μL. Transfused platelets will have a shorter half-life because of circulating antibodies.

*Neonatal Thrombocytopenia*

- In mothers with ITP, placental transfer of the IgG platelet antibodies can result in fetal or **neonatal thrombocytopenia**. Approximately 10% to 15% of neonates will have severe thrombocytopenia (<50,000/μL). The general consensus is that no correlation exists between maternal platelet count (or the presence of maternal platelet antibodies) and fetal platelet count. The most reliable indicator of fetal thrombocytopenia is a history of neonatal thrombocytopenia in a sibling. Fetal platelet count cannot be predicted accurately, and even fetal scalp sampling or percutaneous umbilical blood sampling does not provide reliable estimates. In ITP, the neonatal platelet count declines after delivery, reaching a nadir at 48 to 72 hours of life. Notification of a pediatrician for close monitoring of the neonatal platelet count is very important in preventing the sequelae of neonatal intracranial hemorrhage (ICH), a rare event. Some recommend obtaining umbilical cord platelet counts at delivery.
- **Delivery mode:** Using the fetal platelet count to determine route of delivery is not recommended. This is because ICH appears to be more of a neonatal than an intrapartum event and due to the limitations in obtaining an accurate fetal platelet count. A survey of US perinatologists reported that most prefer not to perform invasive tests to evaluate fetal platelets and support a trial of labor. Unfortunately, no randomized controlled studies have compared delivery mode in these neonates. Previously, the assumption that a fetus with a platelet count lower than 50,000/μL is at significant risk for ICH, coupled with the belief that cesarean delivery is less traumatic than spontaneous vaginal delivery, led to the recommendation of cesarean delivery for severe fetal thrombocytopenia in ITP patients. However, there is no evidence that cesarean section decreases the risk of ICH. Cesarean section should be performed for obstetric indications only.

# THROMBOEMBOLIC DISEASE

Thromboembolic disease is linked with both adverse maternal and fetal/neonatal outcomes. The term **venous thromboembolism (VTE)** encompasses **deep vein thrombosis (DVT)** and **pulmonary embolism (PE)**.

- Pregnant women are four to five times more likely to experience a VTE than age-matched nonpregnant women.
- Incidence of VTE ranges from 0.76 to 2.0 episodes per 1,000 pregnancies. VTEs account for 9% of all maternal deaths in the United States.
- Approximately 80% of VTEs in pregnancy are DVT and 20% are PE.
- Approximately half of all VTEs occur in the antepartum period and appear to be evenly divided among the three trimesters.
- PE occurs more frequently postpartum.
- Cesarean delivery imparts a three to five times greater risk than a vaginal delivery.

## Risk Factors for Venous Thromboembolism

- Pregnancy is considered a hypercoagulable state. Fibrinogen, coagulation factors, and plasminogen activator inhibitor-1 (PAI-1) levels are increased; free protein S levels are decreased, and fibrinolytic activity is decreased. Additionally, VTE risk is increased by anatomic changes in pregnancy including increased venous stasis and compression of the inferior vena cava and pelvic veins by the enlarging uterus.
- One of the most significant risk factors is a personal history of VTE. Maternal medical conditions including heart disease, SCD, lupus, obesity, diabetes, and hypertension increase risk. Other risk factors include recent surgery, family history of VTE, bed rest or prolonged immobilization, smoking, age older than 35 years, multiple gestations, preeclampsia, and postpartum infection.
- **Thrombophilias** may be inherited or acquired.
  - Pregnancy may trigger an event in women with an underlying thrombophilia.
  - Fetal death in utero, severe IUGR, abruption, and severe early-onset preeclampsia have been correlated with underlying thrombophilias that affect uteroplacental circulation; however, this is controversial and recent studies fail to reliably establish causal links between thrombophilias and these adverse pregnancy outcomes.
  - **Inherited thrombophilias** (Table 20-4):
    - Increase the risk of a maternal thromboembolic event approximately eightfold
    - Are present in over half of all maternal thrombotic events.
    - Antithrombin deficiency and homozygosity for factor V Leiden mutation are the most potent of the inherited thrombophilias. Double or compound heterozygotes (for both factor V Leiden and prothrombin G20219A) are also at greater risk of VTE.
  - **Acquired thrombophilias:**
    - Include persistent antiphospholipid antibody syndromes (APS) (lupus anticoagulants or anticardiolipin antibodies). APS is present in 15% to 17% of women with recurrent pregnancy loss.
  - Routine screening for thrombophilias is not recommended in all pregnant women and screening indications are controversial. ACOG no longer recommends thrombophilia testing in women with recurrent fetal loss, placental abruption, IUGR, or preeclampsia. A thrombophilia workup (Table 20-5) should be considered for the following:
    - VTE during pregnancy (workup after delivery) or VTE associated with a non-recurrent risk factor such as prolonged immobilization.

| TABLE 20-4 | Inherited Thrombophilias and Risk of Venous Thromboembolism in Pregnancy |
|---|---|

| Thrombophilia | Odds Ratio |
|---|---|
| Factor V Leiden homozygosity | 34.4 |
| Prothrombin G20210A homozygosity | 26.4 |
| Factor V Leiden heterozygous | 8.3 |
| Prothrombin G20210A heterozygous | 6.8 |
| Protein C deficiency | 4.8 |
| Antithrombin deficiency | 4.7[a] |
| Protein S deficiency | 3.2 |
| Methylenetetrahydrofolate reductase (MTHFR) C677T homozygote | 0.74 |
| Factor V Leiden + prothrombin G20210A (compound heterozygosity)[b] | 88.0 |
| Antiphospholipid antibody syndrome[c] | 15.8 |

[a]Likely an underestimate. Others report 25- to 50-fold increase. Adapted from Robertson L, Greer I. Thromboembolism in pregnancy. *Curr Opin Obstet Gynecol* 2005;17:113–116.
[b]From Gebhardt GS, Hall DR. Inherited and acquired thrombophilias and poor pregnancy outcome: should we be treating with heparin? *Curr Opin Obstet Gynecol* 2003;15:501–506.
[c]From James AH, Jamison MG, Brancazio LR, et al. Venous thromboembolism during pregnancy and the postpartum period: incidence, risk factors, and mortality. *Am J Obstet Gynecol* 2006;194(5):1311–1315.

- Personal or family history of VTE (first-degree relative with VTE before age 50 years in absence of other risk factors).
- APS screening may be appropriate for women with repeated fetal losses (three losses <10 weeks' gestation or one loss >10 weeks' gestation of a morphologically normal fetus).

## Manifestations and Diagnosis of VTE

*Deep Vein Thrombosis*

- Over 70% of **DVTs** in pregnancy develop in the iliofemoral veins, which are more likely to embolize, and the majority are on the left side. **Diagnosis** of DVT is difficult in pregnancy because expected changes in pregnancy may mimic the symptoms of DVT. Additionally, many patients are asymptomatic. If symptoms exist, the most common include calf or lower extremity swelling, pain or tenderness, warmth, and erythema. Homan sign (calf pain with passive dorsiflexion of the foot) is present in <15% of cases, and a palpable cord is present in <10% of cases. Symptoms of an iliac DVT include abdominal pain, back pain, and swelling of the entire leg. In pregnant women with clinical suspicion of DVT, diagnosis is confirmed in <10%.
- **Venous duplex imaging**, including compression ultrasound, color, and spectral Doppler sonography, has replaced contrast venography as the gold standard and is the most commonly available noninvasive diagnostic method, with a sensitivity of 97% and specificity of 94% in symptomatic proximal DVT. If the deep venous system is normal, the presence of a clinically significant thrombus is unlikely. Limitations include poor sensitivity for asymptomatic disease and difficulty in detecting iliac vein thromboses.

| TABLE 20-5 | Thrombophilia Testing |
| --- | --- |

**Primary Tests (Recommended by ACOG)**

Activated protein C resistance screen (95% of positives due to factor V Leiden)
  followed by analysis for factor V Leiden (PCR) if positive
Prothrombin G20210A genotype
Antithrombin functional assay (activity)
Protein C activity
Protein S activity and free and total antigen levels

**Other Tests (Not Recommended by ACOG)**

Activated partial thromboplastin time (aPTT)
Dilute Russell viper venom time (dRVVT)
Anticardiolipin antibodies (IgG and IgM)
Lupus anticoagulant
4G/4G PAI-1 mutation (if not available, plasma PAI-1 activity)
MTHFR mutation screen and/or fasting plasma homocysteine levels
ANA (if early PEC)

Testing should be remote from thrombotic event, not during pregnancy, and while off anticoagulants, except DNA tests.
ACOG, American College of Obstetricians and Gynecologists; PCR, polymerase chain reaction; PEC, preeclampsia; IgG, immunoglobulin G; IgM, immunoglobulin M; MTFHR, methylenetetrahydrofolate reductase; ANA, antinuclear antibody.
Adapted from American College of Obstetricians and Gynecologists. ACOG practice bulletin no. 113: inherited thrombophilias in pregnancy. *Obstet Gynecol* 2010;116:212–222.

- **Magnetic resonance imaging (MRI):** Studies in nonpregnant patients show a sensitivity of 100% and specificity of 98% to 99% for pelvic and proximal DVTs while maintaining a high accuracy in detecting below-the-knee DVTs.
- D-**Dimer test** is a sensitive but nonspecific test for DVT; however, its use in pregnancy is limited, as D-dimer normally increases with gestational age. A normal D-dimer result may be reassuring if clinical suspicion is low.

*Pulmonary Embolism*

- **PE** remains the leading cause of maternal mortality in developed countries. The risk of PE is greatest immediately postpartum, particularly after cesarean delivery, with a fatality rate of nearly 15%. PE most commonly originates from DVT in the lower extremities, occurring in nearly 50% of patients with proximal DVT. Symptoms typically associated with PE are all common in pregnancy, such as shortness of breath, chest pain, cough, tachypnea, and tachycardia. Because of the serious potential consequences of PE and the increased incidence in pregnancy, clinicians must have a low threshold for evaluation. **Diagnosis** starts with a careful history and physical examination, followed by diagnostic tests to rule out other possible etiologies, such as asthma, pneumonia, or pulmonary edema.
  - An arterial blood gas (ABG), electrocardiogram, and chest x-ray should be performed. ABG values are altered in pregnancy and must be interpreted using

pregnancy-adjusted normal values. More than half of pregnant women with a documented PE have a normal alveolar-arterial gradient.

- A chest x-ray helps rule out other disease processes and enhances interpretation of the ventilation-perfusion (V/Q) scan. The risks associated with various radiologic tests indicated for PE workup are minimal compared with the consequences of a missed PE.

- **Pulmonary angiography** is the gold standard for PE diagnosis, but it is expensive and invasive.

- **Computed tomographic (pulmonary) angiography (CTA)** is becoming the recommended imaging test in pregnant women with suspected PE. CTA is easier to perform, more readily available, more cost-effective, and provides a lower dose of radiation to the fetus than a V/Q scan. CTA is also useful in detecting other abnormalities that may be contributing to the patient's symptoms (e.g., pneumonia, aortic dissection). Newer technology, multidetector computed tomography pulmonary angiography, allows visualization of finer pulmonary vascular detail and provides greater diagnostic accuracy.

- Historically, the **V/Q scan** has been the primary diagnostic test for PE. It is interpreted as low, intermediate, or high probability for PE. High-probability scans (i.e., segmental perfusion defect with normal ventilation) confirm PE, with a positive predictive value over 90% when pretest likelihood is high. V/Q scans are limited in their usefulness because of the large proportion of indeterminate results. Most fetal radiation exposure occurs when radioactive tracers are excreted in the maternal bladder. Therefore, exposure can be limited by prompt and frequent voiding after the procedure. If patient is postpartum and breast-feeding, breast milk should not be used for 2 days after a V/Q scan.

- If a pregnant woman has a nondiagnostic lung scan, **bilateral venous duplex** imaging of the lower extremities is recommended to evaluate for DVT. If DVT is found, PE can be diagnosed. If no DVT is seen, **arteriography** may be performed for further evaluation before a commitment to long-term anticoagulation is made, or venous duplex imaging may be repeated in 1 week.

- According to the Centers for Disease Control and Prevention, in all stages of gestation, a dose of <5 rads (0.05 Gy) represents no measurable noncancer health effects. After 16 weeks' gestation, congenital effects are unlikely below 50 rads. The risk for childhood cancer from prenatal radiation exposure is 0.3% to 1% for 0 to 5 rads. Any of the proposed modalities for diagnosis of PE are well below the dose levels that increase congenital abnormalities. Radiation exposure from a two-view chest radiograph is <0.001 rad. A higher dose of fetal radiation is provided with V/Q scan (0.064 to 0.08 rad) compared with CTA (0.0003 to 0.0131 rad). Pulmonary angiography provides approximately 0.2 to 0.4 rad with the femoral approach and <0.05 rad with the brachial approach. Maternal radiation dose is higher with CTA than V/Q scan.

## Treatment of Venous Thromboembolism

- When VTE is suspected, **anticoagulation** with unfractionated heparin (UFH) or low-molecular-weight heparin (LMWH) should be initiated until the diagnosis is excluded. Neither of these anticoagulants cross the placenta nor are secreted into breast milk; thus, there is no risk for teratogenicity or fetal hemorrhage, although bleeding at the uteroplacental junction is possible. Although UFH has been standard treatment for the prevention and treatment of VTE during pregnancy, recent evidence-based clinical practice guidelines now recommend LMWH. Compression stockings and leg elevation should be used for DVT.

- Weight-adjusted **LMWH** should be used for the treatment of VTE (Table 20-6). Advantages of LMWH include fewer bleeding complications, lower risk of heparin-induced thrombocytopenia (HIT) and osteoporosis, longer plasma half-life, and more predictable dose-response relationships. Theoretical concerns have been raised regarding once daily dosing compared to twice daily dosing (i.e., prophylactic or therapeutic) secondary to the increased renal clearance in pregnancy possibly prolonging trough LMWH levels. However, no comparison data of the two regimens are available. Additionally, recent data suggest daily dosing in the treatment of acute VTE is effective. Monitoring of LMWH levels remains controversial. LMWH cannot be monitored using activated partial thromboplastin time (aPTT), as it will likely be normal. Anti–factor Xa activity levels may be measured 4 hours after subcutaneous injection, with a therapeutic peak goal of 0.6 to 1.0 U/mL (slightly higher if once daily dosing is used); however, frequent monitoring is not typically recommended, except at extremes of body weight. If trough levels are evaluated with therapeutic dosing (i.e., 12 hours after dosing), goal level is 0.2 to 0.4 IU/mL. Current guidelines do not provide definitive monitoring recommendations; however, some researchers advocate checking levels periodically (every 1 to 3 months).
- **UFH** is administered either IV or subcutaneously (SC). IV UFH may be a better initial therapeutic option in unstable patients (e.g., large PE with hypoxia or extensive iliofemoral disease) or patients with significant renal impairment (i.e., creatinine clearance <30 mL/min). The goal of the initial bolus dose (typically 80 U/kg) and subsequent maintenance dosing (typically 18 U/kg/hr) is to achieve a midinterval (6 hours postinjection) therapeutic aPTT (often described as an aPTT ratio of 1.5 to 2.5 times normal). Measuring anti–factor Xa heparin levels may assist in evaluating heparin dosing (target level 0.3 to 0.7 IU/mL). Many facilities have standard protocols for heparin titration. IV treatment should be maintained in the therapeutic range for at least 5 days, and therapy may then be continued with either adjusted-dose SC heparin injections or LMWH. If maintained on UFH, the aPTT should be monitored every 1 to 2 weeks. The aPTT response to heparin in pregnant women is often attenuated secondary to elevated heparin-binding proteins and increased factor VIII and fibrinogen. The therapeutic dose may need to be adjusted. Thus, it may be difficult to achieve target aPTT levels late in pregnancy. The major concerns with UFH use during pregnancy are bleeding, osteopenia, and thrombocytopenia. The risk of major bleeding with UFH is approximately 2%. Bone density reductions have been reported in 30% of patients on heparin for over 1 month. HIT occurs in up to 3% of nonpregnant patients and should be suspected when platelet count decreases to <100,000/μL or <50% of baseline value. Typical onset is between 5 and 10 days after starting heparin. In 25% to 30% of patients who develop HIT, onset occurs rapidly (within 24 hours) after starting heparin and is related to recent exposure to heparin. After obtaining a starting platelet level, ACOG recommends checking platelets again on day 5 and then periodically for the first 2 weeks of therapy. Others suggest platelets be monitored at 24 hours and then every 2 to 3 days for the first 2 weeks or weekly for the first 3 weeks. If HIT is acquired and ongoing anticoagulant therapy is required, danaparoid sodium (factor Xa inhibitor, not currently available in the United States) or argatroban (direct thrombin inhibitor) can be used.
- **Warfarin sodium** crosses the placenta and, therefore, is a potential teratogen and may cause fetal bleeding. Warfarin is likely safe during the first 6 weeks' gestation, but between 6 and 12 weeks' gestation, a risk of skeletal embryopathy exists, consisting of stippled epiphyses and nasal and limb hypoplasia. One third of fetuses

| **TABLE 20-6** | Thromboprophylaxis Regimens in Pregnancy |
| --- | --- |

**Prophylactic**

    LMWH

        Enoxaparin 40 mg SC q 24 hr

        Enoxaparin 30 mg SC q 12 hr[a]

        Dalteparin 5,000 U SC q 24 hr

        Tinzaparin 4,500 U SC q 24 hr

    UFH

        UFH 5,000 U SC q 12 hr

Alternative[b]

        UFH 5,000–7,500 U SC q 12 hr in first trimester

        UFH 7,500–10,000 U SC q 12 hr in second trimester

        UFH 10,000 U SC q 12 hr in third trimester (unless aPTT elevated)

**Intermediate dose**

    LMWH

        Enoxaparin 40 mg SC q 12 hr

        Dalteparin 5,000 U SC q 12 hr

    UFH

        UFH SC q 12 hr; doses adjusted to target peak antifactor Xa levels (4 hr after injection) of 0.1 to 0.3 U/mL

**Treatment (weight-adjusted) dose**

    LMWH

        Enoxaparin 1 mg/kg SC q 12 hr (or enoxaparin 1.5 mg/kg SC q 24 hr[c])

        Dalteparin 200 U/kg SC q 24 hr or 100 U/kg SC q 12 hr

        Tinzaparin 175 U/kg SC q 24 hr

    UFH

        UFH SC q 12 hr; doses adjusted to obtain midinterval (6 hr postinjection) therapeutic aPTT (often a ratio of 1.5–2.5)

**Postpartum anticoagulation (for 4–6 wk)**

    Warfarin with a target INR of 2.0–3.0 with initial UFH or LMWH overlap until INR >2.0 for 2 d

    Prophylactic LMWH or UFH

---

[a]Some experts recommend twice daily dosing of enoxaparin secondary to pharmacokinetic properties of LMWH in pregnancy; however, comparison data are lacking. Additionally, women at the extremes of weight may require different dosing.

[b]From James AH, Brancazio LR, Ortel TL, et al. Thrombosis, thrombophilia, and thromboprophylaxis in pregnancy. *Clin Adv Hem Oncol* 2005;3:187–197.

[c]From Chunilal SD, Bates SM. Venous thromboembolism in pregnancy: diagnosis, management and prevention. *Thromb Haemost* 2009;101:428–438.

LMWH, low-molecular-weight heparin; SC, subcutaneous; UFH, unfractionated heparin; aPTT, activated partial thromboplastin time; INR, international normalized ratio.

Adapted from Bates SM, Greer IA, Pabinger I, et al. Venous thromboembolism, thrombophilia, antithrombotic therapy, and pregnancy: American College of Chest Physicians Evidence-Based Clinical Practice Guidelines, 8th ed. *Chest* 2008;133:844S–886S.

exposed to warfarin late in pregnancy develop central nervous system injuries, hemorrhage, or ophthalmologic abnormalities. Warfarin may be used postpartum and may be given to nursing mothers, as it does not enter breast milk. Antepartum use is indicated for women with mechanical heart valves, for which neither Lovenox nor heparin provide adequate anticoagulation.

- Temporary **inferior vena cava filters** are indicated in women in whom anticoagulants are contraindicated. They may be inserted within a week of elective induction or cesarean section and removed postpartum.

## Prophylaxis for Venous Thromboembolism in Pregnancy

*Antepartum*

- Limited data exist regarding the use of prophylactic anticoagulation for VTE during pregnancy. Women need to be stratified by risk and clinical judgment applied when making recommendations for prophylaxis. Although recommendations vary, women at very high risk for VTE probably benefit from UFH or LMWH throughout pregnancy and postpartum. At a minimum, postpartum prophylaxis is usually recommended in women at elevated risk for VTE.

*At Delivery*

- The risk of maternal hemorrhage may be minimized with carefully planned delivery. If possible, induction of labor or scheduled cesarean section should be considered in women on therapeutic anticoagulation dosing regimens, so therapy may be discontinued at an appropriate time. When used in therapeutic doses, LMWH should be discontinued 24 hours before elective induction of labor or cesarean delivery. Epidural or spinal anesthesia should not be administered within 24 hours of the last therapeutic dose of LMWH. A common approach is to transition from LMWH to UFH at 36 to 38 weeks' gestation. If the patient goes into spontaneous labor and is receiving SC UFH, she should be able to receive regional analgesia if the aPTT is normal. If significantly prolonged, protamine sulfate may be administered at 1 mg/100 U of UFH. If the patient is at very high risk for VTE, IV UFH can be started and then discontinued 4 to 6 hours before expected delivery. When receiving LMWH once daily for prophylaxis, regional anesthesia can be administered 12 hours after the last dose. LMWH should be withheld for at least 2 to 4 hours after the removal of an epidural catheter.

*Postpartum*

- Postpartum anticoagulation may be resumed within 12 hours of cesarean delivery and 4 to 6 hours after vaginal delivery. If at high risk of bleeding postpartum, IV UFH may be chosen initially because its effect dissipates more rapidly and may be reversed with protamine sulfate. Once adequate hemostasis is assured, warfarin can be started by initial overlap with UFH or LMWH until international normalized ratio (INR) is 2.0 for 2 consecutive days, with a target INR of 2.0 to 3.0. Anticoagulation should be administered for at least 6 weeks postpartum for DVT and 4 to 6 months for PE.
- Birth control options for women with a history of VTE or those with high-risk thrombophilias:
  - Due to the thrombogenic potential of estrogen-containing contraceptives, progestin-only or nonhormonal contraceptive methods are recommended. Natural family planning, condoms, progestin-only pills, Levonorgestrel-releasing IUD, copper IUD, or tubal ligation/occlusion are methods that can be discussed with patients at high risk for VTE.

## SUGGESTED READINGS

American College of Obstetricians and Gynecologists. ACOG practice bulletin no. 6: clinical management guidelines for obstetrician-gynecologists: thrombocytopenia in pregnancy. *Int J Gynaecol Obstet* 1999;67(2):117–128.

American College of Obstetricians and Gynecologists. ACOG practice bulletin no. 124: inherited thrombophilias in pregnancy. *Obstet Gynecol* 2013;122(3):706–717.

James A; American College of Obstetricians and Gynecologists Committee on Practice Bulletins—Obstetrics. ACOG practice bulletin no. 123: thromboembolism in pregnancy. American College of Obstetricians and Gynecologists. *Obstet Gynecol* 2011;118(3): 718–729.

James AH. Thromboembolism in pregnancy: recurrence risks, prevention and management. *Curr Opin Obstet Gynecol* 2008;20:550–556.

Marik PE, Plante LA. Venous thromboembolic disease and pregnancy. *N Engl J Med* 2008;359: 2025–2033.

Rogers DT, Molokie R. Sickle cell disease in pregnancy. *Obstet Gynecol Clin North Am* 2010; 37(2): 223–237.

Rosenberg VA, Lockwood CJ. Thromboembolism in pregnancy. *Obstet Gynecol Clin N Am* 2007;34:481–500.

Sukenik-Halevy R, Ellis MH, Fejgin MD. Management of immune thrombocytopenic purpura in pregnancy. *Obstet Gynecol Surv* 2008;63(3):182–188.

# 21 Alloimmunization

Berendena I. M. Vander Tuig and Karin J. Blakemore

**Alloimmunization** in pregnancy refers to maternal antibody formation against fetal red blood cell (RBC) or platelet antigens. Antibody-coated erythrocytes or platelets are destroyed by the fetal immune system, leading to fetal anemia or thrombocytopenia. Antibodies are formed after uncrossmatched transfusion or fetomaternal hemorrhage (FMH), when foreign or fetal blood components enter the maternal circulation. Untreated alloimmunization can cause significant fetal and newborn morbidity and mortality from hemolytic anemia (*hydrops fetalis*) or neonatal alloimmune thrombocytopenia.

## RED CELL ALLOIMMUNIZATION

**Red cell alloimmunization** to clinically significant antigens occurs in approximately 25 of 10,000 births. The most common of these antigens is the Rhesus "D" (or Rh D) antigen. Maternal blood type is usually described as ABO$^+$ or ABO$^-$, signifying the presence (+) or absence (−) of the Rh D antigen. The Rhesus system also includes the antigens C, c, E, and e. Other important red cell antigens are the ABO blood group antigens and more than 50 other minor antigens. Only some of these are associated with red cell alloimmunization (Table 21-1).

| TABLE 21-1 | Blood Group Antibodies and Incidence of Hemolytic Disease of the Newborn |
|---|---|

| Frequency of HDN | Antibody |
|---|---|
| Common | c, K1, E |
| Uncommon | e, C, Ce, $Kp^a$, $Kp^b$, cE, k, s, $Fy^a$ |
| Very rare | S, U, M, $Fy^b$, $Co^a$, $Di^a$, $Di^b$, $Jk^a$, $Jk^b$ |
| No occurrence | $Le^a$, $Le^b$, P1, N |

## Rh D Alloimmunization

*Pathophysiology*

- Prevalence of Rh D blood type varies by ethnicity. Fifteen percent of Caucasians and 8% of African Americans and Hispanic Americans are $Rh^-$. The populations with the highest and lowest $Rh^-$ prevalence respectively are Spanish Basque (30%) and Native Americans (1%).
- Exposing an $Rh^-$ woman to Rh D antigen initiates an immune response that produces anti-D immunoglobulin (Ig) M and IgG and results in memory B cells that produce IgG upon reexposure to the antigen. This process is termed **Rh sensitization**.
- During pregnancy, the RBCs of an $Rh^+$ fetus are targeted by maternal IgG, which can cross the placenta. Fetal anemia develops as $Rh^+$ fetal RBCs are sequestered and hemolyzed.
- The fetal response to anemia includes increased erythropoietin production and hematopoiesis. As hemolysis outpaces production, more immature RBCs appear in the fetal circulation, a condition known as *erythroblastosis fetalis*. Extramedullary hematopoiesis may occur.
- If the anemia is left untreated, hydrops fetalis develops. The pathophysiology is not completely understood but is thought to involve heart failure due to anemia, portal hypertension from extramedullary hematopoiesis in the liver, and reduced hepatic protein synthesis leading to hypoalbuminemia.
- **FMH** with transplacental passage of $Rh^+$ fetal erythrocytes into the maternal circulation is the main cause of Rh sensitization. See Table 21-1 for causes of FMH.
  - An immune response can be generated with as little as 20 μL of blood or possibly even less.
  - FMH is most likely to occur at delivery. Cesarean delivery, multifetal delivery, abruption, bleeding previa, or manual placental delivery may increase the quantity of FMH.
  - Fetal RBC antigens are present by 38 days of gestation, so even first-trimester events such as ectopic pregnancy, spontaneous or elective abortion, or threatened abortion can theoretically cause alloimmunization.
  - Invasive prenatal diagnostic procedures such as chorionic villus sampling, amniocentesis, or fetal blood sampling and external cephalic version can lead to FMH and alloimmunization.
  - Maternal trauma can also cause FMH and alloimmunization.

*Prevention*

- Injectable anti-D Ig (RhoGAM) was developed in the 1960s as a means to prevent Rh D alloimmunization. It is made from pooled sterile human IgG antibodies to the Rh D antigen.
- Before RhoGAM's development, 17% of all Rh⁻ women carrying an Rh⁺ fetus developed antibodies during their first incompatible pregnancy.
- Now, with routine screening and use of RhoGAM, only 0.1% to 0.2% of pregnancies in Rh⁻ mothers are complicated by anti–Rh D antibody production.
- RhoGAM prevents alloimmunization by binding to any fetal RBCs that enter the maternal circulation. The fetal cells are then cleared by the mother's immune system. Maternal B-cell immune response is not initiated, so no memory response develops.
- In the United States, RhoGAM is routinely administered to Rh⁻ women at 28 weeks' estimated gestational age (EGA) and again postpartum if neonatal Rh⁺ status is confirmed.
- The standard RhoGAM dose for routine prophylaxis is 300 μg intramuscularly (IM).
- "Mini-dose" RhoGAM (50 μg) IM is sufficient in the first trimester as the fetus' circulating volume is smaller.
- Ten micrograms of RhoGAM IgG "neutralizes" 1 mL of fetal blood. Therefore, the standard dose protects against up to 30 mL of fetal blood entering the maternal system. After an event likely to cause FMH, quantification of FMH with a Kleihauer-Betke (KB) test guides additional RhoGAM dosing.
- The half-life of RhoGAM is 24 days but it can be detected on maternal antibody screens for up to 12 weeks.

## Management of Rh-Unsensitized Patients

- Pregnant patients are screened for antibodies by indirect Coombs test, in which maternal serum is exposed to Rh⁺ red cells.
  - Lack of agglutination signifies the absence of circulating antibody in maternal serum and suggests unsensitized status (Table 21-2).

| TABLE 21-2 | Indications for RhoGAM Administration in Rh⁻, Unsensitized Women with Negative Antibody Screen |
|---|---|

First-trimester spontaneous or elective abortion
Threatened abortion[a]
Ectopic pregnancy
Amniocentesis, fetal blood sampling, or chorionic villus sampling
Second-trimester or third-trimester bleeding (e.g., placenta previa or abruption)
Abdominal trauma
Intrauterine fetal demise
Routine prophylaxis at approximately 28 weeks' EGA
External cephalic version
Birth of an Rh⁺ infant

[a]Use is recommended in the United States, but evidence is limited. RhoGAM is not given to Rh⁺ or sensitized Rh⁻ women.
EGA, estimated gestational age.

- If the indirect Coombs test is positive (i.e., agglutination occurs), the laboratory must distinguish between sensitization and RhoGAM administration earlier in pregnancy.
- $Rh^-$ pregnant patients should be screened at the first prenatal visit. If unsensitized, no intervention is required at that time. If sensitized, see "Management of Rh-Sensitized Patients."
- The antibody screen may be repeated at **28 weeks** of EGA. If the screen is negative, the standard dose of 300 μg of RhoGAM is administered. If the patient is sensitized, see "Management of Rh-Sensitized Patients."
- **At the time of delivery**, both the patient and infant are screened.
  - If the neonate is $Rh^-$, no RhoGAM is necessary.
  - If the neonate is $Rh^+$ and the mother is antibody negative, the standard dose of RhoGAM is given and a KB test is performed to evaluate the need for additional RhoGAM.
  - If the neonate is $Rh^+$ and the mother is antibody positive, no RhoGAM is given and the mother's next pregnancy is managed as Rh sensitized.
- When in question, RhoGAM is given. The risk of giving RhoGAM to a sensitized person is negligible compared with the consequences of permanent sensitization.

## Management of Rh-Sensitized Patients

- An $Rh^-$ patient with anti-D titer $>1:4$ should be considered sensitized.
  - **Accurate gestational dating** is critical for the interpretation of other tests and the timing of interventions.
  - If paternity is absolutely certain, **paternal blood typing** is performed to determine whether the fetus can inherit the Rh D antigen. Paternal zygosity for *RHD* was previously determined by testing the father for products of the closely linked *RHC/E* gene and calculating the probability of heterozygosity from population data. Although this is still used, now quantitative polymerase chain reaction (PCR) techniques are available.
    - If the father is heterozygous for Rh D, the fetus has a 50% chance of being $Rh^+$.
    - If the father is homozygous for Rh D, the fetus will be $Rh^+$ and is at risk.
    - If the father is $Rh^-$, no further testing is indicated.
    - If paternity is unknown or testing is not possible, the fetus is assumed to be $Rh^+$.
  - Follow **serial maternal D antibody titers** monthly until 24 weeks, then every 2 to 4 weeks.
    - Most Rh-sensitized patients have a chronic low D antibody titer. The fetus is not at risk of anemia until a *critical titer* is reached.
    - The critical titer varies by laboratory but is usually between 1:8 and 1:16. An increase of more than one titer dilution (e.g., 1:2 to 1:8) is also considered concerning. The tests should be performed in the same laboratory.
    - The titer represents the maximum dilution that produces a positive Coombs result. A titer of 1:8 would represent 1 part serum to 8 parts diluent. Note that some labs report titers as the denominator only (i.e., titer of 1:2 is reported as "2").
    - Once maternal antibodies exceed the critical titer, the fetus is at risk for the remainder of the pregnancy regardless of subsequent titer values.
    - In the first affected pregnancy, titers correlate well with fetal status. In subsequent pregnancies, the titer may be less predictive.

- If the critical titer is reached and the paternal genotype is unknown or heterozygous, **fetal antigen status** is determined by amniocentesis or free fetal DNA testing.
  - Amniocentesis
    - Fetal blood genotype is determined from amniocyte by PCR. The false-negative rate is up to 1.5%.
    - Both maternal and paternal blood samples should be sent along with the amniotic fluid.
    - Transplacental amniocentesis should be avoided whenever possible to avoid FMH that can worsen the alloimmunization.
    - If the results suggest that the fetus is Rh$^+$, the maternal sample is checked for the Rh pseudogene. Some people, particularly of African descent, are phenotypically Rh$^-$ but have some portions of the *RHD* gene. If these sequences are passed on to the fetus, amniocyte analysis may falsely identify the fetus as Rh$^+$.
    - If the results suggest that the fetus is Rh$^-$, the paternal sample should be analyzed by PCR. Occasionally, spontaneous gene rearrangement results in a fetus mistakenly labeled as Rh$^-$, when in fact, it did inherit the paternal D antigen.
    - If the results suggest that the fetus is Rh$^-$ and a paternal sample is unavailable, the maternal titer is repeated in 4 to 6 weeks. If it remains stable, the fetus is likely Rh$^-$. A rise in the titer should raise suspicion that the fetus is actually Rh$^+$ and the pregnancy should be managed accordingly.
  - Cell-free fetal DNA
    - Fetal DNA can be found in the maternal circulation as early as 38 days of gestation.
    - Cell-free fetal DNA has already been employed as a diagnostic tool for fetal red cell typing, mostly in Europe.
    - A maternal blood sample is obtained and reverse transcriptase PCR is used to amplify *RHD* exons. These exons would not be found in the blood of an Rh$^-$ mother.
      - If the results suggest that the fetus is Rh D$^+$, the result is considered conclusive.
      - If the exons are not found, the presence of fetal DNA must be confirmed.
      - If gene products of the Y chromosome are found, it is an indicator that the fetus is male and the Rh$^-$ result is conclusive.
      - If Y chromosome products are not found, then single nucleotide polymorphism (SNP) analysis must be performed. If >6 of the 92 analyzed SNPs are found to differ between maternal and presumed fetal DNA, then it is assumed that the fetus is female and the Rh$^-$ result is conclusive.
      - If six or fewer of the analyzed SNPs differ, the result is inconclusive. The test may be repeated in 4 to 6 weeks or amniocentesis may be used to determine fetal antigen status.
- Follow **middle cerebral artery (MCA) Doppler** as a noninvasive alternative to amniocentesis to track fetal anemia. Most centers follow Doppler every 1 to 2 weeks to detect evolving anemia. Doppler testing may begin as early as 16 to 18 weeks' EGA.
  - Blood viscosity is decreased in severe anemia, so the peak systolic velocity of blood in the MCA is increased. Additionally, the anemic fetus preferentially shunts blood to the brain, a phenomenon known as "brain sparing," which may also contribute to increased velocity.

- A peak systolic velocity >1.5 multiples of the median (MoM) suggests clinically significant anemia.
- MCA Doppler testing is 88% sensitive and 87% specific. The positive predictive value is 53%, and the negative predictive value is 98%.
- MCA Doppler must be performed in centers with trained, experienced personnel.
- Reliability of MCA Doppler decreases after 35 weeks and after fetal blood transfusion.

- **Amniocentesis** may also be used to follow fetal anemia. In 1961, Liley demonstrated that amniotic fluid bilirubin levels due to fetal hemolysis are directly proportional to the spectrophotometric absorbance at 450 nm ($\Delta OD450$). This measure correlates well with fetal status. Most centers begin serial amniocentesis at 24 to 26 weeks. $\Delta OD450$ trends are more reliable than a single value, so serial amniocenteses should be plotted.
  - The *Liley curve* has three prognostic zones (Fig. 21-1):
    - Zone 1: The fetus is unaffected or only mildly affected; repeat amniocentesis may be performed, usually in 10 to 14 days.
    - Zone 2: The fetus has mild-to-moderate hemolysis. A value in upper zone 2 (>80%) is an indication for fetal blood sampling. A value in the lower zone (<80%) should prompt repeat testing usually in about 10 to 14 days.
    - Zone 3: The fetus is likely to be anemic. Fetal death is highly probable in 7 to 10 days without intervention. Fetal blood sampling is indicated.

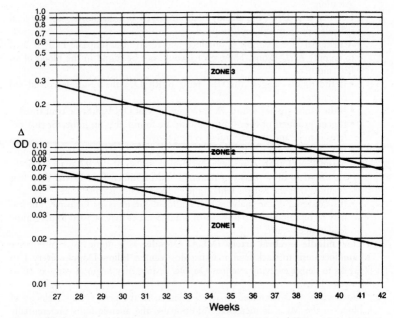

**Figure 21-1.** Liley curve depicting degrees of Rh sensitization. $\Delta OD$, optical density at 450 nm. (From Liley AW. Liquor amnii analysis in management of pregnancy complicated by rhesus sensitization. *Am J Obstet Gynecol* 1961;82:1359–1370.)

○ Exposing the specimen to light or administering maternal corticosteroids will falsely lower the ΔOD450.

○ The *Queenan curve* is an extrapolation of the Liley curve, sometimes used at earlier gestational ages.

• **Fetal blood sampling** via the fetal intrahepatic vein or by cordocentesis (also known as **percutaneous umbilical blood sampling [PUBS]**) allows direct fetal blood sampling. It is performed between 18 and 35 weeks' gestation usually in response to elevated MCA Doppler or concerning ΔOD450 values. Prior to 18 weeks, the anatomic structures of the fetus and umbilical cord are difficult to visualize.

○ If the fetus is found to be anemic at the time of sampling, transfusion of $O^-$ RBCs may be performed. Serial intrauterine transfusions are generally necessary once the fetus is found to be anemic.

○ Fetal blood sampling and fetal intrauterine transfusion should only be performed in a facility with trained personnel and a neonatal intensive care unit capable of caring for the preterm neonate if complications occur.

• **Fetal testing** with serial nonstress tests and/or biophysical profiles may be performed weekly beginning at 28 to 32 weeks' EGA in severe red cell alloimmunization.

• **Delivery** timing is individualized. Per American College of Obstetricians and Gynecologists recommendations, for cases of only mild fetal hemolysis, delivery may be recommended at 37 to 38 weeks or earlier if fetal lung maturity is confirmed. Delivery may be recommended at 32 to 34 weeks in a severely sensitized pregnancy that requires multiple invasive procedures. Alloimmunization alone is not an indication for cesarean section.

• After birth, the neonate may be anemic or jaundiced secondary to **hemolytic disease of the newborn**. Mild cases are treated with red cell transfusion for anemia and phototherapy for hyperbilirubinemia. Intravenous gamma immune globulin (IVIG) or neonatal exchange transfusion may be required for more severe disease.

• **Management of women with a previously affected pregnancy** differs from management of women with their first affected pregnancy. In general, effects of alloimmunization on the fetus or infant become more severe with each subsequent pregnancy.

○ If a patient previously had a significantly affected infant (i.e., hydrops fetalis, need for intrauterine transfusion or neonatal exchange transfusion), titers are less helpful in management, as they may not correlate as well with fetal status.

○ Paternal blood type and fetal antigen status are determined as previously described. If the fetus is $Rh^+$, evaluation for fetal anemia usually begins at 16 to 18 weeks' EGA.

## Other Red Blood Cell Antigens

• Other antigens in the Rh system include **C**, **c**, **E**, and **e**.

  • If the mother is sensitized to any of these, management is generally the same as for Rh D alloimmunization.

• The **Kell** group is the most common minor RBC antigen. At least seven different Kell antigens have been identified. The most common is K.

• Kell alloimmunization more often results from prior maternal transfusion.

• Unlike the other red cell antigens, anti-Kell antibodies cause both hemolysis and suppression of fetal erythropoietin/erythropoiesis.

- Serial titers and ΔOD450 are not helpful; serial MCA Doppler guides clinical management.
- There are many other groups of RBC antigens (Table 21-2). Not all of them cause fetal anemia, and management varies based on the specific antigen.

## PLATELET ALLOIMMUNIZATION

**Neonatal alloimmune thrombocytopenia (NAIT)** is also called fetal alloimmune thrombocytopenia (FAIT) or fetomaternal alloimmune thrombocytopenia (FMAIT). The overall incidence of NAIT is 1 to 2:1,000 deliveries, although this varies by ethnicity. Over 15 platelet antigens have been identified to date, with varying severity of disease. Antibodies to platelet antigen HPA-1a (PLA-1) are implicated in 80% of all NAIT cases and 90% of severe cases.

### Pathophysiology

- The sensitizing process is similar to RBC alloimmunization.
- Antibody-mediated destruction of fetal platelets in the most severe cases can result in fetal intracranial hemorrhage (ICH) or visceral hemorrhage.
- The same alloantigens are found as endothelial cell surface antigens; it is possible that hemorrhage may be exacerbated by immune-mediated damage to the lining of fetal capillaries.
- Maternal antibody transfer can occur as early as the first trimester.
- The fetus of the primary sensitizing pregnancy can develop serious NAIT sequelae.
- Ten percent to 20% of fetuses with NAIT have ICH. Twenty-five percent to 50% of those can be detected in utero by ultrasound. Fetal death in utero occurs in approximately 14% of cases.

### Diagnosis of Neonatal Alloimmune Thrombocytopenia

- **Diagnostic workup** is prompted by clinical suspicion. There is currently no routine screening test for NAIT.
- NAIT evaluation may be initiated for any the following: sonographic detection of in utero fetal hemorrhage, neonatal thrombocytopenia after delivery, or a prior pregnancy affected by NAIT or by fetal hemorrhage. Workup should also be initiated if the mother has a sister whose pregnancy was complicated by NAIT and who is HPA-1a negative.
- The NAIT workup begins with maternal antiplatelet antibody testing. If antigen-specific antibodies are present in maternal blood, then both maternal and paternal platelet genotyping are performed to assess for discordant antigens. Even if antigen-specific antiplatelet antibodies are not present in maternal blood, however, paternal platelet genotype discordance helps to confirm the NAIT diagnosis. Antiplatelet antibodies are not always present or may be only intermittently present.
  - If the paternal genotype is heterozygous for a platelet-specific antigen that the maternal genotype lacks, there is a 50% probability (for each discordant antigen) that the fetus is at risk for NAIT. Platelet genotyping from fetal blood or amniotic fluid should be performed.
  - If the paternal genotype is homozygous for a platelet-specific antigen that the maternal genotype lacks, then all pregnancies are at risk.
  - If the maternal and paternal genotypes are the same, the risk of an affected pregnancy is very low.

- The differential diagnosis for fetal/neonatal thrombocytopenia includes idiopathic thrombocytopenic purpura (ITP). In ITP, maternal platelets are also affected and mothers are thrombocytopenic.

## Management of Neonatal Alloimmune Thrombocytopenia

- **Management** of pregnancies at risk for NAIT varies among centers. There is no consensus on optimal treatment.
- Maternal antibody titers are not useful and do not guide treatment.
- **IVIG** with or without corticosteroids is currently the best noninvasive therapy. **Corticosteroids** are usually reserved for persistent fetal thrombocytopenia despite IVIG treatment. In cases with a history of severe neonatal thrombocytopenia in a previous child, whether or not the child had suffered an ICH, weekly maternal IVIG may be initiated at 12 weeks' EGA and continued throughout the pregnancy.
- **Fetal blood sampling** is the only way to determine fetal platelet count in pregnancies at risk for NAIT. If a patient had a prior pregnancy that was severely affected by NAIT, she can be offered fetal blood sampling at 22 and 28 weeks or later. Antigen-screened platelets can be transfused for severe fetal thrombocytopenia. Cordocentesis or intrahepatic vein (IHV) blood sampling may be used. The IHV site is preferred, as there is a decreased risk of continued bleeding from the sampling site. Furthermore, IHV sampling may avoid the placenta and cause less FMH than cordocentesis, thereby reducing the risk of further sensitization.
  o For possible coincident anemia or acute procedure-related hemorrhage, RBC product is also made available during fetal blood sampling.
  o If fetal thrombocytopenia is severe, weekly transfusions may be required until delivery due to the short half-life of transfused platelets.
  o Fetal sonographic assessment for growth and for any evidence of intrafetal hemorrhage is generally performed.
- **Vaginal delivery** is recommended unless otherwise contraindicated. There is no benefit to cesarean delivery except for the usual obstetric indications. The timing is individualized and is related to fetal status. In severe cases, many centers confirm fetal platelet count before delivery and transfuse as needed prior to induction. At the time of delivery, a complete blood count is obtained on the cord blood.
- After delivery, neonatal platelet counts reach a nadir within the first few days after birth and gradually improve over weeks as maternal antiplatelet antibodies resolve.
- Term infants with platelets <30,000/mL and preterm infants with platelets <50,000/mL are transfused with HPA-compatible platelets ± IVIG.
- Cranial ultrasound is performed to rule out ICH if platelets are <50,000/mL at birth.
- The recurrence rate is high in subsequent pregnancies (85% to 90%). Fetuses may be affected more severely and at an earlier gestational age.

## SUGGESTED READINGS

Aina-Mumuney AJ, Holcroft CJ, Blakemore KJ, et al. Intrahepatic vein for fetal blood sampling: one center's experience. *Am J Obstet Gynecol* 2008;198:387.e1–387.e6.

Althaus J, Blakemore KJ. Fetomaternal alloimmune thrombocytopenia: the questions that still remain. *J Mat Fetal and Neonatal Med* 2007;20(9):633–637.

American College of Obstetricians and Gynecologists. ACOG practice bulletin no. 75: management of alloimmunization. *Obstet Gynecol* 2006;108(2):457–464.

American College of Obstetricians and Gynecologists. ACOG practice bulletin no. 4: prevention of RhD alloimmunization. *Int J Gynaecol Obstet* 1999;66(1):63–70.

Blakemore KJ, Baumgarten A, Schoenfeld-Dimaio MSW, et al. Rise in maternal serum alphafetoprotein concentration after chorionic villus sampling and the possibility of isoimmunization. *Am J Obstet Gynecol* 1986;155(5):988–993.

Bowman, JM. The management of Rh-isoimmunization. *Obstet Gynecol* 1978;52(10):1–16.

Calhoun DA, Christensen RD, Edstrom CS, et al. Postnatal diagnosis and management of alloimmune hemolytic disease of the newborn. UpToDate Web site. http://www.uptodate.com/contents/postnatal-diagnosis-and-management-of-alloimmune-hemolytic-disease-of-the-newborn. Accessed January 4, 2012.

Cunningham FG, Leveno KJ, Bloom SL, et al, eds. Diseases and injuries of the fetus and newborn. In *Williams Obstetrics*, 23rd ed. New York, NY: McGraw-Hill Medical, 2010: 618–625.

Goldsby RA, Kindt TJ, Kuby J, et al. *Immunology*, 5th ed. New York, NY: WH Freeman, 2002.

Moise KJ Jr. Management of pregnancy complicated by Rhesus (Rh) alloimmunization. UpToDate Web site. http://www.uptodate.com/contents/management-of-pregnancy-complicated-by-rhesus-rh-alloimmunization. Accessed November 20, 2012.

Moise KJ Jr. Management of rhesus alloimmunization in pregnancy. *Obstet Gynecol* 2002; 100(3):600–611.

Moise KJ Jr. Overview of Rh(D) alloimmunization in pregnancy. UpToDate Web site. http://www.uptodate.com/contents/overview-of-rhesus-rh-alloimmunization-in-pregnancy. Accessed November 30, 2012.

Moise KJ Jr. Prevention of Rh(D) alloimmunization. UpToDate Web site. http://www.uptodate.com/contents/prevention-of-rh-d-alloimmunization. Accessed January 9, 2013.

Moise KJ Jr, Argoti PS. Management and prevention of red cell alloimmunization in pregnancy. *Obstet Gynecol* 2012;120(5):1132–1139.

Paidas MJ. Prenatal management of neonatal alloimmune thrombocytopenia. UpToDate Web site. http://www.uptodate.com/contents/prenatal-management-of-neonatal-alloimmune-thrombocytopenia. Accessed March 26, 2012.

Peterson JA, McFarland JG, Curtis BR, et al. Neonatal alloimmune thrombocytopenia: pathogenesis, diagnosis and management. *Brit J Haematol* 2013;161(1):3–14

Risson DC, Davies MW, Williams BA. Review of neonatal alloimmune thrombocytopenia. *J Paediatr Child Health* 2012;48(9):816–822.

# 22 Surgical Disease and Trauma in Pregnancy

Emily S. Wu and Nancy A. Hueppchen

## GENERAL CONSIDERATIONS

- One in 500 pregnant women will require nonobstetric surgery.
- The goals for diagnosis and management of surgical disease during pregnancy are to provide definitive treatment and to maintain a successful pregnancy.
- Diagnosis in pregnancy can be difficult due to the physiologic changes of pregnancy; presentation and symptoms may not be typical.
- Always consider and discuss the potential harm to the fetus for any intervention. Similarly, always consider and discuss the potential harm to the mother if intervention is delayed.
- Risks of nonobstetric surgery during pregnancy include preterm labor, preterm delivery, and fetal loss. Overall, there is a 9% risk of preterm delivery with surgery during pregnancy.

### Anatomic and Physiologic Changes in Pregnancy

- The gravid uterus displaces abdominal organs cephalad and brings adnexal structures into the abdomen.
- Uterine compression of the inferior vena cava decreases venous return and may cause supine hypotension syndrome. Whenever possible, the pregnant patient should be placed in the left lateral decubitus position for surgery.
- Increased plasma volume, decreased hematocrit, and generally lower blood pressure make acute blood loss assessment more difficult.
- The hypoalbuminemia of pregnancy predisposes the patient to edema.

### Diagnostic Radiology and the Pregnant Patient

- Pregnancy should not impede the use of necessary imaging studies for critical diagnoses.
- According to consensus statements from multiple professional organizations, the risk of malignancy, miscarriage, or major malformations is negligible in fetuses exposed to 5 rad or less. Potential effects of up to 10 rad are too subtle to be clinically detectable or distinguishable from the background risk. The risk is highest between 8 and 15 weeks' gestation. See Table 22-1 for estimated fetal exposure from common radiologic procedures.
- Iodinated radiographic contrast is rated category B in pregnancy, although it crosses the placenta and poses potential harm to the fetal thyroid, especially at 10 to 12 weeks of gestation. The American College of Obstetricians and Gynecologists recommends avoiding iodinated contrast in pregnancy; in cases where contrast imaging is required, [123]I or technetium 99m (pregnancy category C) should be used in place of [131]I and the newborn should have thyroid function testing in the first week of life.

| TABLE 22-1 | Estimated Conceptus Dose from Common Radiologic Procedures | |
|---|---|---|

| Procedure | Typical Conceptus Dose (rad) | Number of Studies Required to Reach 5 rads |
|---|---|---|
| Cervical spine or extremities x-ray | <0.0001 | >50,000 |
| Chest x-ray (two views) | 0.0002 | 25,000 |
| Abdominal film (single view) | 0.1–0.3 | 17–50 |
| Small bowel study or barium enema | 0.7 | 7 |
| Head CT | 0 | Infinite |
| Chest CT (including PE protocol) | 0.02 | 250 |
| Abdominal CT | 0.4 | 12.5 |
| Abdomen and pelvis CT | 2.5 | 2 |

CT, computed tomography; PE, pulmonary embolism.
Adapted from Wang PI, Chong ST, Kielar AZ, et al. Imaging of pregnant and lactating patients: part 1, evidence-based review and recommendations. *AJR Am J Roentgenol* 2012;198(4):778–784.

- Contrast agents iohexol, iopamidol, iothalamate, ioversol, ioxaglate, and metrizamide do not appear to be teratogenic. In lactating women, it should be safe to continue breast-feeding, but mothers may choose to discard breast milk for 24 hours.
- Gadolinium contrast may be associated with increased risk of pregnancy loss, skeletal abnormalities, and visceral abnormalities. It should be used during pregnancy with extreme caution with full discussion of its risks and benefits.

## SURGICAL DISEASES IN PREGNANCY

- Pregnancy should not preclude any indicated surgery, regardless of trimester.
- Nonurgent surgery is ideally performed in the second trimester. Pelvic surgery during the first trimester carries increased risk of spontaneous abortion from disruption of the corpus luteum. Inadequate operative exposure and risk of preterm delivery complicate third-trimester surgery.
- Elective surgery is generally postponed until after delivery.
- Preoperative and postoperative fetal heart rate monitoring appropriate for gestational age is recommended.
- Intraoperative considerations include the following: positioning in left lateral decubitus, avoiding uterine manipulation, optimizing maternal oxygenation, and avoiding wide variations of blood pressure.
- Intraoperative fetal heart rate monitoring is not routinely recommended but may be appropriate if the fetus is viable, electronic fetal monitoring is physically possible, interventions for fetal indications are available and consent is obtained, and potential interventions for fetal distress will not jeopardize the safety of the planned surgery.

- At standard concentrations, none of the anesthetic agents currently in use have been shown to have a teratogenic effect at any gestational age.
- Current data do not support the routine use of tocolytic agents in the intraoperative setting.

## Acute Appendicitis

- **Acute appendicitis** is the most common surgical complication of pregnancy, occurring in 1/1,700 pregnancies. The incidence of appendicitis is not increased in pregnancy, although appendiceal perforation is more common, particularly in the third trimester. Perforation rates are 43% in pregnancy and only 4% to 19% in nonpregnant patients. This may be related to delayed diagnosis or reluctance to operate on pregnant women.
- **Clinical presentation** includes the following: anorexia, nausea, vomiting, fever, abdominal pain, rebound tenderness, and leukocytosis with bandemia. In the second and third trimesters, the pain is more likely to be diffuse rather than localized to the right lower quadrant.
  - A retrocecal appendix may cause right flank or back pain.
  - Seventy percent of pregnant patients with appendicitis demonstrate rebound, guarding, and referred pain, although these findings are less specific in pregnancy.
  - Some features of appendicitis are similar to normal symptoms of pregnancy, such as leukocytosis and back pain. However, bandemia can be revealing, and careful physical examination can exclude musculoskeletal pain.
- The **differential diagnosis** includes the following: ectopic pregnancy, pyelonephritis, acute cholecystitis, pancreatitis, pulmonary embolism, right lower lobe pneumonia, preeclampsia with liver involvement, pelvic inflammatory disease, preterm labor, abruptio placentae, degenerating myoma, round ligament pain, adnexal torsion, ovarian cyst, and chorioamnionitis. Pyelonephritis is the most common misdiagnosis.
- **Diagnostic evaluation** with ultrasonography is most accurate in the first and second trimesters. In later gestations, positioning the patient in the left lateral decubitus position may assist in identifying the appendix. Magnetic resonance imaging or computed tomography (CT) may be necessary to visualize and evaluate the appendix.
- **Management**
  - Both maternal and perinatal morbidity and mortality are increased for appendicitis in pregnancy. Surgery should not be postponed until the presentation of generalized peritonitis. Treatment is only delayed if the patient is in active labor.
  - For ruptured appendix with active labor, cesarean section may be appropriate. A stable, nonseptic patient with a ruptured appendix in the later stages of labor may have a vaginal delivery.
  - Perioperative antibiotics with a second-generation cephalosporin, extended spectrum penicillin, or triple antibiotic therapy (ampicillin, gentamicin, clindamycin) are administered in all cases and continued postoperatively until 24 to 48 hours afebrile in cases of peritonitis, perforation, or periappendiceal abscess.
  - Laparoscopy may be useful if the diagnosis is uncertain (e.g., with history of pelvic inflammatory disease) and especially in the first trimester. An open laparoscopic entry technique is advisable after 12 to 14 weeks' gestation due to the increased risk of uterine perforation on entering the abdomen.
  - Laparotomy is indicated if suspicion for appendicitis is high, regardless of gestational age. It is also preferred for cases of rupture or generalized peritonitis.

- The role of preoperative or postoperative tocolysis is not well studied and should be used only for standard obstetric indications.
- **Obstetric complications** of appendicitis include preterm labor (10% to 20%), spontaneous abortion, and maternal mortality. For uncomplicated appendicitis, the fetal loss rate is about 5%. Perforated appendicitis increases fetal loss to 20% to 25% and carries a maternal mortality risk of up to 4%.

## Acute Cholecystitis

- **Acute cholecystitis** is common, affecting about 1 in 1,000 pregnant women. The increased gallbladder volume, delayed emptying, and decreased intestinal motility during pregnancy predispose to cholelithiasis. Preexisting gallstones rarely cause acute cholecystitis. However, due to the progesterone-induced decrease in gallbladder contractions, approximately 3% to 10% of pregnant women have asymptomatic cholelithiasis. Cholelithiasis is the main cause of cholecystitis in pregnancy, accounting for more than 90% of cases.
- **Clinical presentation** includes anorexia, nausea, vomiting, fever, and mild leukocytosis, which may also be present at baseline in pregnancy. Symptoms may be localized to the flank, right scapula, or shoulder. Murphy sign is seen less frequently in pregnancy or may be displaced.
- The **differential diagnosis** includes the following: acute fatty liver of pregnancy, abruptio placentae, pancreatitis, acute appendicitis, HELLP syndrome (hemolysis, elevated liver enzymes, and low platelets), peptic ulcer disease, right lower lobe pneumonia, myocardial infarction, and herpes zoster.
- **Diagnostic evaluation** consists of history and physical examination, laboratory tests (leukocyte count, serum amylase, and total bilirubin), and ultrasonography of the right upper quadrant. Magnetic resonance cholangiogram and endoscopic retrograde cholangiopancreatography (ERCP) may be performed in pregnancy.
- **Management**
  - Conservative initial management includes bowel rest, intravenous hydration, analgesia, and fetal monitoring. A short course of indomethacin may be considered to decrease inflammation and relieve pain.
  - Antibiotics are warranted if symptoms persist for 12 to 24 hours or infection develops.
  - Coverage for enteric Gram-negative flora is desired. Typical regimens include piperacillin/tazobactam (Zosyn) or ceftriaxone plus metronidazole.
  - ERCP with sphincterotomy and percutaneous cholecystotomy have been reported for management of more severe cases.
  - Surgical management is required in approximately 25% of cases and is indicated for failure of conservative therapy, recurrence in the same trimester, suspected perforation, sepsis, or peritonitis.
  - Early cholecystectomy, even in uncomplicated cases, decreases the length of hospital stay and the rate of preterm delivery. Some centers proceed to surgery quickly.
  - Although laparoscopic cholecystectomy may be performed in all trimesters, consider scheduling cases in the second trimester if possible.
  - Intraoperative cholangiography may be indicated if gallstone pancreatitis is suspected. It is safe after organogenesis is complete.
- **Complications** of acute cholecystitis in pregnancy include the following: gangrenous cholecystitis, gallbladder perforation, choledocholithiasis, and cholecystoenteric fistulas. Severe complications such as ascending cholangitis and gallstone pancreatitis are associated with 15% maternal mortality and 60% fetal loss.

## Bowel Obstruction

- **Bowel obstruction** during pregnancy is most commonly caused by adhesions (60%) or volvulus (25%).
- Conservative management includes bowel rest, intravenous hydration, and nasogastric suction. Proceed with surgical management if the patient develops an acute abdomen.

## Ovarian Torsion and Ruptured Corpus Luteum

- **Torsion** occurs when an adnexal mass twists on its vascular pedicle. A disproportionate share of these cases occurs in pregnancy (up to one fourth of all torsion cases). Causes of adnexal torsion include corpus luteum cysts, theca lutein cysts, dermoids, other neoplasms, and ovulation induction.
- **Clinical presentation** includes acute pain (usually unilateral) with or without diaphoresis, nausea, and vomiting. An adnexal mass may be palpable.
- **Differential diagnosis** includes acute appendicitis, ectopic pregnancy, degenerating uterine myoma, diverticulitis, small bowel obstruction, pelvic inflammatory disease, and pancreatitis.
- **Diagnostic evaluation** is by history, physical examination, and ultrasonography with Doppler flow to visualize masses, rule out ectopic pregnancy, and observe blood flow to the ovaries.
- **Conservative management** is indicated for ruptured corpus luteum cysts in hemodynamically stable patients. Corpus luteum cysts usually involute by 16 weeks' gestation.
- **Operative management** is indicated for acute abdomen, torsion, or infarction.
  - Cysts that are persistent, larger than 6 cm, or contain solid elements may require surgery. A laparoscopic approach is often used in the management of adnexal masses in pregnancy.
  - If the ovarian corpus luteum is disrupted, progestins can be used up to 10 weeks of pregnancy to prevent miscarriage.
- **Complications** of torsion include adnexal infarction, chemical peritonitis, and preterm labor.

## Breast Mass during Pregnancy

- About 1 in 3,000 pregnant women in the United States is affected by **breast cancer**. Pregnant patients tend to be diagnosed late. The average delay between symptoms and diagnosis is 5 months.
- **Diagnostic evaluation** is similar to that of nonpregnant patient.
  - Mammography, with abdominal shielding, is safe in pregnancy; however, there is a 50% false-negative rate.
  - Breast ultrasonography may differentiate solid and cystic masses without radiation exposure but may also give false-negative results.
  - A clinically suspicious breast mass, even with negative imaging, should be biopsied, regardless of pregnancy status. Fine-needle aspiration and core biopsy are safe in pregnancy.
- **Management** of pregnant patients should avoid external beam radiation and hormonal treatments.
  - Chemotherapy may be used after the first trimester, but the patient should be counseled about risks to the fetus.
  - Methotrexate, tamoxifen, and anthracycline should be avoided during pregnancy.
  - Pregnancy termination should be discussed. However, no survival benefit is shown for first-trimester termination.

## Pregnancy after Bariatric Surgery

- Bariatric surgery is increasingly common among reproductive age women.
- Conception should be delayed for 12 to 24 months after bariatric surgery during the period of most rapid weight loss. In patients who undergo bariatric surgery with a malabsorption component, such as a Roux-en-Y, there is a higher rate of oral contraceptive failure.
- Limited data on pregnancy after bariatric surgery suggest that there is no increase in adverse fetal outcomes. Complications such as gestational diabetes, preeclampsia, and fetal macrosomia may be less common in patients following bariatric surgery than in their obese counterparts but may still occur with greater frequency than the general population.
- Patients who have had gastric banding may need band adjustment during pregnancy.
- Bariatric surgery patients should be appropriately counseled about nutritional goals and risks. Vitamin and mineral deficiencies, including $B_1$, $B_6$, $B_{12}$, folate, vitamin D, iron, and calcium, should be assessed and appropriately treated. In the absence of any deficiencies, blood count, iron, ferritin, calcium, and vitamin D levels can be considered each trimester. Folic acid, $B_{12}$, calcium, vitamin D, and iron supplements are recommended.
- Complications of bariatric surgery, such as anastomotic leak, bowel obstruction, and band erosion, may manifest as nausea, vomiting, and abdominal pain.
- Use of nonsteroidal anti-inflammatory drugs should be avoided.

## TRAUMA IN PREGNANCY

**Trauma** complicates 6% to 7% of all pregnancies and is the leading cause of nonobstetric maternal death during pregnancy, accounting for 40% to 50% of maternal deaths. The leading causes of trauma in pregnancy include motor vehicle accidents (50%), falls (20% to 30%), physical abuse (10% to 20%), gun violence (4%), sexual assault (2%), and thermal injury/burns (1%).

- During the first trimester, the uterus is mostly protected by the bony pelvis.
  - Complications from trauma include preterm labor and delivery, premature rupture of membranes, placental abruption, uterine rupture, fetal–maternal hemorrhage with risk of alloimmunization, direct fetal injury, fetal demise, and maternal bladder rupture.
- Placental abruption is identified in 6% of trauma cases.
- Fetal injury can include skull fractures and intracerebral hemorrhage from blunt pelvic trauma or direct injury from a penetrating wound.
- Fetomaternal hemorrhage occurs in 9% to 30% of trauma cases. Signs include fetal tachycardia, fetal anemia, and fetal demise.
- Due to the risk of fetomaternal hemorrhage, all Rh-negative pregnant women should receive $Rh_o$ (D) immuno globulin, if appropriate, after trauma.

### Trauma Assessment in Pregnancy

- **Assessment of the pregnant trauma patient** is the same as for nonpregnant patients. The mother should be stabilized first, a primary survey conducted, oxygen administered as needed, and intravenous access obtained. Intubation should be performed early, if necessary, to maintain fetal oxygenation and reduce the risk of maternal aspiration.

- **Primary assessment**
  - If the gestational age is >20 weeks, place the patient in the left lateral decubitus position or supine with a wedge under the right hip in order to displace the gravid uterus off the inferior vena cava.
  - Two large-bore intravenous catheters should be placed and crystalloid administered in a volume three times the estimated blood loss.
  - Initiate blood transfusion for estimated blood loss >1 L. Patients may lose up to 1,500 mL of blood before becoming unstable due to the increased blood volume in pregnancy.
  - Avoid vasopressors, if possible, as they depress uteroplacental perfusion. Do not withhold them if they are needed as for cardiogenic or neurogenic shock. See Chapter 3.
- **Secondary assessment** is performed after initial stabilization.
  - Examine the patient's entire body, particularly the abdomen and uterus.
  - Assess fetal well-being and estimate gestational age with ultrasound.
  - Assess fetal heart rate by doptones or continuous monitoring, depending on gestational age, and place a tocodynamometer for uterine contractions.
  - Greater than four contractions per hour during the first 4 hours of monitoring and/or a positive Kleihauer-Betke (KB) test are concerning for abruption. Fewer than four contractions per hour over 4 hours of fetal monitoring and a negative KB are not associated with increased adverse outcomes.
  - Perform a pelvic examination to evaluate for bleeding, ruptured membranes, and cervical change.
- **Diagnostic evaluation**
  - CT scan should be performed if indicated and the patient is stable. It should not be delayed due to pregnancy.
  - Ultrasonography may be used to screen for abdominal injury and to evaluate fetal age and viability. Ultrasound in trauma is 61% to 83% sensitive and 94% to 100% specific in detecting intra-abdominal injury during pregnancy.
  - Diagnostic peritoneal lavage (DPL) is riskier in pregnant patients than in non-pregnant patients but still has a morbidity rate of <1%. Typically, CT and ultrasound are sufficient and DPL is not needed.
  - Laboratory studies include blood type and antibody screen, crossmatch for anticipated needs, complete blood count, KB test, coagulation profile, urinalysis, and toxicology screen including blood alcohol level. Pelvic injuries should be suspected in cases of gross or microscopic hematuria.
  - Cesarean delivery for fetal distress, abruptio placentae, uterine rupture, or unstable pelvic or lumbosacral fracture in labor may be considered if the mother is stable, depending on gestational age, fetal status, and uterine injury.
  - Tocolysis in trauma cases is controversial but not contraindicated. Standard tocolytic agents produce symptoms that can complicate assessments, however, such as tachycardia (betamimetics), hypotension (calcium channel blockers), and altered sensorium (magnesium sulfate).
  - Fetal monitoring protocols after trauma vary among institutions and have not been evaluated rigorously. We typically monitor patients for 2 to 4 hours after any trauma. If contractions are detected, continuous monitoring is extended to 24 hours; injuries that are more serious, significant pain, vaginal bleeding, or nonreassuring fetal monitoring warrant extended observations as well.

## Specific Traumatic Injuries

### Blunt Trauma

- Motor vehicle collision is the most common cause of blunt trauma. Pregnant women should wear seat belts with the lap belt secured as low as possible over the bony pelvis and not across the fundus. The shoulder strap should be placed across the woman's chest.
- Complications include retroperitoneal hemorrhage (more common in the pregnancy from the marked engorgement of pelvic vessels), abruptio placentae, preterm labor, and uterine rupture.
  - Abruptio placentae occurs in up to 38% of major and 3% of minor blunt trauma cases.
  - Uterine rupture occurs in <1% of trauma cases, usually from direct high-energy abdominal impact. It often results in fetal death.
  - Complications are more likely in the presence of pelvic fractures. Pelvic fracture with retroperitoneal hemorrhage in a pregnant woman causes significantly increased blood loss compared to nonpregnant patients.
  - Splenic rupture is the most common cause of intraperitoneal hemorrhage.
  - Direct fetal injury complicates <1% of blunt trauma cases in pregnancy.
- Fetal death is most commonly caused by maternal death and correlates with severity of injury, expulsion from the vehicle, and maternal head injury.

### Penetrating Trauma

- Gunshot and stab wounds are the most common causes of penetrating trauma.
- The health of the mother is of primary concern and takes precedence over the fetus, unless vital signs cannot be maintained in the mother, in which case perimortem cesarean section should be considered.
- Gunshot wounds to the abdomen carry a fetal mortality rate of up to 71%. Evaluation includes thorough examination of all entrance and exit wounds with radiographs or CT to help localize the bullet.
- Stab wounds to the abdomen carry a more favorable prognosis than gunshot wounds to the abdomen and carry a fetal mortality rate of up to 42%. CT may help assess the extent of injuries.
- Exploratory laparotomy is performed for any penetrating trauma to the abdomen. Laparotomy for maternal indications is not considered a reason to perform a cesarean section, unless a fetal indication for cesarean delivery is present or if the gravid uterus prevents appropriate intra-abdominal exploration.
- Tetanus prophylaxis should be considered in eligible candidates.

### Thermal Injuries/Burns

- Both maternal and fetal outcomes after burn injury are related to the extent of burn area, maternal age and health at baseline, and the gestational age of the fetus. As the burn surface area approaches 50%, mortality exceeds 60% to 70%. In general, mortality parallels burn area for term or near-term pregnant patients with extensive thermal injury.

## CARDIOPULMONARY RESUSCITATION IN PREGNANCY

- Fetal survival is improved by restoring maternal circulation.
- Causes of cardiac arrest in pregnant patients include trauma/hemorrhage, pulmonary embolism, amniotic fluid embolism, stroke, maternal cardiac disease, anesthetic complications, and flash pulmonary edema.

- Standard advanced cardiac life support (ACLS) protocols should be followed without modification for pregnancy.
  - Leftward uterine displacement should be used during compressions if it will not compromise the quality of chest compressions.
  - Administer drugs and defibrillation per protocol. Pressors should not be withheld, as fetal outcome depends on successful maternal resuscitation.
  - Intubate early to reduce aspiration risk.
- **Perimortem or emergency cesarean section** is rarely required except in patients with a viable fetus who do not respond to resuscitation. In the latter half of gestation, it can improve maternal resuscitation by increasing venous return and cardiac output.
- **The decision to proceed with postmortem cesarean section** should be made within 4 minutes of cardiac arrest with delivery by 5 minutes for the best outcome. If delivery is delayed more than 10 to 15 minutes, fetal death is likely.
- **Perimortem cesarean** should be performed immediately at the bedside. A sterile field is unnecessary. Generally, a midline vertical skin incision is made with a scalpel and carried down to the uterus. The hysterotomy is also performed by midline vertical incision. After delivery of the fetus and placenta, the uterus is closed using running locked sutures. Continue cardiopulmonary resuscitation throughout the procedure. If maternal survival is possible, start broad-spectrum antibiotics.
  - Infant survival has been reported up to 35 minutes after maternal arrest. Attempt delivery if any signs of fetal life are detected.
  - Delivery does not need to be emergent for maternal brain death unless fetal compromise is present.
  - Careful documentation of the circumstances and indications for the performance of perimortem cesarean is essential.

## SUGGESTED READINGS

American College of Obstetricians and Gynecologists. ACOG committee opinion no. 299: guidelines for diagnostic imaging during pregnancy. *Obstet Gynecol* 2004;104:647–651.

American College of Obstetricians and Gynecologists. ACOG committee opinion no. 474: nonobstetric surgery in pregnancy. *Obstet Gynecol* 2011;117:420–421.

American College of Obstetricians and Gynecologists. ACOG practice bulletin no. 105: bariatric surgery and pregnancy. *Obstet Gynecol* 2009;113:1405–1413.

Brown HL. Trauma in pregnancy. *Obstet Gynecol* 2009;114(1):147–160.

Dietrich CS, Hill CC, Hueman M. Surgical diseases presenting in pregnancy. *Surg Clin N Am* 2008;88:403–419.

Parangi S, Levine D, Henry A, et al. Surgical gastrointestinal disorders during pregnancy. *Am J Surg* 2007;193(2):223–232.

Uzoma A, Keriakos R. Pregnancy management following bariatric surgery. *J Obstet Gynaecol* 2013;33(2):109–141.

Wang PI, Chong ST, Kielar AZ, et al. Imaging of pregnant and lactating patients: part 1, evidence-based review and recommendations. *AJR Am J Roentgenol* 2012;198(4):778–784.

# 23 Postpartum Care and Breast-feeding

Meghan E. Pratts and Shari Lawson

## POSTPARTUM CARE

**Immediate postpartum care** includes monitoring vital signs, managing and relieving pain, and observing for complications. Patients who have had a cesarean section should receive special attention, recognizing that they are postsurgical patients. As the risk of postpartum complications decreases, attention should be turned to education. Important issues to cover include maternal self-care, appropriate sexual and physical activity, breast-feeding, and infant care and nutrition.

### Common Postpartum Complications

- **Postpartum hemorrhage** has various definitions: (a) estimated blood loss of greater than 500 mL for a vaginal delivery or greater than 1,000 mL for a cesarean delivery; (b) a 10% change in hematocrit between admission and the postpartum period; or (c) excessive bleeding that produces symptoms requiring transfusion of packed erythrocytes. Excessive blood loss that occurs within 24 hours of delivery is termed *primary* or *acute* postpartum hemorrhage, whereas bleeding that occurs more than 24 hours after delivery (up to 6 weeks) is termed *secondary* or *late* postpartum hemorrhage. The incidence of postpartum hemorrhage is approximately 4% with vaginal delivery and 6% with cesarean delivery.
- **Postpartum febrile morbidity** is defined as a temperature higher than 38.0°C on at least two occasions at least 4 hours apart after the first 24 hours postpartum. Common causes include breast engorgement, atelectasis, urinary tract infection, endomyometritis, drug reaction (especially with misoprostol use), and wound infection. Less common causes of postpartum fever include **retained products of conception** (especially if bleeding is heavier than normal), **pelvic abscess, infected hematoma, pneumonia** (particularly if the patient received general anesthesia), **ovarian vein thrombosis**, and **septic pelvic thrombophlebitis**. All maternal fevers should be reported to the newborn nursery.
  - **Urinary tract infection** is common in pregnancy and after catheterization; culture should be considered based on clinical examination.
  - **Endomyometritis** complicates 1% to 3% of vaginal deliveries and is up to 10 times more common after cesarean delivery. It presents as fever, uterine fundal tenderness, malaise, or foul-smelling lochia and is usually a polymicrobial infection of Gram-positive aerobes (groups A and B streptococci, enterococci), Gram-negative aerobes (*Escherichia coli*), and anaerobes (*Peptostreptococcus*, *Peptococcus*, *Bacteroides*) from the genital tract. Bacteremia may be present in 10% to 20% of cases. Endomyometritis should be treated with intravenous antibiotics until the patient is clinically improved and afebrile for 24 to 48 hours. The American College of Obstetricians and Gynecologists (ACOG) recommends treatment with gentamicin (1.5 mg/kg every 8 hours) and clindamycin (900 mg

every 8 hours), with the addition of ampicillin (2 g every 4 to 6 hours) if fever persists after initial treatment. Some practitioners simply begin initial therapy with the triple antibiotic regimen. Daily dosing of gentamycin (5 mg/kg every 24 hours) has been shown to be as efficacious and more cost-effective than the low-dose regimen. Further treatment with oral antibiotic therapy is unnecessary once the patient has been afebrile for at least 24 hours and her symptoms have improved. Response to antibiotic treatment is usually prompt. Persistent fever after 48 to 72 hours of antibiotic treatment necessitates further evaluation.

- **Septic pelvic thrombophlebitis (SPT)** is rare and is more frequently associated with cesaren section. It is characterized by high spiking fevers despite appropriate antibiotics. Patients tend to feel well between fevers and have no complaint of pain. Imaging is frequently obtained to look for an abscess, but the pelvic thromboses with SPT are not always seen on computed tomography or magnetic resonance imaging, so the diagnosis is made based on clinical examination and exclusion of other causes. Continuation of intravenous antibiotics and the potential addition of heparin anticoagulation have been suggested for treatment, although this treatment regimen remains controversial.

- **Hypertension** is defined as blood pressure (BP) of 140/90 mm Hg or higher, taken with the patient in a seated position on two or more occasions at least 6 hours apart. Preeclampsia or eclampsia can present postpartum, even in the absence of antenatal complications. Any pressure reading of 140/90 mm Hg or higher should be evaluated by repeating BP measurement, testing urine for protein, and assessing for other signs and symptoms of preeclampsia. In those women who had antenatal preeclampsia, spontaneous postpartum diuresis and normalization of BP are generally expected. Hypertension from preeclampsia can persist for up to 6 weeks, however, and may require further evaluation and treatment.

## Postpartum Immunizations

- **Immunizations/injections** that may be offered postpartum include hepatitis A and B, rubella, rubeola, pertussis, and varicella, all as indicated.
  - **Rh D immunoglobulin:** An unsensitized Rh-negative woman who delivers an Rh-positive infant should receive 300 μg of Rh D immunoglobulin within 72 hours of delivery even if Rh immunoglobulin was given antepartum. If there is laboratory evidence of excessive maternal–fetal hemorrhage, additional doses may be required. The blood bank should perform a rosette test or the Kleihauer-Betke test to assess the amount of maternal–fetal blood mixing and to calculate the additional amount of Rh D immunoglobulin to administer.
  - **Rubella vaccine:** Mothers who are rubella nonimmune should receive the measles-mumps-rubella (MMR) vaccine prior to discharge after delivery. Use of monovalent rubella vaccine (i.e., Rubivax) is generally not appropriate because MMR is more cost-effective and because many women without immunity to rubella also lack immunity to rubeola (measles). Breast-feeding is neither a contraindication to MMR vaccination nor should breast-feeding be discouraged after MMR injection.

## Discharge from Hospital

- When no complications occur, mothers may be discharged 24 to 48 hours after vaginal delivery and 24 to 96 hours after cesaren delivery. The following criteria should be met:
  - Vital signs are stable and within normal limits.
  - Uterine fundus is firm and involuting (within 24 hours, a postpartum uterus without fibroids should decrease to 20-week size).

- The amount and color of lochia are appropriate—red, less than a heavy period, and decreasing.
- Urine output is adequate.
- Perineal pain is adequately controlled with sitz baths, ice packs, and analgesics.
- Any surgical incisions or vaginal repair sites are healing well without signs of infection.
- The mother is able to eat, drink, ambulate, and void without difficulty.
- No medical or psychosocial issues are identified that preclude discharge.
- The mother has demonstrated knowledge of appropriate self-care and care of her infant.
- The issue of contraception has been addressed.
- Appropriate immunizations and Rh D immunoglobulin, if appropriate, have been administered.
- Follow-up care has been arranged for mother and infant.
- Infant nutritional needs have been addressed.

## Outpatient Postpartum Visit

- **The postpartum visit** can be scheduled for 4 to 6 weeks postpartum unless a problem that requires closer follow-up is identified. For example, women with hypertensive complications should have a BP check and brief assessment within 1 week of discharge. For women with a history of postpartum depression or a known mood disorder, closer follow-up is warranted. Immunization status should be reviewed and vaccines that were not given immediately postpartum may be offered. The following are other important elements of routine postpartum visits:

### Physical Exam

- BP, breast, abdomen, and pelvic examination (including vaginal repair assessment)
- At 2 weeks postpartum, the nonmyomatous uterus is usually not palpable abdominally.
- By 6 weeks postpartum, the uterus should return to 1.5 to 2.0 times its nonpregnant size.
- By 6 weeks postpartum, lochia should be essentially absent.
- If lochia is persistent, it should be reevaluated at 10 to 12 weeks. If still bleeding, evaluation is warranted, including measurement of serum human chorionic gonadotropin.

### Sexual Activity and Contraception

- See discussion in "Breast-feeding" section and Chapter 32 for contraception topics.
- When the perineum is healed and bleeding decreased, sexual activity may be safely resumed.
- Any significant dyspareunia should be evaluated.

### Depression Screening

- Assess psychosocial well-being; consider depression screening surveys.
- If there is evidence of depression, antidepressant medication should be considered, and the patient should be referred for mental health care. If you elect to start antidepressant medication, the patient should also be screened for a personal history or a family history of bipolar disorder.
- Thyroid-stimulating hormone level may be determined to evaluate postpartum hypothyroidism.

*Antenatal Complications*

- Patients with preeclampsia should be followed to ensure resolution of symptoms and exclude underlying hypertensive or renal disease.
- Women with gestational diabetes should be screened for diabetes at their postpartum visit due to their increased risk of underlying diabetes outside of pregnancy.

# BREAST-FEEDING

## Recommendations

- The American Academy of Pediatrics advises exclusive breast-feeding for the first 6 months of life and partial breast-feeding (plus complementary foods) for at least 12 months (Table 23-1).

| **TABLE 23-1** | **Benefits of Breast-feeding** |
|---|---|

| **For Newborns** | **For Mothers** |
|---|---|
| - Excellent nutrition matched to needs<br>- Milk content changes with developmental needs (i.e., more protein/minerals after delivery and increased water, fat, and lactose later).<br>- Secretory IgA at high levels in colostrum. Passive immunity passed to infant.<br>- Boosts cellular immunity by promoting phagocytosis by macrophages and leukocytes<br>- Bifidus factor in milk promotes *Lactobacillus bifidus* proliferation, protecting from diarrheal pathogen proliferation.<br>- Decreases the rate and/or severity of bacterial meningitis, bacteremia, diarrhea, respiratory tract infection, necrotizing enterocolitis, otitis media, urinary tract infections, and late-onset sepsis in preterm infants<br>- 21% reduced infant mortality in breast-fed infants in the United States<br>- Breast milk proteins are human specific, thus delaying or reducing some environmental allergies.<br>- May decrease the incidence and severity of eczema | - Supports early bonding between mother and infant<br>- Oxytocin release during milk let-down increases uterine contractions, thereby decreasing postpartum blood loss and facilitating uterine involution.<br>- Decreased lifetime risk of ovarian and premenopausal breast cancer proportional to duration of breast-feeding<br>- Decreased incidence of osteoporosis and postmenopausal hip fracture<br>- Lower cost compared with formula feeding<br>- Facilitates pregnancy spacing due to lactational amenorrhea |

- The World Health Organization recommends continued partial breast-feeding for 2 or more years.
- Breast-feeding should be encouraged as soon as possible after delivery. Infants and mothers who initiate breast-feeding within the first hour after delivery have a higher success rate than those who delay.
- Newborns should be fed every 2 to 3 hours until satiety. Feeding for at least 5 minutes at each breast at each feeding on postpartum day 1 and gradually increasing feeding time over the next few days will allow optimal milk let-down with less nipple soreness.
- Arouse nondemanding infants every 4 hours for feeding. Frequent breast-feeding establishes maternal milk supply, prevents excessive engorgement, and minimizes neonatal jaundice.
- Breast-feeding may be associated with initial minor discomfort. Painful breasts should be assessed and positioning reevaluated. Nursing on the less sore breast first, rotating stress points on nipples, and breaking suction before removing the infant may help. Nipple tenderness can be treated with lanolin cream or all-purpose nipple ointment.
- Breast-feeding increases maternal caloric requirements by 500 to 1,000 kcal/day and increases the risk of deficiencies in magnesium, vitamin $B_6$, folate, calcium, and zinc. Thus, women should be encouraged to continue taking their prenatal multivitamin supplement. Human milk may not provide adequate iron for premature newborns or for infants older than 6 months. These infants, and babies of mothers with iron deficiency, should receive iron supplements. Infants who are breast-fed should also receive vitamin D supplementation because human milk does not provide an adequate supply.
- Women who are not breast-feeding will experience breast engorgement about 3 days postpartum, which is often uncomfortable. Breast binding, ice packs, and avoiding nipple stimulation are recommended.
- Healthy People 2020 goals are 81.9% of all mothers breast-feeding immediately postpartum, 60.6% at 6 months, and 34.1% at 12 months.

### Contraindications to Breast-feeding

- Some structural problems make breast-feeding difficult and sometimes impossible. These include tubular breasts, hypoplastic breast tissue, true inverted nipples (rare), and surgical alterations that sever the milk ducts.
- Contraindications to breast-feeding include the following:
  - Mother actively using drugs of abuse, including excessive alcohol
  - Infant with galactosemia
  - Maternal HIV infection in a developed country. In developing countries, the benefits of breast-feeding may outweigh the small risk of HIV transmission.
  - Maternal active, untreated tuberculosis or women with human T-cell lymphotropic virus type I or II. Women can give their infant expressed breast milk and can breast-feed once their treatment regimen is well established.
  - Active untreated maternal varicella. Once the infant has been given varicella zoster immunoglobulin, expressed milk is allowed if there are no lesions on the breast. Within 5 days of the appearance of the rash, maternal antibodies are produced, making breast milk beneficial for passive immunity.
  - Active herpes simplex lesions on the breast
  - Mothers who are receiving diagnostic or therapeutic radioactive isotopes or have had recent exposure to radioactive materials
  - Mothers receiving antimetabolites or chemotherapeutic agents

*Noncontraindications*

- Healthy term infants with acquired or congenital cytomegalovirus should breast-feed for the benefit of maternal antibodies.
- Babies of mothers with hepatitis A or B may breast-feed as soon as the infant receives appropriate immunoglobulin and the first dose of hepatitis vaccine series. Special attention to avoid broken skin on or around the nipples of mothers with hepatitis B should be advised.
- Mothers with hepatitis C may breast-feed. There is no evidence for hepatitis C transmission via breast milk. Again, advise no breast-feeding if skin on or around nipples is broken.

### Breast-feeding and Maternal Medications

- Nearly all antineoplastic, thyrotoxic, and immunosuppressive medications contraindicate breast-feeding (Table 23-2). In general, breast-feeding can continue during maternal antibiotic therapy. Although all major anticonvulsants are secreted in breast milk, they need not be discontinued unless the infant exhibits excessive sedation (Table 23-3). The Web site of the American Academy of Pediatrics (www.pediatrics.org) contains updated information on medication use in breast-feeding.

### Breast-feeding and Contraception

- Return of fertility: In the non–breast-feeding woman, the average time to first ovulation is 45 days (range 25 to 72 days). The mean time to ovulation is 190 days in women who are breast-feeding exclusively (Fig. 23-1). The **lactational amenorrhea method** is 95% to 99% protective against pregnancy in the first 6 months

| TABLE 23-2 | Medications Contraindicated during Breast-feeding |
|---|---|
| **Medication** | **Reason for Discontinuation** |
| Bromocriptine mesylate | Lactation suppression |
| Cocaine | Cocaine intoxication of the newborn |
| Ergotamine tartrate | Vomiting, diarrhea, convulsions in the newborn |
| Lithium | 10% or more of maternal drug levels found in the newborn |
| Phencyclidine | Potent hallucinogen |
| Radioactive elements | Enter newborn bloodstream |
| Cyclophosphamide | Possible neutropenia and immune suppression in the newborn; unknown effect on growth or association with carcinogenesis |
| Doxorubicin hydrochloride | Same as for cyclophosphamide |

Adapted from Toxicology Network Web site. http://toxnet.nlm.nih.gov/newtoxnet/lactmed.htm. Accessed November 29, 2014; Sachs HC; Committee on Drugs. The transfer of drugs and therapeutics into human breast milk: an update on selected topics. *Pediatrics* 2013;132(3):e796–e809.

| TABLE 23-3 | Common Medications Typically Compatible with Breast-feeding (with No Known Observable Changes in the Nursing Infant When Used) |
|---|---|

- Captopril
- Enalapril
- Hydrochlorothiazide
- Progestins
- Sumatriptan
- Warfarin

Adapted from Toxicology Network Web site. http://toxnet.nlm.nih.gov/newtoxnet/lactmed.htm. Accessed November 29, 2014; Sachs HC; Committee on Drugs. The transfer of drugs and therapeutics into human breast milk: an update on selected topics. *Pediatrics* 2013;132(3):e796–e809.

postpartum if strict criteria are followed. Feedings must be every 4 hours during the day and every 6 hours at night, and supplemental feedings should not exceed 5% to 10%.

- **Contraception during lactation:**
  - **Progestin-only contraceptives** (e.g., mini pill, progestin injectables, progestin implants, and the levonorgestrel intrauterine device) do not affect the quality of and may increase the volume of breast milk. These contraceptives are among the preferred methods of hormonal contraception in the immediate postpartum period. Progestins are detectable in breast milk, but no evidence suggests adverse effects on the infant. The levonorgestrel intrauterine device (Mirena) or the etonogestrel implant (Implanon and Nexplanon) are the progestin-only options with the greatest efficacy; either may be inserted immediately postpartum or at the 6-week postpartum visit without affecting the quality and volume of breast milk.
  - **Nonhormonal methods** of contraception (e.g., condoms, copper intrauterine device, sterilization) will have no impact on milk production and are also among the preferred methods of contraception for lactating mothers.

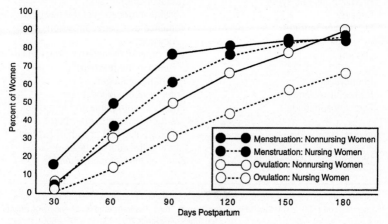

**Figure 23-1.** Postpartum return of menstruation and ovulation.

- The estrogen in **combination estrogen–progestin oral contraceptive pills (OCPs)** can reduce the quantity and duration of breast milk. ACOG recommends that if combination OCPs are preferred, they should not be started before 6 weeks postpartum and should only be started after lactation is well established and the infant's nutritional status is good. Some providers may initiate OCPs earlier if lactation is well established, if the patient declines other forms of contraception, or if the risk of repeat pregnancy is significant. In 2011, the CDC revised its recommendations for combined OCPs postpartum to include that in women without other risk factors for venous thromboembolism, it may be advantageous to begin combined OCPs as early as 21 days postpartum. The WHO recommends waiting at least 6 months before initiating combination OCPs for breastfeeding women worldwide. The U.S. Food and Drug Administration labeling committee recommends not using combination OCPs until the child is completely weaned.

## Mastitis

- **Mastitis** is a breast infection that occurs in 1% to 2% of breast-feeding women, usually between the first and fifth weeks postpartum. It is characterized by a localized sore and reddened, indurated area on the breast and is often accompanied by fever, chills, and malaise.
- Forty percent of mastitis is due to *Staphylococcus aureus* infection. Other common organisms include β-hemolytic streptococci, *E. coli*, and *Haemophilus influenzae*.
- **Treatment** includes continued nursing, nonsteroidal anti-inflammatory pain medication, and antibiotics. Initial antibiotic therapy is often started with dicloxacillin 500 mg orally four times daily for 10 days. Clindamycin 300 mg orally four times per day may be used in patients with an allergy to beta-lactams. Women should continue to express milk, starting on the affected side, to encourage complete emptying. If there is no improvement in 48 hours, antibiotic coverage should be changed to cephalexin or ampicillin with clavulanate (Augmentin). Persistent mastitis, particularly if there is evidence of abscess formation, requires evaluation for the possibility of methicillin-resistant *S. aureus* infection.
- The **differential diagnosis** for mastitis (Table 23-4) includes the following:
  - **Clogged milk ducts:** a tender lump in the breast not accompanied by systemic symptoms that resolves after application of warm compresses and massage.

| TABLE 23-4 | Diagnosis of Postpartum Breast Tenderness | | |
|---|---|---|---|
| **Finding** | **Engorgement** | **Mastitis** | **Plugged Duct** |
| Onset | Gradual | Sudden | Gradual |
| Location | Bilateral | Unilateral | Unilateral |
| Swelling | Generalized | Localized | Localized |
| Pain | Generalized | Intense, localized | Localized |
| Systemic symptoms | Feels well | Feels ill | Feels well |
| Fever | No | Yes | No |

From Beckmann CRB, Ling FW, Barzansky BM, et al. *Obstetrics and Gynecology*, 4th ed. Baltimore, MD: Lippincott Williams and Wilkins, 2002:158, with permission.

Unrelieved, clogged ducts can lead to galactoceles, cysts filled initially with milk that can become a thick cheesy substance that is difficult to drain. Galactoceles may require ultrasound treatment or needle aspiration if conservative methods fail.

- **Breast engorgement while breast-feeding:** bilateral, generalized tenderness of breasts, often occurring 2 to 4 days postpartum and associated with low-grade fevers. May be treated with application of warm compresses followed by hand or pump expression of milk and continued breast-feeding.
- **Inflammatory breast cancer:** a rare disease that presents with breast tenderness and breast skin changes.
- **Breast abscess:** a firm, tender, usually well-circumscribed mass. Breast sonography may be required for diagnosis, and incision and drainage may be necessary for treatment.

## Decreased Milk Supply

- The normal volume of milk produced at the end of the first postpartum week is 550 mL/day. By 2 to 3 weeks, milk production is increased to approximately 800 mL/day. Production peaks at 1.5 to 2.0 L/day. Exclusively breast-fed newborns can be expected to lose 5% to 7% of birth weight in the first week. If the loss is >7% or very rapid, the adequacy of feeding should be assessed. Glycogen stores in full-term infants generally provide sufficient initial nutrition. Therefore, supplemental feeding should be avoided unless medically indicated. Frequent breast-feeding and good maternal nutrition help maintain milk stores. Sheehan syndrome (postpartum pituitary necrosis) can also result in lack of milk production from low prolactin levels. It is characterized by postpartum lethargy, anorexia, weight loss, as well as inability to lactate. See Chapter 13.

## SUGGESTED READINGS

American College of Obstetricians and Gynecologists. ACOG committee opinion no. 361: breastfeeding: maternal and infant aspects. *Obstet Gynecol* 2007;109:279–280.

American College of Obstetricians and Gynecologists. ACOG practice bulletin no. 76: postpartum hemorrhage. *Obstet Gynecol* 2006;108:1039–1047.

Centers for Disease Control and Prevention. Update to CDC's U.S. Medical Eligibility Criteria for Contraceptive Use, 2010: revised recommendations for the use of contraceptive methods during the postpartum period. *MMWR Morb Mortal Wkly Rep* 2011;60:878–873.

French L, Smaill FM. Antibiotic regimens for endometritis after delivery. *Cochrane Database Syst Rev* 2012;(8):CD001067.

Schanler RJ, ed. *Breastfeeding Handbook for Physicians*. Elk Grove Village, IL: American Academy of Pediatrics, 2006.

Truitt ST, Fraser AB, Gallo MF, et al. Combined hormonal versus nonhormonal versus progestin-only contraception in lactation. *Cochrane Database Syst Rev* 2010;(12):CD003988.

# 24 HIV in Pregnancy

Sangini Sheth and Jenell Coleman

The Centers for Disease Control and Prevention (CDC) first reported unusual opportunistic infections in previously healthy gay men in 1981. By 1982, the CDC reported the first case of **AIDS** transmitted from mother to infant. Today, approximately 34 million people are living with **HIV** infection/AIDS worldwide. One half of the infected are women. Over two thirds of infected persons live in sub-Saharan Africa. In 2011, there were an estimated 49,273 new HIV infections in the United States with an incidence of 15.8 per 100,000 people. The number of new HIV diagnoses in women is growing fastest among women of childbearing age. In 2007, the CDC reported HIV as the third leading cause of death in black women from 25 to 44 years of age. Women account for approximately 21% of new HIV infections in the United States annually, and over two thirds are of reproductive age.

With the widespread use of highly active antiretroviral therapy (HAART) in the developed world, people infected with HIV live longer and lead healthier lives. Improved treatment has reduced morbidity, increased survival, and markedly decreased perinatal transmission. Recent data reported a 150% increase in births to HIV-positive women since widespread use of HAART in pregnancy. This chapter summarizes recommendations regarding the care of HIV-infected women during pregnancy; readers are advised that this is a rapidly evolving field and the most current guidelines should be consulted.

## PATHOPHYSIOLOGY OF HIV/AIDS

- HIV is an RNA virus that belongs to the retrovirus (Retroviridae) family and Lentivirus subfamily.
- The most common cause of HIV disease in the United States is HIV-1.
- HIV-2, a related strain, is endemic to Western Africa. It is less virulent than HIV-1 and less transmissible. It has a longer incubation period, is associated with lower viral loads, and progresses to AIDS less often than HIV-1. HIV-2 is primarily seen in the United States in immigrants from West Africa.
- Currently, it is estimated that two thirds to three fourths of new cases of HIV in women in the United States result from heterosexual transmission.
- Without any intervention, maternal-to-child transmission (MTCT) of HIV occurs in 14% to 42% of live births, depending on the setting.
- HIV infection results in progressive depletion of helper T cells.
- The subset of T lymphocytes affected is defined phenotypically by the presence of the CD4 receptor, which is the primary docking protein for HIV.
- Fusion and entry of the virus into the cell are facilitated by coreceptors, including CXCR4 and CCR5.
- Infection results in functional impairment and gradual depletion of CD4 cells, leading to immunodeficiency and subsequent opportunistic infection.

- HIV-RNA level (viral load) reflects active viral replication, and this can be used to track disease progression and therapeutic response. Higher viral loads predict more rapid disease progression.

## COUNSELING AND TESTING

- The American College of Obstetricians and Gynecologists (ACOG) and CDC recommend offering **HIV testing** to all pregnant women:
  - as a routine part of antenatal care, unless the woman declines (opt-out approach).
  - with repeat testing in the third trimester to those in areas with high HIV prevalence, to those known to be at risk, and to those who declined earlier testing.
  - as a rapid screen on presentation to labor and delivery for any pregnant woman of unknown HIV status or any pregnant woman who tested negative in early pregnancy but is at high risk of infection (sexually transmitted infection [STI] diagnosis, illicit drug use, trade of sex for money or drugs, multiple partners, HIV-positive partner, signs/symptoms of HIV, or living in an area with high HIV incidence/prevalence) and was not tested in the third trimester.
- It is important to know individual state law concerning HIV testing in pregnancy, as rules vary widely.
- Studies have shown that the rate of acceptance of HIV testing varies with the approach.
  - When extensive pretest counseling is required and patients must specifically consent to testing (the opt-in approach), testing occurs less frequently. The opt-out approach includes counseling for basic information about HIV, the rationale for testing, the availability of therapeutic and preventive interventions, and recognition of ability to refuse testing.
- Most patients test positive within 1 month of primary infection, however, seroconversion may take up to 6 months.
- The most commonly used HIV screening test is a laboratory serum **enzyme-linked immunosorbent assay (ELISA)**. A positive or indeterminate test is followed by a **Western blot** for confirmation.
- Rapid HIV antibody assays are available and require about 5 to 20 minutes, depending on the test, to obtain a result. Rapid tests use a variety of specimens including blood, plasma, serum or saliva. Many of the simple bedside or office rapid tests are clinical laboratory improvement amendments (CLIA) waived. The sensitivity and specificity of these tests are comparable to the ELISA HIV test. Because the positive predictive value declines with decreasing seroprevalence, a positive result with a rapid HIV test must be confirmed by the Western blot test.
- Appropriate posttest counseling is required. Important issues include:
  - The role of safe sex practices in preventing HIV transmission and limiting other STIs, including superinfection with resistant strains of HIV-1
  - HIV screening of older children who may have been perinatally infected
  - Encouraging substance abuse rehabilitation, if appropriate
  - Encouraging disclosure to sexual partners and health care providers; offer assistance with disclosure and consider issues related to possible domestic violence

## MANAGEMENT OF HIV INFECTION IN PREGNANCY

### Preconception

- Pregnancy intentions and information on effective contraception should be discussed on a routine basis with women of childbearing age. Current data suggest that over 50% of pregnancies in HIV-positive women are unintended. In HIV-positive adolescents, the rate of unintended pregnancy is as high as 83%.

- In pregnancies complicated by HIV disease, the major goals are to optimize maternal health and to reduce the risk of perinatal transmission. Ideally, a treatment plan will be made during preconception counseling that excludes drugs with teratogenic potential. HIV status should be assessed by viral load and CD4 count. Women on antiretroviral therapy should be encouraged to achieve an undetectable HIV-1 RNA viral load prior to conception to decrease the risk of MTCT.
- Women who meet criteria to initiate HAART for maternal viral status should do so prior to pregnancy. Women who do not yet meet HAART criteria are generally not started until after the first trimester. Efavirenz should not be initiated in women who may become pregnant or during the first trimester of pregnancy.
- Appropriate vaccinations to be administered (ideally before conception) include influenza, pneumococcus, hepatitis A, hepatitis B, tetanus. Rubella and varicella vaccine is given prepregnancy if the CD4 count is >200.
- Women should be counseled on the importance of eliminating tobacco, alcohol, and illicit drug use prior to conception.
- Serodiscordant couples that wish to conceive should be referred for expert consultation. Appropriate screening and counseling on safe conception options depending on the gender of the infected partner should be addressed.

## Antepartum

- In the United States, approximately 19% of HIV/AIDS cases are due to injection drug use. Noninjection drug use (e.g., crack cocaine) also contributes to HIV transmission, and illicit drug use has been associated with higher vertical transmission rates. Rehabilitation resources should be provided.
- Screening for domestic violence is important. Approximately two thirds of HIV-positive women have a lifetime or recent history of violence.
- Addressing mental health concerns is paramount. Up to 50% of HIV-positive women experience depression—more than twice as often as HIV-positive men or the general population. HIV-positive women should be screened for depression in pregnancy and managed appropriately. Mental health status can affect medication adherence.
- Variables associated with **increased vertical transmission** include the following:
  - High plasma or genital tract HIV viral load
  - Primary HIV infection or advanced AIDS
  - Low CD4 count
  - Sexually transmitted/genital tract coinfection
  - Placental disruption/abruption, chorioamnionitis
  - Active substance abuse
  - Invasive fetal monitoring or assessment (e.g., fetal scalp sampling, chorionic villus sampling, amniocentesis)
  - Prolonged rupture of membranes
  - Preterm delivery
  - Episiotomy
  - Instrumental delivery
  - Breast-feeding

## Antiretroviral Therapy during Pregnancy

- **All pregnant women should be offered treatment** regardless of CD4 T-cell count or viral load to reduce MTCT (Table 24-1); women should be counseled on the

| TABLE 24-1 | Antiretroviral Therapy and Rates of Perinatal HIV Transmission |
| --- | --- |

| Treatment Category | Vertical Transmission Rate (%) |
| --- | --- |
| Untreated | 20–30 |
| Zidovudine monotherapy | 10 |
| Dual therapy | 4 |
| HAART | 1–2 |

HAART, highly active antiretroviral therapy.

benefits and possible risks of HAART. A combined antiretroviral drug regimen is recommended and adherence must be stressed.
- Initial evaluation should include:
  - History of HIV-related conditions and trend of prior CD4 T-cell counts and HIV viral loads
  - Current CD4 T-cell count and HIV viral load
  - Baseline complete blood cell count and liver function testing
  - Screening for hepatitis C virus and tuberculosis infection
  - Antiretroviral drug resistance studies in all women with HIV-1 RNA viral load levels above the threshold of resistance testing before initiating or changing HAART regimen
  - Appropriate prophylaxis in women at risk for opportunistic infections, as outlined in Table 24-2
- For women who are not on antiretroviral therapy at the beginning of pregnancy, it may be delayed until after the first trimester in women with high CD4 cell count and low HIV viral load. Some evidence has shown that earlier initiation of antiretroviral (ARV) medications may lead to more effective viral suppression and reduce the risk of vertical transmission of HIV.
- Decisions regarding an appropriate regimen should consider:
  - Previous and current ARV treatment and viral resistance. Women who are receiving ARVs for their own health should not discontinue during pregnancy. The current HAART regimen should be continued as long as it is tolerated and effectively leading to viral suppression.
  - Safety and toxicity profiles for specific drugs during pregnancy (considering both mother and fetus)
  - Medical comorbidities that may contraindicate certain medications
  - Patient compliance/adherence to treatment
- Specific drug regimens should be selected in consultation with an HIV specialist.
- To optimally suppress viral replication, minimize the risk of vertical transmission, and minimize the risk of new resistance mutations; strict adherence to the treatment regimen is crucial.
- The use of zidovudine (AZT) alone in the antenatal period is now generally discouraged except in select circumstances including high CD4 count with very low viral load (<1,000), patient refusal of HAART, or patient nonadherence to HAART. Combination therapy should be considered for all pregnant women, regardless of CD4 or HIV viral load.

| TABLE 24-2 | Opportunistic Infection Primary Prophylaxis |

| Opportunistic Infection | Indication | Recommendation |
| --- | --- | --- |
| Pneumocystis jiroveci (formerly called Pneumocystis carinii) pneumonia | CD4 <200 cells/μL | Bactrim DS daily (preferred); dapsone 50 mg bid or 100 mg daily is alternative Aerosol pentamidine 300 mg dose every 4 wk (may be considered in first trimester; may not achieve adequate distribution in lung in later pregnancy) |
| Toxoplasma gondii encephalitis | CD4 <100 | Bactrim DS daily (preferred) OR pyrimethamine 50 mg weekly + dapsone 50 mg daily + leucovorin 25 mg weekly OR dapsone 200 mg + pyrimethamine 75 mg + leucovorin 25 mg all weekly |
| Disseminated Mycobacterium avium complex | CD4 <50 | Azithromycin 1,200 mg weekly OR rifabutin 300 mg by mouth daily (be aware of drug interactions with antiretroviral therapy; rule out active TB) |

Prophylaxis against opportunistic pathogens is indicated at specific CD4 counts, and this treatment should be initiated or maintained in pregnancy. Consult an HIV expert when treatment or secondary prophylaxis/chronic maintenance therapy is needed.

DS, double strength; bid, twice daily; TB, tuberculosis.

Adapted from Kaplan JE, Benson C, Holmes KK, et al; Centers for Disease Control and Prevention; National Institutes of Health; HIV Medicine Association of the Infectious Diseases Society of America. Guidelines for prevention and treatment of opportunistic infections in HIV-infected adults and adolescents. *MMWR Recomm Rep* 2009;58(RR-4);1–207.

- Current **ARV medications** (Tables 24-3 and 24-4) can be divided into five classes:
  - Nucleoside/nucleotide reverse transcriptase inhibitor (NRTI)
  - Nonnucleoside reverse transcriptase inhibitor (NNRTI)
  - Protease inhibitor (PI)
  - Entry inhibitor
  - Integrase inhibitor

## Highly Active Antiretroviral Therapy during Pregnancy

- HAART is the combination of three or four drugs from at least two different classes. It has been shown to dramatically reduce the risk of vertical transmission. Regimens typically include two NRTIs plus a booster PI or an NNRTI for pregnant women who have never received ARV medications (ARV-naïve).

*Nucleoside/Nucleotide Reverse Transcriptase Inhibitors*

- Most extensively studied HIV medication in pregnancy. The preferred NRTI combination among ARV-naïve women is zidovudine and lamivudine based on extensive safe clinical experience in pregnancy and efficacy studies in preventing perinatal transmission.

**TABLE 24-3** Preclinical and Clinical Data on Antiretrovirals in Pregnancy

| Antiretroviral Drug | FDA Pregnancy Category | Placenta Passage | Long-Term Animal Carcinogenicity Studies | Animal Teratogenicity Studies |
|---|---|---|---|---|
| **Nucleoside and nucleotide analogue reverse transcriptase inhibitors** | | | | |
| Abacavir (Ziagen, ABC) | C | Yes (rats) | Positive (malignant and nonmalignant tumors of the liver, thyroid, preputial, and clitoral glands) | Positive (fetal ana-sarca and skeletal malformations) |
| Didanosine (Videx, ddl) | B | Yes (human) | Negative | Negative |
| Emtricitabine, (Emtriva, FTC) | B | Yes (mice and rabbits) | Negative | Negative |
| Lamivudine (Epivir, 3TC) | C | Yes (human) | Negative | Negative |
| Stavudine (Zerit, d4T) | C | Yes (rhesus monkey) | Positive (liver and bladder tumors) | Negative |
| Tenofovir (Viread) | B | Yes (human) | Positive (hepatic adenomas) | Negative |
| Zalcitabine (HIVID, ddC) | C | Yes (rhesus monkey) | Positive (thymic lymphoma) | Positive (hydrocephalus) |
| Zidovudine (AZT) | C | Yes (human) | Positive (noninvasive vaginal epithelial tumors) | Positive (and fetal resorption) |
| **Nonnucleoside reverse transcriptase inhibitors** | | | | |
| Delavirdine (Rescriptor) | C | Unknown | Positive (hepatocellular adenomas, carcinomas) | Positive (VSD) |
| Efavirenz (Sustiva) | D | Yes (monkey, rat, rabbit) | Positive (hepatocellular adeno-mas, carcinomas, pulmonary alveolar/bronchiolar adeno-mas in females) | Positive (anencephaly, anophthalmia, microphthalmia) |

| | | | | |
|---|---|---|---|---|
| Nevirapine (Viramune) | B | Yes (human) | Positive (hepatocellular adenomas and carcinomas) | Negative |
| **Protease inhibitors** | | | | |
| Amprenavir (Agenerase) | C | Minimal/variable (human) | Positive (hepatocellular adenomas and carcinomas) | Negative (but deficient ossification and thymic elongation) |
| Atazanavir | B | Minimal/variable (human) | Positive (hepatocellular adenomas) | Negative |
| Darunavir (Prezista) | B | Unknown | Not completed | Negative |
| Fosamprenavir (Lexiva) | C | Unknown | Positive (benign and malignant liver tumors) | Negative (deficient ossification with amprenavir) |
| Indinavir (Crixivan) | C | Minimal (human) | Positive (thyroid adenomas and carcinomas) | Negative (but extra ribs) |
| Lopinavir/ritonavir (Kaletra) | C | Yes (human) | Minimal/variable (human) | Positive (hepatocellular adenomas and carcinomas) |
| Nelfinavir (Viracept) | B | Minimal/variable (human) | Positive (thyroid follicular adenomas and carcinomas) | Negative |
| Ritonavir (Norvir) | B | Minimal (human) | Positive (liver adenomas and carcinomas) | Negative (but cryptorchidism) |
| Saquinavir (Fortovase) | B | Minimal (human) | Negative | Negative |
| Tipranavir (Aptivus) | C | Unknown | In progress | Negative (decreased ossification and weights) |

*(Continued)*

**TABLE 24-3** Preclinical and Clinical Data on Antiretrovirals in Pregnancy *(Continued)*

| Antiretroviral Drug | FDA Pregnancy Category | Placenta Passage | Long-Term Animal Carcinogenicity Studies | Animal Teratogenicity Studies |
|---|---|---|---|---|
| **Entry inhibitor** | | | | |
| Enfuvirtide (Fuzeon) | B | Unknown | Not done | Negative |
| Maraviroc (Selzentry) | B | Unknown | In progress | Negative |
| **Integrase inhibitors** | | | | |
| Raltegravir (Isentress) | C | Yes (rats) | In progress | Negative (extranumerary ribs) |

FDA, U. S. Food and Drug Administration; VSD, ventricular septal defect.
Adapted from Benson CA, Kaplan JE, Masur H, et al; Centers for Disease Control and Prevention; National Institutes of Health; HIV Medicine Association of the Infectious Diseases Society of America. Treating opportunistic infections among HIV-infected adults and adolescents. *MMWR Recomm Rep* 2004;53(RR-15);1–112.

- Pregnancy does not alter the pharmacokinetic profile.
- Maternal/fetal safety considerations:
  - **Lactic acidosis/hepatic steatosis** is a life-threatening complication related to mitochondrial toxicity. Associated with long-term use of NRTIs, particularly in combination of didanosine/stavudine.
    - Clinical manifestations include malaise, weakness, nausea/vomiting, abdominal pain, liver function abnormalities. Can proceed to multiorgan failure. May be confused with pregnancy complications such as HELLP syndrome or acute fatty liver of pregnancy.
    - Monitor liver function tests and electrolytes monthly in last trimester. Evaluate new symptoms thoroughly. Check lactic acid levels with concerning clinical picture, not routinely.
  - **Mitochondrial toxicity** in NRTI-exposed infant can be associated rarely with neurologic defects.
  - **Anemia** is most associated with zidovudine. Monitor hemoglobin/hematocrit and supplement iron and folate.
    - The increased mean corpuscular volume typical of zidovudine use does not indicate folate or $B_{12}$ deficiency.

*Protease Inhibitors*

- Most PIs are now used with low-dose ritonavir "boost" to achieve a better pharmacokinetic profile. Lopinavir and atazanavir are the preferred PIs in ARV-naïve women.
- Minimal transplacental passage.
- Drug–drug interactions are common. Consult drug interaction tables for patients on any other medications.
- Pharmacokinetic studies suggest lower blood levels of some PIs in pregnancy with standard dosing.
- Maternal/fetal safety considerations:
  - **Hyperglycemia/diabetes** is an increased risk in general population taking PIs but this group does not have an increased risk in gestational diabetes. Standard glucose screening recommended at 24 to 28 weeks. Consider earlier screening in women with:
    - PI-based antiretroviral therapy started before pregnancy or with other risk factors for glucose intolerance.
  - Preterm delivery: There is conflicting data on the risk of preterm birth with combination antiretroviral therapy, particularly PIs. Recent meta-analysis of 14 clinical studies in the United States and Europe found no increase in preterm delivery in treated recipients compared to no therapy.

*Nonnucleoside Reverse Transcriptase Inhibitors*

- Nevirapine (NVP) and efavirenz (EFV), the commonly used NNRTIs, have long half-lives.
  - If a combination regimen NNRTI is stopped, there will be a period of functional monotherapy as the other drugs are metabolized and excreted while NNRTI levels persist. Significant NVP levels have been found up to 3 weeks after a single dose of NVP. This increases risk for NNRTI resistance.
  - If an NNRTI regimen is used during pregnancy with a plan to discontinue after delivery, an NRTI "tail" should be prescribed for approximately 7 days after the final NNRTI dose to reduce resistance risk. Another option is to switch the NNRTI to a PI 3 to 4 weeks before delivery, although this is less studied.

- Maternal/fetal safety considerations:
  - NVP (Viramune) is associated with 12-fold increased risk of symptomatic **hepatotoxicity** when started in women with CD4 counts >250/μL.
  - Death from fulminant hepatic failure has been reported.
    - Most cases occur within the first 18 weeks of therapy; onset can be abrupt. Women who become pregnant while on NVP-containing regimens and have immune reconstitution with higher CD4 counts are at lower risk. NVP naïve women with CD4 counts >250/μL should not be started on NVP as part of combination therapy unless benefit clearly outweighs risk.
    - When NVP multidrug therapy is initiated, close clinical and laboratory monitoring is advised.
    - Hepatotoxicity has not been reported with single-dose NVP for peripartum prophylaxis.
  - NVP carries risk for drug rash as high as 17%. Severe hypersensitivity and Stevens-Johnson syndrome have been reported. Two-week introduction dosing of 200 mg NVP daily, increasing to 200 mg twice daily may be helpful.
- EFV (Sustiva) is pregnancy category D.
  - Serious teratogenic effects in primates and neural tube defects in humans with early in utero exposure are reported.
  - EFV should be avoided in sexually active HIV-positive women who are not using effective consistent contraception.
  - EFV should also be avoided in pregnancy, particularly in the first trimester.
  - However, if a woman is on EFV when she conceives, she does not need to discontinue it during the first trimester, as long as EFV is part of a regimen providing effective virologic suppression.

*Entry Inhibitors, Integrase Inhibitors*
- There is little data on the use of these newer drugs in pregnancy.

## Intrapartum
- Combination HAART regimen should be continued intrapartum.
- **Intravenous (IV) zidovudine** should be administered to women with an HIV viral load >400 copies/mL or unknown viral load near delivery regardless of antepartum regimen or mode of delivery. For women on an antepartum regimen that includes oral zidovudine, the oral zidovudine should be stopped while they receive the IV infusion.
- Women on HAART and with HIV viral load <400 copies/mL near delivery do not require IV zidovudine; their HAART regimen should be continued during labor and delivery regardless of mode of delivery.
- A scheduled cesarean section at 38 weeks is recommended for women with an HIV viral load >1,000 copies/mL near delivery. When C-section is planned, IV zidovudine should be administered for at least 3 hours prior to C-section to ensure therapeutic blood levels (1-hour IV loading dose followed by continuous IV dose for 2 hours) to minimize risk of vertical transmission.
- IV zidovudine should be started immediately in women presenting in labor with a positive rapid HIV test; CD4 T lymphocyte and HIV-1 RNA viral load should accompany confirmatory HIV antibody testing in the postpartum period.
- Single-dose NVP has not been shown to decrease transmission further in women on combination antiretroviral therapy.

**TABLE 24-4** Pharmacokinetics and Toxicity of Antiretroviral Drugs and Recommendations for Use in Pregnancy

| | ARV (Abbreviation), Trade Name | Pharmacokinetics in Pregnancy | Concerns in Pregnancy | Rationale for Use in Pregnancy |
|---|---|---|---|---|
| | **NRTI-recommended agents** | | | |
| **Preferred Agents** | **Zidovudine** (AZT, ZDV), Retrovir | Not significantly altered in pregnancy, no change in dose indicated | No evidence for human teratogenicity. Well-tolerated short-term safety demonstrated. | Preferred NRTI for use in combination therapy |
| | **Lamivudine** (3TC), Epivir | Not significantly altered in pregnancy, no change in dose indicated | No evidence for human teratogenicity. Well-tolerated short-term safety demonstrated. | Because of extensive experience with lamivudine in pregnancy in combination with zidovudine, lamivudine plus zidovudine is the recommended dual NRTI backbone. |
| **Alternative Agents** | **Abacavir** (ABC), Ziagen | Not significantly altered in pregnancy, no change in dose indicated | No evidence for human teratogenicity. Hypersensitivity reaction in 5%–8% nonpregnant patients. HLA-B*5701 testing should be conducted and negative prior to initiation. | Alternative NRTI for dual NRTI backbone |

*(Continued)*

**TABLE 24-4** Pharmacokinetics and Toxicity of Antiretroviral Drugs and Recommendations for Use in Pregnancy *(Continued)*

| ARV (Abbreviation), Trade Name | Pharmacokinetics in Pregnancy | Concerns in Pregnancy | Rationale for Use in Pregnancy |
|---|---|---|---|
| **Emtricitabine** (FTC), Emtriva | Slightly lower levels in third trimester; no need to increase dose | Risk of renal toxicity—monitor renal function. No evidence for human teratogenicity. Clinical studies show bone demineralization with chronic use (significance unknown). | Alternative NRTI for dual NRTI backbone |
| **Tenofovir** (TDF), Viread | AUC lower in third trimester but trough levels adequate. | | Alternative NRTI for dual NRTI backbone. Preferred in combination with 3TC or FTC in women with chronic HBV. |
| **Use in Special Circumstances** | | | |
| **Didanosine** (ddI), Videx EC | Not significantly altered in pregnancy, no change in dose indicated | Increased risk of birth defects compared to general population after first trimester and later exposure—clinical relevance uncertain | Need to administer on empty stomach and potential toxicity—only use in circumstances where preferred and alternative NRTIs cannot be used. |
| | | Lactic acidosis, potentially fatal, noted in pregnant women taking ddI and d4T together | Do not use with d4T. |

| | | |
|---|---|---|
| **Stavudine** (d4T), Zerit | Not significantly altered in pregnancy, no change in dose indicated | No evidence for human teratogenicity. Lactic acidosis, potentially fatal, noted in pregnant women taking ddI and d4T together. | Only use in circumstances where preferred and alternative NRTIs cannot be used. Do not use with ddI or ZDV. |
| **Zalcitabine** (ddC), HIVID | Not recommended | | |
| **NNRTIs** | | | |
| **Nevirapine** (NVP), Viramune | Not significantly altered in pregnancy, no change in dose indicated | No evidence for human teratogenicity. Increased risk of symptomatic liver toxicity (often rash-associated and potentially fatal) among women with CD4 counts >250/μL when first starting treatment. | Nevirapine should be initiated in pregnant women with CD4 >250/mm$^3$ only if benefits outweigh risks. |
| **Preferred Agents** | | | |

*(Continued)*

**TABLE 24-4** Pharmacokinetics and Toxicity of Antiretroviral Drugs and Recommendations for Use in Pregnancy (Continued)

| | ARV (Abbreviation), Trade Name | Pharmacokinetics in Pregnancy | Concerns in Pregnancy | Rationale for Use in Pregnancy |
|---|---|---|---|---|
| Use in Special Circumstances | **Efavirenz** (EFV), Sustiva | AUC decreased in third trimester but target exposure generally exceeded and no dose is change recommended. | FDA pregnancy class D; anencephaly, anophthalmia, cleft palate noted in primate studies of first trimester use | EFV should not be used in women planning to become pregnant or those that are sexually active and not using effective contraception; alternative regimens should be considered. EFV may be continued in women presenting for antenatal care in first trimester if they have virologic suppression on EFV. |
| Insufficient Data | **Etravirine** (ETR), Intelence | | | |
| | **Rilpivirine** (RPV), Endurant | | | |
| | **Protease Inhibitors** | | | |

| Preferred Agents | | | |
|---|---|---|---|
| **Atazanavir** (ATV), Reyataz | Standard dosing in pregnancy may result in decreased plasma concentrations. Some experts recommend increased dosing in second and third trimesters for all pregnant women; ATV package recommends increase dose with TDF or H2 receptor blocker. | No evidence for human teratogenicity | Preferred PI to use in combination ARV regimens. Should combine with low-dose RTV boosting. |
| **Lopinavir/Ritonavir** (LPV/r), Kaletra | Consider increasing dose from two tablets twice daily to three tablets twice daily during the third trimester, with return to standard dosing postpartum. Data from older capsule formulation suggest lower blood levels with standard dosing in third trimester. Once daily LPV/r dosing is not recommended in pregnancy. | No evidence for human teratogenicity. Well-tolerated short-term safety demonstrated. | Pharmacokinetic studies of new tablet formation are underway but insufficient data to make a definitive recommendation regarding dosing in pregnancy. |
| **Ritonavir** (RTV), Norvir | Lower levels in pregnancy. | No evidence for human teratogenicity. Limited experience with full dose and should only be used as low-dose boost. | Should be used as low-dose RTV "boost" in combination with second PI |

*(Continued)*

**TABLE 24-4** Pharmacokinetics and Toxicity of Antiretroviral Drugs and Recommendations for Use in Pregnancy *(Continued)*

| | ARV (Abbreviation), Trade Name | Pharmacokinetics in Pregnancy | Concerns in Pregnancy | Rationale for Use in Pregnancy |
|---|---|---|---|---|
| **Alternative Agents** | **Darunavir** (DRV), Prezista (must combine with low-dose RTV boosting) | PK data in pregnancy limited. | Safety data in pregnancy limited in humans. | Use when preferred or other alternative agents cannot be used. Combined with low-dose RTV boost. |
| | **Saquinavir** (SQV), Invirase (must combine with low-dose RTV boosting) | Limited data suggest 1,000 mg SQV capsules/100 mg RTV twice daily results in sufficient drug levels in pregnant women. | Safety data in pregnancy limited in humans. Well-tolerated, short-term safety demonstrated. | Must combine with low-dose RTV boost. Baseline ECG needed due to risk of PR and/or QT prolongation; contra-indicated in those with preexisting cardiac conduction system abnormalities. |
| **Use in Special Circumstances** | **Indinavir** (IDV), Crixivan (must combine with low-dose RTV boosting) | Insufficient levels without RTV boost. | No evidence for human teratogenicity. | Only use when preferred and alternative regimen options are not available due to pill burden, twice daily dosing, and risk of renal stones. Must combine with low-dose RTV boost. |

| | | | |
|---|---|---|---|
| | | Levels variable in late pregnancy at 1,250 mg bid dosing (do not use 750 mg tid dosing in pregnancy) | Consider use in women not otherwise requiring therapy in whom other regimens are not available. |
| | | No evidence for human teratogenicity. Well-tolerated, short-term safety demonstrated. | |
| **Insufficient Data** | **Fosamprenavir** (FPV), Lexiva | | |
| | **Tipranavir** (TPV), Aptivus | | |
| | *Insufficient data to recommend entry inhibitors and integrase inhibitors* | | |

ARV, antiretroviral; NRTI, nucleotide reverse transcriptase inhibitor; AUC, area under the curve; HBV, hepatitis B virus; NNRTI, nonnucleoside reverse transcriptase inhibitor; FDA, U.S. Food and Drug Administration; PI, protease inhibitor; PK, pharmacokinetics; ECG, electrocardiogram; bid, twice a day; tid, three times a day.
Adapted from Panel on Treatment of HIV-Infected Pregnant Women and Prevention of Perinatal Transmission. Recommendations for use of antiretroviral drugs in pregnant HIV-1-infected women for maternal health and interventions to reduce perinatal HIV transmission in the United States, Table 5 (pp. 14–29). http://aidsinfo.nih.gov/contentfiles/lvguidelines/PerinatalGL.pdf. Accessed April 6, 2013.

## Postpartum

- Continuation of ARV treatment in the postpartum period is dependent on a number of factors as listed below and is a decision that should involve the patient and her primary HIV care provider.
  - CD4 count: Randomized control data demonstrates a benefit in treatment for those women with a CD4 count <500 cells/mm$^3$. There is growing data that there may be clinical benefit in treating patients with CD4 cell counts >500 cells/mm$^3$. A multicenter trial (PROMISE study) investigating the risks and benefits of discontinuing combination ARV regimens in postpartum women with high CD4 cell count is underway.
  - Patient preference
  - Partner HIV status
  - Compliance and risk of viral resistance with suboptimal adherence
  - Drug toxicity
  - Cost
- Infants should receive zidovudine starting 6 to 12 hours after birth and continuing for 6 weeks. Infants born to women who did not receive antepartum ARV medication (and with or without intrapartum maternal prophylaxis) should receive zidovudine for 6 weeks plus three doses of NVP in the first week of life—at birth, 48 hours later, 96 hours after the second dose. No studies are available to determine whether additional ARVs are beneficial for those infants delivered by cesarean section to mothers who received antenatal ARV treatment but had high viral loads (HIV RNA >1,000 copies/mL) near delivery. Among infants of women with high viral loads near delivery who deliver vaginally, zidovudine combined with NVP should be administered. If the mother's HIV status is unknown at the time of delivery, immediate rapid HIV antibody testing of mother or baby is recommended and the infant should receive zidovudine and NVP prophylaxis if the rapid test is positive.

## Perinatal HIV Transmission: Mode of Delivery

- **Evidence does NOT support cesarean delivery for patients on combination therapy with viral load <1,000 copies/mL.**
- Evidence is mixed regarding C-section in patients with viral load >1,000 copies/mL who present in labor or with ruptured membranes. Mode of delivery should be selected based on duration of rupture, labor progress, HIV viral load, current antiretroviral therapy, and other clinical factors. Augmentation to shorten the time to vaginal delivery may be considered for some patients.
- HIV-infected women have higher **complication rates** (mostly infectious) from scheduled cesarean deliveries than from vaginal deliveries but less than those associated with urgent or emergent C-sections. They also have more complications than uninfected women after cesarean delivery, particularly with lower CD4 counts. The complications with cesarean section are not of sufficient frequency or severity to outweigh the potential benefit for women with increased risk of vertical transmission.
- More studies are needed to determine the optimal management of preterm premature rupture of membrane with HIV infection and for patients with newly diagnosed HIV in labor (Table 24-5).
- Early data indicated that transmission risk increased with low maternal CD4 counts and rupture of membrane for longer than 4 hours. However, more recent data have found that duration of membrane rupture does not increase MTCT if the patient is taking HAART, has a low viral load, and receives zidovudine intrapartum.

**TABLE 24-5** Treatment Recommendations Based on Clinical Scenario in the United States

| Clinical Scenario | Testing | Treatment |
|---|---|---|
| HIV-infected pregnant woman on HAART | If detectable viremia, resistance testing | • Continue current regimen if successfully suppressing viremia<br>• Continuous infusion of zidovudine intrapartum to women with HIV viral load >400 copies/mL (or unknown) near delivery and continue HAART during labor (hold oral zidovudine if part of antepartum regimen and VL >400 copies/mL while receiving intravenous ZDV infusion)<br>• Zidovudine for 6 wk postpartum for infant<br>• Assess need for continuing HAART after delivery; recommendations for continuing postpartum HAART are the same as in nonpregnant patients. |
| HIV-infected pregnant woman who are ARV naïve | Resistance testing prior to therapy and once on therapy if suboptimal viral suppression (<1 log drop after 4 wk of ARVs) | • Initiate HAART (avoid EFV in first trimester)<br>• Delayed initiation may be considered in women with high CD4 counts and low viral load; earlier initiation may lead to better viral suppression. Risk of potential fetal effects should be weighed against benefits of antiretrovirals in the first trimester<br>• Use one or more NRTIs with good placental passage (ZDV, 3TC, ABC, TFV, FTC) in regimen if feasible<br>• Use NVP in ARV regimen only if CD4 count <250 cells/mm$^3$<br>• Continuous infusion of zidovudine intrapartum to women with HIV viral load >400 copies/mL (or unknown) near delivery and continue HAART during labor (hold oral zidovudine if part of antepartum regimen and VL >400 copies/mL while receiving intravenous ZDV infusion)<br>• Zidovudine for 6 wk postpartum for infant<br>• Assess need for continuing HAART after delivery; recommendations for continuing postpartum HAART are the same as in nonpregnant patients. |

*(Continued)*

**TABLE 24-5** Treatment Recommendations Based on Clinical Scenario in the United States *(Continued)*

| Clinical Scenario | Testing | Treatment |
|---|---|---|
| HIV-infected pregnant women who are ARV experienced but not currently receiving ARVs | Full antiretroviral history, resistance testing prior to initiating ARV and if suboptimal response on treatment | • Initiate HAART based on resistance testing and history.<br>• Delayed initiation may be considered in women with high CD4 counts and low viral load; earlier initiation may lead to better viral suppression. Risk of potential fetal effects should be weighed against benefits of antiretrovirals in the first trimester.<br>• Use one or more NRTIs with good placental passage (ZDV, 3TC, ABC, TFV, FTC) in regimen if feasible.<br>• Use NVP in ARV regimen only if CD4 count <250 cells/mm$^3$.<br>• Continuous infusion of zidovudine intrapartum to women with HIV viral load >400 copies/mL (or unknown) near delivery and continue HAART during labor (hold oral zidovudine if part of antepartum regimen and VL >400 copies/mL while receiving intravenous ZDV infusion)<br>• Continuous infusion of zidovudine intrapartum to women with HIV viral load >400 copies/mL (or unknown) near delivery and continue HAART during labor (hold oral zidovudine if part of antepartum regimen and VL >400 copies/mL while receiving intravenous ZDV infusion)<br>• Zidovudine 6 wk postpartum for infant<br>• Assess need for continuing HAART after delivery; recommendations for continuing postpartum HAART are the same as in nonpregnant patients. |

| HIV-infected women who received no antiretroviral therapy prior to labor | — | • Continuous infusion zidovudine intrapartum<br>• Infants born to HIV-infected mothers who did not receive antepartum antiretrovirals should be started on combination ARV prophylaxis immediately after birth. ZDV for 6 wk with NVP three doses (at birth, 48 hr later, and 96 hr after second dose) is equally effective and less toxic than three drug regimens.<br>• Assess need for continuing HAART after delivery; recommendations for continuing postpartum HAART are the same as in nonpregnant patients. |

HAART, highly active antiretroviral therapy; VL, viral load; ZDV, zidovudine; ARV, antiretroviral; EFV, efavirenz; NRTI, nucleotide reverse transcriptase inhibitor; 3TC, lamivudine; ABC, abacavir; TFV, tenofovir; FTC, emtricitabine; NVP, nevirapine; IV, intravenous.

Adapted from Panel on Treatment of HIV-Infected Pregnant Women and Prevention of Perinatal Transmission. Recommendations for use of antiretroviral drugs in pregnant HIV-1-infected women for maternal health and interventions to reduce perinatal HIV transmission in the United States, Table 6 (pp. 30–33). http://aidsinfo.nih.gov/contentfiles/lvguidelines/PerinatalGL.pdf. Accessed April 7, 2013.

- **In general, amniotomy, fetal scalp electrodes for fetal monitoring, and operative vaginal delivery or episiotomy should be avoided.**
- Uterotonic medications typically used in the management of postpartum hemorrhage due to uterine atony may interact with a patient's ARV regimen:
  - Protease inhibitors are cytochrome P (CYP) 3A4 enzyme inhibitors, and therefore, Methergine should be used only if benefit from use outweighs risks and there are no alternative options available. The lowest effective dose should be administered when use is necessitated.
  - CYP3A4 enzyme inducers such as NVP, EFV, or etravirine may make Methergine less effective, requiring additional uterotonic medications.

## Management in Resource-Limited Areas

- Management of HIV-positive pregnancies in resource poor countries can be very different from the recommendations presented here. With limited medications, poor health infrastructure, reduced bottle feeding options, and less laboratory testing availability, these recommendations cannot always apply.

## POSTPARTUM CONTRACEPTION

The postpartum period is an important time to discuss safe sex practices and provide comprehensive family planning services. Contraception counseling, when initiated during prenatal care, is associated with more effective contraception use postpartum.

- A dual protection strategy using barrier protection such as condoms and another effective contraception method should be considered in HIV-infected women.
- Long-term reversible contraception (LARC) methods such as injectables, implants, and intrauterine devices may serve as options.
- Drug interactions between oral contraceptive pills and ARV medications have been observed in pharmacokinetic studies. Studies are ongoing to investigate clinical implications and alternative contraception methods are recommended in cases of known drug interactions.
- Although conflicting results have been published regarding possible increased risk of HIV transmission in women using hormonal contraception (HC), the World Health Organization and CDC recommend HC may be used in women with HIV who do not have other contraindications.

## COINFECTION WITH VIRAL HEPATITIS

Some women with HIV are coinfected with hepatitis B (HBV) or hepatitis C (HCV) virus. Antepartum screening is recommended. The hepatitis B vaccine series should be initiated for those women screening negative. Women with chronic HBV should be screened for hepatitis A antibodies and receive the hepatitis A virus vaccine series if they screen negative.

### Hepatitis B/HIV Coinfection

- Consultation with an expert is recommended for management of pregnant women with HIV/HBV coinfection.
- Treatment with interferon alpha or pegylated interferon alpha is not recommended during pregnancy.
- Women with chronic HBV who require HAART or HBV treatment should receive a three-drug regimen including a dual NRTI/nucleotide analogue reverse transcriptase

inhibitor (NtRTI) backbone of tenofovir plus lamivudine or emtricitabine. These drugs show activity against HBV. Triple therapy is indicated to prevent HBV drug resistance.

- An elevation of hepatic enzymes may occur following antiretroviral therapy initiation due to an immune-mediated flare in HBV disease from immune reconstitution syndrome, particularly in women with a low CD4 cell count.
- HBV may increase the hepatotoxicity of certain agents, specifically PIs and NVP. Women with HIV/HBV coinfection should be counseled about signs and symptoms of liver toxicity.
  - Liver function tests should be obtained 1 month after starting treatment and then at least every 3 months.
  - Discontinuation of ARVs postpartum may result in exacerbation of HBV infection; liver function tests should be monitored and treatment reinitiated for HIV and HBV if a flare is suspected.
- Infants should receive hepatitis B immunoglobulin and the first dose of the HBV vaccine series within 12 hours of birth. The second dose of the HBV series should be administered at 1 month; the third dose at 6 months.

## Hepatitis C/HIV Coinfection

- The seroprevalence of HCV in HIV-positive pregnant women is 17% to 54%.
- Pegylated interferon alpha is not recommended, and ribavirin is contraindicated during pregnancy.
- Coinfection significantly increases perinatal HCV transmission. Maternal HCV/HIV coinfection may also increase risk for perinatal HIV transmission.
- Effective combination therapy with three drugs should be considered for all HCV/HIV-infected women regardless of CD4 count and viral load.
- These women can also experience a transient worsening in symptoms due to immune-mediated flare in HCV disease.
- HCV may increase the hepatotoxicity of certain agents, specifically PIs and NVP. See recommendations for HBV for testing protocol (as mentioned earlier).
- Intrapartum management of HIV/HCV-coinfected women is no different from management of HIV infection alone. Decisions concerning mode of delivery in HCV/HIV-coinfected pregnant women should be based on HIV considerations alone.
- Infants should receive HCV antibody testing after 18 months of age. If earlier testing is indicated or desired, HCV RNA testing can be performed between 3 and 6 months of age.

## SUGGESTED READINGS

American College of Obstetricians and Gynecologists. ACOG committee opinion no. 234: scheduled cesarean delivery and the prevention of vertical transmission of HIV infection. *Int J Gynecol Obstet* 2001;73:279–281.

American College of Obstetricians and Gynecologists. ACOG committee opinion no. 313: the importance of preconception care in the continuum of women's health care. *Obstet Gynecol* 2005;106(3):665–666. http://www.ncbi.nlm.nih.gov/pubmed/16135611. Accessed April 5, 2013.

Apetrei C, Marx PA, Smith SM. The evolution of HIV and its consequences. *Infect Dis Clin North Am* 2004;18(2):369–394.

Branson BM, Handsfield HH, Lampe MA, et al. Revised recommendations for HIV testing of adults, adolescents, and pregnant women in health-care settings. *MMWR Recomm Rep* 2006;55(RR-14):1–17; quiz CE1–CE4. http://www.ncbi.nlm.nih.gov/pubmed/16988643. Accessed April 5, 2013.

Cohen MS, Chen YQ, McCauley M, et al. Prevention of HIV-1 infection with early antiretro-viral therapy. *N Engl J Med* 2011;365(6):493–505.

Cooper ER, Charuat M, Mofenson L, et al. Combination antiretroviral strategies for the treat-ment of pregnant HIV-1-infected women and prevention of perinatal HIV-1 transmission. *J Acquir Immune Defic Syndr* 2002;29(5):484–494.

Dao H, Mofenson LM, Ekpini R, et al. International recommendations on antiretroviral drugs for treatment of HIV-infected women and prevention of mother-to-child HIV transmis-sion in resource limited settings: 2006 update. *Am J Obstet Gynecol* 2007;197(3)(suppl): S42–S55.

Hammer SM. Clinical practice. Management of newly diagnosed HIV infection. *N Engl J Med* 2005;353(16):1702–1710.

Panel on Treatment of HIV-Infected Pregnant Women and Prevention of Perinatal Transmission. Recommendations for use of antiretroviral drugs in pregnant HIV-1-infected women for maternal health and interventions to reduce perinatal HIV transmission in the United States. http://aidsinfo.nih.gov/contentfiles/lvguidelines/PerinatalGL.pdf. Accessed April 5, 2013.

# 25 Obstetric Anesthesia

Abigail D. Winder and Jamie Murphy

Labor and delivery is a time of intense pain, often influenced by the psychological, emotional, social, cultural, and physical state of the parturient. Multiple techniques and procedures for pain relief during the birthing process are available. With appro-priate counseling of risks and benefits, patients can choose their preferred analgesic treatments.

## PAIN PATHWAYS

- In the first stage of labor (cervical dilation), the pain is visceral, produced by the distention of the lower uterus and cervix and ischemia of the uterine and cervical tissues. Visceral pain signals traverse T10 to L1 white *rami communicantes* and enter the spinal cord.
- The second stage involves both visceral and somatic pain. The parturient experiences more somatic pain in the late first stage of labor (7 to 10 cm cervical dilation), entering into the second stage from distention of the vagina, perineum, and pelvic floor. Somatic pain signals traverse the pudendal nerve (S2 to S4) and enter into the anterior spinal cord. The parturient also experiences rectal pressure. See Chapter 30 for more on biologic basis of pain perception.

## OVERVIEW OF OBSTETRIC ANALGESIA/ANESTHESIA

- Local, regional, and systemic methods of analgesia and anesthesia are used in obstetrics. Local and regional methods include local injection, peripheral nerve block, and regional block. Systemic methods can be administered intramuscularly, intravenously, or by inhalation. General anesthesia is often used in cases where total motor and sensory loss is necessary (Table 25-1) or when contraindications to neuraxial anesthesia are present.

- During the first stage of labor, visceral pain is mollified by the preferred use of regional anesthesia, such as an epidural, spinal, or a combination of both.

- In **vaginal deliveries**, the goal is to block nociceptive pathways while preserving motor function so that the parturient is comfortable but can participate actively with second stage expulsive effort. Local anesthesia or peripheral nerve block with pudendal injection or more systemic analgesia with intravenous (IV) pain medication or spinal/epidural block can be used during the second stage of labor.

- In **cesarean delivery**, anesthetic selection is often determined by the condition of the mother and fetus, the urgency of the procedure, and physician preference. Operative anesthesia requires a denser motor and sensory block than that used for a vaginal delivery. Neuraxial anesthesia is often the preferred method used because it provides adequate pain control while minimizing the maternal risk of aspiration or unanticipated difficult airway. In addition, neuraxial anesthesia decreases systemic catecholamine release and systemic response to surgery, avoids the side effects of postoperative IV narcotics, and allows the mother to interact with the newborn soon after delivery. Effective neuraxial anesthesia can be achieved by epidural, spinal, or combined spinal epidural approaches. General anesthesia is appropriate when the patient presents with contraindications to neuraxial anesthesia, medical indications, or in emergency cases where neuraxial anesthesia cannot be administered in a timely manner. Supplemental local anesthesia can be used by the obstetrician on the operative field as well.

| TABLE 25-1 | Use of Anesthesia in Obstetric Situations |

| Situation | Local | Peripheral Nerve Blocks | Regional | Systemic | General | Oral Analgesics |
|---|---|---|---|---|---|---|
| Labor—first stage | | X (Paracervical) | X | X | | |
| Vaginal delivery | X | X (Pudendal) | X | X | | |
| Cesarean section | X | | X | | X | |
| Urgent | X | | X | | X | |
| Postpartum pain | | | X | X | | X |
| Postoperative pain | | X | X | X | | X |

X, marks usual options for obstetric anesthesia.

For more information on practice patterns for obstetric anesthesia, see Bucklin BA, Hawkins JL, Anderson JR, et al. Obstetric anesthesia workforce survey. *Anesthesiology* 2005;103:645–653.

# TYPES OF OBSTETRIC ANALGESIA/ANESTHESIA

## Local Injection (Field Block)

*Indications*

- Used before cutting or repairing episiotomies or lacerations during and after the delivery
- Common agents include **lidocaine** (1% to 2%) or **2-chloroprocaine** (1% to 3%), which provide anesthesia for 20 to 40 minutes. The maximum allowed dose of injected lidocaine is 4.5 mg/kg.

*Advantages*

- Can provide pain relief without special equipment or personnel
- Local block can relieve most of the pain of simple laceration repair.
- Minimal systemic effect if administered correctly

*Limitations*

- May not cover entire field well or may not entirely block pain perception.

*Risks/Complications*

- Inadvertent IV injection can lead to serious systemic complications.
- Hypotension, arrhythmias, and seizures are rare complications.

## Peripheral Nerve Block (Pudendal, Paracervical)

*Indications*

- **Paracervical block** may be considered for the first stage of labor in patients for whom an epidural or spinal is contraindicated, unavailable, or undesired.
- **Pudendal block** may be used as analgesia during the second stage of labor or before operative vaginal deliveries if neuraxial anesthesia has not been provided or in supplement if there is inadequate pain relief.

*Technique*

- Paracervical: Five to 10 mL of local anesthetic (e.g., 2% chloroprocaine) is injected in the lateral vaginal fornices at the 4 and 8 o'clock positions to a depth of 3 to 4 mm.
- Pudendal: Five to 10 mL of local anesthetic (e.g., 1% lidocaine) is injected transvaginally about 1 cm medial and posterior to the ischial spine along the sacrospinous ligament at a depth of about 1 cm bilaterally. Care must be taken to avoid injecting directly into the pudendal vessels.

*Advantages*

- Peripheral nerve block is highly effective and may offer relief in up to 75% of cases.

*Limitations*

- Total anesthetic injection limits apply, as mentioned earlier.
- In some cases, relief may be inadequate. Twenty to 30 minutes are required before full effect. Pudendal block may be ineffective in up to 50% of patients and is frequently unilateral.

*Risks/Complications*

- Intravascular injection can result in systemic effects including medication toxicity, hematoma formation, and pelvic infection; these are recognized complications.

- Fetal bradycardia is a known side effect of paracervical block, occurring in approximately 15% of cases. Direct fetal injection is also a risk with paracervical block, resulting in fetal cardiac toxicity. Except in select cases in which other analgesia is not available, paracervical block is usually avoided.

## Regional Anesthesia (Epidural, Spinal)

- **Epidural and spinal anesthesia** are the preferred methods for obstetric pain control in the United States. They may be administered separately or as a combined spinal-epidural (CSE). Analgesia occurs at or below the T8 to T10 dermatomes, with varying degrees of motor blockade.

### Indications

- Neuraxial anesthesia is the preferred method of pain control because of its effectiveness and safety. General anesthesia is associated with increased maternal morbidity associated with increased risk of maternal aspiration and unanticipated difficult intubation.
- May be used when there is anticipated difficulty with intubation, a history of malignant hyperthermia, cardiovascular or respiratory disorders, or a need to prevent autonomic hyperreflexia in women with high spinal cord lesions.
- Regional anesthesia is preferred in women with preeclampsia because it may increase intravillous blood flow and reduce the need for general anesthesia if cesarean delivery is indicated.
- Maternal request alone is sufficient reason to give regional anesthesia.

### Technique

- Table 25-2 lists agents commonly used for obstetric regional anesthesia.
- **Epidural** (Fig. 25-1): A catheter is introduced into the lumbar epidural space through an epidural needle. The catheter is secured to the patient's back with adhesive tape. Medication is administered via continuous infusion pump (preferred) or intermittent bolus to provide consistent pain relief. Local anesthetic, neuraxial opioid, or a combination of both is used. A test dose (typically 3 mL of

| TABLE 25-2 | Epidural/Spinal Anesthetics | |
|---|---|---|
| **Class** | **Action** | **Examples** |
| Local anesthetics | Block conductance through sodium channels in axons. Reversible effect | Amides: lidocaine, bupivacaine, ropivacaine<br>Ester: chloroprocaine |
| Opioids | Act on opioid receptors in dorsal horn of spinal cord | Morphine, fentanyl, sufentanil, alfentanil, meperidine |
| Adrenergic agonists | Bind to alpha-2 receptors in the spinal cord | Epinephrine, clonidine, dexmedetomidine |
| Cholinergic agonists | Increase cholinergic effect via muscarinic receptors in the dorsal horn of spinal cord | Neostigmine |

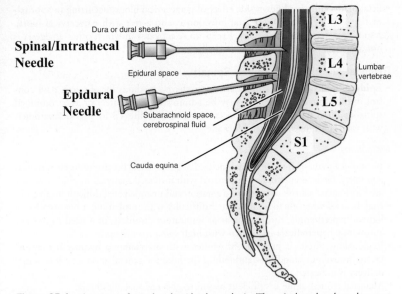

**Figure 25-1.** Placement of spinal and epidural anesthesia. The spinal cord ends at the conus medullaris near lumbar vertebral bodies L1/L2 in adults, with the cauda equina nerves extending below. Spinal anesthesia is injected directly into the cerebrospinal fluid of the subarachnoid space, whereas epidural anesthesia is deposited in the epidural space (near L3/L4). Combined spinal–epidural analgesia can be administered with a single needle that allows intrathecal injection followed by epidural catheter placement. L, lumbar; S, sacral. (Adapted from Taylor C, Lillis CA, LeMone P. *Fundamentals of Nursing,* 2nd ed. Philadelphia, PA: JB Lippincott, 1993, with permission.)

1.5% lidocaine with 1:200,000 epinephrine in bolus) should be given to rule out intrathecal or intravascular catheter placement and avoid complications. Patient-controlled epidural anesthesia allows the patient to self-administer small bolus doses by pressing a dose-demand button. Pain relief may be further improved by a combination of continuous plus patient-controlled dosing. Breakthrough pain is addressed by increasing the continuous infusion rate or giving a second bolus dose.

- **Spinal:** A local anesthetic, often in combination with an opioid, is injected into the subarachnoid space. The onset of action is rapid. Continuous spinal anesthesia can be given via an intrathecal catheter, although there is a risk for transient neurologic syndrome especially with infusions of high-dose lidocaine anesthetics.
- **CSE:** This is the needle-through-needle approach in which a smaller bore spinal needle (i.e., −24G to 27G) is placed inside the epidural needle. The spinal medication is injected, then the small needle is withdrawn and an epidural catheter threaded into the epidural space as mentioned earlier. A single spinal bolus of opioid, sometimes with local anesthetic, is injected into the subarachnoid space. This method combines the rapid onset of spinal anesthesia with the longer lasting relief of an epidural.

*Advantages*

- Regional analgesia provides excellent pain control but allows the patient to participate actively in the labor and delivery process.

- Increased use of neuraxial anesthesia and the reduction in general anesthesia during delivery has led to significant decreases in anesthesia-associated maternal morbidity and mortality related to aspiration pneumonia and inability to intubate.

## Limitations

- Regional anesthesia cannot be placed in every case due to time limitations, anatomic considerations, comorbidities, or contraindications.
- Twenty to 30 minutes are required for full effect of an epidural.
- Spinal anesthesia lasts only 30 to 250 minutes depending on the drug injected.
- CSE is associated with a higher incidence of fetal bradycardia, with emergency cesarean delivery occurring in 1% to 2% of cases.
- Failure of the spinal component may occur in 4% of cases in which CSE is used.

## Contraindications

- Patient refusal
- Coagulopathy
- Thrombocytopenia
- Infection at injection site
- Sepsis
- Hemodynamic instability or refractory hypotension
- Increased intracranial pressure caused by a mass lesion

## Risks/Complications

- **Infection:** meningitis, epidural abscess, reactivation of latent herpes simplex virus (HSV) (associated with neuraxial morphine use), and maternal fever
- **Neurologic complications:** epidural hematoma, neural injury, spinal headache, catheter- and needle-related complications, back pain, and nerve palsies
  - **Spinal headache:** If the subarachnoid space is entered by the epidural needle, a spinal headache may result in up to 70% of patients. Management includes analgesics, supine positioning, hydration, caffeine, and abdominal binding. A **blood patch** can be offered if conservative management fails and the patient desires it.
  - **Back pain:** There is no evidence implicating epidural anesthesia as a cause of chronic back pain.
  - **Nerve palsies:** Injuries to the lumbosacral trunk, lateral femoral cutaneous, femoral, and common peroneal nerves have been reported.
- **Adverse drug reactions:** Local anesthetic toxicity, high spinal block/respiratory distress, allergic reaction, and transient neurologic impairment are possible complications.
  - **Local anesthetic toxicity:** Symptoms include tinnitus, disorientation, and seizures; cardiovascular symptoms include hypotension, dysrhythmias, and cardiac arrest.
  - **High spinal:** Respiratory compromise may result if the block progresses above the C6 dermatome level.
  - **Motor block:** Motor impairment can reduce maternal expulsive efforts and alter the birthing process and parturient experience.
  - Intrathecal opioids can cause **maternal respiratory depression** and hypoxemia.
- **Hypotension:** Low blood pressure can result with regional anesthesia from sympathetic blockade–induced vasodilation or position-dependent decreased venous return. Hypotension is significant when symptoms develop, such as maternal light-headedness or fetal bradycardia. Episodes can be treated with bolus IV fluids or low-dose ephedrine (5 mg) or phenylephrine (100 μg). Adequate IV hydration must occur before epidural or spinal access is placed.

- **Fetal complications**
  - **Nonreassuring fetal monitoring:** Bradycardia and transient heart rate decelerations may occur. Hydration is usually adequate treatment, although pressor support (as mentioned earlier) may be indicated. Repositioning should also be attempted.
  - **Instrumentation:** There is mixed evidence for increased rates of forceps or vacuum delivery with regional anesthesia, with challenges in demonstrating causation versus association.
  - When compared to IV systemic opioid analgesia, early neuraxial anesthesia does not increase the risk of cesarean delivery.

## Systemic Analgesia

Opioids (morphine, fentanyl, meperidine) or mixed opioid agonist-antagonists (butorphanol, nalbuphine) are used for systemic pain relief (Table 25-3). They can be administered by intramuscular or IV injection depending on the onset and duration of relief desired.

*Indications*
- Maternal request

*Advantages*
- Rapid onset and ease of administration
- Can be administered via IV patient-controlled anesthesia

*Limitations*
- Randomized controlled trials demonstrated higher pain scores during labor for parenteral compared with regional anesthesia.

| TABLE 25-3 | Parenteral Agents for Labor Pain | | | | |
|---|---|---|---|---|---|
| Agent | Class | Usual Dose | Frequency | Onset | Duration |
| Meperidine (Demerol) | Opioid | 25–50 mg IV | q1–2 hr | 5 min IV | 2–3 hr |
| | | 50–100 mg IM | q2–4 hr | 30–45 min IM | |
| Fentanyl | Opioid | 50–100 μg IV | q1 hr | 1–3 min IV | 3–4 hr |
| | | 100 μg IM | | 7–10 min IM | |
| Morphine | Opioid | 2–5 mg IV | q4 hr | 3–5 min IV | 3–4 hr |
| | | 5–10 mg IM | | 20–40 min IM | |
| Nalbuphine (Nubain) | Mixed opioid agonist/ antagonist | 5–10 mg IV or IM | q3 hr | 2–3 min IV | 3–6 hr |
| | | | | 10–15 min IM | |
| Butorphanol (Stadol) | Mixed opioid agonist/ antagonist | 1–2 mg IV or IM | q4 hr | 5–10 min IV | 3–4 hr |
| | | | | 10–30 min IM | |

IV, intravenous; IM, intramuscular.
Adapted from Althaus J, Wax J. Analgesia and anesthesia in labor. *Obstet Gynecol Clin N Am* 2005;32:231–244.

- It is difficult to obtain adequate pain control throughout labor with only narcotic analgesia.

*Risks/Complications*
- Maternal respiratory depression requires close monitoring.
- Sedative effects may increase aspiration risk.
- All opiates cross the placenta, affecting both fetal and newborn status. Fetal tracings may show decreased variability with maternal narcotic analgesia. Newborns may require extra assistance after delivery including supplemental oxygen and ventilatory support.

## General Anesthesia
*Indications*
- General anesthesia is useful in urgent situations in which epidural/spinal is not available, in cases where regional anesthesia is contraindicated, and in parturients with medical problems that require general anesthesia.

*Technique*
- Before intubation, the patient receives a nonparticulate antacid, such as sodium citrate, to neutralize gastric pH and decrease aspiration risk. One hundred percent oxygen is administered for 3 to 5 minutes before induction and intubation to fortify oxygen reserve.
- IV agents are used in a rapid sequence induction to minimize aspiration from the abdominal distention/pressure of the gravid uterus.
- The trachea is intubated quickly with a cuffed endotracheal tube as cricoid pressure is applied to reduce aspiration risk.

*Advantages*
- Intubation can be performed rapidly in emergent cases.
- Inhaled fluorinated anesthetics cause rapid uterine relaxation which may be used to correct uterine inversion or to facilitate internal/external version or release fetal head entrapment.
- The patient remains still throughout the procedure and does not remember an extensive or prolonged procedure.

*Limitations*
- The parturient is unable to witness the birth of her child.
- All inhalational agents cross the placenta and can affect the fetus, leading to brief neonatal respiratory depression after delivery; the time from intubation to delivery should be as brief as feasible and safe.

*Risks/Complications*
- Given the decreased functional residual capacity and increased oxygen requirements of pregnancy, in addition to increased airway edema and friability, there is an **increased maternal morbidity** associated with general anesthesia/intubation.
- **Aspiration** and hypoxemia can lead to postoperative medical complications.
- **Neonatal respiratory depression** occurs as a result of fetal perfusion of the anesthetics
- Uterine relaxation can increase surgical **blood loss**. Pitocin, Methergine, and misoprostol should all be on hand at the time of obstetric general anesthesia.

## SUGGESTED READINGS

American College of Obstetricians and Gynecologists. ACOG practice bulletin no. 36: obstetric analgesia and anesthesia. *Obstet Gynecol* 2002;100:177–191.

Gaiser R. Chapter 2: physiologic changes of pregnancy. In Chesnut DH, Polley LS, Tsen LC, et al, eds. *Chesnut's Obstetric Anesthesia: Principles and Practice*, 4th ed. Philadelphia, PA: Mosby Elsevier, 2009.

Kopp SL, Horlocker TT. Anticoagulation in pregnancy and neuraxial blocks. *Anesthesiol Clin* 2008;26:1–22.

Santos AC, Bucklin BA. Chapter 13: local anesthetics and opioids. In Chesnut DH, Polley LS, Tsen LC, et al, eds. *Chesnut's Obstetric Anesthesia: Principles and Practice*, 4th ed. Philadelphia, PA: Mosby Elsevier, 2009.

Wong CA, Nathan N, Brown DL. Chapter 12: spinal, epidural, and caudal anesthesia. In Chesnut DH, Polley LS, Tsen LC, et al, eds. *Chesnut's Obstetric Anesthesia: Principles and Practice*, 4th ed. Philadelphia, PA: Mosby Elsevier, 2009.

# III  Gynecology

# 26  Anatomy of the Female Pelvis

Lauren Owens and Isabel Green

## ABDOMINAL WALL

The **anterior abdominal wall** lies ventrally and is outlined superiorly by the lower edge of the rib cage; caudally by the iliac crests, inguinal ligaments, and pubic bone; and dorsolaterally by the lumbar spine and adjacent muscles.

### Layers of the Anterior Abdominal Wall
- **Skin**
- **Subcutaneous layer:** This consists of fat globules in a meshwork of fibrous septa. **Camper fascia** is the more superficial aspect of the subcutaneous layer.

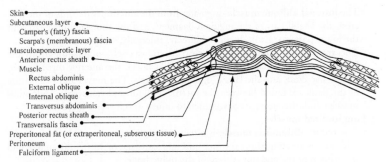

**Figure 26-1.** Layers of the anterior abdominal wall cephalad to the arcuate line.

**Scarpa fascia** is the deeper portion and has a more organized consistency than Camper fascia secondary to more fibrous tissue.

- **Musculoaponeurotic layer:** Located immediately below the subcutaneum, the musculoaponeurotic layer consists of layers of fibrous tissue and muscles that hold the abdominal viscera in place.
  - **Rectus sheath:** The aponeuroses of the external oblique, internal oblique, and transversus abdominis muscles comprise the rectus sheath.
  - The anterior rectus sheath is anatomically different above and below the **arcuate line.** The arcuate line (linea semicircularis, semilunar fold of Douglas) is located midway between the umbilicus and symphysis pubis. It marks the lower edge of the posterior rectus sheath.
    - **Above the arcuate line**, the anterior rectus sheath is composed of the aponeuroses of the external oblique and ventral half of the internal oblique muscles. The posterior rectus sheath is composed of the aponeuroses of the dorsal half of the internal oblique and transversus abdominis muscles (Fig. 26-1).
    - **Below the arcuate line**, the anterior rectus sheath is composed of the aponeuroses of all the muscles previously mentioned (Fig. 26-2).
    - The **linea alba** is the midline between the rectus abdominis muscles. Above the arcuate line, the linea alba marks the fusion of the anterior and posterior rectus sheaths.
- **Abdominal wall muscles**
  - **Oblique flank muscles** lie lateral to the rectus abdominis muscles.
    - The **external oblique muscle** originates from the lower eight ribs and iliac crest and runs obliquely, anteriorly, and inferiorly.

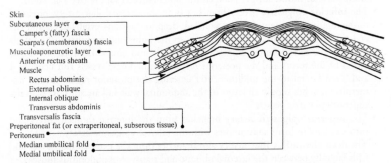

**Figure 26-2.** Layers of the anterior abdominal wall caudal to the arcuate line.

- The **internal oblique muscle** originates from the anterior two thirds of the iliac crest, the lateral part of the inguinal ligament, and the thoracolumbar fascia in the lower posterior flank. It runs obliquely, anteriorly, and superiorly.
  - The **transversus abdominis muscle** runs transversely, originating from the lower six costal cartilages, the thoracolumbar fascia, the anterior three fourths of the iliac crest, and the lateral inguinal ligament. The nerves and vasculature of the flank are found between the internal oblique and transversus abdominis muscles and, therefore, are susceptible to injury in transverse incisions.
- **Longitudinal muscles**
  - The **rectus abdominis muscle** is a paired muscle, found on either side of the midline, originating from the sternum and cartilage of ribs 5 through 7 and inserting into the anterior surface of the pubic bone.
  - The **pyramidalis muscle** is a vestigial muscle with a variable presence among individuals. It arises from the pubic bone and inserts into the linea alba several centimeters cephalad to the symphysis ventral to the rectus abdominis muscle.
- The **transversalis fascia** is a layer of fibrous tissue, located underneath the abdominal wall muscles and outside the peritoneum. The transversalis is separated from the peritoneum by a variable layer of adipose tissue.
- **Peritoneum:** A single layer of serosa lines the posterior aspect of the anterior abdominal wall. Five vertical folds converge toward the umbilicus.
  - The **median umbilical fold** is a single fold created by the **median umbilical ligament** or **obliterated urachus**.
    - The apex of the bladder blends into the median umbilical ligament and is highest in the midline. This relationship should be considered when entering the peritoneal cavity.
  - The **medial umbilical folds** are paired folds lateral to the median umbilical fold, remnants of the obliterated umbilical arteries; they converge at the umbilicus.
  - The **lateral umbilical folds** are paired folds caused by the inferior epigastric vessels.

## Vasculature of the Abdominal Wall

- **Subcutaneous vascular supply** (Fig. 26-3)
  - The **superficial epigastric artery** branches from the femoral artery after it descends through the femoral canal. It runs superomedially, approximately 5 cm lateral to the midline.
  - The **superficial circumflex iliac artery** branches from the femoral artery and runs laterally toward the flank.
- **Musculofascial blood supply** parallels the subcutaneous supply (see Fig. 26-3).
  - The **inferior epigastric artery** branches from the external iliac artery, proximal to the inguinal ligament. It runs cephalad, deep to the transversalis fascia and lateral to the rectus muscle. Midway between the pubis and umbilicus, the vessels intersect the lateral border of the rectus muscle and course between the dorsal aspect of the rectus and the posterior rectus sheath. These vessels run between 4 and 8 cm lateral to the midline. After entering the posterior rectus sheath, numerous branches supply all layers of the abdominal wall and anastomose with the superior epigastric vessels.
  - The **superior epigastric artery** branches from the internal thoracic artery and runs caudally to form anastomoses with the inferior epigastric artery.
  - The **deep circumflex iliac artery** also branches from the external iliac artery and runs laterally between the internal oblique and transversus abdominis muscles.

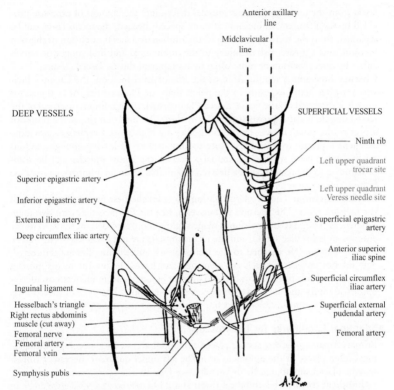

**Figure 26-3.** Vasculature and laparoscopic landmarks of the anterior abdominal wall. (Original drawing by Alice W. Ko from Bankowski BJ, Hearne AE, Lambrou NC, eds. *The Johns Hopkins Manual of Gynecology and Obstetrics*, 2nd ed. Philadelphia, PA: Lippincott Williams & Wilkins, 2002.)

## Abdominal Wall Incisions

- **Vertical:** A midline incision provides optimal exposure to the abdomen. The incision is made from the symphysis to below the umbilicus, depending on how much space is needed. A small incision or "mini-lap" may offer excellent visualization and improved cosmesis. The incision can always be extended more cephalad and then circumferentially around the umbilicus to the left to avoid the ligamentum teres. The anterior rectus sheath is incised longitudinally. The peritoneum is entered taking care to avoid the superior aspect of the bladder.

- **Pfannenstiel incision:** This is one of the most common incisions in obstetrics and gynecology. A transverse incision is made approximately two fingerbreadths (3 to 4 cm) above the pubic symphysis. Transverse incisions are generally less painful and more cosmetic than longitudinal incisions as they run along Langer lines. The incision is continued through the rectus sheath, and then the rectus muscles are dissected cephalad and caudad off the posterior aspect of the rectus sheath. Then, the rectus muscles are separated in the midline to gain entry to the peritoneum through a midline longitudinal incision. The degree of separation of the rectus fascia from the underlying rectus muscles determines the amount of exposure provided by the Pfannenstiel incision. If more space is needed, the rectus fascia can be separated from the rectus muscle up to the umbilicus. Lateral extension of the skin incision runs a greater risk of injury to the ilioinguinal and iliohypogastric nerves either by direct incision or more often by entrapment during fascial closure.

- **Cherney incision:** A modification of the Pfannenstiel incision, the Cherney incision provides better exposure to the pelvis than the Pfannenstiel. After the rectus muscle is dissected off the fascia, as in a Pfannenstiel, the tendinous insertion of the rectus muscle is cut approximately 0.5 cm above the insertion site at the posterior aspect of the pubic bones. The rectus bellies are then moved cephalad, providing excellent exposure to the pelvis. Note the importance of leaving enough tendons on the pubic bone so that the caudal aspect of the rectus muscles can be reapproximated to the tendon with a delayed absorbable suture in a horizontal mattress fashion during closure.

- **Maylard incision:** The Maylard incision provides the best pelvic exposure of all the incision types. This incision is transverse, like the Pfannenstiel, with two main differences. The Maylard incision is made slightly more cephalad (at the level of the anterior superior iliac spine), and the rectus muscles are not dissected off the fascia. Rather, they are left attached to the rectus sheath and the muscles are transected. The inferior epigastric vessels are identified and ligated before the rectus muscles are transected completely. This helps to prevent blood loss from inadvertent inferior epigastric injury and also serves to preserve blood supply. This type of incision has the potential for greater blood loss but also for better pelvic exposure.

## Abdominal Landmarks for Laparoscopy

- Primary laparoscopic trocars are placed for initial access. In gynecology, these are most often placed at the umbilicus or in the left upper quadrant. Accessory trocars may be placed suprapubically or laterally (see Fig. 26-3).
  - **Umbilical trocar:** The umbilical trocar should be placed at a 45-degree angle in thin women in order to avoid hitting the aorta or common iliacs. In an obese patient, the trocar can be placed at a more perpendicular angle due to the amount of adipose tissue that must be traversed.
  - **Left upper quadrant trocar:** A trocar may be placed at Palmer point, 3 cm below the left costal margin in the midclavicular line. Prior to trocar insertion, the stomach should be emptied with a nasogastric tube. This location is preferred in patients with prior midline surgery to avoid potential visceral adhesions.
  - **Suprapubic trocar:** The suprapubic trocar is placed two fingerbreadths above the pubic symphysis. It is placed under direct visualization and after Foley insertion in order to assure that the bladder is not in line of the trocar path.
  - **Lateral trocars:** The lateral trocars are placed at least 5 cm cephalad to the pubic symphysis and 8 cm lateral to the midline in order to avoid the inferior epigastric vessels. The trocar is placed under direct visualization lateral to the lateral umbilical folds to avoid injury to the inferior epigastric vessels.

# PELVIC VISCERA

## Vagina

- The **vagina** is shaped like a flattened tube, starting at the distal hymenal ring and ending at the fornices surrounding the proximal cervix. Its average length is 8 cm; this varies greatly with age, parity, and surgical history.

- The vaginal epithelium is nonkeratinized, stratified squamous epithelium lacking mucous glands and hair follicles.
- Deep to the epithelium is the vaginal muscularis or endopelvic fascia. The term *fascia* is misleading because this is actually fibromuscular tissue that includes fibroblasts, smooth muscle cells, and elastin, in addition to type I and III collagen, all loosely arrayed to create an elastic supportive layer. At the vaginal apex, this fibromuscular layer coalesces to create the **cardinal** and **uterosacral** ligaments. The fanshaped cardinal ligament creates a sheath that envelops the uterine artery and vein, fusing medially with the paracervical ring. The uterosacral portion inserts into the posterior and lateral aspect of the paracervical ring and then curves laterally along the pelvic sidewall to attach to the presacral fascia that overlies the second, third, and fourth sacral vertebrae. Together, the cardinal and uterosacral ligaments pull the vagina proximally toward the sacrum, suspending it over the muscular levator plate.
- The endopelvic fascias of the anterior and posterior vaginal wall are known as the **pubocervical fascia** and **rectovaginal fascia**, respectively. Again, these layers are not true fasciae but composed of fibromuscular sheets. Superiorly, the pubocervical fascia attaches to the cervix and the cardinal/uterosacral support of the vaginal apex. Laterally, it coalesces with the fascia of the obturator internus muscle to create the **arcus tendineus fascia pelvis (ATFP)** or "white line." Inferiorly, it attaches to the pubic symphysis. The rectovaginal fascia in the upper vagina coalesces with the lateral support of the anterior vaginal wall and fuses with the ATFP. The lower half of the rectovaginal fascia fuses with the aponeurosis of the levator ani muscles along a line referred to as the **arcus tendineus fascia rectovaginalis**. At its most inferior point, the rectovaginal septum fuses with the perineal body (Fig. 26-4).

## Uterus

- The **uterus** is a fibromuscular organ composed of the corpus and the cervix.
- **Corpus:** The **endometrium** is the innermost lining of the uterus made up of columnar epithelium and specialized stroma. The superficial layer of the endometrium contains hormonally sensitive spiral arterioles, which shed with each cycle. The **myometrium** contains interlacing smooth muscle fibers, and the **serosal** surface of the uterus is formed by peritoneal mesothelium. The **fundus** is the portion of the uterus cephalad to the endometrial cavity. The **cornua** are located where the fallopian tubes insert into the uterine cavity, lateral to the fundus.
- **Cervix:** The cervix is generally 2 to 4 cm in length and has two parts: the **portio vaginalis** (protruding into the vagina) and the **portio supravaginalis** (lying

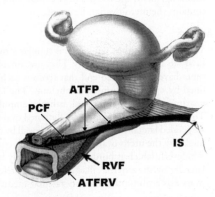

**Figure 26-4.** Illustration of attachment of rectovaginal fascia (RVF) and arcus tendineus fascia pelvis (ATFP) to the pelvic sidewall. RVF represents the ideal line of suture placement during lateral defect repair. PCF, pubocervical fascia; ATFRV, arcus tendineus fascia rectovaginalis; IS, ischial spine. (From Leffler KS, Thompson JR, Cundiff GW, et al. Attachment of the rectovaginal septum to the pelvic sidewall. *Am J Obstet Gynecol* 2001;185:43, with permission.)

above the vagina). The cervix is made up of dense fibrous connective tissue and is surrounded in a circular fashion by a small amount of smooth muscle into which the cardinal and uterosacral ligaments and pubocervical and rectovaginal fascia insert. The cervix contains a central longitudinal canal connecting the endometrial cavity with the vagina, called the **endocervical canal**. The **internal os** of the cervix is at the junction of the endocervical canal and the endometrial cavity. The **external os** is the distal opening of the cervical canal to the vagina. The **squamocolumnar junction** is located at the external os. It marks the transition from the squamous epithelium of the ectocervix to the columnar epithelium of the endocervical canal at the external os. The squamocolumnar junction is sampled with Pap smears and is a common site for cervical dysplasia and cancer. The **ectocervix** is the outer portion of the cervix.

## Ligaments of the Uterus

- These ligaments are formed by thickening of the endopelvic fascia or folds of peritoneum.
- The **round ligament** courses from the anterolateral aspect of the uterine corpus through the inguinal canal to insert into the labia majora. It has a fibromuscular element and can give rise to leiomyomas. It contains the **artery of Sampson**. This ligament provides no support for the uterus.
- The **utero-ovarian ligament** contains the anastomotic vasculature of the uterine and ovarian vessels and connects the uterus and ovaries.
- The **cardinal ligaments (Mackenrodt ligaments)** extend from the lateral pelvic walls and insert into the lateral portion of the vagina, uterine cervix, and isthmus. These contain both the uterine artery and vein and play an important role in support of the pelvic organs.
- The **infundibulopelvic ligament (IP ligament, suspensory ligament of the ovary)** contains the ovarian vessels. The ovarian arteries branch directly off the aorta. The right ovarian vein feeds into the inferior vena cava, whereas the left vein drains into the left renal vein.
- The **uterosacral ligaments** extend from the sacral fascia and insert into the posterior portion of the uterine isthmus and endopelvic fascia. They are composed of connective tissue and smooth muscle and contain the autonomic sympathetic and parasympathetic nerves of the pelvic organs. Together, the cardinal and uterosacral ligaments form the parametrium and play an important role in pelvic organ support.
- The **broad ligament** is the peritoneum that covers the uterus and fallopian tubes. It forms a mesentery around the uterine structures: The mesoteres surrounds the round ligament, the mesosalpinx contains the fallopian tube, and the mesovarium contains the utero-ovarian ligament.

## Adnexa

- The **fallopian tubes** are bilateral tubular structures that connect the endometrial cavity to the peritoneal cavity. They are, on average, 10 cm in length. Distally, the tubes have a fimbriated end that receives each ovum after ovulation. The lumen is lined by ciliated columnar epithelium. The fallopian tube has four regions (from proximal to distal): interstitial, isthmic, ampullary, and infundibular.
- The **ovaries** are bilateral, white, flattened oval structures that store ova. The ovary is suspended laterally from the pelvic sidewall by the IP ligament and medially from the uterus by the utero-ovarian ligament. Each ovary rests in the ovarian fossa (fossa of Waldeyer), which is bordered dorsomedially by the hypogastric artery and ventrolaterally by the external iliac artery. The ureter runs at the base of this fossa. The ovary has a fibromuscular and vascular medulla and an outer cortex that contains

specialized stroma with follicles, corpora lutea, and corpora albicantia. The ovary is covered by cuboidal epithelium.

## Ureter

- The **ureter** courses from the kidneys retroperitoneally, crosses the pelvic brim at the level of the bifurcation of the common iliac artery, and continues in the medial leaf of the broad ligament. It enters the tunnel of Wertheim as it passes under the uterine artery 1.5 cm lateral to the cervix at the level of the internal cervical os and enters the trigone of the bladder. The three most common areas of ureteral injury during gynecologic surgery are at the pelvic brim during clamping of the IP ligaments, during clamping of the uterine artery at time of hysterectomy, and near the trigone when mobilizing the bladder off the lower uterine segment.

## SURGICAL SPACES OF THE PELVIS

The reproductive, urinary, and gastrointestinal organs found in the pelvis have the ability to change their size and shape independently of each other, which is made possible by their loose attachments via connective tissue planes composed of fat and areolar tissue. These planes are potential spaces that can be entered with surgical dissection. The neurolymphovascular supply to the organs remains in the connective tissue septae, permitting blunt and bloodless dissection of the surgical spaces. Eight avascular spaces are described: prevesical, vesicovaginal, paravesical (2), pararectal (2), rectovaginal, and retrorectal (Fig. 26-5).

- The **prevesical space**, also known as the **space of Retzius** or **retropubic space**, is separated ventrally from the rectus abdominis by the transversalis fascia. Laterally, the muscles of the pelvic wall, cardinal ligament, and attachment of the pubocervical fascia to the ATFP border the prevesical space. Important structures within the space of Retzius include the dorsal clitoral vessels, obturator nerves and vessels, nerves of the lower urinary tract, iliopectineal line, ATFP, and the arcus tendineus levator ani. Burch urethropexies are performed in this space.

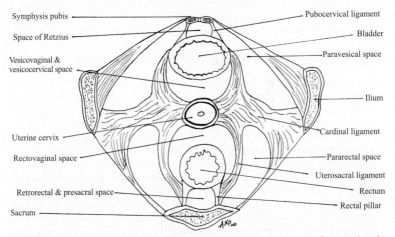

**Figure 26-5.** Surgical spaces of the pelvis. (Original drawing by Alice W. Ko from Bankowski BJ, Hearne AE, Lambrou NC, eds. *The Johns Hopkins Manual of Gynecology and Obstetrics*, 2nd ed. Philadelphia, PA: Lippincott Williams & Wilkins, 2002.)

- The **vesicovaginal spaces (also called vesicocervical)** are separated by a thin supravaginal septum. The spaces are bound caudally by the fusion of the junction of the proximal one third and distal two thirds of the urethra with the vagina, ventrally by the urethra and bladder, cephalad by the peritoneum, forming the vesicocervical reflection. This is the space entered when developing a "bladder flap" during cesarean delivery or hysterectomy.

- The **paravesical spaces** are paired spaces adjacent to the bladder. They are bordered medially by the bladder and obliterated umbilical artery, laterally by the obturator internus, dorsally by the cardinal ligament, ventrally by the pubic symphysis, and caudally by the levator ani. The ureter can be found in the tissue between the paravesical and vesicovaginal spaces. Parametrial tissue obtained in a radical hysterectomy is located between the paravesical and pararectal spaces.

- The **pararectal spaces** are paired spaces adjacent to the rectum. The space is bordered medially by the ureter, uterosacral ligament, and rectum; laterally by the hypogastric vessels and pelvic wall; ventrolaterally by the cardinal ligament; and dorsally by the sacrum. The coccygeus forms the floor of this space. Bleeding can be encountered from the lateral sacral and hemorrhoidal vessels if dissection is carried to the pelvic floor. These spaces allow access to the sacrospinous ligaments, as well as identification of the ureter for ureterolysis when indicated.

- The **rectovaginal space** is bordered caudally by the apex of the perineal body; laterally by the uterosacral ligament, ureter, and rectal pillars; ventrally by the vagina; and dorsally by the rectum. The **pouch of Douglas** or **posterior cul-de-sac** is the space between the uterus and rectum bounded inferiorly by the peritoneum. The rectovaginal space is below this peritoneum and cul-de-sac and is developed by incising the peritoneal fold between the uterus and rectum.

- The **retrorectal space** is caudal to the presacral space and bordered ventrally by the rectum, posteriorly by the sacrum, and laterally by the uterosacral ligaments. The **presacral space** is bordered laterally by the internal iliac arteries, cephalad by the bifurcation of the aorta, dorsally by the sacrum, and ventrally by the colon. It contains the presacral nerve (superior hypogastric plexus), the middle sacral artery and vein (originating from the dorsal aspect of the aorta and vena cava), and the lateral sacral vessels. This space is entered for sacrocolpopexy for pelvic organ prolapse, presacral neurectomy for pelvic pain, and para-aortic lymph node dissection.

## VASCULATURE OF THE ABDOMEN AND PELVIS

- **Aorta:** From cephalad to caudad, the arteries that stem from the aorta below the diaphragm are inferior phrenic, celiac trunk, suprarenal, superior mesenteric, renal, lumbar, ovarian, inferior mesenteric, and median sacral. The aorta then bifurcates into the common iliac arteries at the level of the fourth lumbar vertebra.

- **Celiac trunk:** The celiac trunk has three main branches: the **left gastric**, the **splenic**, and the **common hepatic** arteries. The **left gastric artery** divides into the esophageal branches and branches that supply the lesser curvature of the stomach. The **splenic artery** divides into pancreatic branches: **short gastric arteries**, which supply the fundus of the stomach, and the **left gastroepiploic artery**, which supplies the greater omentum and the greater curvature of the stomach. The left gastroepiploic artery anastomoses with the right gastroepiploic, which is a terminal branch of the common hepatic. The **common hepatic artery** has two main divisions: the **proper hepatic artery** and the **gastroduodenal artery**. The proper hepatic artery divides into the **right gastric artery** and enters the lesser omentum to anastomose with the **left gastric artery** and terminates into the **right and left hepatic arteries**. The **cystic**

**artery** often branches from the right hepatic artery and supplies the gallbladder. The **gastroduodenal artery** branches into the **supraduodenal artery**, the **right gastroepiploic artery**, and the **superior pancreatoduodenal artery**. The **right gastroepiploic artery** enters the greater omentum and anastomoses with the left gastroepiploic artery along the greater curvature of the stomach. The **superior pancreatoduodenal artery** supplies the second part of the duodenum and the head of the pancreas.

- The **superior mesenteric artery** branches into the **jejunal** and **ileal artery** branches, the **ileocolic artery**, the **right colic artery**, and the **middle colic artery**.
- The **inferior mesenteric artery** branches into the **left colic artery**, the **sigmoid branches**, and the **superior rectal artery**.
- **Ovarian vessels:** The ovarian arteries originate from the anterior aspect of the aorta and course toward the pelvis, crossing laterally over the **ureters** at the level of the pelvic brim and passing branches to the ureters and fallopian tubes. They then cross medially over the proximal external iliac vessels and run medially in the infundibulopelvic ligaments. The left ovarian vein drains into the left renal vein, whereas the right ovarian vein drains directly into the inferior vena cava.
- The aorta bifurcates into the **common iliac arteries** at the level of the fourth lumbar vertebra. The common iliac then bifurcates into the **external and internal** (hypogastric) **arteries**. The hypogastric artery divides into an anterior and posterior division 3 to 4 cm after the branching off of the common iliac artery. The **ureter** courses anteriorly to the division of the hypogastric and external iliac arteries.
  - **Anterior division of the hypogastric artery:** Some variance exists in the branching pattern. The branches include the obturator, uterine, vaginal, inferior, and superior vesicals; middle rectal; internal pudendal; and inferior gluteal arteries. The **ureter** passes laterally under the **uterine artery** at the level of the internal cervical os. During hypogastric artery ligation, the anterior division of the hypogastric artery should be doubly ligated with 1-0 silk (do not divide) 2.5 to 3.0 cm distal to the bifurcation of the common iliac. The dissection is done laterally to medially to avoid damaging the hypogastric vein.
  - **Posterior division of the hypogastric artery:** The branches include the iliolumbar, lateral sacral, and superior gluteal arteries, all of which have anastomosing channels in the pelvis.
- **External iliac artery:** The deep epigastric and deep circumflex iliac arteries branch from the external iliac artery before it travels under the inguinal ligament and into the femoral canal, where it becomes the femoral artery.
- **Anastomoses:** The **superior rectal artery** branches off the inferior mesenteric artery, the **middle rectal artery** branches off the anterior division of the hypogastric artery, and the **inferior rectal artery branches** off the pudendal artery (a branch of the hypogastric). This allows for redundant blood flow to the pelvis.

## VULVA AND PERINEUM

### External Anatomy

- The bony pelvic outlet is bordered anteriorly by the ischiopubic rami and posteriorly by the coccyx and sacrotuberous ligaments. The outlet can be divided into anterior and posterior triangles sharing a common base along a line between the ischial tuberosities.
- **Skin and subcutaneous layer** (Fig. 26-6). The subcutaneous tissue has two nondiscrete layers: Camper fascia and Colles fascia.
  - **Camper fascia** includes the continuation of this layer from the anterior abdominal wall.
  - **Colles fascia** is similar to Scarpa fascia of the anterior abdominal wall. It fuses posteriorly with the perineal membrane and laterally with the ischiopubic rami.

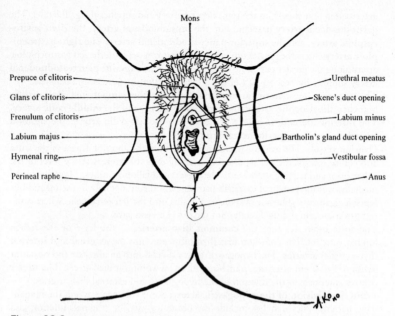

**Figure 26-6.** Vulva and perineum. (Original drawing by Alice W. Ko from Bankowski BJ, Hearne AE, Lambrou NC, eds. *The Johns Hopkins Manual of Gynecology and Obstetrics*, 2nd ed. Philadelphia, PA: Lippincott Williams & Wilkins, 2002.)

- The **mons (mons pubis, mons veneris)** is hair-bearing skin overlying adipose tissue that lies on the pubic bones.
- The **labia majora** extend posteriorly from the mons and contain similar hair-bearing skin. The labia majora contain the insertion of the round ligaments.
- The **labia minora** are hairless skin folds that split anteriorly to form the prepuce and frenulum of the clitoris. They overlie loosely organized connective tissue rather than adipose tissue.
- **Gland duct openings**
  - The **greater vestibular (Bartholin) gland** duct opening is seen on the posterolateral aspect of the vestibule 3 to 4 mm lateral to the hymenal ring.
  - The **minor vestibular gland** duct opening is seen in a line above the greater vestibular gland duct opening toward the urethra.
  - The **Skene ducts** are located inferolateral to the urethral meatus at approximately 5 and 7 o'clock.
- **Specialized glands**
  - **Holocrine sebaceous glands** are located in the labia majora and are associated with hair shafts.
  - **Apocrine sweat glands** are located lateral to the introitus and anus. **Hidradenitis suppurativa** can occur if these glands become chronically infected. **Hidradenomas** are neoplastic enlargements of these glands.
  - **Eccrine sweat glands** are also located laterally to the introitus and anus. They can enlarge and form a **syringoma**.

## Superficial Compartment of the Vulva

- This compartment lies between the subcutaneous layer and the perineal membrane (Fig. 26-7).
- The **clitoris** consists of the glans, a shaft that is attached to the pubis by a subcutaneous suspensory ligament, and paired crura that stem from the shaft and attach to the inferior aspect of the pubic rami.
- **Ischiocavernosus muscles** overlie the crura of the clitoris. They originate at the ischial tuberosities and free surfaces of the crura and insert into the upper crura and clitoral shaft.
- **Bulbospongiosus muscles** originate in the perineal body and insert into the clitoral shaft. They overlie the centrolateral aspects of the vestibular bulbs and Bartholin gland.
- **Superficial transverse perineal muscles** originate from the ischial tuberosities and insert into the perineal body.
- The **perineal body (central tendon of the perineum)** is connected anterolaterally with the bulbocavernosus muscle and anteriorly with the perineal membrane, which attaches the perineal body to the inferior pubic rami. The perineal body is attached laterally to the superficial transverse perineal muscles, posteriorly to the external anal sphincter, and superiorly to the distal rectovaginal fascia.
- The **vestibular bulbs** are paired erectile tissues that lie immediately under the skin of the vestibule and under the bulbocavernosus muscles.
- **Bartholin glands** lie between the bulbocavernosus muscles and the perineal membrane at the tail end of the vestibular bulb. Their ducts empty into the vestibular mucosa.

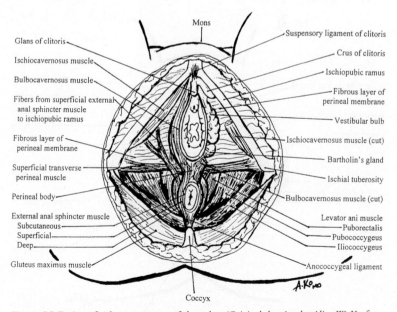

**Figure 26-7.** Superficial compartment of the vulva. (Original drawing by Alice W. Ko from Bankowski BJ, Hearne AE, Lambrou NC, eds. *The Johns Hopkins Manual of Gynecology and Obstetrics*, 2nd ed. Philadelphia, PA: Lippincott Williams & Wilkins, 2002.)

## Pelvic Floor

- The **pelvic floor** comprises the perineal membrane and the muscles of the pelvic diaphragm. It helps support the pelvic contents above the pelvic outlet.
- The **perineal membrane** is a triangular sheet of dense fibromuscular tissue that spans the anterior triangle. It provides support by attaching the urethra, vagina, and perineal body to the ischiopubic rami. The perineal membrane contains the dorsal and deep nerves and vessels to the clitoris.
- The **muscles of the pelvic diaphragm** comprise the levator ani and coccygeal muscles. These are covered by the superior and inferior fascias (Fig. 26-8).
  - **Levator ani muscles**
  - The **puborectalis** arises from the inner surface of the pubic bones and inserts into the rectum. Some fibers form a sling around the posterior aspect of the rectum.
  - The **pubococcygeus** arises from the pubic bones and inserts into the anococcygeal raphe and superior aspect of the coccyx.
  - The **iliococcygeus** arises from the **arcus tendineus levator ani** and inserts into the anococcygeal raphe and coccyx.
  - The **coccygeus muscle** arises from the ischial spine and inserts into the coccyx and lowest area of the sacrum. It lies cephalad to the sacrospinous ligament.

## Posterior Triangle

- This area is bounded bilaterally by the ischial tuberosities and posteriorly by the coccyx.
- **External anal sphincter**
  - The superficial portion is attached anteriorly to the perineal body and posteriorly to the coccyx.

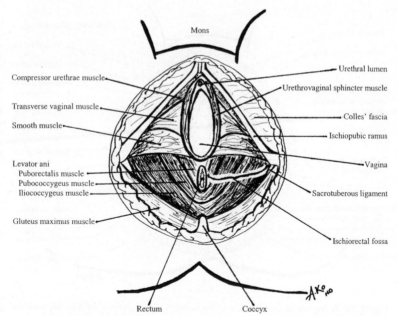

**Figure 26-8.** Pelvic diaphragm. (Original drawing by Alice W. Ko, from *The Johns Hopkins Manual of Gynecology and Obstetrics*, 2nd Ed. Philadelphia, PA: Lippincott Williams and Wilkins, 2002.)

- The deep portion encircles the rectum and blends in with the puborectalis muscle.
- **Internal anal sphincter:** This sphincter is a smooth muscle that is separated from the external sphincter by the intersphincteric groove as well as fibers from the longitudinal layer of the bowel.
- The **ischioanal fossa** contains the pudendal neurovascular trunk; it is bordered medially by the levator ani muscles and laterally by the obturator internus muscles. It has an anterior recess that lies above the perineal membrane and a posterior portion that lies above the gluteus maximus. This space allows for physiologic expansion of the rectum.

*Levels of Pelvic Support*

- The pelvic muscles and connective tissue are the primary support for the pelvic organs. The pelvic muscles consist of the **levator ani plate** (i.e., puborectalis, pubococcygeus, and ileococcygeus) and the coccygeus muscle. The **connective tissue attachments** (uterosacral/cardinal ligament complex and the endopelvic fascia) stabilize the pelvic organs in the correct position to receive support from the pelvic muscles. With pelvic muscle weakness or damage secondary to obstetric injury, the endopelvic fascia becomes the primary mechanism of support. This stress can attenuate, stretch, or break the endopelvic fascia resulting in failure of support of the pelvic organs and pelvic organ prolapse.
- There are three levels of support, as described by DeLancey:
  - **Level I** is the upper vertical axis or uterosacral/cardinal ligament complex. The uterosacral/cardinal ligament complex supports the cervix and upper vagina to maintain vaginal length and to keep the upper vaginal axis nearly horizontal so that it rests on the rectum and can be supported by the levator plate.
  - **Level II** is the horizontal axis or paravaginal supports. The pubocervical fascia and rectovaginal fascia spread over the vagina and condense into the ATFP to support the midvagina and create the anterior lateral vaginal sulci.
  - **Level III** is the lower vertical axis or perineal body, perineal membrane, and the superficial muscles (bulbocavernosus, ischiocavernosus, superficial and deep transverse perineal muscles). This supports and maintains the normal position of the distal one third of the vagina and introitus, which is nearly vertical in a standing female.
- Levels I, II, and III are connected through continuation of the endopelvic fascia.

# NERVES OF THE PELVIS AND PERINEUM

## Pelvic Diaphragm

- The **pudendal nerve** supplies the external anal sphincter and the urethral sphincter.
- The **anterior branch of the ventral ramus of S3 and S4** innervates the levator ani and coccygeal muscles.

## Perineum

- The **pudendal nerve** is the sensory and motor nerve of the perineum.
  - The pudendal nerve originates from the sacral plexus (S2 to S4), exits the pelvis through the greater sciatic notch, hooks around the ischial spine and sacrospinous ligament, and enters the pudendal canal **(canal of Alcock)** in the lesser sciatic notch. The pudendal nerve has several terminal branches:
    ○ The **clitoral nerve** runs along the superficial aspect of the perineal membrane to supply the clitoris.
    ○ The **perineal nerve** runs along the deep aspect of the perineal membrane. Its branches supply the muscles of the superficial compartment; subcutaneum; and skin of the vestibule, labia minora, and medial aspect of the labia majora.

○ The **inferior hemorrhoidal nerve (inferior rectal)** innervates the external anal sphincter and the perianal skin.

• A pudendal block is performed by injecting anesthetic just inferior to the ischial spine; this provides local analgesia for vaginal deliveries. This block may also be performed in cases of nerve injury or compression and resulting pudendal neuralgia.

## Nerve Injuries in Gynecologic Surgery

• Nerve injuries are encountered from positioning, incisions, use of retractors, and dissection (Table 26-1).

| TABLE 26-1 | Nerve Injuries in Gynecologic Surgery | | |
|---|---|---|---|
| **Nerve** | **Injury** | **Motor Loss** | **Sensory Loss** |
| Femoral L2–L4 | Deep retraction on psoas muscle, excessive hip flexion | Hip flexion, knee extension, knee DTR, leg adduction | Anteromedial thigh, anteromedial leg and foot |
| Lateral femoral cutaneous L2–L3 | Deep retraction on psoas muscle, excessive hip flexion | None | Anterolateral and posterolateral thigh |
| Genitofemoral branch L1–L2 | Pelvic sidewall dissection | None | Mons, labia majora, anterior superior thigh |
| Obturator L2–L4 | Retroperitoneal surgery, lymph node dissection, paravaginal defect repair | Leg abduction | Anteromedial thigh |
| Sciatic L4–S3 | Extensive endopelvic resection | Hip extension, knee flexion | Lateral calf, dorsomedial foot |
| Common peroneal L4–S2 | Compression from stirrups on lateral calf | Foot dorsiflexion and eversion | Lateral calf, dorsomedial foot |
| Tibial L4–S3 | Compression from stirrups on lateral calf | Foot plantar flexion and inversion | Toes, plantar foot |
| Iliohypogastric T12 | Transverse abdominal incision | None | Mons, labia, inner thigh |
| Ilioinguinal L1 | Transverse abdominal incision | None | Groin, symphysis pubis |

DTR, deep tendon reflex.
Adapted from Irvin W, Anderson W, Rice L. Minimizing the risk of nerve injury in gynecologic surgery. *Obstet Gynecol* 2004;103:374–382.

## LYMPHATIC DRAINAGE OF THE PELVIS

- The vulva and lower vagina drain to the **inguinofemoral lymph nodes** and then to the **external iliac nodes**. See Chapter 44.
- The cervix drains through the cardinal ligaments to the **pelvic nodes (hypogastric, obturator, and external iliac)** and then to the **common iliac and para-aortic lymph nodes**.
- The **uterus** drains through the broad ligament and intraperitoneal ligament to the **pelvic and para-aortic lymph nodes**.
- The **ovaries** drain to the **pelvic and para-aortic lymph nodes**.

## SUGGESTED READINGS

Ashton-Miller JA, DeLancey JO. Functional anatomy of the female pelvic floor. *Ann NY Acad Sci* 2007;1101:266–296.

DeLancey JO. Anatomic aspects of vaginal eversion after hysterectomy. *Am J Obstet Gynecol* 1992;166:1717–1728.

DeLancey JO. Structural anatomy of the posterior pelvic compartment as it relates to rectocele. *Am J Obstet Gynecol* 1999;180:815–823.

Law YM, Fielding JR. MRI of pelvic floor dysfunction: review. *Am J Roentgenol* 2008;191: S45–S53.

Weber AM, Walters MD. Anterior vaginal prolapse: review of anatomy and techniques of surgical repair. *Obstet Gynecol* 1997;89:311–318.

# 27 Perioperative Care and Complications of Gynecologic Surgery

Khara M. Simpson and Stacey A. Scheib

## PREOPERATIVE CARE

The main objectives of the **preoperative assessment** are:
- Completion of a thorough history and physical examination
- Selection of the ideal surgery
- Identification of potential limitations
- Optimization of the patient's medical condition

The goal is to decrease perioperative morbidity and complications and to optimize outcomes.

## Informed Consent

- **Informed consent** should include the rationale and explanation of the procedure as well as alternatives such as expectant management, nonsurgical interventions, and other surgical options. An interactive dialogue should occur between physician and patient. When more than one option is available, the surgeon should provide education and guidance without coercion. Ultimately, the patient must determine which of the options is appropriate.

- Risk discussion should address the specific procedure as well as general surgical risks and should be accompanied by a discussion of interventions intended to minimize those risks. These risks include, but are not limited to, bleeding and possible blood transfusion (Table 27-1), organ injury (bladder, ureter, bowel, vessel, or nerve), unanticipated organ removal, need for additional surgery, myocardial infarction, congestive heart failure, thromboembolic complications, infection, and perioperative death. Injury and failure rates should be cited based on personal data and current literature when available. Discussion of interventions such as perioperative antibiotics, deep vein thrombosis (DVT) prophylaxis, and postoperative incentive spirometry should be included. Possible changes in plans due to intraoperative surgical findings should be included in the consent document, as well as the possibility of a change in mode of access (e.g., laparoscopic to open procedure, vaginal to abdominal procedure). Documentation of the preoperative discussions and the patient's response and acceptance of risk, including informed refusal, is crucial.

## Medical Evaluation and Optimization

*Preoperative Evaluation*

- **Preoperative evaluation:** History and physical examination are essential for evaluating surgical eligibility and the need for further testing or consultation. Identifying occult disease and optimizing preexisting conditions are of utmost importance. Abnormal findings and comorbid conditions need to be evaluated appropriately. Routine health maintenance evaluation and screening should be considered especially in the absence of regular medical care. It may be beneficial for patients with complex preexisting conditions to be comanaged with a medical specialist. Preoperative consultation with an anesthesiologist is important for the medically

| TABLE 27-1 | Risks of Blood Transfusion |
|---|---|
| Bacterial contamination of platelet components | 1:12,000 |
| Bacterial contamination from packed red cells | 1:5 million |
| Hepatitis C virus | 1:1.6 million |
| Hepatitis B virus | 1:180,000 |
| HIV | 1:1.9 million |
| Fatal red cell hemolytic reaction | 1:250,000–1.1 million |
| Delayed red cell hemolysis | 1:1,000–1,500 |
| Transfusion-related acute lung injury (TRALI) | 1:5,000 |
| Febrile red cell nonhemolytic reaction | 1:100 |
| Allergic urticarial reaction | 1:100 |
| Anaphylactic reaction | 1:150,000 |

From Jones HW, Rock WA. Control of pelvic hemorrhage. In Rock JA, Jones HW, eds. *Te Linde's Operative Gynecology*, 9th ed. Philadelphia, PA: Lippincott Williams & Wilkins, 2003, with permission.

complicated patient, those with known difficult airways, and those with a history of anesthesia complications.

- **Preoperative testing and imaging:** Preoperative testing should be based on risk factors for abnormal physiology, including comorbid conditions, tobacco use, exercise intolerance, and irregular examination findings. Mild and even asymptomatic conditions that may be exacerbated by medical and surgical interventions should be anticipated. Guidelines are available from the American Society of Anesthesiologists (ASA) and American Heart Association (AHA)/American College of Cardiology.
  - Gynecologic patients are strongly advised to have current Pap smear and mammography results. Red blood cell type and screen should be performed on most patients, with exceptions made for very minor outpatient procedures. **A pregnancy test will be required on all reproductive age women (<50 years), and endometrial biopsy is recommended by the American College of Obstetricians and Gynecologists for women with abnormal uterine bleeding older than the age of 45 years.** Imaging should be individualized, but computed tomography (CT), magnetic resonance imaging (MRI), and pelvic ultrasound are helpful for illustrating anatomy and extent of disease, thereby optimizing surgical planning.
- **Preoperative cardiac evaluation:** The preoperative cardiac evaluation should be directed toward the detection of symptoms using directed questioning looking for conditions such as angina, heart failure, and arrhythmias. **For women older than the age of 50 years, general preoperative workup includes detailed history and physical examination, as well as electrocardiogram (ECG).** Additional cardiac workup depends on the planned surgery and the patient's functional status.
  - In low-risk procedures (minimally invasive, minimal blood loss and fluid shifts), no additional workup or treatment is needed, and most patients can proceed directly to surgery.
  - Major intraperitoneal surgery is considered intermediate risk with a reported cardiac risk of 1% to 5%. These patients should be assessed by their functional status.
  - Functional status is based on a patient's ability to perform 4 metabolic equivalents (METs) of activity or greater without chest pain, dyspnea, or fatigue.
    - A MET is a unit equal to the metabolic equivalent of oxygen uptake while quietly seated. Four METs is equal to walking on a flat surface or climbing a flight of stairs. If the patient can perform 4 METs of activity without dyspnea or fatigue, she is considered to have a normal functional status and may proceed to intermediate-risk surgery without further cardiac testing. If her functional status is <4 METs, additional evaluation may be indicated based on clinical risk factors that include history of ischemic heart disease, history of compensated or prior heart failure, history of cerebrovascular disease (stroke), diabetes mellitus, and chronic kidney disease (defined as a creatinine >2 mg/dL).
  - For gynecologic surgeries that are considered high risk (prolonged surgeries that involve large fluid shifts), patients with a functional capability <4 METs and one to three risk factors may warrant further cardiac testing, such as cardiac stress test or echocardiogram.

### Preoperative Management

- **Thromboembolic prophylaxis:** The approximate risk of DVT in hospitalized patients after major gynecology procedures is 10% to 40%. It is the standard of care to offer DVT prophylaxis (Table 27-2).
- **Antibiotic prophylaxis:** See Table 27-3 for preoperative antibiotic prophylaxis. Evidence supports the use of antibiotics in cases of hysterectomy, with data on abdominal and vaginal routes generalized to laparoscopic hysterectomy. Single-dose

**TABLE 27-2** Thromboprophylaxis for Gynecologic Procedures

| Procedure | Risks | Recommended Thromboprophylaxis |
|---|---|---|
| Minor procedures | No additional risk factors | Early and frequent ambulation |
| Entirely laparoscopic | No additional risk factors | Early and frequent ambulation |
| Entirely laparoscopic | VTE risk factors are present. | One or more of LMWH, LDUH, IPC, or GCS |
| Major gynecologic surgery | No additional risk factors | LMWH, LDUH, or IPC started just before surgery and used continuously while the patient is not ambulating |
| Major gynecologic surgery | VTE risk factors are present. | LMWH or LDUH three times daily or IPC started just before surgery and used continuously while the patient is not ambulating. Alternatives include combined LMWH or LDUH plus mechanical thromboprophylaxis with GCS or IPC, or fondaparinux. |
| Extensive surgery for malignancy | | Same as above for major surgery with VTE risks |

For major gynecologic procedures, recommend that thromboprophylaxis continue until discharge from hospital. For selected high-risk gynecology patients, including some of those who have undergone major cancer surgery or have previously had venous thromboembolism (VTE), consider continuing thromboprophylaxis after hospital discharge with LMWH for up to 28 days.

LMWH, low-molecular-weight heparin; LDUH, low-dose unfractionated heparin; IPC, intermittent pneumatic compression; GCS, graduated compression stockings.

Adapted from Geerts WH, Bergqvist D, Pineo GF, et al. Prevention of venous thromboembolism: American College of Chest Physicians Evidence-Based Clinical Practice Guidelines (8th ed.). *Chest* 2008;133(6)(suppl 1):381S–453S.

prophylaxis appears to be as effective as multiple doses, with less risk of adverse events and microbial resistance. To reduce surgical site infections (SSI), first-generation or second-generation cephalosporins are preferred for most patients or clindamycin with gentamicin for those with severe penicillin allergy.

- Antibiotics should be administered prior to incision. Antibiotics should be re-dosed according to half-life and blood loss (e.g., cefazolin is redosed every 3 to 4 hours or if >1,500 mL of blood loss).
- Postoperative antibiotic prophylaxis has not been shown to be effective.
- Preoperative treatment of bacterial vaginosis (BV) is recommended. BV is a known risk factor for SSI, and treatment with metronidazole 4 days prior to surgery has been demonstrated to decrease the risk of cuff cellulitis.
- **Antibiotic prophylaxis for subacute bacterial endocarditis:** The AHA no longer recommends routine prophylaxis for bacterial endocarditis for routine genitourinary (GU) or gastrointestinal (GI) tract procedures. One exception is in patients undergoing a GU or GI procedure in the setting of active infection.

**TABLE 27-3** Antibiotic Prophylaxis for Gynecologic Procedures

| Procedure | Antibiotic | Dose |
|---|---|---|
| Hysterectomy *or* Urogynecologic procedure, including those involving mesh | Cefazolin[1] | 1 or 2 g IV[2] |
| | Clindamycin[3] plus | 600 mg IV |
| | Gentamycin *or* | 1.5 mg/kg IV |
| | Aztreonam *or* | 400 mg IV |
| | Quinolone[4] | 600 mg IV |
| | Metronidazole plus | 1.5 mg/kg IV |
| | Gentamycin *or* | 600 mg IV |
| | Quinolone[4] | 400 mg IV |
| Laparoscopy[5] | None | |
| Laparotomy | None | |
| Hysteroscopy[6] | None | |
| Hysterosalpingogram[7] *or* chromopertubation[7] | Doxycycline | 100 mg BID PO × 5 days |
| D&C for induced abortion | Doxycycline | 100 mg 1 hr before procedure and 200 mg PO after *or* |
| | Metronidazole | 500 mg BID PO × 5 days |
| IUD insertion | None | |
| Endometrial biopsy | None | |
| Urodynamics | None | |

IV, intravenous; PO, by mouth; D&C, dilation and curettage; IUD, intrauterine device; BID, twice daily.
[1]Acceptable alternatives include cefotetan, cefoxitin, cefuroxime or ampicillin-sulbactam.
[2]A 2 g dose is recommended in women with a BMI ≥35 or weight greater than 100 kg or 220 lbs.
[3]Regimen of choice in patients with a history of immediate hypersensitivity to penicillin.
[4]Ciprofloxicin or levofloxacin or moxifloxacin.
[5]Including diagnostic and operative procedures (e.g., sterilization).
[6]Including diagnostic and operative procedures (e.g., endometrial ablation, sterilization).
[7]Only in cases with dilated fallopian tubes.
Adapted from American College of Obstetricians and Gynecologists. ACOG practice bulletin no. 104: antibiotic prophylaxis for gynecologic procedures. *Obstet Gynecol* 2009;113:1180–1189, with permission.

- For patients with a prosthetic cardiac valve, previous history of endocarditis, unrepaired cyanotic congenital heart defect including palliative shunts and conduits, completely repaired congenital heart defect with prosthetic material or device during the first 6 months after the procedure, repaired congenital heart defect with residual defect at the site or adjacent to the site of a prosthetic patch or device, cardiac transplant, or cardiac valvulopathy, it may be reasonable to use an antibiotic regimen that covers organisms known to cause endocarditis, particularly *enterococci*. Preferred agents include penicillin, ampicillin, piperacillin, or vancomycin.
- **Bowel preparation:** Mechanical bowel preparation has not been shown to improve visualization or outcomes. A clear liquid diet for 24 hours on the day before surgery is a safe alternative to a mechanical bowel preparation that can cause electrolyte abnormalities and dehydration.
- **Medications:** Antihypertensive, cardiac, reflux, psychiatric, asthma, and antiseizure medications should be taken on the morning of surgery, with a sip of water.

- Diabetic patients should take one third of the long-acting insulin, and those with an insulin pump should be on their basal rate. Oral hypoglycemics should not be taken on the day of surgery. Metformin should be stopped 2 days before surgery and not restarted for at least 48 hours after surgery due to the risk of lactic acidosis.
- Aspirin and Plavix should be discontinued 7 days before surgery; other nonsteroidal anti-inflammatory drugs should be stopped 3 days before surgery. Patients on an anticoagulant will require a detailed plan of management. Coumadin therapy should be discontinued 4 to 5 days prior to surgery and converted to subcutaneous low-molecular-weight heparin (LMWH). On the day of surgery, the morning dose of heparin is held and coagulation studies are drawn immediately before surgery to avoid operating with a hypocoagulable state.
- Patients who were treated with steroids within the last year on a long-term basis (e.g., prednisone >5 mg/day for >3 weeks) should receive intraoperative stress doses of steroids. Two options are hydrocortisone 50 or 100 mg intravenously or methylprednisolone 100 mg intravenously at the time of surgery. The steroids are continued for 24 hours postsurgery.
- Herbal supplements are discontinued 1 to 2 weeks prior to surgery, as many have anticoagulant or coagulopathic effects.
- These medication adjustments should be arranged in coordination with the patient's primary care physician. Postoperative instructions should address resumption of any discontinued medications.
- **Perioperative beta-blockade** should be continued for patients who are already on them to prevent cardiac events associated with surgery.

## INTRAOPERATIVE COMPLICATIONS

### Hemorrhage

- Incidence of **pelvic hemorrhage** in major gynecologic surgery is reported as 1% to 2% in abdominal hysterectomy and 0.7% to 2.5% for vaginal hysterectomy. Other procedures associated with higher rates of hemorrhage are Burch colposuspension, abdominal sacrocolpopexy, and lymph node dissection. Previous surgery, large malignant or benign masses, history of pelvic inflammatory disease, and endometriosis can cause anatomic distortion predisposing a patient to injury and pelvic hemorrhage.
  - Control of pelvic bleeding starts with **preventive measures**, such as proper patient positioning, choosing an appropriate incision to ensure adequate exposure, meticulous surgical technique, and limited blunt dissection. Once hemorrhage is encountered, communication with anesthesia and operating room staff is essential.
  - Hemorrhage management is centered on four basic actions: (a) assess vital signs, (b) obtain adequate intravenous access, (c) resuscitate with judicious use of fluid or blood components, and (d) achieve hemostasis.
    - **Direct pressure** should be applied to sites of bleeding, allowing time for proper identification and control with electrocautery, ligation, or surgical clips. Bleeding in the presacral area can also be managed with **bone wax** or **sterile tacks**.
    - **Hypogastric artery ligation** may be used for uncontrolled venous bleeding, as it lowers pulse pressure.
    - Topical hemostatic agents, such as fibrin glue, Gelfoam, and Surgicel, can be applied to small venous bleeding sites.
    - **Pelvic packing**, using moist laparotomy pads, may be used temporarily for continued hemorrhage or left intra-abdominally with postoperative intensive care

unit monitoring. The patient is usually returned to the operating room in 48 to 72 hours to remove the packs, irrigate, and close the abdomen.
- See also Chapter 3.
- **Postoperative bleeding** may be detected through changes in vital signs consistent with hypovolemia, patient restlessness, disproportionate pain relative to surgery or analgesics, abdominal ecchymosis, and abdominal distention. A larger than anticipated reduction in postoperative hematocrit should raise suspicion. These findings should prompt further evaluation to determine whether active bleeding is present. Orthostatic blood pressures, serial blood counts, and imaging studies (i.e., ultrasound or CT) should be performed as indicated. A stable hematoma can often be managed conservatively. Active bleeding requires blood replacement, and reexploration is often necessary. With the availability of interventional radiology, **pelvic artery embolization** has clinical success rates of 90% for postsurgical and posttraumatic hemorrhage and avoids the additional morbidity of reoperation.

## Ureteral Injury

- **Ureteral injury** rates have been reported from 0.4% to 2.5% during benign pelvic surgery, and only one third are recognized intraoperatively. Most commonly reported rates of injury are 0.1% to 1.7% during abdominal hysterectomy and 0% to 0.1% for vaginal hysterectomy. The highest rates are seen in laparoscopic surgery, with an odds ratio of 2.6 when compared to the abdominal route. During vaginal hysterectomy, the ureter can be traumatized at its entry point at the trigone. Laparoscopic procedures, especially ablation of endometriosis, carry an increased risk of ureteral injury near the uterosacral ligament.
- **Prevention and detection:** Steps taken to avoid ureteral injury during hysterectomy include development of the vesicouterine space, skeletonization of the uterine arteries, and cephalad traction on the uterus, all of which deflect the ureters laterally and downward. These measures are equally important in laparoscopic and abdominal surgery. The ureter can be visualized in the pararectal space on the medial leaf of the broad ligament. The pelvic ureter approaches within 1 cm of the infundibulopelvic ligament, lies approximately 1.5 cm lateral to the internal cervical os, and approaches within 0.9 cm of the upper third of the vagina. These distances are important during dissection, clamp placement, and in the consideration of thermal injury with the use of electrosurgery. Preoperative intravenous pyelograms (IVP) and ureteral stenting have a questionable role in decreasing ureter injury risk.
- **Intraoperative cystoscopy** with indigo carmine is an excellent test for assessing ureteral integrity and allows immediate corrective surgery to be undertaken if injury is detected. This technique is recommended for all urogynecologic surgery and major gynecologic surgery to identify and prevent sequelae of intraoperative urinary tract injury, as well as decrease liability from an undetected injury.
- **Management:** In cases of crush injury without transection, stenting the ureter for an extended period and placing a drain at the site of injury may be sufficient therapy. Complete transection above the pelvic brim or partial transection is repaired by suturing the defect end-to-end (**uretero-ureterostomy**). Reimplantation into the bladder (**uretero-neocystostomy**) is performed if the injury is within 6 cm of the ureterovesical junction. Mobilization of the bladder along the external iliac vessels with attachment to the psoas tendon (**psoas hitch**) can be used to bridge the gap and decrease tension at the anastomotic site when necessary. In cases of insufficient residual ureteral length, a Boari flap or ileal interposition can be performed. **Transuretero-ureterostomy** for injuries high in the pelvis is no longer recommended. Drains should be placed near the anastomosis to prevent urinoma

formation and detect leakage. Delayed diagnosis of a ureteral injury may require retrograde pyelography with cystoscopy and stent placement or percutaneous nephrostomy with antegrade stent placement. The recovery potential of the kidney depends on the duration of the obstruction, the degree of obstruction, the degree of backflow, the presence or absence of infection, and the extent to which each kidney was functional before the injury.

## Bladder Injury

- The rate of **bladder injury** in benign gynecologic surgery is 0.5% to 1%. The rate during abdominal hysterectomy is 0.2% to 2.3%, which is increased compared to the vaginal hysterectomy rate of 0.3% to 1.5%. Major lacerations may require mobilization of the bladder for tension-free repair. Multiple cystotomies may be joined into one defect. A two-layer closure with 2-0 or 3-0 synthetic absorbable suture is recommended, and the seal assessed by placing sterile milk, indigo carmine, or methylene blue retrograde into the bladder. A Foley or suprapubic catheter is left in place for 7 to 14 days. A small cystotomy that occurs with a trocar during placement of a mid-urethral sling requires catheterized bladder decompression for only 24 to 48 hours.
- A missed bladder or ureteral injury usually results in postoperative urinary ascites or urinoma, abdominal or flank pain, and distention with fever, chills, oliguria, nausea, and vomiting. These patients may have elevated blood urea nitrogen and creatinine levels and may respond to aggressive hydration and bladder rest. Unrecognized surgical injuries are the most common cause of GU fistulas in the developed world.

## Bowel Injury

- Inadvertent **bowel injury** occurs most often in gynecologic surgeries from an abdominal approach and is reported in 0.1% to 1% of abdominal hysterectomies and 0.1% to 0.8% of vaginal hysterectomies.
- A systematic evaluation of the bowel should be performed at the end of procedures where extensive lysis of adhesions is performed. Serosal injuries can be closed with permanent or delayed absorbable 3-0 suture. Gastrostomies, enterotomies, or colostomies may be closed in two layers using a continuous mucosal repair with 2-0 absorbable suture and an imbricating seromuscular interrupted 2-0 permanent suture.
  - Suture lines should be perpendicular to the longitudinal axis of the lumen to avoid luminal constriction. In cases of multiple enterotomies, the bowel may be resected and anastomosed. A nasogastric tube can be used for decompression in stomach and small bowel injuries. Distal colonic injury does not warrant colostomy except in cases of previous radiation or infection.

## Nerve Injury

- Malpositioning or retractor placement is the usual cause of **nerve injury** in gynecologic surgery. However, hematoma formation, a foreign body, or transection can also be complicating factors.
  - **Common peroneal nerve** injury is most often caused by compression at the lateral epicondyle from the stirrups and may result in a transient, postoperative foot drop.
  - **Lateral femoral cutaneous nerve** injury can result from placement of self-retaining retractors or hyperflexion of the hips in lithotomy position and results in anterior lateral thigh paresthesia and pain. One should be aware of the location, depth, and the exact pressure exerted by the lateral sidewall retractors on the iliopsoas muscle.

- **Femoral nerve** injury can result in motor or sensory injury, or both, and may occur when the deep retractors rest on the psoas muscle or when the thighs are severely flexed on the abdomen in the lithotomy position. Passing below the relatively firm inguinal ligament, the femoral nerve is vulnerable to compression at that point. Postoperatively, the patient may experience weakness in the quadriceps muscle and difficulty walking.
- The **sciatic nerve** can be injured when the surgical assistant rests on the dorsal aspect of the thigh during vaginal surgery or when the hip is flexed and the knee is suddenly straightened. This tends to happen more commonly with free hanging ("candy cane") stirrups. As with common peroneal nerve injury, this injury typically leads to foot drop.
- The **obturator nerve** may be injured during dissection or with leg positioning. Excessive external rotation at the hip may result in a stretch injury. Patients may complain of difficulty walking and will have weakness of the internal compartment muscles and demonstrate deficiency in adduction.
- The **iliohypogastric and ilioinguinal nerves** are at risk for injury or entrapment when a Pfannenstiel incision extends beyond the lateral margin of the inferior rectus abdominis muscle or during trocar placement and port site closure. Typically, patients report a sharp or burning pain radiating from the incision to the suprapubic area or paresthesias in this area.
- Most compression and stretch injuries resolve completely over several weeks to months. Physical therapy is required in cases with motor deficits. In cases of ilioinguinal or iliohypogastric injury, infiltration of local anesthesia in this area can help in diagnosis of this type of nerve injury and provide temporary relief of the symptoms. Neurectomy is usually indicated if a local nerve block is found to be effective. The key to treatment is prevention: proper patient positioning, periodic reassessment during long surgeries, proper retractor placement, and careful dissection.

## Complications Specific to Laparoscopy

- One analysis of 70,000 cases in Finland reported complication rates (per 1,000) as follows: overall, 3.6; major complications, 1.4; intestinal injury, 0.6; ureteral injury, 0.3; bladder injury, 0.3; and vascular injuries, 0.1.
- **Port placement:** The majority of injuries during laparoscopy occur during access. A recent Cochrane review found that Veress entry technique had an increased risk of preperitoneal insufflation and false tracking. However, open entry may be prudent in patients with a history of multiple lower abdominal surgeries or inflammatory bowel disease. The left upper quadrant or "Palmer point" is an alternate site for insertion of the Veress needle for creation of a pneumoperitoneum and primary trocar insertion when significant periumbilical adhesions are suspected. The gastric contents must be aspirated with a nasogastric or oral gastric tube prior to using this method. The skin incision is made between the left midclavicular and anterior axillary lines approximately two fingerbreadths below the left costal margin to avoid the superior epigastric vessels. The Veress needle is inserted perpendicularly and shallowly into the peritoneal cavity to allow insufflation; then, a 5-mm trocar can be inserted. This approach offers two advantages: (a) short distance between layers of the anterior abdominal wall and (b) less chance of adhesions in the left upper quadrant in patients with a history of prior abdominal surgery. During primary port placement, the small bowel, iliac artery, and colon are the most commonly injured structures. With secondary ports, abdominal wall vessels, iliac arteries, and aorta are at most risk for injury. A systematic review of the field should be performed in every case

after gaining primary access prior to Trendelenburg positioning. All secondary ports should be inserted under direct visualization.

- **Extraperitoneal insufflation of $CO_2$:** Misplacement of a Veress needle in the preperitoneal space causes this complication and can impair visualization due to peritoneal tenting. In most cases, $CO_2$ can be allowed to escape and needle placement attempted again. If this is not successful, open laparoscopy is performed. Mediastinal emphysema is an uncommon complication that requires observation for respiratory compromise and, in severe cases, may require ventilation.

- **Vessel injury:** The Veress needle or trocar may traumatize omental, mesenteric, major abdominal, or pelvic vessels. Trendelenburg position should never be obtained prior to trocar placement; the table should be flat. The sacral promontory should be palpated as a landmark of the aortic bifurcation. In thin patients, the Veress needle is directed at 45 degrees and in obese patients, at 90 degrees. The most accurate confirmation of peritoneal access is an opening pressure of <10 mm of Hg.

  - The *superficial epigastric* vessels may be identified by transillumination, especially in thinner patients; however, the deeper *inferior epigastric* vessels should be identified intra-abdominally prior to accessory trocar placement. The inferior epigastric vessels begin their cephalad course between the medial umbilical ligament and the entry point of the round ligament into the inguinal canal. The secondary trocars are inserted perpendicularly, lateral to the edge of the rectus muscles. Maintaining the perpendicular insertion until the peritoneal cavity is entered is essential to prevent damage to the inferior epigastric vessels.

  - Management of inferior epigastric vessel injury includes balloon tamponade with a Foley or suture ligature using a Carter-Thomason or Endo Close device. Consider enlarging the incision at the trocar site or proceeding to laparotomy to improve visualization. Damage to major retroperitoneal vessels generally requires emergent laparotomy and consultation with a vascular surgeon.

- **Bowel injury:** Intestinal injuries have been reported at a rate of <0.5%. Approximately half of these injuries occur on entry and half occur as a result of electrocautery, either direct thermal injury or due to coupling. Most bowel injuries are not recognized at the time of surgery. If bowel perforation with the Veress needle is suspected, the needle should be withdrawn and insufflation attempted at another site. If the laparoscope enters the bowel lumen, it should be left in place to limit contamination and to facilitate identification of the injured site. Generally, puncture sites from the pneumoperitoneum needle can be managed conservatively. Repair may be accomplished by routine laparoscopic or open techniques. A thermal injury is often treated by resection or oversewing of the bowel in cases of smaller injury. Monopolar energy has been shown to have a thermal spread up to several centimeters away; therefore, extreme caution should be used when using electrosurgery on strands of tissues attached to bowel. Symptoms of bowel injury can range from increased pain at the trocar site to abdominal distention and diarrhea to sepsis. CT scan is the best imaging study to confirm the diagnosis. Access injuries or traumatic injuries often present early, in the first hours or days postoperatively. Thermal injury may present late (3 to 7 days after surgery) due to delayed necrosis at the site of injury and subsequent bowel perforation. Unrecognized bowel injury is one of the most common causes of postoperative death from laparoscopy.

- **Bladder injury:** Prevention is best achieved by decompression of the bladder with a Foley, avoiding low suprapubic ports and with direct visualization during trocar placement. Bladder injury is not restricted to port placement and also occurs during dissection of the vesicouterine space. Low anterior fibroids and history of prior cesarean section increase that risk. Injury may be detected by the presence of air or blood in the drainage bag of an indwelling Foley catheter. The size of the injury dictates treatment. Needle perforations can be managed expectantly. Lacerations <10 mm long will heal spontaneously if the bladder is drained continuously with a Foley catheter for 3 to 4 postoperative days. Larger injuries require suturing, as described earlier. This can be performed laparoscopically by surgeons experienced in laparoscopic suturing technique.

- **Ureteral injury:** Laparoscopic-assisted vaginal hysterectomy is the leading gynecologic procedure in which ureteral injury occurs. Electrosurgical instruments are also associated with injuries during laparoscopic surgery. Careful exposure and identification of anatomy is the best way to reduce risk of injury to the ureter. If ureteral injury is suspected, intravenous indigo carmine should be administered and cystoscopy performed intraoperatively.

- **Dehiscence and hernia:** The overall incidence of incisional dehiscence and hernia is approximately 0.02% and is greater with trocar-cannula systems >10 mm in diameter. Richter hernias, which typically have a delayed diagnosis, contain a portion of the intestinal wall in a peritoneal defect. General recommendations for fascial closure are to close all defects >10 mm and defects >5 mm that are lateral to the rectus sheath after significant tissue extraction or peritoneal stretch. Both fascia and peritoneum should be closed.

## Complications Specific to Hysteroscopy

- **Fluid overload:** Fluids can be delivered into the uterine cavity with sufficiently high pressure to allow intravasation of the distention media into the vascular system. Serious complications can occur if intravasation is excessive. The risks and allowable fluid deficits vary according to type of distention media used. Absorption is increased as a function of increasing flow pressure, uterine size, and operative time. Automated fluid-monitoring systems have made the exact measurements of input and output of the distending medium much easier. The surgeon should be aware of the deficit at all times and should be updated frequently by operating room staff (Table 27-4).
  - Electrolyte-containing media (normal saline and lactated Ringer) are relatively safe, but fluid overload is still possible. These media can be used with bipolar instruments. Alternative fluid media carry increased risk of overload.
  - Three percent sorbitol and 1.5% glycine are low-viscosity, hypotonic, electrolyte-free solutions. When absorbed into the bloodstream, they cause hyponatremia, arrhythmias, cerebral edema, coma, and death.
  - Mannitol 5% is an iso-osmolar media that can also cause hyponatremia.
  - Hyskon, a high-viscosity 32% solution of dextran 70, provides a clear field because it does not mix with blood. In the bloodstream, it acts as a volume expander, potentially leading to acute noncardiogenic pulmonary edema. Dextran molecules can trigger disseminated intravascular coagulation and anaphylaxis. In an acute setting, dextran molecules must be removed from the circulation with plasmapheresis.

- **Uterine perforation** may be managed conservatively, particularly with a blunt instrument, with close monitoring, or overnight hospitalization. In cases of active bleeding or perforation with electrosurgical instruments, conversion to laparoscopy or laparotomy is required.

| TABLE 27-4 | Guidelines for Fluid Management during Hysteroscopy |

Fluid input and output should be monitored preoperatively and intraoperatively by an individual assigned to this task. Results should be reported to the surgical team at regular intervals.

Low-viscosity, electrolyte-poor fluids: A fluid deficit of 750 mL implies excessive intravasation of fluid. Surgeon should consider termination of procedure in patients with high cardiovascular risk or comorbid conditions.

Nonelectrolyte solutions: A fluid deficit of 1,000–1,500 mL implies excessive intravasation of fluid but depends on patient weight and other factors. The infusion should be stopped, procedure concluded, and electrolyte and fluid status assessed. Diuretics and other interventions should be initiated as needed.

Electrolyte solutions: A fluid deficit of 2,000 mL implies excessive intravasation of fluid. Management is same as previous.

Discontinuing the infusion at lower thresholds should be considered in outpatient settings, with limited acute care and laboratory services.

Automated fluid monitoring systems facilitate early recognition of fluid imbalance.

Adapted from Loffer FD, Bradley LD, Brill AI, et al. Hysteroscopic fluid monitoring guidelines. The ad hoc committee on hysteroscopic training guidelines of the American Association of Gynecologic Laparoscopists. *J Am Assoc Gynecol Laparosc* 2000;7:167–168, with permission; American College of Obstetricians and Gynecologists. ACOG technology assessment in obstetrics and gynecology, number 4, August 2005: hysteroscopy. *Obstet Gynecol* 2005;106(2):439–442, with permission.

## POSTOPERATIVE COMPLICATIONS

### Postoperative Fever

- A commonly accepted diagnosis of **fever** requires a temperature at or above 38°C (100.4°F) on two occasions at least 4 hours apart. Febrile morbidity within the first 48 hours of surgery has been estimated to occur in up to 50% of gynecologic surgery patients. Atelectasis, an often cited reason for low-grade febrile illnesses, has not been shown to be causal for fever during this period in the literature. Noninfectious etiologies, such as medications, malignant hyperthermia, thrombotic or embolic events, ureteral injuries, cardiovascular events, endocrine abnormalities, and transfusion reactions, should be included in the differential diagnosis and workup for postoperative fever.
- **Evaluation:** Evaluation should include a review of the patient's history and a thorough examination, with specific attention to sites as follows: pulmonary examination; palpation of the suprapubic region and costovertebral angles; evaluation of incisions, catheter and line sites, and extremities; and pelvic examination to evaluate the vaginal cuff for cellulitis, hematoma, or abscess.
- **Testing:** Initial laboratory and radiologic assessment should be tailored to the individual patient. Complete blood count with differential, urinalysis, and urine culture should be performed. Urinalysis will be of limited value in patients with bladder catheters. Blood cultures seldom yield positive results except in patients with high fever or risk factors for endocarditis and are most sensitive when drawn at the time of the fever. Imaging studies may include chest and abdominal radiographs, IVP,

ultrasonography of the pelvis and kidneys, contrast bowel studies, and CT scan. Chest CT or ventilation-perfusion (V/Q) scan should also be considered to rule out pulmonary embolism (PE).

## Postoperative Infection

- **Urinary tract infection:** The bladder is a common site of infection in surgical patients, largely due to contamination with indwelling Foley catheters. Pyelonephritis is a rare complication. The treatment is hydration and antibiotic therapy tailored to the pathogen.
- **Respiratory infection:** Preventive measures are early ambulation and intensive respiratory therapy (i.e., incentive spirometry, chest physical therapy) for reversal of hypoventilation and atelectasis. Patient education prior to surgery has an important role in compliance with postoperative incentive spirometry. Patients at risk of postoperative pneumonia include those with an ASA status of 3 or higher, preoperative hospital stay of 2 days or longer, surgery lasting 3 hours or longer, surgery in the upper abdomen or thorax, nasogastric suction, postoperative intubation, or a history of smoking or obstructive lung disease. Smoking cessation should be encouraged preoperatively, not only for respiratory complications but also for wound healing.

## Wound Infection

- **Prevention:** Risk factors for SSI include age, nutritional status, diabetes, smoking, obesity, coexistent infections at a remote body site, colonization with microorganisms, altered immune response, and length of preoperative stay.
- **Surgical closure:** Studies in cesarean section patients have shown closure of the subcutaneous fat compared with nonclosure reduces wound complications (defined as hematoma, seroma, wound infection, wound separation). In women with fat thickness >2 cm, suture closure of subcutaneous fat decreases the risk of wound disruption. Further trials are justified to investigate suturing materials and techniques. Whether these findings can be extrapolated to gynecologic surgery is unclear. Recent meta-analyses have failed to show that the routine use of closed suction drains prevents surgical infections.
- **Wound care:** Wound care has recently shifted away from an aggressive cleaning approach to one that emphasizes a clean but moist environment and minimizes the mechanical irritation caused by frequent dressing changes. Hydrogel applications play an important role, and vacuum systems can aid in wound drainage and facilitation of blood flow to the wound, resulting in a seemingly more rapid closure.

## Incisional or Vaginal Cuff Cellulitis

- Fever, leukocytosis, and pain localizing to the pelvis may accompany a severe cellulitis in which adjacent pelvic tissues are involved. Broad-spectrum antibiotic therapy should be initiated. If an abscess is suspected at the cuff or incision, drainage is indicated in the operating room or under ultrasound guidance. Intra-abdominal abscesses are characterized by persistent fever and leukocytosis. Radiologic confirmation with ultrasonography or CT scan is usually needed for diagnosis.
- Treatment involves parenteral antibiotics, with possible drainage in cases of large collections or failure to improve on antibiotics alone. Sonographic or CT scan–guided drain placement has obviated the need for surgical exploration in many circumstances. Reexploration in cases of active infection or abscess is approached with reservation due to associated high morbidity.

## Necrotizing Fasciitis

- Group A *Streptococcus* can cause a progressive, inflammatory infection of the deep fascia, with necrosis of the subcutaneous tissues. Surgeons must be acutely aware of this potentially life-threatening complication in any patient with a wound infection. Clinically, the infection results in extensive soft tissue destruction, including necrosis of skin, subcutaneous tissue, and muscle. Erythema and induration around the wound should be marked and followed closely. Extensive and aggressive surgical debridement and broad-spectrum antibiotic therapy are warranted at first suspicion. Treatment delay and obesity increase an already high mortality rate.

## Venous Thromboembolism

- **DVT:** DVT can cause unilateral lower extremity swelling, pain, and erythema. A palpable cord may be detected. Duplex Doppler ultrasonographic imaging has replaced venography as the gold standard for diagnosing DVT.
- **PE:** The signs and symptoms of PE include anxiety, shortness of breath, tachypnea, chest pain, hypoxia, tachycardia, and mental status changes. Symptoms should prompt a thorough evaluation; chest radiograph, ECG, and arterial blood gas assessment are the first-line tests. The chest radiograph helps distinguish between pneumonia and embolism. ECG findings are usually nonspecific except for tachycardia, but they help rule out an ischemic cardiac event. Laboratory evaluation with arterial blood gas test may show hypoxemia, hypocapnia, respiratory alkalosis, and an increased arterial-alveolar gradient.

### Imaging

- Radionucleotide imaging (V/Q scan) and contrast-enhanced CT arteriography are the current studies available for the evaluation of a suspected PE. V/Q scans have a high sensitivity but a low specificity. Contrast-enhanced CT arteriography is rapid, easily accessible in most large hospitals, and less prone to interference from other underlying pulmonary disease. Its sensitivity is greatest for detecting emboli in the main, lobar, or segmental pulmonary arteries. In most institutions, the CT arteriography has replaced the V/Q scan as the first-line diagnostic imaging study.

### Therapy

- Intravenous unfractionated heparin (UFH) has been the traditional treatment for DVT and PE. Recent studies have established that LMWH and the pentasaccharide fondaparinux are equivalent to UFH. The half-life of LMWH is longer, the dose response is more predictable, and less bleeding may occur while producing an equivalent antithrombotic effect. When using UFH, oral therapy with Coumadin is started as early as possible, and the patient can discontinue UFH when a therapeutic international normalized ratio value is reached. Placement of a vena caval filter may be necessary in patients with acute thromboembolism and active bleeding or a high potential for bleeding, patients who are on medical therapy with a history of multiple venous thrombi, and patients with a history of heparin-induced thrombocytopenia. Bleeding that occurs after the use of heparin-related compounds can be reversed with protamine sulfate; Coumadin-related bleeding can be reversed with vitamin K or with plasma or factor IX concentrates. The most effective treatment is prevention. See also Chapter 20.

## Ileus and Bowel Obstruction

- **Diagnosis:** Infection, peritonitis, electrolyte disturbances, extensive manipulation of the GI tract, and prolonged procedures may cause postoperative ileus. Postoperative adhesions occur in about 25% but can be up to 90% of patients who undergo major gynecologic surgery and represent one of the most common causes of intestinal obstruction. The prevalence of ileus or small bowel obstruction following hysterectomy is 0.2% to 2.2%. Nausea, vomiting, and distention may be present with both. Absent and hypoactive bowel sounds are more likely to occur with ileus, whereas borborygmi, rushes, and high-pitched tinkles are more characteristic of postoperative obstruction. Abdominal radiographs show distended loops of large and small bowel, with gas present in the rectum in the setting of ileus. Single or multiple loops of distended bowel with air-fluid levels are seen in postoperative obstruction. These findings may be difficult to distinguish in the early postoperative period. In prolonged cases, it may be helpful to obtain a study with oral contrast to identify a transition point.

- **Treatment:** Ileus is treated with bowel rest, intravenous fluids, electrolyte repletion, and nasogastric suction in cases of persistent vomiting. Most cases of partial obstruction will respond to conservative management with bowel rest and nasogastric decompression. Increasing abdominal pain, progressive distention, fever, leukocytosis, or acidosis should increase the suspicion for complete bowel obstruction, which may require reexploration. In cases with delayed improvement, a CT scan may help identify bowel perforation or abscess. Parenteral nutrition should also be considered in patients with prolonged GI compromise.

## Diarrhea

- **Diarrhea** is not uncommon after abdominal and pelvic surgery. Prolonged or multiple episodes, however, may represent a pathologic process, such as impending small bowel obstruction, colonic obstruction, or pseudomembranous colitis. *Clostridium difficile*–associated colitis may result from exposure to any antibiotics; stool testing can confirm clinical suspicions. Extended oral metronidazole therapy and hydration are needed for adequate treatment, and oral vancomycin may be necessary in refractory cases.

## Genitourinary Fistulae

- In the United States, most **GU fistulae** are the result of pelvic surgery, usually after an abdominal hysterectomy for benign conditions. In the developing world, most fistulas are due to obstetric trauma secondary to absent or poor obstetric care. Patients may present with persistent vaginal discharge or recurrent urinary tract infections.
- The simplest initial test for a GU fistula is the tampon test. A tampon is inserted into the vagina. The bladder is then filled with methylene blue or indigo carmine through a Foley catheter. The patient is given an oral dose of Pyridium. The appearance of blue dye on the tampon suggests a vesicovaginal fistula. An orange tampon is suggestive of a ureteral-vaginal fistula. Fluid pooling in the vagina can also be sent for a creatinine level. Further workup may include IVP, cystoscopy, voiding cystourethrogram, retrograde ureteral studies, and MRI. Simple fistulas often resolve with drainage by either Foley catheter or percutaneous nephrostomy tube placement to allow healing and decreased inflammation. Surgical repair is necessary if this is unsuccessful.

## SUGGESTED READINGS

American College of Obstetricians and Gynecologists. ACOG practice bulletin no. 104: antibiotic prophylaxis for gynecologic procedures. *Obstet Gynecol* 2009;113:1180–1189.

Douketis JD, Berger PB, Dunn AS, et al. The perioperative management of antithrombotic therapy: American College of Chest Physicians Evidence-Based Clinical Practice Guidelines (8th ed.). *Chest* 2008;133(6)(suppl 1):299S–339S.

Jones HW, Rock WA. Control of pelvic hemorrhage. In Rock JA, Jones HW, eds. *Te Linde's Operative Gynecology*, 9th ed. Philadelphia, PA: Lippincott Williams & Wilkins, 2003.

Tapson VF. Acute pulmonary embolism. *N Engl J Med* 2008;358(10):1037–1052.

Wilson W, Taubert KA, Gewitz M, et al. Prevention of infective endocarditis: guidelines from the American Heart Association. *Circulation* 2007;116(15):1736–1754.

# 28 Infections of the Genital Tract

Sangini Sheth and Jean M. Keller

## INFECTIONS OF THE LOWER GENITAL TRACT

Symptoms caused by **infections of the lower genital tract** are among the most common presenting complaints of gynecologic patients. This chapter reviews the following: vulvar infections, parasitic infections, ulcerative lesions, vaginitis, cervicitis, and pelvic inflammatory disease (PID). Urinary tract infections are covered in Chapter 16.

### Vulvar Infections

*Human Papillomavirus*

- Human papillomavirus (HPV) infection is the most common sexually transmitted disease (STD) in the United States, with an estimated 80% of sexually active women having acquired genital HPV by the age of 50 years. Most HPV infection is asymptomatic or subclinical, with the majority of patients clearing the infection within 2 years.

- There are over 100 types of HPV, of which approximately 30 are mucosal and can infect the lower genital tract in women. HPV types 6 and 11 cause ***condyloma acuminata*** or genital warts. HPV can be classified as low-, intermediate-, and high-risk for the development of **squamous cell carcinoma**, with the majority of cervical cancer caused by HPV types 16 and 18 (see Chapter 45).

- HPV prevalence is highest among 20- to 24-year-olds. Risk factors for HPV infection include number of sexual partners, history of other sexually transmitted infections (STIs), smoking, and immune deficiency such as HIV or use of immunosuppressive medications.

- **Signs and symptoms** of genital warts include soft, sessile, and/or verrucous lesions on any mucosal or dermal surface that range in size and formation. Lesions are usually multifocal and asymptomatic, although itching, burning, bleeding, vaginal discharge, and pain can occur.

- **Diagnosis:** Genital warts are usually diagnosed by gross inspection, and colposcopic examination may aid in the identification of cervical or vaginal lesions. HPV testing is not warranted for the diagnosis of genital warts and results would not alter management. Biopsy is recommended if there is no response to standard therapy; the lesions worsen with therapy; there are hyperpigmented, indurated, fixed, ulcerated, bleeding, or atypical lesions; if the patient is immunocompromised; or if the diagnosis is uncertain. Condyloma acuminatum must be differentiated from the lesion of secondary syphilis, condyloma lata.

- **Treatment:** Treatment is indicated for cosmetic benefit and to address symptoms. There are multiple modalities for the treatment of genital warts, including surgical excision, application of topical cytotoxic or keratolytic agents, cytodestructive techniques, and immune modulators. No single treatment method has been shown to be optimal and therefore treatment should be based on patient preference and provider experience. Clinical factors to consider in choosing a treatment modality include anatomic location, size, morphology, and number of lesions. Additional factors that might influence treatment choice include cost of treatment, convenience, and side effects. Lesions may spontaneously regress and recur. A combination of approaches may be required. No therapy can ensure complete eradication of the virus and it remains unclear whether treatment reduces further transmission (Table 28-1). Most lesions resolve within 3 months of treatment; however, recurrence rates range from 30% to 70%.

  - Complications from treatment include hypo- or hyperpigmentation of treated areas with ablative or immune-modulating modalities. Rarely, abnormal scarring or chronic pain can occur.

- **Prevention:** Two types of HPV vaccine are licensed by the U.S. Food and Drug Administration (FDA). Cervarix is a bivalent vaccine that protects against HPV types 16 and 18, which accounts for 70% of all cervical cancer. Gardasil is a quadrivalent vaccine against types 16 and 18, as well as types 6 and 11 found in 90% of genital warts. The HPV vaccine is recommended for female patients 9 to 26 years old and male patients 9 to 21 years old but can be given up to 26 years of age. Vaccination does not replace routine cervical cancer screening. See also Chapters 45 and 46.

*Molluscum Contagiosum*

- **Molluscum** is a benign poxvirus infection of the skin found worldwide but is most common in the developing world. It is spread by skin contact (sexual or nonsexual), autoinoculation, and fomites. The incubation period ranges from several weeks to months.

- **Signs and symptoms** include the appearance of dome-shaped papules with central umbilication ranging from 2 to 5 mm in diameter. Multiple lesions may arise but generally are fewer than 20. The lesions are usually asymptomatic but occasionally pruritic and may become inflamed and swollen. They are usually self-limited, lasting for 6 to 12 months, but may take as long as 4 years to resolve.

- **Diagnosis:** The characteristic appearance of molluscum contagiosum lends itself to clinical diagnosis by gross inspection. When in doubt, a crush preparation (i.e., microscopic examination of white, waxy material expressed from a nodule) can be performed. Intracytoplasmic eosinophilic inclusion bodies (molluscum bodies) inside keratinocytes confirm the diagnosis. Immunocompromised patients with

**TABLE 28-1    Treatment Options for Genital Warts**

| Therapy | Application | Clearance Rate (%) | Recurrence Rate (%) | Use in Pregnancy |
|---|---|---|---|---|
| **Patient applied** | | | | |
| Imiquimod 5% cream | Apply three times a week at bedtime for up to 16 wk. Wash the area with soap and water 6–10 hr after application. | 40–77 | 5–19 | Contraindicated |
| Podofilox 0.5% solution or gel | Apply bid for 3 d, no treatment for 4 d; repeat the cycle for up to four times. Do not exceed 10 cm$^2$ area of treatment or 0.5 mL volume of podofilox per day. | 68–88 | 16–34 | Contraindicated |
| Sinecatechins 15% ointment | Apply three times daily (0.5 cm strand to each wart) until complete resolution of warts (do not exceed 16 wk of treatment). Do not use in immunosuppressed patients or those with clinical genital herpes or open wounds. | 54–57 | 10 | Contraindicated |
| **Provider administered** | | | | |
| Podophyllin resin at 10%–25% in benzoin | Can be repeated one or two times weekly, as needed | 38–79 | 21–65 | Contraindicated |
| 5-Fluorouracil epinephrine gel | Intralesion injection weekly for up to 6 wk | 61 | 50–60 | |

| Interferons | Inject at the edge of and beneath the wart with a 26- to 32-gauge needle. | 36–53 | 21–25 | Not recommended |
| Topical trichloroacetic acid or bichloroacetic acid (80%–90% solution) | Apply small amount one or two times weekly until the wart sloughs off. Typical course is six treatments. | 81 | 36 | Permitted |
| Excisional procedures | Electrocautery or sharp excision may be employed. | 89–93 | 19–22 | Only if obstructing vaginal delivery |
| Cryotherapy with liquid nitrogen | Can be repeated one or two times weekly until resolved | 70–96 | 25–39 | Permitted |
| $CO_2$ laser excision | | 72–97 | 6–49 | Not recommended |

bid, twice a day.
From Workowski KA, Berman S; Centers for Disease Control and Prevention. Sexually transmitted diseases treatment guidelines, 2010. *MMWR Recomm Rep* 2010;59(RR-12):1–110, with permission.

HIV/AIDS or other conditions can develop giant lesions (>15 mm in diameter) and large numbers of lesions that may be resistant to standard therapy.

- **Treatment:** Molluscum contagiosum is usually self-limited. Multiple regimens have been evaluated in clinical trials, with none being convincingly efficacious. Many practitioners employ watchful waiting. Treatment should be considered, however, in immunosuppressed individuals and those with sexually transmitted lesions that risk infecting their partners. Lesion visibility and patient preference may prompt therapy, which consists of evacuation of the core material with cryofreezing, curettage, or laser ablation.

## Parasites

### Pediculosis Pubis

- An ectoparasite, *Phthirus pubis* is usually restricted to the pubic, perineal, and perianal areas but may infect the eyelids and other body parts. It can be transmitted sexually or via close contact through shared bedding or clothing. The parasite deposits eggs at the base of the hair follicle. The incubation period is 1 week and the crab louse lives for about 6 weeks but dies within 24 hours without blood.
- **Symptoms** of infection include intense pruritus in the affected area, sometimes accompanied by maculopapular lesions. Occurrence of a large number of bites over a short period may lead to systemic manifestations, such as mild fever, malaise, or irritability.
- **Diagnosis** is made by gross visualization of lice, larvae, or nits in the pubic hair or microscopic identification of crablike lice under oil.

### Scabies

- **Scabies** is caused by the mite *Sarcoptes scabiei* var. *hominis*. It is transmitted via prolonged close contact (sexual or nonsexual) and may infect any part of the body, especially flexural surfaces of the elbows, wrists, finger webs, axilla, genitals, and buttocks.
- Fomite transmission is considered possible through clothing, bedding, or towels. The adult female burrows beneath the skin, lays eggs, and travels quickly across the skin. Crusted or Norwegian scabies is highly infectious and is an aggressive infestation in immunodeficient, debilitated, or malnourished persons, and is associated with increased treatment failure.
- **Symptoms** include the insidious onset of severe intermittent pruritus approximately 3 to 6 weeks after the initial exposure. Subsequent infections can become symptomatic within 24 hours of reinfection. The intense pruritus may worsen at night and include most of the body. The characteristic lesion is the burrow, a 1- to 10-mm curving track that serves to house the mite. Other lesions include papules and vesicles.
- **Diagnosis** can often be made clinically based on history and gross appearance of the burrows. Skin scrapings can be obtained for microscopic examination under oil.
- **Treatment** (Table 28-2) for pediculosis pubis and scabies requires an agent that kills both adult organisms and eggs. Treatment should include decontamination of clothing and bed linens with dry cleaning or machine washing and drying with hot cycle. Treat pruritus with antihistamines.
  - Toxic effects of lindane include seizures and aplastic anemia. This agent is not recommended for use in pregnant or lactating women, children younger than age 2 years, or patients with extensive dermatitis.

| TABLE 28-2 | Treatment Options for Parasites | |
| --- | --- | --- |
| | Pediculosis Pubis | Scabies |
| Permethrin (Nix) cream—*safe in pregnancy* | Apply 1% cream rinse to the affected areas, wash off after 10 min, and comb the infested areas with a fine-toothed comb. | Apply 5% cream to all areas of the body from the neck down and wash off after 8–14 hr. |
| Pyrethrins with piperonyl butoxide—*safe in pregnancy* | Apply to the affected area and wash off after 10 min. | — |
| Ivermectin | 250 μg/kg orally, repeated in 2 wk | 200 μg/kg orally, repeated in 2 wk |
| Malathion | 0.5% lotion applied for 8–12 hr and washed off | — |
| Lindane 1% (Kwell) lotion, cream, or shampoo—*not for use in pregnancy* | — | Not first line due to toxicity. Apply 1 oz of lotion or 30 g of cream in a thin layer to all areas of the body from the neck down and thoroughly wash off after 8 hr. |

- Treat pruritus with antihistamines.
- Clothes and linens should be laundered in hot water and heat dried or removed from body contact for at least 72 hr.
- Sexual partners should be treated. Infected individuals should be tested for other sexually transmitted infections.

From Workowski KA, Berman S; Centers for Disease Control and Prevention. Sexually transmitted diseases treatment guidelines, 2010. *MMWR Recomm Rep* 2010;59(RR-12):1–110, with permission.

## Genital Ulcers

- The most common infectious causes of genital ulcers in young, sexually active women are herpes simplex virus (HSV) and *Treponema pallidum* (syphilis). Less common causes include chancroid and donovanosis. Genital herpes is the most prevalent. All of these lesions are associated with increased risk of HIV acquisition. A patient presenting with genital ulcers should be evaluated for syphilis, herpes, and *Haemophilus ducreyi* in areas where chancroid is prevalent, as well as HIV if status is unknown.

### Genital Herpes

- At least 50 million people in the United States have HSV-2 genital herpes, a chronic STI. Multiple types of herpesvirus have been identified. Historically, HSV-2 accounts for the majority of genital infections; however, HSV-1 now accounts for up to 50% of first-episode cases. HSV-1 genital infections are less likely to recur and less commonly result in asymptomatic viral shedding. The majority of persons infected with HSV-2 remain undiagnosed and intermittent viral shedding accounts for most HSV transmission.

- **Clinical diagnosis** of genital herpes is both insensitive and nonspecific. The classic presentation of multiple, painful, vesicular, or ulcerative lesions is absent in many patients. Herpetic outbreaks can last as long as 2 to 6 weeks in a first-episode primary infection and up to 7 days in recurrent outbreaks. Classically, lesions are preceded by vulvar paresthesias or pruritus, followed by the formation of multiple vesicles that coalesce into ulcerations, which may be painful. Outbreaks are self-limiting, and lesions heal without scar formation. The prodrome of itching or burning in the affected area is important for counseling patients on when to start antiviral therapy because systemic symptoms are usually absent. The majority of patients with HSV-2 will experience recurrent outbreaks in the first year with declining frequency over time. Patients should be counseled that asymptomatic shedding of virus with possible transmission to sexual partners can occur in the absence of outbreaks.

- **Diagnosis:** Clinical suspicion is based on history and the appearance of lesions. Obtain laboratory confirmation with type-specific virologic and serologic testing. Documentation of HSV-1 or HSV-2 is useful for prognosis and counseling.

  - **Virology:** Cell culture and polymerase chain reaction (PCR) testing are preferred for diagnosis of HSV. Sensitivity of cell culture is low, especially with recurrent lesions or those that have begun to heal. PCR is becoming more common due to its increased sensitivity. Viral culture isolates should be typed to determine HSV-1 or HSV-2; lack of HSV detection by culture or PCR does not prove absent infection because viral shedding is intermittent.

- **Serology** can confirm clinical suspicion in the absence of a positive culture; antibodies develop within weeks of infection. Type-specific assays that differentiate glycoprotein 1 (HSV-1) from glycoprotein 2 (HSV-2) are recommended. The presence of HSV-2 antibodies is predominantly seen in genital infections and patients should therefore be counseled as such. HSV-1 antibodies, however, may be the result of childhood transmission although genital transmission is growing.

- **Treatment** (Table 28-3)
  - Systemic antiviral therapy for HSV may reduce symptoms and complications of infection. Medical management does not eradicate the virus or reduce the frequency or severity of recurrences after medication is stopped. Primary genital herpes outbreaks should be treated with antiviral therapy, as patients are at increased risk for severe or prolonged symptoms.
  - Episodic treatment for recurrent herpes should be initiated within 1 day of lesions or during prodromal period.
  - Suppressive therapy can reduce recurrence in up to 80% of patients. Daily suppressive therapy with valacyclovir 500 mg a day has been shown to decrease HSV-2 transmission in discordant, heterosexual couples.
  - Recurrences will decrease over time regardless of suppressive therapy, so providers should address continued suppressive therapy yearly.
  - Severe or complicated disease should be treated with intravenous acyclovir (5 to 10 mg/kg every 8 hours for 2 to 7 days or until clinical improvement is observed followed by oral therapy to complete 10-day course).
  - Topical antiviral therapy has not shown any benefit and is not recommended.
  - The virus cannot be completely eradicated and remains latent in the cell bodies of sacral nerves S2, S3, and S4.

| TABLE 28-3 | Treatment for Genital Herpes | |
|---|---|---|
| Stage | Treatment | Duration |
| Primary outbreak— outpatient | Acyclovir, 400 mg PO tid | 7–10 d |
| | Acyclovir, 200 mg PO five times a day | |
| | Famciclovir, 250 mg PO tid | |
| | Valacyclovir, 1 g PO bid | |
| Episodic recurrences (begin treatment with prodrome or within 1 d of lesion outbreak) | Acyclovir, 400 mg PO tid | 5 d |
| | Acyclovir, 800 mg PO tid | 2 d |
| | Acyclovir, 800 mg PO bid | 5 d |
| | Famciclovir, 125 mg PO bid | 5 d |
| | Famciclovir, 1 g PO bid | 1 d |
| | Valacyclovir, 1 g PO qd | 5 d |
| | Valacyclovir, 500 mg PO bid | 3 d |
| Daily suppression therapy | Acyclovir, 400 mg PO bid | Per day |
| | Famciclovir, 250 mg PO bid | |
| | Valacyclovir, 500 mg PO qd | |
| | Valacyclovir, 1 g PO qd | |
| Recommended regimens in persons with HIV | Acyclovir, 400 mg PO tid | 5–10 d |
| | Famciclovir, 500 mg PO bid | 5–10 d |
| | Valacyclovir, 1 g PO bid | 5–10 d |

PO, orally; tid, three times a day; bid, twice a day; qd, every day.
From Workowski KA, Berman S; Centers for Disease Control and Prevention. Sexually transmitted diseases treatment guidelines, 2010. *MMWR Recomm Rep* 2010;59(RR-12):1–110, with permission.

- An effective HSV vaccine is not yet available.
- All women with genital herpes should be counseled on the natural history of HSV, sexual and perinatal transmission risks, and ways to reduce transmission.
- **Complications** include herpes encephalitis (rare but potentially life-threatening) and urinary tract infection (which can cause urinary retention or severe pain).
- **Counseling:** Patients should be advised to remain abstinent from the onset of prodromal symptoms until complete reepithelialization of lesions. Couples should discuss the role of suppressive therapy in decreasing transmission risk. Counseling should be appropriate to the HSV type.
- **During pregnancy**, women with primary HSV should be treated with antiviral therapy. Perinatal transmission is possible, and therefore, cesarean delivery is recommended for women with active lesions or prodromal symptoms of genital HSV at delivery. The risk of perinatal HSV transmission is high among women who acquire HSV near time of delivery and low for those with recurrent herpes. Many providers prescribe suppressive therapy for pregnant women with a history of genital herpes beginning at 36 weeks' gestation. Also see Chapter 11.

### Syphilis

- The spirochete *T. pallidum* causes the systemic disease syphilis. The disease is contagious only when mucocutaneous lesions are present. This occurs through contact with a chancre, condyloma lata, or mucosal lesion. The organism can penetrate skin or mucous membranes, incubating over a period of 10 days to 3 months. Syphilis has a complex course characterized by the immunologic response to the spirochete.

- Syphilis is divided into overlapping stages: primary, secondary, neurologic, and tertiary based on clinical findings to guide treatment and follow-up. Latent infections without clinical manifestations is detected with serologic testing and characterized as early latent, infection acquired in the previous year or late latent, and infection of greater than 1 year duration or latent syphilis of unknown duration. Determination of early latent versus late latent or latent infection of unknown duration guides duration of therapy.
  - **Primary syphilis** usually presents as a hard, painless, solitary chancre appearing on the vulva, vagina, or cervix, although extragenital lesions may occur. Lesions that occur on the cervix or in the vagina often go unrecognized. Nontender inguinal lymphadenopathy is frequently present. The primary chancre resolves spontaneously within 2 to 6 weeks.
  - **Secondary syphilis** occurs after hematogenous spread of the spirochete and is characterized by protean manifestations including generalized nonpruritic papulosquamous rash typically on the palms and soles, irregular rash, mucous patches, patchy alopecia, condyloma lata, and generalized lymphadenopathy. Systemic symptoms such as fever, headache, and malaise also occur.
  - **Latent syphilis** is defined by seropositivity without evidence of clinical manifestations. Latent syphilis documented as acquired during the previous year is referred to as early latent. All other latent syphilis is either late latent or latent syphilis of unknown duration. The late latent phase (>1 year) is not infectious by sexual transmission, but the spirochete may transplacentally infect the fetus.
  - **Tertiary syphilis** develops in up to one third of the untreated or inadequately treated patients and refers to gummas, locally destructive lesions of the bone, skin, or other organs. Cardiovascular involvement in tertiary syphilis includes aortic aneurysm and aortic valvular insufficiency.
  - **Neurosyphilis** can occur during any stage of syphilis and is not synonymous with tertiary syphilis. All patients with clinical evidence of central nervous system involvement, evidence of active tertiary syphilis, or serologic treatment failure should have examination of the cerebrospinal fluid (CSF) performed. CSF should be tested for fluorescent treponemal antibody absorption (FTA-ABS) reactivity.
  - **Diagnosis:** *T. pallidum* cannot be cultured in vitro. The diagnosis is made definitively by identifying the spirochete through dark-field microscopy or by direct fluorescent antibody tests of lesion exudate or tissue. The majority of syphilis infection is diagnosed presumptively with nontreponemal serologic tests, such as the Venereal Disease Research Laboratory (VDRL) or rapid plasma reagin (RPR) and treponemal tests. A positive VDRL or RPR requires confirmation with treponemal testing. These are FTA-ABS, *T. pallidum* passive particle agglutination assay (TP-PA assay), various enzyme immunoassays, and chemiluminescence immunoassays. False-positive nontreponemal tests are associated with pregnancy, autoimmune disorders, chronic active hepatitis, intravenous drug use, febrile illness, and immunization. Serologic tests become positive 4 to 6 weeks after exposure, usually 1 to 2 weeks after the appearance of the primary chancres. The specific FTA-ABS test remains positive indefinitely. Some laboratories have begun screening with treponemal tests which will be positive in individuals with previously treated syphilis as well as those with untreated or incompletely treated syphilis. A positive result must be followed by a nontreponemal test with titer. If the nontreponemal test is negative,

a different treponemal test should be performed to verify the results of the first test. If the second treponemal test is positive, those without a history of prior treatment should be offered treatment.

- The diagnosis of neurosyphilis cannot be made with a single test but requires a combination of reactive serologic tests, CSF analysis, and reactive VDRL-CSF with or without clinical symptoms.
- The diagnosis of syphilis should prompt HIV testing and if negative repeated again in 3 months for those living in high HIV-risk areas (prevalence >1% of the population).
- **Pregnancy:** All women should be screened for syphilis in early pregnancy, and this is mandated in most states. In high-risk patients or in high-prevalence areas, syphilis testing should be repeated twice in the third trimester (i.e., at 28 to 32 weeks' gestation and again at delivery).
- **Treatment** options are listed in Table 28-4. Penicillin G is the recommended treatment for all stages of infection; however, the choice of preparation should be based on stage and clinical symptoms of disease. Individuals with an allergy to penicillin may be desensitized and treated with benzathine penicillin. Intravenous penicillin G is the only treatment with documented efficacy in pregnancy.
- **Follow-up:** Definitive criteria for treatment cure or failure have not been established. Clinical follow-up and serologic VDRL or RPR titers should be obtained (preferably at same lab) every 6 months for 1 year or at 3, 6, 9, 12, and 24 months if HIV-positive. If signs or symptoms persist, or there is a fourfold increase in titer, then treatment has failed or the patient has been reinfected. If initial high titer >1:32 remains stable or does not decrease fourfold (two dilutions) in 6 months, treatment failure may have occurred. These patients should undergo repeat HIV testing, lumbar puncture for CSF evaluation, and retreatment. For patients with neurosyphilis, if CSF pleocytosis is noted initially, a repeat CSF evaluation should occur every 6 months until the cell count normalizes. If the cell count is not decreasing by 6 months or has not normalized by 2 years, retreatment should be considered.

### Other Ulcerative Lesions

- **Chancroid** is rare in the United States and appears to be declining worldwide as well but may still occur in regions of Africa and the Caribbean. Definitive diagnosis is with detection of *H. ducreyi* on special culture media not widely available and has a sensitivity of 80%. Probable diagnosis can be made if the following criteria are met: (a) One or more painful genital ulcers are present, (b) no evidence of *T. pallidum* by dark-field examination or serologic testing 7 days after the onset of ulcers, (c) HSV testing of the ulcer is negative, and (d) the clinical appearance of genital ulcers and regional lymphadenopathy (if present) is typical for chancroid. Successful treatment with antibiotics resolves clinical symptoms but in some cases, scarring can result. Recommended treatment is azithromycin 1 g orally (PO) single dose, ceftriaxone 250 mg intramuscularly single dose, ciprofloxacin 500 mg PO twice a day (bid) (contraindicated in pregnancy) × 3 days, or erythromycin 500 mg PO three times a day × 7 days.
- **Granuloma inguinale (donovanosis)** also occurs rarely in the United States but is endemic in some tropical and developing areas. The genital ulcer is caused by the intracellular bacterium *Klebsiella granulomatis*. The disease is a slowly progressive ulcerative lesion on the perineum or genitals without regional lymphadenopathy. The lesion is highly vascular and subcutaneous granulomas may occur. The organism is

**TABLE 28-4** Recommended Treatment for Syphilis

| Phase | Medication | Dosage | Duration |
|---|---|---|---|
| Primary, secondary, and early latent syphilis (<1 yr) | Benzathine penicillin G | 2.4 million U IM | 1 dose |
| Penicillin allergy (nonpregnant) | Doxycycline or tetracycline | 100 mg PO bid<br>500 mg PO qid | 14 d<br>14 d |
| Late latent syphilis (>1 yr) and secondary syphilis without neurosyphilis | Benzathine penicillin G | 2.4 million U IM<br>(7.2 million U total) | q wk for 3 wk |
| Penicillin allergy (nonpregnant) | Doxycycline or tetracycline | 100 mg PO bid<br>500 mg PO qid | 28 d<br>28 d |
| Neurosyphilis | Aqueous crystalline penicillin G | 3–4 million U IV q4h<br>(18–24 million U per day) | 10–14 d |
| Alternate regimen (if compliance assured) | Procaine penicillin PLUS probenecid | 2.4 million U IM qd plus<br>500 mg PO qid | 10–14 d<br>10–14 d |
| Tertiary syphilis (gumma, cardiovascular syphilis) | Benzathine penicillin G | 2.4 million U IM<br>(7.2 million U total) | q wk for 3 wk |
| Syphilis during pregnancy | Penicillin<br>Desensitize if allergic | Parenteral regimen appropriate for the stage of syphilis | — |
| Primary or secondary syphilis in HIV-positive patients | Benzathine penicillin G<br>Desensitize if allergic | 2.4 million U IM | 1 dose |
| Latent syphilis in HIV-positive patients | Benzathine penicillin G<br>Desensitize if allergic | 2.4 million U IM<br>(7.2 million U total) | q wk 3 wk |

IM, intramuscular; PO, orally; bid, twice a day; qid, 4 times a day; IV, intravenous; qd, every day.
From Workowski KA, Berman S; Centers for Disease Control and Prevention. Sexually transmitted diseases treatment guidelines, 2010. *MMWR Recomm Rep* 2010;59(RR-12):1–110.

difficult to culture and no FDA-cleared DNA detection tests exist. The diagnosis is made by dark stain and visualization of Donovan bodies. Extragenital infection can occur with extension to the pelvis and dissemination to abdominal organs, bones, or the mouth. Treatment with antimicrobials halt progression of the lesion but relapse can occur 6 to 18 months after effective therapy. Recommended treatment is for 3 weeks or until lesions have completely healed and include doxycycline 100 mg bid × 3 weeks (recommended), alternatively azithromycin 1 g PO q week × 3, ciprofloxacin 750 mg PO bid, erythromycin 500 mg four times a day (qid), or trimethoprim-sulfamethoxazole double strength 1 tablet PO bid.

- **Lymphogranuloma venereum (LGV)** is caused by *Chlamydia trachomatis* serovars L1, L2, or L3 and presents with tender inguinal and/or femoral lymphadenopathy that is usually unilateral. A self-limited genital ulcer or papule may occur at the site of inoculation. Rectal exposure can result in proctitis or colitis with mucoid hemorrhagic discharge, anal pain, tenesmus, fever, and constipation and if left untreated can result in chronic colorectal fistulas and strictures. Both genital and colorectal lesions can develop secondary bacterial inflectional coinfection including sexually and nonsexually transmitted pathogens.
  - Diagnosis is based on clinical suspicion, epidemiologic information, and exclusion of other etiologies with clinical symptoms similar to LGV. Chlamydial testing of genital and lymph node specimens with culture, direct immunofluorescence, or nucleic detection can be used for diagnosis but rectal specimens using nucleic acid amplification tests (NAATs) for *C. trachomatis* are not FDA cleared. PCR-based genotyping to differentiate LGV from non-LGV *C. trachomatis* are not widely available. In the absence of specific LGV diagnostics, patients with clinical suspicion of LGV should be treated. Doxycycline for 21 days is the preferred treatment and alternative treatment is erythromycin 500 mg PO qid × 21days.

## Vaginitis

- **Vaginitis** is characterized by pruritus, discharge, odor, dyspareunia, and dysuria. The most common causes are bacterial vaginosis, vulvovaginal candidiasis, and trichomoniasis. The vagina is normally colonized by several organisms, including *Lactobacillus acidophilus*, diphtheroids, *Candida albicans*, *Gardnerella vaginalis*, *Escherichia coli*, group B streptococci (GBS), genital Mycoplasmatales and other flora. Its physiologic pH is approximately 4.0, with peroxide-producing *L. acidophilus* inhibiting overgrowth of pathogenic bacteria. Vaginal fluid is typically white, odorless, and seen in dependent areas of the vagina.
- **Diagnosis** of vaginitis must begin with a focused history on the constellation of vaginal symptoms, location, duration, relation to menstrual cycle, use of prior treatment, douching, and sexual history. Physical examination should start with inspection of the vulva and include speculum examination to obtain samples for vaginal pH, amine ("whiff") test, saline wet mount, and potassium hydroxide (KOH) microscopy. DNA amplification tests for *Neisseria gonorrhoeae* and *C. trachomatis* may be indicated. The three major types of vaginitis and their distinguishing characteristics are described in Table 28-5.

### Bacterial Vaginosis

- **Bacterial vaginosis (BV)** is the most common cause of vaginitis although most women with BV are asymptomatic. No single infectious agent is responsible; rather, there is a shift in the composition of vaginal flora, with up to a 10-fold increase in facultative anaerobic bacteria such as *G. vaginalis*, *Mycoplasma hominis*, *Atopobium*

| TABLE 28-5 | Distinguishing Characteristics of Vaginitis | | |
|---|---|---|---|
| | Bacterial Vaginosis | *Trichomonas* Vaginitis | Candidal Vaginitis |
| **Vaginal pH** | >4.5 | 5.0–7.0 | — |
| **Vaginal secretions** | Thin, white, adherent; amine (fishy) odor with potassium hydroxide (KOH) | Thin, frothy, white, gray, yellow; copious | Thick, white, curdlike |
| **Wet preparation** | Clue cells, few WBCs | Trichomonads, WBCs | Hyphae and buds, WBCs (best seen with KOH prep) |

WBCs, white blood cells.
From Amsel R, Totten PA, Spiegel CA, et al. Nonspecific vaginitis. Diagnostic criteria and microbial and epidemiologic associations. *Am J Med* 1983;74(1):14–22.

*vaginae* and *Prevotella*, *Bacteroides*, *Peptostreptococcus*, and *Fusobacterium* species, with a decrease in the concentration of *Lactobacillus* species. It has been implicated as a risk factor for preterm premature rupture of membranes and preterm delivery. The microbial alterations associated with BV are not completely understood or whether it is associated with a sexually transmitted pathogen; however, it has been associated with multiple male and female partners, new sex partner, lack of condom use, douching, decrease in vaginal lactobacillus, increased risk of STIs, PID, and postprocedural gynecologic infections. Treatment of BV prior to an abortion or hysterectomy decreases the risk of postoperative infection.

- **Diagnosis:** BV is diagnosed by the presence of at least three of the Amsel clinical criteria: (a) homogenous thin white discharge coating the vaginal walls, (b) vaginal pH >4.5, (c) more than 20% of epithelial cells appearing to be clue cells on microscopic examination, and (d) fishy odor before or after the addition of 10% KOH to the sample (amine test). Detection of three of these criteria has been correlated to Gram stain, considered the gold standard for BV diagnosis, which determines the concentration of lactobacillus to other organisms. Commercially available point-of-care card tests to detect elevated pH and trimethylamine are now available and may be useful when a microscope is not available.
- **Treatment:** Treatment regimens are shown in Table 28-6 and are recommended for women with symptoms. Benefits of treatment in nonpregnant include amelioration of the signs and symptoms of BV and reduction in the risk of acquisition of HIV, *N. gonorrhoeae*, *C. trachomatis*, and other viral STIs.
  - BV has been associated with adverse pregnancy outcomes, including premature rupture of membranes, preterm labor, preterm birth, intra-amniotic infection, and postpartum endometritis, although the only established benefit in pregnant women is the reduction of symptoms. Currently, treatment is recommended for

| TABLE 28-6 | Treatment for Bacterial Vaginosis | | |
|---|---|---|---|
| **Medication** | **Dosage** | **Duration** | **Use in Pregnancy** |
| Metronidazole | 500 mg PO bid | 7 d | Recommended |
| Clindamycin phosphate cream 2% | 1 full applicator (5 g) intravaginally qhs | 7 d | Not recommended |
| Metronidazole gel 0.75% | 1 full applicator (5 g) intravaginally daily | 5 d | Not recommended |
| **Alternative regimens**[a] | | | |
| Clindamycin ovules | 100 g intravaginally qhs | 3 d | Not recommended |
| Clindamycin hydrochloride | 300 mg PO bid | 7 d | Recommended |
| Tinidazole | 2 g PO daily | 2 d | Not recommended |
| Tinidazole | 1 g PO daily | 5 d | Not recommended |

[a]Extended-release metronidazole (750 mg) and single-dose clindamycin intravaginal cream are also available. Metronidazole 250 mg PO tid for 7 days is also recommended in pregnancy.
PO, orally; bid, twice a day; qhs, at bedtime; tid, three times a day.
From Workowski KA, Berman S; Centers for Disease Control and Prevention. Sexually transmitted diseases treatment guidelines, 2010. *MMWR Recomm Rep* 2010;59(RR-12):1–110.

symptomatic pregnant women only. Treatment of male partners is not necessary or beneficial in preventing recurrence.

- **Follow-up:** Recurrence of BV is common, recurring in up to 30% of women within 3 months. Either retreatment with the same therapy or a different treatment option is acceptable for early treatment failure. Women with multiple recurrences may benefit from metronidazole gel twice weekly for 4 to 6 months after completing a treatment course. Follow-up in 1 month for asymptomatic pregnant women at high risk for preterm delivery should be considered.

*Trichomoniasis*

- **Trichomoniasis** is an STI with 7.4 million cases in the United States annually and is caused by the unicellular protozoan *Trichomonas vaginalis*. Trichomonads can survive on wet towels and other surfaces and thus can be nonsexually transmitted. Its incubation period ranges from 4 to 28 days.
- **Diagnosis:** Vaginal exam may reveal a frothy, malodorous yellow-green discharge with vulvar irritation and the cervix may appear erythematous and friable. However, many women have minimal or no symptoms. A wet smear preparation that is promptly reviewed may reveal the flagellated, mobile protozoon with a sensitivity of approximately 60% to 70%. Trichomonas culture tests have 90% sensitivity. Point-of-care tests are available and have higher sensitivity than vaginal examination, but false-positives can occur. Culture of secretions is sensitive and highly specific and should be obtained when microscopic evaluation is negative in women who have clinical suspicion for trichomonas. An FDA-cleared test for gonorrhea and chlamydia has been modified to detect *T. vaginalis* in vaginal, endocervical, or urine specimens and sensitivity range from 88% to 97% and specificity of 98% to 99% is another diagnostic option. Liquid-based testing Pap tests have increased

sensitivity for *T. vaginalis*; however, false positives have occurred and confirmatory testing may be needed.

- **Treatment** consists of one 2-g dose of either metronidazole or tinidazole PO. Alternatively, metronidazole 500 mg PO bid for 7 days can be used. Metronidazole gel has an efficacy of <50% and is not recommended. Patients with allergy to metronidazole should be referred for desensitization and subsequent treatment with metronidazole. The patient's sexual partners should be treated as well. Although trichomoniasis has been associated with premature rupture of membranes and preterm delivery, treatment of the infection has not been shown to reduce these risks. An earlier study suggested that treatment of asymptomatic trichomoniasis in pregnant women was associated with increased preterm delivery rate in the treatment group. However, a more recent analysis from a randomized trial in Africa concluded that there was no difference in risk of preterm or low birth weight in women with trichomoniasis who were treated versus those who were not.

- **Follow-up:** High rates of reinfection have been found after initial diagnosis and treatment of trichomonas so rescreening after 3 months is a considerable option, although the benefit of this has not been evaluated. Most organisms respond well to standard treatment but low-level resistance to metronidazole has been documented for 2% to 5% of vaginal trichomoniasis. If treatment failure occurs, most infections will respond to retreatment with either 2 g of tinidazole or metronidazole 500 mg PO bid for 7 days. High-level metronidazole resistance is rare but if it occurs, further management should be discussed with a specialist.

## Vulvovaginal Candidiasis

- Vulvovaginal candidiasis (VVC) is usually caused by *C. albicans* and accounts for 80% to 92% of the cases. Lifetime incidence of VVC is 75%, with 40% to 45% of women having repeated infections. The majority of women with uncomplicated VVC have no identifiable precipitating factors. Complicated or recurrent VVC occurs in 5% of women. These are often nonalbicans species and are most often found in immunocompromised women, uncontrolled diabetics, or pregnant women.

- **Diagnosis:** The presence of vulvar pruritus, pain, swelling, external dysuria, and redness are clinically suggestive of VVC. Signs include vulvar fissures or excoriations, erythema, and vulvar edema. The diagnosis of uncomplicated VVC can be made based on signs and symptoms of VVC with the presence of hyphae and spores on saline or 10% KOH wet preparation, Gram stain of vaginal secretions positive for yeasts, hyphae, or pseudohyphae, or culture or other diagnostic test yields positive yeast results. Empiric treatment with negative wet mount can be administered to women with clinical signs and symptoms of VVC.

  - Diagnosis should be classified as uncomplicated versus complicated VVC to guide treatment. Features of uncomplicated VVC include sporadic or infrequent episodes and mild to moderate symptoms with *C. albicans* infection. Complicated VVC is defined as four or more episodes of infection in 1 year and impacts a small percentage of women. Recurrent VVC is not well understood and most women impacted have no predisposing conditions although women who are immunocompromised with diabetes or treatment with corticosteroids do not respond well to short-term treatments and VVC occurs more frequently in pregnancy. The incidence of VVC in HIV is unknown but colonization rates are higher among HIV-infected women and correlate to severity of immunosuppression. Systemic azole exposure is associated with nonalbicans *Candida*. Culture should be performed in women not responding to treatment, in cases where a nonalbicans species is suspected, or with recurrent VVC to establish species and sensitivity.

| TABLE 28-7 | Treatment for Uncomplicated Yeast Infections |
|---|---|

**Intravaginal agents**
**Butoconazole** 2% cream 5 g intravaginally for 3 d[a]
**Butoconazole** 2% cream 5 g (sustained release), single application
**Clotrimazole** 1% cream 5 g intravaginally for 7–14 d[a]
**Clotrimazole** 2% cream 5 g intravaginally for 3 d[a]
**Clotrimazole** 100 mg vaginal tablet for 7 d
**Miconazole** 2% cream 5 g intravaginally for 7 d[a]
**Miconazole** 4% cream 5 g intravaginally for 3 d[a]
**Miconazole** 100 mg vaginal suppository, one suppository for 7 d[a]
**Miconazole** 200 mg vaginal suppository, one suppository for 3 d[a]
**Miconazole** 1200 mg vaginal suppository, 1 suppository for 1 d
**Nystatin** 100,000-unit vaginal tablet, one tablet for 14 d
**Tioconazole** 6.5% ointment 5 g intravaginally in a single application[a]
**Terconazole** 0.4% cream 5 g intravaginally for 7 d
**Terconazole** 0.8% cream 5 g intravaginally for 3 d
**Terconazole** 80 mg vaginal suppository, one suppository for 3 d

**Oral agent**
**Fluconazole** 150 mg oral tablet, one tablet in single dose

---

[a]Over-the-counter (OTC) preparations.
From Workowski KA, Berman S; Centers for Disease Control and Prevention. Sexually transmitted diseases treatment guidelines, 2010. *MMWR Recomm Rep* 2010;59(RR-12):1–110.

- **Treatment:** Symptomatic patients, including pregnant women, should be treated. See Table 28-7. Medications available over-the-counter include butoconazole, clotrimazole, miconazole, and tioconazole. Only topical therapies are recommended in pregnancy. For severe VVC, extended treatment with topical azoles up to 14 days or fluconazole 150 mg in two doses 72 hours apart is recommended. Maintenance therapy with 150 mg of fluconazole or clotrimazole 200 mg twice a week or 500 mg once a week is recommended. Maintenance therapy is effective in reducing recurrence in up to 50% of women.
- **Follow-up:** If symptoms persist or recur within 2 months, patients should return for follow-up.
- **Treatment of male partners** is not indicated unless the partner has symptoms of yeast balanitis or in cases of recurrent VVC.

## Cervicitis

- **Cervicitis** is characterized by two major diagnostic signs: a purulent or mucopurulent cervical exudate and/or sustained cervical bleeding in response to manipulation by an examining swab. Patients may be asymptomatic but commonly report abnormal vaginal discharge and intermenstrual bleeding. The primary pathogens of mucopurulent cervicitis are the two sexually transmitted organisms *C. trachomatis* and *N. gonorrhoeae*; however, trichomoniasis and genital herpes infections can also be associated with cervicitis. In the majority of cases, no etiologic agent is identified; limited data has implicated BV, *Mycoplasma genitalium*, and frequent douching as other causes of cervicitis. Leukorrhea (>10 white blood cell per high-power field on microscopy) of vaginal fluid may be associated with chlamydial or gonorrheal infections. Patients with symptoms of cervicitis should also be evaluated for PID, *C. trachomatis*, *N. gonorrhoeae*, *T. vaginalis*, and BV.

*Chlamydia*

- **Chlamydia trachomatis** is the most frequently reported sexually transmitted bacterial disease in the United States. Risk factors include age younger than 25 years old, low socioeconomic status, multiple sex partners, and unmarried status. Sequelae of *C. trachomatis* infection in women may include PID, ectopic pregnancy, chronic pelvic pain, and infertility.
- **Microbiology:** *C. trachomatis* is an obligate intracellular organism that preferentially infects the squamocolumnar cells in the transition zone of the cervix.
- **Signs and symptoms:** Chlamydial cervicitis is asymptomatic in about 75% of cases. Patients with *C. trachomatis* infection may complain of abnormal vaginal discharge, burning with urination, spotting, or postcoital bleeding. A yellow mucopurulent discharge may be present.
- **Diagnosis:** NAAT using PCR is the preferred method of diagnosis for chlamydial and gonorrheal cervicitis and can be performed on vaginal, cervical, or urine samples. Screening programs have shown reduction in the rate of chlamydia infection and incidence of PID; therefore, annual screening is recommended for all sexually active women younger than the age of 25 years and in women older than 25 years who present with risk factors. Women with cervicitis should also be evaluated for trichomoniasis and BV (Table 28-8).
- **Treatment:** Presumptive therapy can be initiated based on clinical findings and STD risk assessment (Table 28-9). Treatment for coinfection with gonorrhea is recommended if local prevalence is >5%. Concomitant treatment for BV or trichomoniasis should be given if detected. Sexual partners should be referred to a clinic for treatment.

| TABLE 28-8 | Testing for Gonorrhea and Chlamydia Infection | | | |
|---|---|---|---|---|
| | *N. gonorrhoeae* | | *C. trachomatis* | |
| | Sensitivity | Specificity | Sensitivity | Specificity |
| Endocervical culture | 70–85 | 100 | 60–70 | 100 |
| Immunoassay | >80 | 97–100 | Not reliable | |
| Nucleic acid probe | 77–97 | 96–100 | 92 | 99.7 |
| PCR/LCR | 95 | 100 | 96.7 | 99.7 |

Values are in percentages.
PCR, polymerase chain reaction; LCR, ligase chain reaction.
Adapted from Black CM. Current methods of laboratory diagnosis of *Chlamydia trachomatis* infections. *Clin Microbiol Rev* 1997;10(1):160–184; Van Dyck E, Ieven M, Patten S, et al. Detection of *Chlamydia trachomatis* and *Neisseria gonorrhoeae* by enzyme immunoassay, culture, and three nucleic acid amplification tests. *J Clin Microbiol* 2001;39(5):1751–1756; Koumans EH, Johnson RE, Knapp JS, et al. Laboratory testing for *Neisseria gonorrhoeae* by recently introduced nonculture tests: a performance review with clinical and public health considerations. *Clin Infect Dis* 1998;27: 1171–1180.

| TABLE 28-9 | Treatment for *Chlamydia trachomatis* | | |
|---|---|---|---|
| **Medication** | **Dosage** | **Duration** | **Use in Pregnancy** |
| **Recommended** | | | |
| Azithromycin | 1 g PO | 1 dose | Recommended |
| Doxycycline | 100 mg PO bid | 7 d | Contraindicated |
| Amoxicillin (in pregnant women) | 500 mg PO tid | 7 d | Acceptable regimen for pregnancy only |
| **Alternative** | | | |
| Erythromycin base | 500 mg PO qid | 7 d | Alternative |
| Erythromycin ethylsuccinate | 800 mg PO qid | 7 d | Alternative |
| Ofloxacin | 300 mg PO bid | 7 d | Contraindicated |
| Levofloxacin | 500 mg PO qd | 7 d | Contraindicated |

PO, orally; bid, twice a day; tid, three times a day; qid, four times a day; qd, every day.
From Workowski KA, Berman S; Centers for Disease Control and Prevention. Sexually transmitted diseases treatment guidelines, 2010. *MMWR Recomm Rep* 2010;59(RR-12):1–110.

- **Follow-up:** Test of cure is not recommended except in pregnancy (4 to 5 weeks after treatment) unless noncompliance or reinfection is suspected or if symptoms persist. Both patient and partner should sustain from intercourse for 1 week after treatment to avoid reinfection. Retesting 3 months after treatment is recommended in order to assess for reinfection.

*Gonorrhea*
- Risk factors for **gonorrhea** are essentially the same as those for *C. trachomatis*.
- **Microbiology:** *N. gonorrhoeae* is a Gram-negative diplococcus that infects columnar or pseudostratified epithelium. Genital, pharyngeal, and disseminated infections may occur. The incubation period is 3 to 5 days.
- **Signs and symptoms:** In women, symptoms often go unrecognized until complications (PID) have occurred. When present, symptoms include vaginal discharge, dysuria, or abnormal uterine bleeding. The most commonly infected site is the endocervix.
- **Diagnosis:** Culture, nucleic acid hybridization tests, and NAATs are available for the diagnosis of urogenital *N. gonorrhea*. Culture and nucleic acid hybridization tests require endocervical specimens, whereas NAATs allows the widest variety of specimen sites including endocervical, vaginal, urethral, and urine. NAATs have greater sensitivity than culture; however, culture is the most widely available option for detection in the nongenital sites and is used when antibiotic sensitivity testing is indicated (see Table 28-8). Targeted screening of women younger than 25 years old or those at risk for infection (multiple sexual partners, prior history of gonorrhea or other STI, inconsistent barrier protection use, those with a history of commercial sex work or drug use, women living in areas of high prevalence) is recommended. All women positive for gonorrhea should be tested for other STIs such as chlamydia, HIV, and syphilis.

- **Treatment** options are listed in Table 28-10. Due to increasing resistance, fluoro-quinolones are no longer recommended for the treatment of *N. gonorrhea*; cephalo-sporins are the only recommended class of antimicrobials. Because coinfection with *C. trachomatis* is common, treatment of both is recommended unless the NAAT is negative. Sexual partners should be referred for treatment. Although azithromycin 2 g PO is effective against uncomplicated gonorrhea, concerns about resistance development, expense, and gastrointestinal upset should limit its use.
- Follow-up with a test of cure several weeks after treatment for uncomplicated gon-orrhea is not required. Retesting 3 months after treatment is recommended in order to assess for reinfection.

---

**TABLE 28-10**    Treatment for *Neisseria gonorrhoeae*

**Uncomplicated gonococcal infections of the cervix, urethra, and rectum[a]**
*Recommended regimens*
**Ceftriaxone** 250 mg intramuscular (IM) in a single dose
   OR
**Cefixime** 400 mg orally once or 400 mg by suspension (200 mg/5 mL)
   OR
   Single-dose injectable **cephalosporin**
   *PLUS*
Treatment for chlamydia unless ruled out

**Uncomplicated gonococcal infections of the pharynx[a]**
*Recommended regimens*
**Ceftriaxone** 125 mg IM in a single dose
   *PLUS*
Treatment for chlamydia unless ruled out

**Disseminated gonococcal infection (DGI)**
*Recommended regimen*
**Ceftriaxone** 1 g IM or IV every 24 hr
  *Alternative regimens*
  **Cefotaxime** 1 g IV every 8 hr
   OR
  **Ceftizoxime** 1 g IV every 8 hr
*Oral follow-up regimen*
**Cefixime** 400 mg orally twice daily
  OR
**Cefixime** 400 mg suspension (200 mg/5 mL) twice daily
Any regimen should be continued for 24–48 hr after clinical improvement
   then switch to oral medicines to complete 1 wk of therapy.

---

[a]These regimens are recommended for all adult and adolescent patients, regardless of travel history or sexual behavior.
IV, intravenous.
From Workowski KA, Berman S; Centers for Disease Control and Prevention. Sexually transmitted diseases treatment guidelines, 2010. *MMWR Recomm Rep* 2010;59(RR-12):1–110.

# INFECTIONS OF THE UPPER GENITAL TRACT

## Pelvic Inflammatory Disease

- **PID** is an inflammatory disorder of any combination of the endometrium, fallopian tubes, ovaries, myometrium, parametrium, and pelvic peritoneum.
- **Pathophysiology and microbiology:** PID is caused by the spread of infection via the cervix. PID is often associated with STIs such as *N. gonorrhoeae* and *C. trachomatis*; however, numerous exogenous and endogenous microorganisms may be involved, including anaerobes, *G. vaginalis*, *Haemophilus influenza*, Gram-negative rods, *Streptococcus agalactia*, and enteric species. Other organisms include *Mycoplasma* spp., *Ureaplasma* spp., and cytomegalovirus. Diagnosis of PID should include testing for *N. gonorrhea* and *C. trachomatis* and screening for HIV.
- **Prevention:** There are no signs and symptoms pathognomic for PID, and the clinical picture does not accurately predict the extent of tubal involvement. A high degree of suspicion for PID and treatment based on minimal or subtle signs may help reduce the incidence of long-term sequelae. Episodes of PID may have unrecognized or absent symptoms; delays in diagnosis and treatment contribute to serious sequelae. One in four women with PID will experience tubal infertility, an ectopic pregnancy, or chronic pelvic pain. Treatment of sexual partners and education is important in reducing the rate of recurrent infections.
- **Risk factors** include a previous history of PID, multiple sex partners, adolescence, BV, and current infection by a sexually transmitted organism. A woman's risk of PID is not increased by intrauterine device (IUD) use. See Chapter 32.
- **Signs and symptoms:** The most common presenting symptom is abdominopelvic pain. Other symptoms include vaginal discharge, dyspareunia, abnormal bleeding, right upper quadrant pain, fever and chills, nausea, and dysuria.
- **Diagnosis** of PID is difficult because the presenting signs and symptoms vary widely. Health care providers should maintain a low threshold for the diagnosis of PID based on minimal clinical criteria.
  - **Minimal criteria:** Empiric treatment should be initiated in sexually active young women and other women at risk for STDs if they are experiencing pelvic or lower abdominal pain, if no other cause can be identified, and if one or more of the following are present on pelvic examination:
    - Cervical motion tenderness
    - Uterine tenderness
    - Adnexal tenderness
  - **Additional criteria for diagnosis, which increase specificity**
    - Oral temperature >101°F (>38.3°C)
    - Abnormal cervical or vaginal mucopurulent discharge
    - Predominance of white blood cells on saline microscopy of vaginal secretions
    - Elevated erythrocyte sedimentation rate
    - Elevated C-reactive protein
    - Laboratory documentation of cervical infection with *N. gonorrhoeae* or *C. trachomatis*
  - **PID specific criteria**
    - Endometrial biopsy with histopathologic evidence of endometritis
    - Transvaginal sonography or magnetic resonance imaging techniques showing thickened, fluid-filled tubes with or without free pelvic fluid or tuboovarian complex
    - Laparoscopic abnormalities consistent with PID

- **Treatment** goals for PID are the prevention of tubal damage that leads to infertility and ectopic pregnancy and prevention of chronic infection. Many patients can be successfully treated as outpatients, and early ambulatory treatment should be the initial therapeutic approach once a presumptive diagnosis has been established. Antibiotic choice should provide broad empiric coverage targeting the major etiologic organisms (*N. gonorrhoeae* and *C. trachomatis*) but should also address the polymicrobial nature of the disease (Table 28-11). Negative endocervical screening for *N. gonorrhoeae* and *C. trachomatis* does not rule out possibility of upper reproductive tract infection. Patients with tuboovarian abscesses should be admitted for at least 24 hours direct inpatient observation and should receive clindamycin or metronidazole with doxycycline for continued oral therapy after transition from parenteral therapy for adequate anaerobic coverage. Due to quinolone resistance in *N. gonorrhoeae*, quinolone-based regimens are not recommended except in situations where cephalosporins are not feasible. Among women with an IUD in place, there is not enough evidence to recommend IUD removal with acute PID; however, close clinical follow-up is necessary.
- **Criteria for hospitalization**
  - Surgical emergencies (e.g., appendicitis) cannot be excluded.
  - Pregnancy
  - Failure to respond clinically to oral antimicrobial therapy
  - Inability to follow or tolerate an outpatient oral regimen
  - Severe illness, nausea and vomiting, or high fever
  - Suspected tuboovarian abscess (at least 24 hours of direct inpatient observation recommended)
- **Follow-up:** Clinical improvement should be noted within 3 days of initiating treatment; those not improving will typically require hospitalization, diagnostic tests, and possible surgical intervention.
- **Sequelae:** Approximately 25% of PID patients experience long-term sequelae. Infertility due to tubal occlusion affects anywhere from 6% to 60% of women following an episode of PID, depending on severity, whereas the risk of ectopic pregnancy is approximately 6 to 10 times the normal. Chronic pelvic pain and dyspareunia have also been reported and are associated with the presence of adhesive disease and the number of episodes. Fitz-Hugh-Curtis syndrome is the development of fibrous perihepatic adhesions resulting from the inflammatory process of PID that may result in acute right upper quadrant pain and tenderness.

## Endometritis (Nonpuerperal)

- **Pathophysiology:** Endometritis is caused by the ascension of pathogens from the cervix to the endometrium. Pathogens include *C. trachomatis*, *N. gonorrhoeae*, *Ureaplasma urealyticum*, and *M. genitalium*. Chronic endometritis is often linked to common bacteria such as streptococci, staphylococci, and *E. coli*. Organisms that produce BV may also produce histologic endometritis, even in women without symptoms. Endometritis is also an important component of PID and may be an intermediate stage in the spread of infection to the fallopian tubes.
- **Signs and symptoms:**
  - With **chronic endometritis**, many women are asymptomatic. The classic symptom of chronic endometritis is intermenstrual vaginal bleeding. Postcoital bleeding, menorrhagia, and a dull, constant lower abdominal pain are other complaints.
  - In **acute endometritis**, uterine tenderness is common.

**TABLE 28-11** Treatment for Pelvic Inflammatory Disease

**Parenteral treatment for severe PID**

Transition to oral therapy, which usually can be initiated within 24–48 hr of
clinical improvement, should be guided by clinical experience.
*Recommended parenteral regimen A*
**Cefotetan** 2 g IV every 12 hr
  OR
**Cefoxitin** 2 g IV every 6 hr
  PLUS
**Doxycycline** 100 mg orally or IV every 12 hr (IV and oral administration have
similar bioavailability; administer orally when possible)
*Recommended parenteral regimen B*
**Clindamycin** 900 mg IV every 8 hr
  PLUS
**Gentamicin** loading dose IV or IM (2 mg/kg body weight) followed by mainte-
nance dose (1.5 mg/kg) every 8 hr. Single daily dosing (3–5mg/kg) may be
substituted.
  *Alternative parenteral regimen*
  **Ampicillin/sulbactam** 3 g IV every 6 hr
    PLUS
  **Doxycycline** 100 mg orally or IV every 12 hr
  *Transition from parenteral to oral regimen*
  **Doxycycline** 100 mg PO bid
    OR
  **Clindamycin** 450 mg qid
  **To complete a 14-day treatment course. Clindamycin preferred oral agent in
  setting of tuboovarian abscess.**

**Oral treatment for mild to moderate PID**

Parenteral and oral therapies have similar efficacy in treatment of women with
mild to moderate PID. Women who do not respond to oral therapy within
72 hr should be reevaluated to confirm the diagnosis and should be admin-
istered parenteral therapy on either an outpatient or inpatient basis.
*Recommended oral regimen*
**Ceftriaxone** 250 mg IM in a single dose
  PLUS
**Doxycycline** 100 mg orally twice a day for 14 d
  WITH OR WITHOUT
**Metronidazole** 500 mg orally twice a day for 14 d
  OR
**Cefoxitin** 2 g IM in a single dose and
**Probenecid** 1 g orally administered concurrently in a single dose
  PLUS
**Doxycycline** 100 mg orally twice a day for 14 d
  WITH OR WITHOUT

*(Continued)*

| TABLE 28-11 | Treatment for Pelvic Inflammatory Disease *(Continued)* |
|---|---|

**Metronidazole** 500 mg orally twice a day for 14 d
  **OR**
Other parenteral **third-generation cephalosporin** (e.g., **ceftizoxime** or
  **cefotaxime**)
  **PLUS**
**Doxycycline** 100 mg orally twice a day for 14 d
  **WITH OR WITHOUT**
**Metronidazole** 500 mg orally twice a day for 14 d

For full details and alternative oral treatment regimens, see updated Centers for Disease Control and Prevention guidelines.
IV, intravenous; IM, intramuscular; PO, orally; bid, twice a day; qid, four times a day.
Adapted from Workowski KA, Berman S; Centers for Disease Control and Prevention. Sexually transmitted diseases treatment guidelines, 2010. *MMWR Recomm Rep* 2010;59(RR-12):1–110.

- **Diagnosis:** The diagnosis of chronic endometritis is established by endometrial biopsy and culture. The classic histologic findings of chronic endometritis are an inflammatory reaction of monocytes and plasma cells in the endometrial stroma (five plasma cells per high-power field). A diffuse pattern of inflammatory infiltrates of lymphocytes and plasma cells throughout the endometrial stroma or even stromal necrosis is associated with severe cases of endometritis.
- **Treatment:** The treatment of choice for chronic endometritis is doxycycline, 100 mg PO bid for 10 days. Broader coverage of anaerobic organisms may also be considered, especially in the presence of BV. When endometritis is associated with acute PID, the treatment should focus on the major etiologic organisms, including *N. gonorrhoeae* and *C. trachomatis*, and should also include broader polymicrobial coverage.
- See Chapter 23 for puerperal **endomyometritis**.

## SUGGESTED READINGS

American College of Obstetricians and Gynecologists. ACOG practice bulletin no. 57: gynecologic herpes simplex virus infections. *Obstet Gynecol* 2004;104:1111–1117.

American College of Obstetricians and Gynecologists. ACOG practice bulletin no. 72: vaginitis. *Obstet Gynecol* 2006;107:1195–1206.

Biggs WS, Williams RM. Common gynecologic infections. *Prim Care Clin Office Pract* 2009; 36:33–51.

Leone PA. Scabies and pediculosis pubis: an update of treatment regimens and general review. *Clin Infect Dis* 2007;44:S153–S159.

Mers D, Wolff T, Gregory K, et al. USPSTF recommendations for STI screening. *Am Fam Physician* 2008;77(6):819–824.

Soper DE. Pelvic inflammatory disease. *Obstet Gynecol* 2010;116:419–428.

Wiley D, Masongsong E. Human papillomavirus: the burden of infection. *Obstet Gynecol Surv* 2006;61(6):S3–S14.

# Ectopic Pregnancy

Virginia Mensah and Melissa Yates

An **ectopic pregnancy (EP)** occurs when a fertilized ovum implants outside of the uterine cavity.

## EPIDEMIOLOGY OF ECTOPIC PREGNANCY

- Two percent of all first-trimester pregnancies and 6% of all pregnancy-related deaths
- EP is the leading cause of death in the first trimester.
- At least one third of pregnancies that occur after tubal sterilization procedures are EPs.
- Women who use an intrauterine device (IUD) have an overall decreased risk of both intrauterine and extrauterine pregnancies. However, when pregnancy does occur, risk of EP is higher than in women not using an IUD.
- In assisted reproductive technology (ART), the incidence of EP is approximately 3% to 5%. These pregnancies tend to be recognized at an earlier stage due to close monitoring in these patients.
- Ninety-seven percent of ectopic pregnancies are implanted within the fallopian tube, although implantation can occur within the abdomen, cervix, ovary, or uterine cornua. Other rare locations for implantation include previous hysterotomy scars and the rudimentary horn of a uterus. EPs also occur following hysterectomy.
- **Risk factors for EP** include pelvic inflammatory disease, previous tubal surgery, infertility, current or previous use of an IUD, two or more pregnancy termination procedures, diethylstilbestrol exposure, age >40 years, smoking, greater than three previous spontaneous abortions, and assisted reproduction.
- **Risk factors for recurrent EP** include previous EP (even if previous EP was treated by salpingectomy), previous spontaneous miscarriage (with likelihood increasing with each miscarriage), and a history of pelvic surgery. No significant increase exists in women with a history of pelvic infections when these patients are compared to those with a primary presentation of EP.
- Etiology of EPs is often multifactorial, and an estimated 40% to 50% of EPs have an unknown etiology.

## DIAGNOSIS OF ECTOPIC PREGNANCY

### Clinical Presentation

- The **Classic triad** (present in less than 50% of patients) is amenorrhea followed by abnormal vaginal bleeding and abdominal or pelvic pain.
- **Pain** is present in 95% of patients with rupturing EP. It is usually located in the lower quadrants but can be anywhere within the abdomen. Cervical motion tenderness (CMT) is present in 75% of patients with ruptured EP.
- **Vaginal spotting** is present in 60% to 80% of patients and is usually scant, dark brown bleeding, either intermittent or continuous.
- EP may present as a surgical emergency, and timely diagnosis is essential (Fig. 29-1).

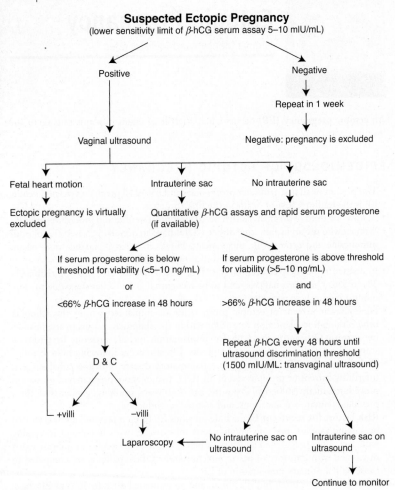

**Suspected Ectopic Pregnancy**
(lower sensitivity limit of β-hCG serum assay 5–10 mIU/mL)

Positive

Negative

Repeat in 1 week

Vaginal ultrasound

Negative: pregnancy is excluded

Fetal heart motion

Intrauterine sac

No intrauterine sac

Ectopic pregnancy is virtually excluded

Quantitative β-hCG assays and rapid serum progesterone (if available)

If serum progesterone is below threshold for viability (<5–10 ng/mL)

or

<66% β-hCG increase in 48 hours

If serum progesterone is above threshold for viability (>5–10 ng/mL)

and

>66% β-hCG increase in 48 hours

D & C

Repeat β-hCG every 48 hours until ultrasound discrimination threshold (1500 mIU/ML: transvaginal ultrasound)

+villi

−villi

Laparoscopy ← No intrauterine sac on ultrasound

Intrauterine sac on ultrasound

Continue to monitor

**Figure 29-1.** Evaluation of the stable patient with suspected EP. Hormonal parameters can vary depending on the assay technique and reference standard used. The discriminatory threshold for sonographic detection of an intrauterine gestational sac is established by each institution. (Reused with permission from Damario MA, Rock JA. Ectopic pregnancy. In Rock JA, Jones HW III, eds. *TeLinde's Operative Gynecology*, 9th ed. Philadelphia, PA: Lippincott Williams & Wilkins, 2003:516.)

## Differential Diagnosis

- **Salpingitis** presents with similar signs and symptoms as EP, but negative pregnancy test results, and an elevated white blood cell (WBC) and temperature.
- **Threatened abortion:** In this condition, bleeding is usually heavier, pain is localized to the lower mid abdomen, and CMT is generally absent.

- **Appendicitis:** Persistent right lower quadrant pain, with fever and gastrointestinal (GI) symptoms, suggests appendicitis. CMT, if present, is usually less severe than with EP. Pregnancy test results are negative, and amenorrhea or abnormal vaginal bleeding is usually absent.
- **Ovarian torsion:** Pain is initially intermittent and later becomes constant as vascular supply is compromised. Findings may include an elevated WBC and a palpable adnexal mass, but pregnancy test results are negative.
- **Other conditions** in the differential should include normal intrauterine pregnancy, heterotopic pregnancy (especially in the case of ART), ruptured ovarian cyst, bleeding corpus luteum, endometriosis, diverticulitis, and dysfunctional uterine bleeding. Gastroenteritis, urinary tract infection, or renal calculus early in pregnancy may also mimic an EP.

## Physical Examination

- **Ruptured unstable EP** is a surgical emergency. If unstable, patients may have signs of hypovolemic shock, including tachycardia, hypotension, and confusion. Abdominal exam may reveal peritonitis, including guarding, rigidity, or rebound tenderness. Up to 15% of women complain of shoulder pain, secondary to diaphragmatic irritation from hemoperitoneum.
- **Hemodynamically stable EP:** Tenderness in patients with EP may be generalized (45%), located bilaterally in the lower quadrants (25%), or located unilaterally in a lower quadrant (30%). Rebound tenderness may or may not be present. CMT, resulting from peritoneal irritation, is usually present but is not specific for EP. A palpable adnexal mass or mass in the cul-de-sac is reported in approximately 40% of cases; absence of a palpable mass does not rule out EP.

## Laboratory Evaluation

- If EP is diagnosed before rupture, a laboratory diagnosis may be made and conservative treatment offered.

### Quantitative Gonadotropin Levels

- **Quantitative beta-human chorionic gonadotropin ($\beta$-hCG):** The titer climbs in a linear fashion from 2 to 4 weeks after ovulation in normal pregnancy, frequently doubling every 48 to 72 hours until it reaches 10,000 mIU/mL.
- Minimum rise in $\beta$-hCG for a viable intrauterine pregnancy (IUP) is typically 53% in 48 hours. Thus, $\beta$-hCG that increases less than 50% in 48 hours is almost always associated with an abnormal pregnancy. Serial serum hCG values that increase or decrease more slowly than expected when compared to viable IUPs or spontaneous abortions, respectively, are suggestive of EP; however, the entire clinical picture must be considered.
  - Levels of $\beta$-hCG are more likely to plateau (<15% change) with an EP than with a spontaneous abortion.
  - A $\beta$-hCG level of <1,500 mIU/mL accompanied by pain and vaginal bleeding increases the likelihood of an EP by 2.5 times.
  - Patients with a single $\beta$-hCG of 2,000 mIU/mL and no identifiable gestational sac on transvaginal ultrasound (TVUS) should have a repeat $\beta$-hCG in 12 to 24 hours. A rapidly falling $\beta$-hCG can indicate a completed spontaneous abortion. However, careful consideration of last menstrual period and the possibility of a multifetal gestation should be considered.
  - Seventeen percent of patients with EP will have normal $\beta$-hCG doubling time (greater than 53% rise in 48 hours).

*Hemoglobin and Hematocrit*

- Baseline blood counts should be obtained. Serial measurements are useful if the diagnosis of ruptured EP is uncertain. An acute drop in **hemoglobin or hematocrit** over the first few hours of observation is more revealing than the initial reading. After acute hemorrhage, initial readings may be at first unchanged or only slightly decreased; a subsequent decline represents restoration of depleted blood volume by hemodilution.

*Metabolic Panel*

- Baseline creatinine and liver transaminases should be obtained in preparation for methotrexate (MTX) treatment for EP. Any signs of renal, hepatic, or hematologic dysfunction are a contraindication to MTX treatment.

*Progesterone*

- A normal IUP should be associated with a serum progesterone value of 20 ng/mL or greater. A value of <5 ng/mL indicates a nonviable pregnancy.
- Of limited use in diagnosing EP, as many patients with EP will have serum progesterone levels between 10 and 20 ng/mL. A progesterone level may be used to predict viability of a pregnancy of unknown location but is insufficient for EP diagnosis.

## Diagnosis by Imaging: Transvaginal Ultrasound

- **Most common sites of EP:** ampullary (70%), isthmic (12%), fimbrial (11.1%), ovarian (3.2%), interstitial and cornual (2.4%), abdominal (1.3%), and cervical (0.15%).
- **The discriminatory zone** is the lowest β-hCG level in which ultrasound should detect evidence of an IUP. Depending on the institution, this β-hCG level ranges from 1,500 to 2,000 mIU/mL for detection via TVUS.
- When the β-hCG level is below 2,000, ultrasound diagnosis of EP should be based on visualization of an adnexal mass rather than absence of intrauterine gestational sac.
- Heterotopic pregnancy (combined intrauterine and extrauterine pregnancy) is rare, although less so among women conceiving through in vitro fertilization (IVF). Serial hCG concentrations are not interpretable in the presence of both a viable IUP and EP. On ultrasound examination, the diagnosis is suggested by visualization of both an ectopic and an IUP or the presence of echogenic fluid in the cul-de-sac in the presence of an IUP. Surgery (e.g., salpingostomy or salpingectomy) is the standard treatment of heterotopic pregnancy with a tubal component because the IUP is a contraindication to medical therapy.
- Sensitivity of TVUS in the diagnosis of EP ranges from 70% to 90%. Despite relative accuracy in detection of EPs, there remain some cases where results of TVUS are inconclusive regarding location of pregnancy in the setting of a positive pregnancy test. These are deemed pregnancy of unknown location (PUL). An EP is eventually diagnosed in 7% to 20% of women with PUL. It is important to note that PUL is a classification scheme and not a final diagnosis.
- PUL is a term provided by a classification scheme which was designed to "improve objective comparison of research outcomes in the diagnosis of EP and to reduce clinical heterogeneity." Using this scheme, there are five classifications depending on sonographic findings: definite EP, probable EP, PUL, probable IUP, and definite IUP.
- For women with PUL, final outcome is classified as visualized EP, visualized IUP, spontaneously resolved PUL, and persisting PUL. In the category of persisting

PUL, further final outcomes are classified as nonvisualized EP, treated persistent PUL, resolved persistent PUL, or histologic IUP.

- **Radiologic signs of EP** include an empty uterus, cystic or solid adnexal masses, dilated and thick-walled fallopian tubes, free echogenic fluid in pelvis, hematosalpinx, extrauterine gestational sac that contains a yolk sac (with or without an embryo), and increased blood flow to the adnexa which contains the EP (using Doppler technology).
- **Pseudosac:** Ten percent of ectopic pregnancies have a pseudosac in the uterus that lacks the "double decidual" sign of an IUP. A pseudosac tends to be oval in shape with irregular margins in contrast to the smooth margins of an IUP. It also tends to appear centrally in the intrauterine cavity.
- An EP greater than 2 cm in size can be visualized with TVUS.
- Adnexal cardiac activity may be seen when the β-hCG titer is greater than 15,000 mIU/mL.

## Diagnosis by Pathology: Dilation and Curettage

- When β-hCG concentration is above 1,500 to 2,000 mIU/mL and TVUS fails to confirm an IUP, dilation and curettage (D&C) should be considered to distinguish between an abnormal IUP and an EP.
- In a recent study of patients with a β-hCG level above 2,000 mIU/mL and no visible IUP on ultrasound, 45.7% had an EP as compared with 54.3% who had a spontaneous abortion. Of the patients with a β-hCG level below 2,000 mIU/mL with similar findings, 68.8% had an EP, whereas 31.2% had a spontaneous abortion.
- Women with abnormally rising or plateauing β-hCG <2,000 should undergo curettage before initiation of MTX to ensure that a patient with a spontaneous abortion is not treated unnecessarily.
- Absence of chorionic villi in a curettage specimen suggests the presence of EP; however, the sensitivity is only 70%, as it may represent a completed spontaneous abortion. β-hCG values should continue to be followed.
- If the β-hCG level is rising or has reached a plateau after D&C, MTX treatment should be initiated.

# TREATMENT FOR ECTOPIC PREGNANCY

Initial management is based on the patient's stability. During initial workup, blood should be obtained for a serum hCG, type and screen (with crossmatch as needed), complete blood count (CBC), prothrombin time, partial thromboplastin time, and complete metabolic panel (especially if MTX treatment is being considered). Patients in shock or with a surgical abdomen should be resuscitated with intravenous fluids, using two large-bore intravenous cannulas, have an indwelling catheter placed to monitor urine output, and be taken to the operating room as soon as possible. For the stable patient with an EP, various medical or surgical therapeutic options may be considered.

## Medical Management: Methotrexate

- **Mechanism of action:** As a folic acid antagonist, MTX inactivates dihydrofolate reductase, causing depletion of tetrahydrofolate, which is necessary for DNA and RNA synthesis. The result is inhibition of growth of the rapidly dividing trophoblast cells of an EP.

| TABLE 29-1 | Criteria for Methotrexate Therapy |
|---|---|

**Stovall and Ling, 1993[a]**

   Hemodynamic stability

   Increase in β-hCG titers after curettage

   Transvaginal sonogram showing an unruptured EP of <3.5 cm in greatest diameter

   Desire for future fertility

**American College of Obstetricians and Gynecologists, 1990[b]**

   Gestational sac size of <3 cm

   Desire for future fertility

   Stable or rising β-hCG levels with peak values of <15,000 mIU/mL

   Intact tubal serosa

   No active bleeding

   EP fully visible at laparoscopy

   Cervical and cornual pregnancy (in selected cases)

---

β-hCG, beta-human chorionic gonadotropin; EP, ectopic pregnancy.

[a]Adapted from Stovall TG, Ling FW. Single-dose methotrexate: an expanded clinical trial. *Am J Obstet Gynecol* 1993;168:1759–1762.

[b]From American College of Obstetricians and Gynecologists. Ectopic pregnancy. ACOG technical bulletin no. 150. *Int J Gynaecol Obstet* 1992;37(3):213–219.

- **Criteria for MTX therapy** are listed in Table 29-1.
- **Absolute and relative contraindications to MTX therapy** are listed in Table 29-2.
- **Prior to administration of MTX**
  - Determine patient's blood type and give RhoGAM, if necessary.
  - Obtain a CBC and metabolic panel including liver and renal function studies.
- **Drug side effects** of MTX include nausea, vomiting, stomatitis, dermatitis, diarrhea, gastric distress, dizziness, elevated liver transaminases, pneumonitis, neutropenia (rare), and reversible alopecia (rare).
  - In one meta-analysis, 36.2% of patients experienced side effects that correlated with effectiveness of treatment in both single-dose and multidose protocols.
  - The most common side effects are elevated transaminases, mild stomatitis, and GI upset.
- **Treatment side effects**
  - Perhaps the most significant side effect is abdominal pain that arises 2 to 3 days after treatment, presumably from the cytotoxic effect of the drug causing tubal abortion. This pain may complicate the diagnosis of ruptured ectopic and require hospital admission for close observation. Nonsteroidal anti-inflammatory drugs should be avoided for analgesia due to risk of interaction with MTX.
  - Increase in β-hCG levels during first 1 to 3 days of treatment
  - Vaginal bleeding or spotting
  - 10% risk of tubal rupture

## TABLE 29-2 Contraindications to Methotrexate Therapy

### American College of Obstetricians and Gynecologists, 2008[a]

*Absolute contraindications*

Breast-feeding

Overt or laboratory evidence of immunodeficiency

Alcoholism, alcoholic liver disease, or other chronic liver disease

Preexisting blood dyscrasia, such as bone marrow hypoplasia, leukopenia, thrombocytopenia, or significant anemia

Peptic ulcer disease

Hepatic, renal, or hematologic dysfunction

*Relative contraindications*

Gestational sac larger than 3.5 cm

Embryonic cardiac motion

### American Society for Reproductive Medicine, 2006[b]

*Absolute contraindications*

Breast-feeding

Evidence of immunodeficiency

Moderate to severe anemia, leukopenia, or thrombocytopenia

Sensitivity to MTX

Active pulmonary or peptic ulcer disease

Clinically important hepatic or renal dysfunction

IUP

*Relative contraindications*

Ectopic mass >4 cm on TVUS

Embryonic cardiac activity on TVUS

Patient declines blood transfusion

Patient is unable to follow-up

High initial hCG (>5,000)

MTX, methotrexate; IUP, intrauterine pregnancy; TVUS, transvaginal ultrasound; hCG, human chorionic gonadotropin.
[a]Adapted from American College of Obstetricians and Gynecologists. Medical management of ectopic pregnancy. ACOG practice bulletin no. 94. *Obstet Gynecol* 2008;111:1479–1485.
[b]From Practice Committee of the American Society for Reproductive Medicine. Medical treatment of ectopic pregnancy. *Fertil Steril* 2006;86(5)(suppl 1):S96–S102.

- **MTX dosing regimens**
  - **Single-dose versus multidose treatment:** Treatment protocols that involve single or multiple injections of MTX have been developed (Table 29-3). Benefits of a single dose include decreased cost, better side effect profile, improved patient compliance, and no need for leucovorin rescue treatment. The benefit of the multidose regimen is a lower failure rate. A systematic review reported a failure

| TABLE 29-3 | Methotrexate Treatment Protocols for Ectopic Pregnancy |
|---|---|

|  | Single-Dose Regimen[a] | Two-Dose Regimen[b] | Fixed Multidose Regimen[c] |
|---|---|---|---|
| **Schedule** | Day 1, repeat if necessary | Days 0 and 4 | Days 1, 3, 5, 7 |
| **Medication** | | | |
| Methotrexate | 50 mg/m$^2$ IM | 50 mg/m$^2$ IM | 1 mg/kg IM |
| Leucovorin | None | None | 0.1 mg/kg IM (days 2, 4, 6, 8) |
| **Surveillance** | Measure hCG on days 4 and 7, checking for 15% decrease from days 4–7. | Measure hCG on days 4 and 7, checking for 15% decrease from days 4–7. | Measure hCG on MTX dose days and continue until 15% decrease between values. |
|  | If <15% decrease, repeat dosing (50 mg/m$^2$) on day 7 and measure hCG on days 11 and 14. | If <15% decrease, repeat dosing (50 mg/m$^2$) on days 7 and 11, measuring hCG levels. | If <15% decrease or increase, consider repeating MTX regimen. |
|  | If >15 % decrease, measure hCG levels weekly until reaching nonpregnant level. | | |

IM, intramuscular; hCG, human chorionic gonadotropin; MTX, methotrexate.

[a]From Stovall TG, Ling FW. Single-dose methotrexate: an expanded clinical trial. *Am J Obstet Gynecol* 1993;168:1759–1762.

[b]From Barnhart K, Hummel AC, Sammel MD, et al. Use of "2-dose" regimen to treat ectopic pregnancy. *Fertil Steril* 2007;87:250.

[c]From Rodi IA, Sauer MV, Gorril MJ, et al. The medical treatment of unruptured ectopic pregnancy with methotrexate and citrovorum rescue: preliminary experience. *Fertil Steril* 1986;46:811–813.
Adapted from American College of Obstetricians and Gynecologists. ACOG practice bulletin no. 94: medical management of ectopic pregnancy. *Obstet Gynecol* 2008;111:1479–1485.

rate of 14.3% or higher with single-dose MTX when pretreatment β-hCG levels are higher than 5,000 mIU/mL, compared with a 3.7% failure rate for hCG levels less than 5,000 mIU/mL. If hCG levels are higher than 5,000 mIU/mL, the two-dose regimen may be appropriate while avoiding the need for leucovorin rescue and improving patient compliance.

• The overall success rate for MTX is 89%. The success rate of single-dose treatment is reported to be 88.1% versus 92.7% for the multidose regimen ($p = .035$).

- Patients with previous EPs are four times more likely to fail MTX treatment.
- **Special indications for MTX treatment** include known EP in difficult locations, such as cervical, ovarian, or cornual pregnancies in which the risk of surgical management outweighs the risk of attempted medical management.
- **Treatment monitoring:** Concentration of β-hCG often rises after the initial MTX injection. The level of β-hCG should drop by at least 15% from day 4 to day 7 following administration. TVUS is not an appropriate modality for determining treatment failure. Enlargement of the ectopic mass and/or free fluid in the pelvis are common findings after MTX injection and may prompt unnecessary interventions.
- **Treatment failure** is generally defined as a need for subsequent surgical intervention, although some studies use the term to describe the failure of a single MTX injection to lower β-hCG concentration by at least 15%.

## Surgical Management

- Surgical management is the appropriate course of treatment in hemodynamically unstable patients or patients who have failed MTX therapy. Surgical management is also indicated in patients who have had a previous ectopic in the same fallopian tube.
- The surgical techniques should be tailored to the specific findings and situation, and they include salpingostomy, salpingectomy, partial salpingectomy, segmental resection, cornual resection, and possible hysterectomy for interstitial pregnancy.
  - **Salpingostomy** is the preferred treatment for women who desire future fertility and have a compromised contralateral fallopian tube. A linear incision is made on the antimesenteric border over the pregnancy, which usually extrudes from the incision and is removed. Bleeding points are cauterized with laser or needlepoint cautery, and the incision is left to heal by secondary intention. EPs located in the ampulla are ideal candidates.
  - **Salpingectomy** involves the removal of the entire tube on the affected side. Consideration must be given to tubal damage at the time of surgery, especially in the case of a second EP in the same tube. Candidates for salpingectomy include women who have failed salpingostomy, completed childbearing, and patients with uncontrolled bleeding.
  - EP after tubal ligation is most often located in the fimbriated end of the tube. In this case, both fimbriae should be surgically removed and the proximal segments of the tube cauterized to prevent recurrent EP.

### Laparoscopy

- Minimally invasive laparoscopy is the preferred surgical approach in the hemodynamically stable patient. It usually provides a definitive diagnosis, although early EPs are missed 4% to 8% of the time. Not all patients are ideal candidates (e.g., patients with large body habitus or previous abdominal surgeries). Surgical approaches include linear salpingostomy and salpingectomy.
- **Contraindications to laparoscopy** may include pelvic adhesions, hemoperitoneum, pregnancy >4 cm, and hemodynamic instability.
- Linear salpingostomy requires postoperative MTX in 15% of cases, often due to presence of persistent trophoblastic tissue. Serial β-hCG levels must be followed weekly.
- Tubal rupture is not an absolute indication for salpingectomy, especially if the rupture site is linear and small. The rupture site can be used to evacuate the pregnancy and preserve the tube.
- Salpingectomy is indicated when the tube continues to bleed after linear salpingostomy, when an EP occurs in a tube with previous damage, or when an EP occurs

in a tube with a previously identified hydrosalpinx in a patient who is currently undergoing IVF.
- Copious irrigation of the pelvis is indicated to prevent adhesions and trophoblastic implants.

*Laparotomy*
- Laparotomy is indicated for a patient with obvious hemorrhage and hemodynamic compromise. After hemostasis is obtained, the treatment of choice is complete or partial salpingectomy. With a ruptured interstitial or cornual pregnancy, cornual resection may be required. Laparotomy is also indicated when adhesive disease precludes adequate visualization through the laparoscope.

*Complications of Surgical Management*
- Persistent trophoblastic tissue and persistent EP are considered surgical failures. Levels of β-hCG should be followed weekly after salpingostomy, until nonpregnant levels are reached. Surgically managed EPs can be given a dose of MTX for eradication of persistent trophoblastic tissue if β-hCG levels are found to plateau, in lieu of reoperation.

## FOLLOW-UP AND PROGNOSIS

- After one EP, approximately 60% of patients conceive spontaneously.
- The recurrence risk ranges from 10% to 27%, which is 5 to 10 times greater than the risk for EP in the general population. The risk of recurrence increases in patients who have had two or more EPs. Only one out of three will conceive, and 20% to 57% of these will have EPs.
- Subsequent tubal patency rates are similar (80% to 85%) for patients treated medically or with salpingostomy.
- Patients with badly damaged fallopian tubes and those whose tubes have been removed can conceive through IVF.
- Patients should be advised to use reliable contraceptive methods until initial inflammation resolves (6 to 12 weeks). Contraception will avoid confusion between rising β-hCG levels from a new pregnancy and those from a persistent EP if conception occurs in the immediate postoperative period.
- Patients should undergo extensive counseling regarding their risk for recurrent EP and the necessity for early medical attention for subsequent pregnancies. The latter includes serial determinations of β-hCG levels until an early ultrasound examination can document an IUP or EP.
- Postoperative RhoGAM must be given to an Rh-negative woman to prevent Rh alloimmunization in a future pregnancy.

## SUGGESTED READINGS

Barnhart KT. Ectopic pregnancy. *N Engl J Med* 2009;361:379–387.
Barnhart KT, Gosman G, Ashby R, et al. The medical management of EP: a meta-analysis comparing "single-dose" and "multidose" regimens. *Obstet Gynecol* 2003;101:778–784.
Barnhart KT, Van Mello NM, Bourne T, et al. Pregnancy of unknown location: a consensus statement of nomenclature, definitions, and outcome. *Fertil Steril* 2011;95(3):857–866.
Bouyer J, Coste J, Shojaei T, et al. Risk factors for EP: a comprehensive analysis based on a large case-control, population-based study in France. *Am J Epidemiol* 2003;157:185–194.

Gerton GL, Fan XJ, Barnhart K, et al. Presumed diagnosis of EP. *Obstet Gynecol* 2002;100: 505–510.

Lipscomb GH, McCord ML, Stovall TG, et al. Predictors of success of methotrexate treatment in women with tubal ectopic pregnancies. *N Engl J Med* 1999;341:1974–1978.

Lipscomb GH, Stovall TG, Ling FW. Nonsurgical treatment of EP. *N Engl J Med* 2000;343:1325–1329.

Marion LL, Meeks GR. Ectopic pregnancy: history, incidence, epidemiology and risk factors. *Clin Obstet Gynecol* 2012;55(2):376–386.

Van Mello NM, Femke M, Ankum WM, et al. Ectopic pregnancy: how the diagnostic and therapeutic management has changed. *Fertil Steril* 2012;98(5):1066–1073.

# Chronic Pelvic Pain

Khara M. Simpson and Wen Shen

**Chronic pelvic pain (CPP)** is a common and often difficult problem, with direct medical costs estimated at $1 to $2 billion per year in the United States. CPP affects quality of life, increases work absenteeism, decreases overall productivity, and limits normal physical, social, emotional, and sexual function. The differential diagnosis is extensive and the cause is often multisystem and multifactorial. CPP is the diagnosis for 10% to 20% of gynecology office referrals. Up to 90% of patients with CPP will undergo one or more unsuccessful, and often unnecessary, gynecologic procedures. At least 40% of gynecologic laparoscopies are performed for CPP, but only 30% to 60% of those surgeries reveal a cause. Ten percent to 20% of hysterectomies are performed with the primary indication of CPP, but relief is not universal.

## TYPES OF PELVIC PAIN

There are no standard diagnostic criteria, but a reasonable **definition of CPP** is cyclic or noncyclic pain in the lower abdomen, pelvis, lower back, or buttocks of at least 6 months duration that causes functional disability and motivates the patient to seek medical help. Because of varied definitions, the epidemiology and natural history of CPP are not well described. **Acute pelvic pain** can be defined with the same criteria but lasts <30 days.

- CPP is most common in younger adult women. Four percent to 15% of reproductive age women are affected, similar to other common disorders such as asthma, migraine headache, and lower back pain.
  - **Dysmenorrhea** (pain associated with menstrual cycles) occurs in up to 90% of women. Risk factors include age <30 years; body mass index <20; tobacco use; early menarche; menometrorrhagia; and history of pelvic inflammatory disease (PID), tubal ligation, and physical/sexual assault.
  - **Dyspareunia** (pain during sexual activity) occurs in 1% to 40% of women. Risk factors include female circumcision, history of PID, anxiety, depression, sexual assault, and postmenopausal status.

- **Noncyclic pelvic pain** (with no relation to menses) occurs in 4% to 40% of women. Risk factors include anxiety, depression, prior cesarean section, pelvic adhesions, endometriosis, menorrhagia, and history of miscarriage or physical/sexual abuse.

## BIOLOGY AND CLASSIFICATION OF PAIN PERCEPTION

Acute **pain perception** is an evolutionary protective mechanism causing reflexive withdrawal from noxious stimuli. Individuals with congenitally impaired pain sensation have shorter lifespans.

- **Pain receptors** respond to intense mechanical stress or local inflammatory/pain mediators (e.g., histamine, bradykinin, substance P). That stimulus is transduced to an electrical impulse that is transmitted via A-delta (fast myelinated) and C-fiber (slow unmyelinated) dorsal root ganglion neurons to synapse in the dorsal horn of the spinal cord. Second-order pain neurons then cross the anterior commissure and travel via the lateral spinothalamic tract to the thalamus where they synapse again. Third-order pain neurons project from the thalamus to the insular cortex (emotional content), the anterior cingulate cortex (planning/motivational function), and the primary sensory cortex (primary pain perception).
- **Pain afferent pathways** can be modulated in the brain and spinal cord by descending pathways that can augment or diminish pain sensation. The possible interactions between acute pain perception, chronic pain pathway activation, and higher level/emotional modulation of pain circuitry underlie the complex pathophysiology of CPP. Normal descending inhibition of dorsal horn synaptic activity, for example, is decreased in chronic pain syndromes such as irritable bowel syndrome. Emotional factors such as depression and anxiety also decrease the pain threshold.
- **Nociceptive somatic pain** (e.g., postoperative pain, trauma, inflammation) is produced by heat, cold, mechanical, and chemical stimuli. Deep somatic pain is detected within muscles, ligaments, and bone. Deep visceral pain from internal organs is poorly localized and has some overlap with somatic sensory tracts in the spinal cord, causing "referred pain." The T10 to L1 afferent visceral pain fibers that innervate the uterus, adnexa, and cervix also supply the lower ileum, sigmoid colon, and rectum. Pelvic pain sensations can originate in any of those closely related structures.
- **Neuropathic pain** (e.g., postherpetic neuralgia, diabetic neuropathy, nerve entrapment, Taxol chemotherapy–induced peripheral neuropathy) is due to peripheral or central nerve damage causing a malfunction in pain detection. It is commonly perceived as a chronic burning or tingling pain and produced from both local and systemic processes.
- Current **pain theory** incorporates the Descartean concept of sensory specificity (i.e., a single stimulus is conducted along a dedicated pain pathway) and more recent ideas regarding the modulating influence of emotional, cognitive, cultural, attentive, and suggestive factors on both initial transmission and ultimate perception.
- **Psychogenic pain** (e.g., somatization) is another possible etiology in a complete biopsychosocial model, representing the physical manifestation of unresolved emotional or psychological conflict.
- It can be difficult to determine whether a patient has a symptom of nociceptive stimulation or an ongoing malfunction of pain perception or both. Acutely painful

processes, for example PID, may eventually resolve but leave permanently remodeled pelvic structures (e.g., adhesions) that can cause chronic pain. An extended inflammatory stimulus (e.g., inflammatory bowel disease) can lead to higher order pain sensitization and hyperesthesia. Pain associated with intense emotional content (e.g., childhood sexual abuse) can alter neurocognitive development, leading to hypervigilance and heightened pain sensation.

- Although gynecologists often think of CPP as originating from either gynecologic or nongynecologic sources, it may be more helpful to take a broader view. Anatomic localization (e.g., abdominal wall, bowel, bladder, perineum), affected organ system (e.g., gastrointestinal, genitourinary, musculoskeletal, psychiatric), and type of pain (e.g., somatic, visceral, neuropathic, psychogenic) are possible diagnostic paradigms.

## EVALUATION OF CHRONIC PELVIC PAIN

The **evaluation of CPP** starts with a complete medical history and the goal of establishing an enduring therapeutic physician–patient relationship.

### History and Physical Exam

- **Prior records** (including past history, test results, operative notes, and pathology reports) should be reviewed to avoid redundant tests or procedures and to gauge the effectiveness of prior interventions and progress over time.
- **Pain inventory questionnaires** can be helpful in recording subjective and objective data and may increase the efficiency of initial data gathering. Useful resources are available from the International Pelvic Pain Society (IPPS) at www.pelvicpain.org. Pain questionnaires are helpful in allowing the patient to develop a coherent and relevant narrative before appearing at the office and allow rapid review of symptoms, permitting the interview to focus on pain issues. A personal body pain map is extremely helpful in focusing the differential and examination.
- Adequate time should be allotted for a **complete medical and psychosocial history** without rushing the patient. A detailed review of systems, including genitourinary, gastrointestinal, musculoskeletal, and psychoneurologic questions, is important.
  - Establish a detailed understanding of the intensity, location, character, and duration of the pain and any association with intercourse, menstruation, defecation, recent or distant surgery, radiation treatments, or abdominopelvic infections. Precipitating and relieving factors should be reviewed.
  - Screening for physical or sexual abuse, domestic violence, and other psychosocial stressors (e.g., death of loved one, divorce) should be completed. Twenty percent to 60% of patients with CPP report a history of sexual or childhood abuse. A complete mental health history and depression screening are helpful; mood and personality disorders are frequently comorbid with CPP. It is not clear whether these problems are a cause or result of pain. Increased depression scores, however, correlate with increased pain scores, so simultaneous treatment is most effective.
  - Current, usual, and worst pain can be recorded using a pain scale (e.g., visual analogue scale). Associated symptoms such as weight loss, hematochezia, and perimenopausal/postmenopausal bleeding should prompt a thorough investigation for malignancy.

- The **physical exam** begins with a general and neurologic assessment. Fully explain the plan and exam techniques to relieve anxiety and promote patient cooperation and comfort. The IPPS physical exam form or similar tools may be useful for recording the complete assessment. The exam should help narrow the differential, rule out systemic disease or neoplasm, and suggest additional testing.
  - Evaluate the **general appearance**, including dress, nutrition, posture, apparent age, gait, and pain behaviors. Evaluate **posture** (both seated and standing) and **gait** (for any hip height and leg length discrepancy).
  - Ask the patient to **indicate the precise location** of her pain. If she is able to use a single finger, a discrete source is more likely than if she uses a broad sweeping motion of the entire hand.
  - Note the presence of **scars** or **hernias** on abdominal exam. Gently attempt to elicit pain with palpation of the skin, fascia, or muscle. Especially note any reproducible tenderness. Appropriate **trigger point mapping** should be performed if fibromyalgia is in the differential.
  - Look for **Carnett sign** (i.e., increased abdominal tenderness when the patient lifts her head and shoulders in the supine position) suggesting abdominal wall rather than intra-abdominal pathology. Pain with the **Beatty maneuver** (i.e., thigh abduction against resistance) may suggest piriformis syndrome. The **obturator sign** (i.e., pain with flexion and internal rotation of the hip while lying supine) and the **psoas sign** (i.e., pain with hip flexion against resistance) can indicate inflammation or dysfunction within those muscles. The **straight leg raise test** evaluates radiculopathy or intervertebral disc disease. The **FABER test** (i.e., pain with flexion/abduction/external rotation of the hip) assesses hip and sacroiliac joint pathology.
  - A thorough **neurologic examination**, including sensation, muscle strength, and reflexes, may be required. Examine the spine for scoliosis while the patient is sitting, standing, walking, and bending at the waist.
  - The **gynecologic exam** starts with external observation and then palpation with cotton swabs to define hyperesthetic areas (even if the skin appears normal). Colposcopic examination of the vulva and vestibule may be helpful. Light touch and pinprick sensation testing of the vulva is required.
    - Start the internal examination with a single-digit vaginal exam. Assess the vestibule, vaginal walls, rectum, urethra, bladder trigone, pubic arch, pelvic floor muscles, cervix, and vaginal fornices. Initial assessment of the uterus and adnexa are performed with a single digit as well.
    - Visual inspection of the vaginal vault can begin with a single speculum blade. Assess the vaginal cuff or cervix, cervical os, paracervix, and vaginal mucosa.
    - Finally, perform a bimanual exam of the uterus, adnexa, and other pelvic contents followed by rectovaginal exam. Fecal occult blood testing may be indicated. The bimanual exam, being the most invasive part of the evaluation, should be performed last. Some patients will be unable to tolerate any additional evaluation following the bimanual exam.

## Imaging and Laboratory Testing

- **Imaging and diagnostic testing** are tailored to the differential.
  - Pelvic ultrasonography is of little benefit unless uterine or adnexal pathology is suspected. Transvaginal imaging may better assess the pelvic structures than the transabdominal approach.

- Magnetic resonance imaging can be helpful in selected cases, especially if adenomyosis is suspected.
- Plain x-ray of the chest, spine, abdomen, or joints or computed tomography scan is rarely indicated.
- Colonoscopy can assess colorectal cancer, inflammatory bowel disease, diverticulosis, and invasive endometriosis. It is indicated in cases with persistent diarrhea or hematochezia.
- Cystoscopy and evaluation for interstitial cystitis/bladder pain syndrome are frequently indicated early in the workup.
- **Laboratory testing** is guided by the history and physical and may include urine pregnancy test, vaginal pH and wet mount, gonorrhea and chlamydia polymerase chain reaction, complete blood count, erythrocyte sedimentation rate, thyroid-stimulating hormone, rapid plasma reagin, hepatitis B surface antigen, HIV test, urinalysis/microscopy, and urine culture. There is no standard laboratory panel for CPP. Serum cancer antigen 125 testing is not useful unless a cancer workup is initiated. Endocrine testing for follicle-stimulating hormone, estradiol, and gonadotropin-releasing hormone (GnRH) stimulation test may be indicated for suspected ovarian remnant syndrome.

## Laparoscopy and Consults

- Although **pelviscopy** is performed for more than 40% of CPP cases, it should be employed only when noninvasive evaluation is completed and for cases in which a diagnosis can be reasonably anticipated. Laparoscopy is not a substitute for a complete history and physical or for diagnoses that can be made without a procedure. Most causes of CPP are *not* detectable by laparoscopy. It is most commonly performed when endometriosis or other structural pathology is suspected.
- Selected evaluation by neurology, gastroenterology, anesthesiology, urology, psychiatry, or physical therapy **consultants** can provide important multidisciplinary perspective and assist in forming a complete treatment plan. Often, patients have been through a long, tedious, and piecemeal evaluation by multiple providers followed by redundant diagnostic and treatment failures. Performing a complete and multidisciplinary assessment from the start may reach a successful outcome more efficiently and reassure a demoralized and anxious patient. In addition, some tests are only appropriately obtained via consultation, such as nerve conduction studies or electromyography, if they are necessary.

## DIFFERENTIAL DIAGNOSIS OF PELVIC PAIN

The **differential diagnosis** of pelvic pain is extensive, and many patients deserve multiple diagnoses.

- Selected **causes of CPP** are listed in Table 30-1. Previously undiagnosed medical illness should also be considered, such as neoplasia, sickle cell disease, hyperparathyroidism, urolithiasis, lead/mercury intoxication, lactose intolerance, chronic constipation, chronic appendicitis, and chronic fatigue syndrome.
- The clinical satisfaction of applying Occam razor and assigning only one unifying diagnosis after a thorough workup for CPP is not likely; management of multiple disease processes is often required. The following disorders, in addition to being primary etiologies, are frequently comorbid with CPP and deserve special consideration.

- **Dysmenorrhea** is reported in up to 80% of women with CPP. It is characterized by cramping pelvic or suprapubic pain that radiates to the lower back or thighs, often with mood or behavioral changes. Nausea/vomiting, diarrhea, irritability, and fatigue may be present. The pathophysiology is inflammatory prostaglandin release upon progesterone withdrawal at the end of the menstrual cycle. Patients with hyperalgesia may experience significantly longer and more intense menstrual pain. Managing "normal menstrual pain" can be an important consideration for patients with CPP.

- **Endometriosis** is diagnosed in up to 70% of pelvic pain patients, although biopsy-proven disease is present in perhaps only 30%. See Chapter 38. Up to 80% of patients treated with laparoscopic excision of endometriosis have short-term pain relief, but less than half of those continue to report improved pain scores at 1 year.

- **Irritable bowel syndrome (IBS)** is a primary or secondary diagnosis in 40% to 60% of patients with CPP. Associated symptoms of IBS include abdominal distention, bloating, fatigue, and headache. Symptoms are sometimes worse before menses. Although often comorbid with CPP, this is often a diagnosis of exclusion when considering a primary etiology for CPP.

- **Pelvic adhesions** are eventually diagnosed in about 25% of women with CPP, but a causal relationship is debatable. Pain localization, but not intensity, correlates with the presence of isolated adhesions detected during pelviscopy. Adhesiolysis has not been proven to provide dramatic relief.

- **Interstitial cystitis/bladder pain syndrome** is a chronic inflammatory disorder with aspects of a chronic visceral pain syndrome that frequently coexists with other causes of CPP. Diagnosis is made by cystoscopy and hydrodistention under anesthesia, with findings of glomerulations or Hunner ulcers. Treatment is with oral pentosan sulfate (Elmiron), antihistamines, and low-dose tricyclic antidepressants (e.g., amitriptyline). Bladder installation of an anesthetic cocktail of lidocaine, heparin, steroids, and sodium bicarbonate can provide pain relief on an intermittent or continuous basis.

- **Pelvic congestion syndrome** (symptomatic varicose veins of the pelvis) can be objectively diagnosed by transcervical pelvic venogram. Randomized trials show correlation between venogram scores and pain, with improvement after treatment. Treatment options include hormonal therapy (progestins, combined oral contraceptives), pelvic vein embolization, and hysterectomy.

- **Myofascial pain** is comorbid with 10% to 20% of CPP. Physical therapy is the mainstay of treatment. Selective serotonin reuptake inhibitors (SSRIs) and muscle relaxants may be useful adjuncts.

- **Dyspareunia** can be a primary or secondary symptom in CPP. Additionally, the psychological effect of CPP on relationships and sexual function should be addressed in the evaluation and treatment plan.

- **Low back pain** is often a separate treatable problem that can exacerbate CPP.

## MANAGEMENT OF CHRONIC PELVIC PAIN

**Management of CPP** depends on the etiology and comorbidities (see Table 30-1). The best outcomes may come from a rehabilitation approach with a consistent provider, personalized multidisciplinary treatment, extensive patient education and counseling, and regular office visits. The physician must be open-minded and supportive but offer realistic and explicit goals for therapy. The patient may be desperate for a

**TABLE 30-1    Differential Diagnosis of Chronic Pelvic Pain**

| Category | Etiology | Mechanism | Testing/Diagnosis | Treatment |
|---|---|---|---|---|
| Cyclic/ recurrent gynecologic | **Endometriosis** | Ectopic endometrial tissue infiltration and inflammation. Can progress from cyclic to noncyclic pain as adhesions develop. | H&P, ± imaging, laparoscopy with biopsy | Ovulation suppression (i.e., OCPs, progestins, GnRH agonists), surgical ablation, excision of endometriomas |
| | **Endosalpingiosis Adenomyosis** | Ectopic fallopian tube epithelium Endometrial stroma and glands deeper than 2 mm within the myometrium results in menorrhagia and dysmenorrhea by uncertain mechanism. | Biopsy, pelvic washings MRI | Ablation, GnRH agonists NSAIDs, OCPs, GnRH agonists, progesterone IUD, hysterectomy |
| | **Primary/ secondary dysmenorrhea** | Primary = uterine menstrual pain Secondary = menstrual pain due to structural pathology | H&P, rule out other causes | NSAIDs, OCPs, GnRH agonists, LUNA procedure, transcutaneous electrical nerve stimulation, treatment of secondary causes |
| | **Ovarian remnant syndrome** | FSH stimulation of inadequately excised ovarian tissue at time of oophorectomy. Similar mechanism if ovaries are purposefully conserved at hysterectomy. | Surgical history, serum FSH, and estrogen in premenopausal range | Adhesiolysis and removal of all ovarian tissue may cure >90%. |
| | **Cervical stenosis** | Blocked cervical os results in hematometra, retrograde menstruation. | Pelvic exam, ultrasound | Dilation of cervical os in the office or under sedation in operating room |

*(Continued)*

**TABLE 30-1** Differential Diagnosis of Chronic Pelvic Pain *(Continued)*

| Category | Etiology | Mechanism | Testing/Diagnosis | Treatment |
|---|---|---|---|---|
| *Noncyclic gynecologic* | **Abdominopelvic adhesions** | Scar tissue from infection, trauma, endometriosis. Left-sided sigmoid adhesions are a frequent finding. | H&P, laparoscopy | Laparoscopy/laparotomy and adhesiolysis |
| | **Uterine retroversion** | Rare cause of deep dyspareunia and dysmenorrhea. Very rare cause of uterine pelvic incarceration in early pregnancy. | Pelvic exam, ultrasound, pessary test for symptom relief | Hodge pessary or laparoscopic uterine suspension |
| | **Chronic endometritis/ chronic PID** | Pelvic tuberculosis, tubo-ovarian abscess, chronic chlamydial endometritis, inflammation. More frequent in populations with high rates of STDs. | Cervical chlamydia PCR, endometrial biopsy, ultrasound, laparoscopy | Antibiotic therapy; erythromycin or doxycycline 2–4×/wk |
| | **Chronic vulvovaginitis** | Recurrent or chronic yeast, *Trichomonas*, or fungal infections | H&P, wet prep, culture | Antibiotics, boric acid vaginal suppositories |
| | **Vaginal cuff pain** | Posthysterectomy chronic low-grade cuff cellulitis, seroma, neuroma, or nerve entrapment | H&P, pelvic exam, anesthetic blocks | Cuff resection/revision, cuff anesthesia injection, chemical neurolysis |
| | **Contact vulvitis** | Contact irritant from lotion, soaps, clothing, etc. | H&P | Eliminate offending agents, ± apply topical steroids |
| | **Vulvodynia** | Vulvar hyperalgesia due to neuropathic and pelvic floor pain | Exam, ± biopsy | Vaginal physical therapy, biofeedback, TCA |
| | **Vulvar vestibulitis** | Subset of vulvodynia. Nonspecific vestibular inflammation; severe entry dyspareunia. | H&P, ± vulvar skin biopsy | Vestibulectomy/perineoplasty if conservative management fails |

| | | | |
|---|---|---|---|
| **Pudendal neuralgia** | Pudendal nerve injury or entrapment | H&P, nerve block | Avoid sitting for prolonged periods of time. Pain medications, nerve block, or surgical decompression for severe cases. |
| **Pelvic congestion syndrome** | Pelvic vein insufficiency from pelvic ttissue edema. Pain with increased intra-abdominal pressure, prolonged standing. Increased risk with collagen vascular disease (e.g., Ehlers-Danlos). | History of postcoital aching pain + ovarian point tenderness; pelvic venography (transuterine contrast injection with real-time radiography) | Medroxyprogesterone acetate, endovascular embolization, hysterectomy |
| **Pelvic organ prolapse** | Trauma or intrinsic laxity of vaginal or uterine-supporting tissues causing discomfort or pain | Exam, POP-Q measurements | See Chapter 31. |
| *Gastrointestinal* **Irritable bowel syndrome** | Functional bowel disorder | H&P, rule out other causes | Increase dietary fiber, loperamide, stool softeners, dicyclomine |
| **Inflammatory bowel disease (ulcerative colitis and Crohn disease)** | Chronic bowel inflammation | Cramping lower abdominal pain and bloody diarrhea, stool studies, colonoscopy, biopsies | Anti-inflammatory drugs, steroids. Refer to gastroenterology. |

*(Continued)*

**TABLE 30-1** Differential Diagnosis of Chronic Pelvic Pain *(Continued)*

| Category | Etiology | Mechanism | Testing/Diagnosis | Treatment |
|---|---|---|---|---|
| *Gastrointestinal (continued)* | **Diverticular disease** | Colonic outpouchings of mucosal/submucosa due to muscularis weakness at sites of higher pressure; present in >10% of women older than age 40 yr. Can become infected/inflamed. | AXR, barium enema, colonoscopy | Antibiotics for infection, increased dietary fiber and hydration |
| | **Intermittent bowel obstruction** | Mechanical partial obstruction, usually secondary to adhesions | AXR (upper GI with small bowel follow-through study), CT scan, biopsy of any mass | Bowel decompression and conservative management or surgical adhesiolysis |
| *Urologic* | **Interstitial cystitis/bladder pain syndrome(IC/BPS)** | Chronic noninfectious cystitis and hyperesthesia | H&P, potassium sensitivity testing, cystoscopy, hydrodistention | Hydrodistention, intravesical DMSO, oral pentosan polysulfate, low-dose TCA, antihistamines |
| | **Chronic/recurrent urinary tract infection** | Bacterial or fungal infection, often due to anatomic abnormalities, causes irritative voiding symptoms. Increases with age and PMP status. | Urinalysis, urine culture, test of cure | Antibiotics, ± prophylactic suppression |
| | **Urethral syndrome** | Chronic urethral inflammation, infection, or obstruction, similar to IC/BPS | History of dysuria, frequency, urgency, and slow painful urine stream; exam, cystoscopy, urine culture, chlamydia PCR | Hormone replacement therapy in PMP women, biofeedback, DMSO, NSAIDs, muscle relaxants, and alpha antagonists may be useful. |

| | | |
|---|---|---|
| **Urethral diverticulum** | Herniation of the urethral lining; pocket may become infected/inflamed. It is a rare cause of chronic pain. | History of dysuria, dyspareunia, and postvoid dribbling. Anterior vaginal wall mass. Urinalysis, urine culture, ± cytology, voiding cystourethrography, double-balloon positive pressure urethrography, ultrasound, MRI, urethroscopy. | Antibiotics for infection, surgical excision |
| **Detrusor-sphincter dyssynergia** | Urethral sphincter relaxation does not occur in coordination with detrusor activity causing increased bladder pressure and urine retention. Often from CNS injury or multiple sclerosis. | Urodynamics, EMG study | Urethral stent, transurethral sphincterotomy, botulinum toxin injection, and catheterization are possible treatments. |
| *Musculoskeletal* **Levator ani syndrome** | Pelvic floor muscle spasm; chronic or recurrent rectal or vaginal pain or dyspareunia | Pain reproduction or trigger point detection on vaginal or rectal exam | Heat packs, muscle relaxants, massage, physical therapy, relaxation techniques |
| **Osteoarthritis** | Referred pelvic pain from chronic degenerative loss of cartilage especially at the hip, knee, sacroiliac, and vertebral joints | Musculoskeletal exam, joint x-rays | Weight loss, lifestyle modification, NSAIDs, physical therapy, joint replacement surgery |

*(Continued)*

**TABLE 30-1** Differential Diagnosis of Chronic Pelvic Pain *(Continued)*

| Category | Etiology | Mechanism | Testing/Diagnosis | Treatment |
|---|---|---|---|---|
| *Musculoskeletal (continued)* | **Thoracolumbar syndrome** | Hypermobility of thoracolumbar junction in patients with lumbar fusion; referred anterior abdominal and lateral hip pain | Musculoskeletal exam, spinal/hip x-rays | Physical therapy, NSAIDs, and orthopedic referral may be appropriate. |
| | **Myofascial pain syndrome** | Irritability, spasm, pain of pelvic floor or abdominal muscles | H&P, pelvic exam, EMG testing | Physical therapy, trigger point injection, muscle relaxant |
| | **Fibromyalgia** | Global myofascial pain syndrome due to abnormal pain processing/signaling | 11 of 18 painful diagnostic trigger points | Exercise, physical therapy, warm packs, massage, NSAIDs, biofeedback, relaxation techniques, low-dose SSRIs, muscle relaxants, trigger point injections |
| | **Coccydynia** | Trauma to the coccyx can cause S1–S4 nerve pain referred to pelvic floor. | Dynamic spine/coccygeal x-rays, MRI, diagnostic local anesthetic injection | Local anesthetic or steroid injections, NSAIDs, TCAs, physical therapy, rarely coccygectomy |
| | **Hernia** | Inguinal, obturator, spigelian, umbilical, etc. | Exam, CT scan | Manual reduction, binders, avoiding increased intra-abdominal pressure, surgical correction |

| | | | | |
|---|---|---|---|---|
| | **Lumbar vertebral compression fracture** | Osteoporosis, trauma, malignancy; lumbar spine fractures | Spinal x-ray, CT or MRI, DEXA scan | Referral for treatment, physical therapy, rehabilitation, lumbar orthotic brace, occupational therapy, pain medication; surgery for neurologic impairment |
| | **Piriformis syndrome** | Sciatic nerve impingement by piriformis muscle spasm or overuse syndrome; buttock, thigh, and leg pain. Running and biking can exacerbate. | Rule out lumbar disk herniation (i.e., sciatic root impingement), complete neurologic exam, spinal imaging | NSAIDs, muscle relaxants, physical therapy, local steroid/anesthetic/botulinum toxin injection |
| *Neurologic* | **Nerve entrapment** | Surgical injury of ilioinguinal or iliohypogastric nerve can cause neuroma formation. Obturator internus can press on obturator nerve. Mechanical nerve impingement or stretch can lead to neuropathy. | History, anatomic correlation, and diagnostic nerve block | Transcutaneous neurolysis, myofascial release procedure, local anesthetic injection, or surgical neurectomy if medical therapy fails |
| | **Peripheral neuropathy/ neuritis/ neuralgia** | Numerous local and systemic processes that damage peripheral nerves; persistent numbness, burning, tingling pain | H&P, evaluate for systemic disease and infectious causes (e.g., herpes zoster) | TCAs, gabapentin, pregabalin, valproate, transcutaneous electrical nerve stimulation |
| | **Abdominal migraine** | Neuronal hyperexcitation; paroxysmal abdominal pain ± nausea/vomiting/flushing. Usually in children, rare in adults. | H&P, family history, rule out other causes, consider neuroimaging | Sleep, antiemetics, TCAs, refer to neurology |

*(Continued)*

**TABLE 30-1** Differential Diagnosis of Chronic Pelvic Pain *(Continued)*

| Category | Etiology | Mechanism | Testing/Diagnosis | Treatment |
|---|---|---|---|---|
| *Psychiatric[a]* | **Posttraumatic disorders** | Sexual or physical abuse, especially in childhood | History, psychiatric assessment, rule out organic pathology | Psychotherapy, treat depression, SSRIs, antidepressants |
| | **Somatization disorder** | Internal psychological conflict and hypersensitivity to pain stimuli | Four different sites of pain plus two GI, one sexual, and one pseudoneurologic symptom (per diagnostic criteria). Rule out organic pathology. | Psychiatry referral, cognitive behavioral therapy, antidepressants |

This list is not exhaustive but represents the multiple systems and variety of diagnoses in the workup of CPP. General treatments are listed only to indicate possible therapies used for each condition.

[a]Also include a broader psychiatric differential such as bipolar disorders, personality disorders, depression, and substance abuse.

H&P, history and physical; OCPs, oral contraceptive pills; GnRH, gonadotropin-releasing hormone; NSAIDs, nonsteroidal anti-inflammatory drugs; IUD, intrauterine device; LUNA, laparoscopic uterosacral nerve ablation; FSH, follicle-stimulating hormone; MRI, magnetic resonance imaging; PID, pelvic inflammatory disease; STD, sexually transmitted disease; PCR, polymerase chain reaction; TCA, tricyclic antidepressants; POP-Q, pelvic organ prolapse quantification; AXR, abdominal x-ray; GI, gastrointestinal; CT, computed tomography; DMSO, dimethyl sulfoxide; PMP, postmenopausal; CNS, central nervous system; EMG, electromyography; SSRI, selective serotonin reuptake inhibitors; DEXA, dual energy x-ray absorptiometry.

diagnosis and may have exaggerated, nonanatomic pain or nonphysiologic sensations. Tailor treatments to the patient and address the underlying etiology, associated pain syndrome, psychological needs, and physical therapy concerns. Develop an accurate problem list and plan of management for each pain component. There is no strong evidence to support medical versus surgical management. At 1 year, about half of surgical patients report improved pain, whereas the rest report no change or worsening symptoms; similar proportions have been reported with medical treatment.

## Medical Therapy

- **Medical therapies** are selected to correct or arrest underlying pathology and to relieve pain symptoms. Analgesics should be dosed on noncontingent schedules with additional breakthrough pain treatment as needed. Acetaminophen is a good first-line analgesic.
  - **Nonsteroidal anti-inflammatory drugs (NSAIDs)** (e.g., ibuprofen, aspirin, naproxen) are a mainstay of pain treatment, especially if inflammation is present. Contraindications to NSAID treatment (e.g., liver disease for acetaminophen, renal failure or peptic ulcer disease for NSAIDs) must be excluded. Prescribe medications with adequate dosing and frequency. Higher than usual doses may be required.
  - **Opioid analgesia** with oral tramadol, codeine, oxycodone, and hydrocodone may be indicated. Intravenous medications are rarely indicated for CPP. Combination long- and short-acting opioids can be beneficial. A chronic pain specialist can be helpful when initiating or titrating drug therapy.
  - **Hormonal treatment** is frequently used for endometriosis and dysmenorrhea.
    - Continuous oral contraceptive pills and GnRH agonists (e.g., goserelin, Lupron Depot) prevent ovulation and may help pain associated with menses, including endometriosis.
    - There is good evidence that **medroxyprogesterone** 50 mg orally each day helps control endometriosis symptoms. Depot medroxyprogesterone acetate 150 mg intramuscularly every 3 months is another option.
  - **Thiamine (vitamin $B_1$)** 100 mg orally daily, **vitamin E** supplementation, and oral **magnesium** supplementation are possible nutritional approaches to dysmenorrhea, although effectiveness of data is limited.
  - **SSRI antidepressants** (e.g., fluoxetine, sertraline) have not been shown to work well for pain, but they are useful for treatment of comorbid depression or anxiety disorders that can increase pain perception. Serotonin norepinephrine reuptake inhibitors (e.g., duloxetine, venlafaxine, milnacipran) are effective for depression, anxiety, and neuropathic pain.
  - **Tricyclic antidepressants** (e.g., amitriptyline, nortriptyline) are the most effective neuropathic pain medications; they may act by lowering the pain threshold (see Table 30-1). **Antiseizure medications** (e.g., gabapentin, pregabalin, carbamazepine) are useful for neuropathic pain.
  - **Muscle relaxants** (e.g., cyclobenzaprine, baclofen) are sometimes useful for muscle spasm, but they should be used as adjuncts or second-line agents with nonsteroidal drugs until a course of physical therapy can be completed.

## Surgical Treatment

- **Surgical therapies** are indicated for specific diagnoses or for patients who do not improve with medical treatments.
  - Surgical treatment of severe endometriosis or adhesions (i.e., **adhesiolysis**) can be curative in some cases. Patients should understand that there is a strong possibility

that additional therapies or medication may be required and that the surgical procedure can lead to unforeseen complications.

- **Laparoscopic uterosacral nerve ablation (LUNA)** has been used for dysmenorrhea in patients with endometriosis who desire to maintain fertility, but several controlled clinical trials show that it is ineffective.
- The superior hypogastric plexus is excised with **presacral neurectomy**. There is some evidence showing modest pain reduction for patients with midline pelvic pain due to dysmenorrhea/endometriosis. The procedure can lead to complications such as ureteral injury and uncontrolled bleeding and should be performed by experienced surgeons only.
- **Pudendal nerve release** from Alcock canal by transgluteal or transperineal approach is performed for some patients with pudendal nerve entrapment, although there are only limited data by which to judge the procedure.
- **Hysterectomy** can be performed for patients with evidence of uterine pain (e.g., adenomyosis, some cases of endometriosis) who have completed their childbearing and have not responded well to medical management. Sixty percent to 80% of appropriately selected patients report pain improvement.

## Other Treatment Options

- Neurologic/pain anesthesia therapies are useful for CPP that can be discretely localized or is due to a specific peripheral nerve injury. Local anesthetic (e.g., lidocaine) can be injected for **cutaneous nerve or trigger point block**. Longer acting **peripheral nerve blocks** can benefit some patients. **Botulinum toxin** injection can improve unresponsive spasmodic muscular disorders. Referral to an anesthesia pain specialist may be warranted.
- **Physical therapy** by a provider with expertise in pelvic floor disorders can be helpful in both evaluation and treatment of CPP. Stretching, strengthening, hot/cold applications, pelvic floor training, transcutaneous electrical nerve stimulation, and biofeedback can be used.
- **Psychotherapy** is almost always beneficial for a patient with chronic pain. Psychological disorders can be diagnosed and managed, and cognitive behavioral therapy, psychotherapy, or counseling can benefit almost all CPP patients. If abuse is reported, the patient should be referred for psychological counseling regardless of the degree to which that history contributes to her pain. In some cases, referral for family or relationship counseling may be indicated as well.
- **Alternative/holistic therapies** such as massage, relaxation techniques, and acupuncture may be appropriate adjunctive interventions for many patients and enhance the effectiveness of traditional medical or surgical therapy. These should be discussed with the patient and integrated in her treatment plan early on.

## SUGGESTED READINGS

American College of Obstetricians and Gynecologists. ACOG practice bulletin no. 51: chronic pelvic pain. *Obstet Gynecol* 2004;103:589–605.

Bettendorf B, Shay S, Tu F. Dysmenorrhea: contemporary perspectives. *Obstet Gynecol Surv* 2008;63(9):597–603.

Bhutta HY, Walsh SR, Tang TY, et al. Ovarian vein syndrome: a review. *Int J Surg* 2009;7: 516–520.

Hillis SD, Marchbanks PA, Peterson HB. The effectiveness of hysterectomy for chronic pelvic pain. *Obstet Gynecol* 1995;86(6):941–945.

Howard FM. Chronic pelvic pain. Clinical gynecologic series: an expert's view. *Obstet Gynecol* 2003;101:594–611.

Lamvu G, Williams R, Zolnoun D, et al. Long-term outcomes after surgical and nonsurgical management of chronic pelvic pain: one year after evaluation in a pelvic pain specialty clinic. *Am J Obstet Gynecol* 2006;195:591–600.

Latthe P, Mignini L, Gray R, et al. Factors predisposing women to chronic pelvic pain: systematic review. *Br Med J* 2006;332(7544):749–755.

# Urogynecology and Reconstructive Pelvic Surgery

Jennifer L. Hallock and Chi Chiung Grace Chen

**Urogynecology** is the subspecialty of obstetrics and gynecology that addresses aspects of pelvic floor dysfunction in women including urinary incontinence (UI), anal incontinence (AI), and pelvic organ prolapse (POP). Symptomatic pelvic floor disorders are common, ranging from 25% to 50% in American women and increasing with age.

- Little is known about the natural history of pelvic floor disorders. For instance, not all women with prolapse are symptomatic, and symptoms do not necessarily correlate with physical exam findings.
- Pelvic floor disorders such as POP are the indication for more than 300,000 surgeries annually in the United States at a cost of $1 billion. Up to 11% of women have surgery for POP or stress urinary incontinence (SUI) by the age of 80 years. Twenty-nine percent of patients will require repeat surgery.

## NORMAL ANATOMY AND FUNCTION

- **Anatomy of the bladder:** The bladder is both an elastic muscular reservoir and a pump for urination. The urethra serves as the conduit, but micturition requires coordination of urethral and bladder functions. Urethral muscular components which affect urinary continence include an outer layer of striated muscle arranged in a circular pattern (external urethral sphincter [EUS]). Internal to the striated component of the urethral sphincter is a circular layer of smooth muscle, which in turn surrounds a well-developed layer of inner longitudinal muscle (internal urethral sphincter [IUS]). Deep to these layers is a prominent vascular plexus that is believed to contribute to continence by forming a watertight seal via coaptation of the mucosal surfaces. Distally, the fibers of the compressor urethrae pass over the urethra to insert into the urogenital diaphragm near the pubic ramus. Urethral function

| TABLE 31-1 Neuroanatomy of the Bladder and Urethra | | |
|---|---|---|
| **Muscle** | **Innervation** | **Neurotransmitter Rreceptors** |
| External urethral sphincter (EUS) | Perineal branch of pudendal nerve | Nicotinic acetylcholine |
| Internal urethral sphincter (IUS) | Sympathetic fibers from hypogastric plexus | Muscarinic acetylcholine, alpha- and beta-adrenergic, and others |
| Detrusor relaxation | Sympathetic fibers | Beta-adrenergic |
| Detrusor contraction | Parasympathetic fibers from sacral plexus | Muscarinic acetylcholine |

Adapted from de Groat WC. Integrative control of the lower urinary tract: preclinical perspective. *Br J Pharmacol* 2006;147(S2):S25–S40.

is also impacted by the relatively static supportive layer beneath the vesical neck, which provides a backstop against which the urethra is compressed during increased intra-abdominal pressure.

- **Neurophysiology of the lower urinary tract (Table 31-1)**
- **Micturition cycle:** The bladder has two basic functions: storing urine (sympathetic) and, when socially appropriate, evacuating urine (parasympathetic). Bladder filling occurs with relaxation of the detrusor muscle and contraction of the IUS. With bladder filling, afferent activity via baroreceptors triggers the storage reflex to maintain sympathetic tone in the IUS. When the bladder is full, afferent activity in the pelvic nerve stimulates the micturition reflex.
- **Anatomy of the pelvic floor:** See Chapter 26.
- **Anatomy of the anal sphincters:** The internal anal sphincter (IAS) is smooth muscle innervated by the parasympathetic nervous system and is tonically contracted, whereas the external anal sphincter (EAS) is striated muscle innervated by sympathetic nervous system and can only sustain voluntary contraction for a few minutes. The puborectalis muscle and the EAS function together.
- **Anal continence** is the end result of orchestrated functioning of the cerebral cortex, along with sensory and motor fibers innervating the colon, rectum, anus, and pelvic floor. The distension of the rectum by stool entering from the sigmoid colon causes the urge to defecate, and the IAS to relax while the EAS contracts (known as the rectoanal inhibitory reflex). At an appropriate time, the anorectal angle is straightened, the rectum is contracted, the EAS is inhibited, and the rectal contents are released. Rectal filling beyond 300 mL results in the sensation of urgency.

## ETIOLOGY OF PELVIC FLOOR DISORDERS

- Most women with pelvic floor disorders have multiple risk factors.
  - **Race:** Epidemiologic studies have not consistently demonstrated any racial or ethnic difference in the prevalence of pelvic floor disorders. Some studies address variables such as knowledge and perception about pelvic floor disorders and access to care.

- **Age:** The prevalence of POP, UI, and AI has been observed to increase with age. Although bladder capacity, ability to postpone voiding, bladder compliance, and urinary flow rate decrease with age in both sexes, overactive bladder symptoms and incontinence are not a normal result of aging.
- **Hypoestrogenism:** Estrogen deficiency can result in urogenital atrophy with resultant thinning of the submucosa and a decrease in the functional urethral length. The literature is unclear as to the association of estrogen deficiency and lower urinary tract symptoms (LUTS).
- **Parity and childbirth:** The incidence of pelvic floor disorders such as UI, POP, and AI are higher among parous than nulliparous women. Damage to the pelvic tissues during a vaginal delivery is thought to be a key factor in the development of these disorders, which may be more significant with operative delivery. In addition, lacerations of the internal and external anal sphincters at the time of vaginal delivery can result in impaired anal sphincter strength and AI.
- **Underlying medical conditions** such as diabetes, obesity, dementia, stroke, depression, Parkinson, or multiple sclerosis may be risk factors for pelvic floor disorders.
- **Previous pelvic surgery** may increase the risk of pelvic floor disorders.
- **Pharmacologic agents**, such as diuretics, caffeine, anticholinergics, and alpha-adrenergic blockers, may affect urinary tract function.
- Chronically **increased intra-abdominal pressure** (chronic obstructive pulmonary disease [COPD], chronic constipation, obesity) may be a risk factor for LUTS and POP.

## PATIENT EVALUATION IN UROGYNECOLOGY

### History and Physical Examination

- Any patient evaluation in urogynecology should include a thorough medical, surgical, gynecologic, and obstetric history. The clinical evaluation should elicit the patient's complaints, defining the location and severity of support defects and evaluating other potential etiologies of pelvic floor symptoms. Pelvic floor defects are rarely localized to one anatomic compartment and are often multifactorial. The clinician should gain an understanding of the duration, frequency, severity, precipitating factors, social impact, effect on hygiene, effect on quality of life, and measures used to avoid bothersome symptoms. Patients may be reluctant to volunteer symptoms of pelvic floor disorders.
- Symptoms of pelvic floor disorders including LUTS, POP, or AI can be grouped into four main categories:
  - **Bulge:** Patients may complain of pelvic pressure, heaviness, protruding tissues, or bulging.
  - **Voiding dysfunction or incontinence:** Patients may complain of day- or nighttime involuntary loss of urine, with or without Valsalva or urgency. Patients may have symptoms associated with urethral obstruction secondary to prolapse, especially with anterior compartment prolapse. They may have urinary hesitancy, incomplete emptying, or the need for vaginal splinting or Valsalva before successfully passing urine. Patients may have associated recurrent or persistent urinary tract infections (UTIs) secondary to urinary retention. They may also report irritative voiding symptoms such as urgency, frequency, and urge incontinence. They may demonstrate occult stress incontinence when prolapse is reduced (e.g., after surgery or with pessary placement).

- **Defecatory⁺ dysfunction:** Patients may have symptoms of defecatory dysfunction, especially with apical and posterior compartment prolapse. These include symptoms of incomplete defecation, required splinting or straining, constipation, and pain with defecation. Women with anal sphincter defects may present with AI of flatus, liquid, or formed stool.
- **Altered sexual functioning and body image:** Patients may complain of dyspareunia, avoidance of intercourse, decreased libido, and decreased self-image.
- There are many validated and reliable questionnaires that can aid in eliciting a symptom history from patients, such as the Pelvic Floor Distress Inventory, the Pelvic Floor Impact Questionnaire, and the Pelvic Organ Prolapse/Urinary Incontinence Sexual Questionnaire.
  - **Urinary diary:** The patient records the volume and frequency of fluid intake and voiding as well as symptoms of frequency and urgency and episodes of incontinence over 24 hours, ideally for 3 days. This will allow the practitioner to better characterize the patient's symptoms as well as enable the patient to use it as a therapeutic tool to modify her behavior.
- A comprehensive **physical examination** should be performed at the first visit, including:
  - A screening **neurologic examination** to evaluate overall mental status and sensory and motor function of the lower extremities.
  - A **pelvic exam**, including a systematic evaluation of all components of the pelvic floor, including innervation, vulvar architecture, muscular and connective tissue support, and perineal scars. Particular attention should be given to urethral anatomy and hypermobility (see Q-tip test in the succeeding text).
    - **Speculum exam**, using a Sims speculum or the posterior blade of a Graves speculum, is helpful to assess support, the presence of scarring, and any associated findings.
    - The **bimanual exam** investigates the location, size, and tenderness of the bladder, uterus, cervix, and adnexa. The strength of the levator ani muscles is assessed by placing one or two fingers in the vagina and asking the patient to squeeze. The firm muscular sling of the posterior puborectalis should be readily palpable.
  - **Sacral nerve roots** and the **sacral reflex** (also called the bulbocavernosus reflex) should be evaluated. When the clitoris or the area lateral to the anus is lightly scratched, an ipsilateral contraction of the anal sphincter should occur. In older patients, this reflex may be absent. In obese patients, this reflex may be difficult to evaluate.
  - The **Q-tip test** evaluates urethral support. A cotton swab is placed in the urethra to the level of the urethrovesical junction, and the change in axis from rest to strain is measured to assess urethral hypermobility. Angular measurements of >30 degrees are generally considered hypermobile. **Urethral hypermobility** is thought to occur due to loss of integrity of the fibromuscular tissue that supports the bladder neck and urethra.
  - A **rectal examination** can further assess pelvic pathology as well as evaluate the presence of fecal impaction. The exam should include an inspection of the perineal area for evidence of skin irritation or stool on the skin as well as digital examination of the anal sphincter for resting and squeeze pressure. One should also note the presence of a gaping anus or scarring.
- To evaluate POP, four specific anatomic components should be assessed: (a) anterior vaginal wall, (b) uterus and vaginal apex, (c) posterior vaginal wall, and (d) presence or absence of an enterocele. These compartments should be assessed with a standardized

system. The International Continence Society (ICS), American Urogynecologic Society, Society of Gynecologic Surgeons, and the National Institutes of Health recommend the standardized **Pelvic Organ Prolapse Quantification (POPQ)** system for grading support defects (Fig. 31-1). Many staging systems exist, but the POPQ system is widely accepted and published, easily learned, and reproducible. Additionally, pelvic muscle function can be assessed using scales such as Brink.

- The POPQ uses the hymen as a fixed point of reference and describes six specific topographic points on the vaginal walls (Aa, Ba, C, D, Bp, and Ap) and three distances (genital hiatus, perineal body, total vaginal length).
- The prolapse of each segment is measured in centimeters during Valsalva relative to the hymenal ring with points inside the vagina reported as negative numbers and outside as positive. The numeric values are then translated to a stage as described in Table 31-2.
- The perineal body is normally at the level of the ischial tuberosities. Descent of >2 cm below this level with flattening of the intergluteal sulcus indicates **perineal descent**.
- To fully evaluate POP, the patient may need to perform a Valsalva maneuver in lithotomy or strain while seated or standing while being examined by the provider. Pelvic floor muscle strength can be assessed, as outlined earlier.
  - Examination of the anterior vaginal wall should include evaluation of the support of the urethra. With a speculum (or half of the speculum) used to depress the posterior vaginal wall, the patient is asked to strain, and any descent of the anterior vaginal wall is noted.

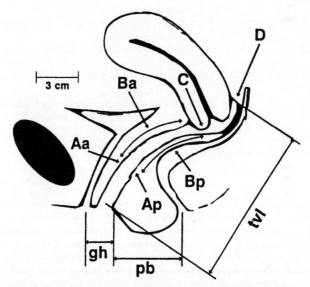

**Figure 31-1.** The Pelvic Organ Prolapse Quantification (POPQ) system components and anatomic reference points. For explanation of terms, see Table 31-2. (From Bent AE, Ostergard DR, Cundiff GW, et al, eds. *Ostergard's Urogynecology and Pelvic Floor Dysfunction*, 5th ed. Philadelphia, PA: Lippincott Williams & Wilkins, 2003:97, with permission.)

| TABLE 31-2 | Description and Staging of the Pelvic Organ Prolapse Quantification System |
|---|---|

| Point/Distance | Description |
|---|---|
| Aa | Midline anterior vaginal wall, 3 cm proximal to the urethral meatus |
| Ba | Anterior vaginal wall, most distal point between Aa and anterior fornix (cuff) |
| C | Edge of the cervix (or vaginal cuff in posthysterectomy patients) |
| D | Posterior fornix. Not used in patients with hysterectomy |
| Ap | Midline posterior vaginal wall, 3 cm proximal to the hymenal ring |
| Bp | Posterior vaginal wall, most distal point between Ap and posterior fornix (cuff) |
| Genital hiatus | Middle of the urethral meatus to posterior midline hymenal ring |
| Perineal body | Posterior margin of genital hiatus to the middle anus |
| Total vaginal length | Greatest depth of vagina with C or D reduced to its normal position |
| **Staging of the POPQ system** | |
| **Stage 0** | Perfect support; Aa, Ap at $-3$. C or D within 2 cm of TVL from introitus. |
| **Stage 1** | Most distal portion of prolapse is $-1$ (or more negative) proximal to introitus. |
| **Stage 2** | Most distal portion within 1 cm of the hymenal ring (between $-1$ and $+1$). |
| **Stage 3** | Most distal portion $>+1$ cm but $<$(TVL-2) cm distal to introitus. |
| **Stage 4** | Complete prolapse; most distal portion between TVL and (TVL-2) cm distal to introitus. |

POPQ, Pelvic Organ Prolapse Quantification; TVL, total vaginal length.

- Isolated evaluation of the posterior vaginal wall demonstrates rectoceles and enteroceles. With a speculum retracting the anterior vaginal wall, the posterior wall of the vagina can be inspected. A **rectocele** is present when the posterior vaginal wall and underlying rectum protrude toward the hymenal ring on straining. Rectovaginal examination helps demonstrate anterior displacement of the anterior rectal wall. An **enterocele** is suspected with a bulging of the apical posterior vaginal wall outward or when peristalsis is seen. On rectovaginal examination, small bowel can be palpated between the vagina and rectum with the patient straining.
- A positive result on a **stress test** is essential to the diagnosis of SUI. The stress test is performed by looking for urine leakage from the urethral meatus when

abdominal pressure is increased. It can be done while standing or in the dorsal lithotomy position, with different bladder volumes and maximum capacity, and is very specific for SUI. As mentioned in the following text, it is important to exclude transient pathology that may predispose a patient to UI such as UTI. False-negative results can be explained by low bladder volume or lack of patient effort.

## Diagnostic Tests

- Diagnostic tests can be ordered if indicated.
- **Urinalysis** can be used to exclude other pathology, such as microscopic hematuria. **Urine culture** can evaluate for UTI.
- **Postvoid residual (PVR)** measurement can aid in diagnosing overflow incontinence. Most consider PVR to be abnormal if >1/3 of void volume or >150 mL.
- **Cystourethroscopy** can be used to assess the anatomy of bladder and urethra interior.
- **Urodynamic studies** can be used to assess the physiologic function of the bladder during filling and voiding. Simple cystometric testing can be performed in the office using a straight catheter and syringe to fill the bladder with a known volume of sterile water. At various bladder volumes, the patient is asked to cough and Valsalva in an attempt to demonstrate SUI or induce a detrusor contraction. Multichannel cystometrics, using one catheter in the bladder and the other either in the vagina or rectum, can be used for patients with complex symptoms or voiding complaints.
  - **Anorectal manometry** provides quantitative information regarding function of the rectum, anus, and anal sphincter. It can also be used therapeutically in conjunction with biofeedback.
  - **Endoanal ultrasonography:** The value of endoanal ultrasound lies in its ability to locate defects in the internal or external sphincter to facilitate planning for surgical correction.
  - **Magnetic resonance imaging** can provide detailed soft tissue evaluation without radiation. This imaging modality may be useful if one suspects an enterocele that is not clearly palpable or if the patient's symptoms do not appear consistent with her anatomy on physical examination. It is also the gold standard for evaluating urethral diverticulum.
  - **Defecography:** During a defecating proctogram, the patient's pelvis is imaged using fluoroscopy as she defecates while sitting after an enema is used to infuse contrast material. This test may be especially useful in patients with defecatory complaints.
  - **Anoscopy**, **proctoscopy**, **sigmoidoscopy**, or **colonoscopy** may be indicated in patients in whom anatomic abnormalities are suspected, such as cancer or inflammatory bowel disease.

## LOWER URINARY TRACT SYMPTOMS

Disorders of the lower urinary tract are categorized by storage or voiding symptoms. LUTS include overactive bladder and UI, described separately in the following text. For most LUTS, the first line of management is conservative. Definitions of some common LUTS include:

- **Frequency**—the complaint of voiding too often. In some populations, a cutoff for normal is seven voids during waking hours.

- **Urgency**—the complaint of a sudden compelling desire to pass urine that is difficult to defer. Urgency can occur with or without urge incontinence.
- **Nocturia**—the complaint of waking at night one or more times to void.
- **Nocturnal enuresis**—the complaint of loss of urine occurring during sleep.

## Overactive Bladder

- **Overactive bladder (OAB)** is a clinical diagnosis to describe bothersome symptoms of urinary urgency with daytime frequency or nocturia, with or without urge incontinence. OAB often results from inappropriate detrusor contraction. When spontaneous or provoked involuntary detrusor contractions are demonstrated on urodynamic testing, OAB is referred to as **detrusor overactivity (DO)**. DO may be neurogenic (associated with an underlying neurologic process) or idiopathic.
  - The estimated overall prevalence of OAB in adult American women is 15% to 27%, which increases with age and in institutionalized women.
  - Treatment of OAB includes the first-line methods of lifestyle modifications, behavioral therapy with pelvic floor physical therapy, and pharmacotherapy. If these methods provide unsatisfactory results, second-line methods can be tried. These therapies include sacral nerve stimulation, botulinum toxin A, and urinary diversion.

*Lifestyle Modifications and Behavioral Management of Overactive Bladder*

- **Lifestyle modifications** include weight loss, caffeine intake reduction, smoking cessation, and manipulation of daily fluid intake.
- **Bladder retraining drills** involve scheduled voiding with progressive increases in the interval between voids.
- **Biofeedback** is a form of patient reeducation in which a closed feedback loop is created so that one or more of the patient's normally unconscious physiologic processes is made accessible to her by auditory, visual, or tactile signals.
- **Pelvic floor muscle exercise (PFME)**, requiring repeated voluntary pelvic floor muscle training (Kegel exercises), may be used in conjunction with bladder retraining.
- **Functional electrical stimulation** and **weighted vaginal cones** may be used during PFME although the evidence is unclear if there is additional benefit.

*Medical Management of Overactive Bladder*

- Oral and transdermal medications are available and can be combined with behavioral therapies to improve efficacy.
  - **Anticholinergics** inhibit involuntary detrusor contractions and are the first-line pharmacotherapy for OAB due to their safety and efficacy. Dry mouth is the most common side effect. There are minimal differences found in efficacy or side effects between the various anticholinergics available. These medications are not recommended in patients with closed angle glaucoma or impaired gastric emptying.
    - Of the five subtypes of muscarinic receptors, M2 is the most common in the bladder followed by M3.
    - Oxybutynin (Ditropan) and tolterodine tartrate (Detrol) do not differ in outcomes. Oxybutynin is relatively selective for M3 and M1 receptors, and common side effects include dry mouth, constipation, blurred vision, and gastritis. Tolterodine tartrate targets M3 and M2 receptors and is better tolerated than the short-acting form of oxybutynin. In general, long-acting varieties are better tolerated but are more expensive.

    o Anticholinergic medications with potentially fewer side effects are available. Trospium (Sanctura) is hydrophilic and theoretically does not cross the blood–brain barrier, limiting central nervous system side effects. Darifenacin (Enablex) binds to M3 receptors, whereas solifenacin (VESIcare) binds M3 and M1 relatively selectively and are thought to cause less frequent dry mouth, a principal reason for noncompliance with treatment.

- **Tricyclic antidepressants** such as imipramine improve bladder hypertonicity and compliance, suppressing involuntary detrusor contractions through multiple sites of action including Onuf nucleus.
  - o Mirabegron (Myrbetriq) is a beta$_3$ agonist also used for the treatment of OAB symptoms. It relaxes the detrusor muscle during storage phase and increases bladder capacity by augmenting the sympathetic nervous system stimulation of the bladder.

*Surgical Management of Overactive Bladder*

- Surgical management of DO is reserved for intractable cases that have already failed multiple attempts at nonsurgical management. Procedures include **sacral nerve root neuromodulation**, **augmentation cystoplasty**, and **urinary diversion** via an ileal conduit. There is level I evidence supporting intradetrusor **botulinum toxin injections** in women with neurogenic and idiopathic DO; however, there is a high rate of associated urinary retention and UTI, as well as the need for repeat injections to maintain efficacy over time.

# URINARY INCONTINENCE

The ICS defines **UI** as any involuntary leakage of urine. In the United States, the prevalence of UI in adult women is approximately 50%.

## Types of Urinary Incontinence

- **SUI**, or urodynamic stress incontinence, is the most common type of UI among ambulatory incontinent women, accounting for 50% to 70% of cases. SUI occurs when abdominal pressure exceeds bladder pressure, for example, with coughing, sneezing, or laughing.
- **Urge UI** is involuntary leakage accompanied by or immediately preceded by the urge to void. Many patients complain of inability to reach the toilet in time. Involuntary detrusor contractions are typically the cause.
- **Mixed incontinence** describes symptoms of both stress and urge UI.
- **Functional incontinence** is associated with cognitive, psychological, or physical impairments that make it difficult to reach the toilet or interfere with appropriate toileting. A useful mnemonic is **DIAPPERS**: **D**elirium, **I**nfection, **A**trophy, **P**harmacology, **P**sychology, **E**ndocrinopathy, **R**estricted mobility, and **S**tool impaction.
- **Bypass incontinence** may be caused by urogenital fistulae or by congenital or acquired anatomic abnormalities.
  - In the United States, gynecologic surgery is the most common cause of **urogenital fistulae** (0.1% of all hysterectomies). Other causes include radiation, trauma, and severe pelvic pathology. In developing countries, obstetric injuries are the most common cause. Patients often report painless and continuous vaginal leakage of urine, usually within the context of recent pelvic surgery (1 to 2 weeks). Instillation of methylene blue dye into the bladder will stain a vaginal pack if a

vesicovaginal fistula is present which can be confirmed on cystourethroscopy. Intravenous pyelography (IVP) or computed tomography scan can be performed to evaluate for possible ureterovaginal fistula. The preferred surgical route for correction of a vesicovaginal fistula is vaginal; however, in certain instances, an abdominal route may be optimal. The vaginal Latzko procedure is commonly used for postsurgical vesicovaginal fistulae. Treatment of ureterovaginal fistulae depends on location. Often, simply stenting the involved ureter can correct the fistula. If the ureterovaginal fistula persists and is close to the ureterovesical junction, ureteroneocystostomy can be performed. A psoas bladder hitch or Boari flap can be used to alleviate tension on this anastomosis. The interposition of vascular flaps may aid in the surgical success of fistula correction.

- **Suburethral diverticulum** is an outpouching of the urethra, and patients often complain of dysuria, recurrent UTIs, dyspareunia, and postvoid dribbling.

## Treatment of Stress Urinary Incontinence

- **Pharmacologic:** The limited available medications for SUI are aimed toward increasing urethral sphincter tone. The efficacy for these interventions is unclear.
- **Pelvic muscle exercise:** Limited long-term prospective studies of this low-risk intervention suggest effectiveness, which is dependent on patient adherence.
- **Continence pessaries:** A prospective study comparing continence pessary to behavior therapy for SUI found that they have comparable results at 12 months (~50% satisfaction rate).
- **Surgery:** The etiology of SUI may be multifactorial and may not be completely corrected by surgery. Reported cure rates after surgery are usually high although can vary widely depending on parameters used to define cure of SUI. The most common techniques currently used for the treatment of SUI are retropubic colposuspension, suburethral sling, and urethral bulking agents.

### Surgical Procedures for Stress Urinary Incontinence

- **Retropubic urethropexy** procedures are indicated for women with SUI and a hypermobile proximal urethra and bladder neck.
  - The **Burch retropubic colposuspension** is a well-established surgery for SUI. Through a Pfannenstiel or Cherney incision, or laparoscopically, permanent sutures are placed in the fibromuscular tissue lateral to the bladder neck and proximal urethra, and the urethrovesical junction is supported by attaching these sutures to the iliopectineal line (i.e., Cooper ligament). Reported 5-year success rates have been over 80%.
  - The **Marshall-Marchetti-Krantz (MMK)** procedure supports the bladder neck and urethra similar to the Burch, except the permanent sutures are placed through the periosteum of the pubic symphysis instead of Cooper ligament. This technique is seldom used now due to the risk of osteitis pubis.
- **Suburethral slings** are indicated for SUI with urethral hypermobility, although data also suggests some efficacy in patients with limited urethral mobility. The sling can be placed at the midurethra or bladder neck. It supports the urethra or bladder neck, providing static stabilization of the urethra at rest and dynamic compression of the urethra with increases in abdominal pressure. Suburethral slings can be created using various biologic and synthetic materials. The slings can be placed via retropubic versus transobturator approach. Cochrane analysis suggested improved cure rates compared to Burch at the cost, however, of a more invasive surgery.

- **Tension-free vaginal tape (TVT):** A polypropylene mesh is placed without tension at the midurethra through the retropubic space or space of Retzius. Success rates of TVT are similar to that of Burch colposuspension. Bladder perforation is the most common complication (5%), with bowel or vascular injuries being the most serious complications (both <1%). Cystoscopy is warranted to evaluate for bladder perforation by the placement of TVT trocars, which is most likely to occur between 10 and 2 o'clock if the bladder is viewed as a clock face. Postoperative risks include graft exposure and urinary retention.
- **Tension-free transobturator tape (TOT):** A polypropylene mesh is placed without tension at the midurethra through the obturator foramen, instead of through the retropubic space. The TOT avoids the possibility of vascular injury in the space of Retzius and potential bowel injury. Bladder perforation is less likely (less than 0.1%) but cystoscopy is still warranted. Other postoperative risks include thigh pain and abscess. These procedures may be less successful for certain patient populations.
- **Urethral bulking agent injections** may be appropriate in patients with SUI without urethral hypermobility (i.e., less than 30 degrees). Various agents are approved by the U.S. Food and Drug Administration (FDA) to improve urethral coaptation after cystoscopic administration, although in the literature, one agent is not superior to another. These agents include autologous fat, calcium hydroxylapatite particles (Coaptite), and polydimethylsiloxane (Macroplastique). Although collagen has been studied extensively, it is no longer commercially available for urethral bulking. Symptomatic improvement at 1 year ranges from 60% to 80%, although recurrence of symptoms requiring reinjection within months or years is common. Complications are less frequent than with other surgical techniques for treating SUI but include transient urinary retention.
- Other surgical methods that have been shown to be less effective and are less commonly performed for SUI includes **cystocele repair**, described by Howard Kelly in 1913 as a surgical treatment for SUI, as well as **needle suspension procedures** such as the Stamey technique.

## URINARY RETENTION

- **Neurogenic lower urinary tract or pelvic floor dysfunction** is diagnosed after confirming pathology that is neurologic in nature. There may be overdistention of the bladder, or neurogenic acontractile detrusor, with resultant involuntary urinary retention. Patients may have absent or delayed sensation to void, increased bladder capacity, and high PVRs. They may complain of overflow incontinence, dribbling, hesitancy, frequency, or nocturia. The condition may be associated with central or peripheral neurologic disorders such as diabetes, multiple sclerosis, or spinal cord injury.
- **Detrusor sphincter or pelvic floor dyssynergia** is a lack of coordination between bladder contraction and urethral sphincter and pelvic floor relaxation and can result in incomplete bladder emptying and voiding dysfunction. This condition is commonly associated with neurologic disease.
- **Bladder outlet obstruction** may occur as a result of previous anti-incontinence surgery, anterior vaginal wall prolapse, or other anatomic abnormalities such as urethral diverticulum, fibroid, or malignancy.

- **Treatment for urinary retention:**
  - **Intermittent self-catheterization** is safe and can be used for transient or long-term conditions.
  - **Pessaries** can relieve urinary retention caused by obstruction due to prolapse. In women fitted with pessaries for prolapse, 50% of urinary symptoms improved, but occult SUI (SUI with prolapse reduction) was a common side effect.
  - **Urethrolysis** can be performed after anti-incontinence surgery has resulted in voiding dysfunction and urinary retention secondary to obstruction.
  - **Sacral root neuromodulation** is approved for idiopathic voiding dysfunction.
  - **Resection of urethral diverticula** and correction of other anatomic abnormalities usually results in relief of obstructive or irritative voiding symptoms.
  - **Botox** can be injected into the urethral sphincter to relax a neurogenic outlet obstruction.

## PAINFUL BLADDER SYNDROME

**Painful bladder syndrome (PBS)** or **interstitial cystitis (IC)** is a chronic inflammatory condition that is poorly understood. The ICS differentiates PBS from IC. The former is a clinical diagnosis of exclusion when a patient presents with the irritative voiding symptoms of urgency, frequency, and pelvic or lower urinary tract pain (70% of cases). Dyspareunia, sleep disturbance, and UI may be present. In contrast, IC is diagnosed based on cystoscopic findings such as urothelial glomerulations, petechial hemorrhages, or Hunner ulcer after hydrodistention or histologic findings such as a proliferation of mast cells.

- The prevalence of PBS in the United States is 5 to 500 per 100,000, as estimates may vary based on diagnostic criteria or definition used. PBS is more common in young, Caucasian (91%) women in their 40s. It is a frequent cause of chronic pelvic pain (see Chapter 30).
- The clinical presentation is highly variable. Irritative urinary symptoms and pain may be present. These patients may often complain of pain with bladder fullness which is relieved with bladder emptying.
- **Treatment** is oriented to symptom control because no cure currently exists.
  - **Conservative** therapy helps some women. This includes **behavior modification** (e.g., timed voiding, bladder retraining), **diet modification** (e.g., avoid caffeine, acidic foods, alcohol), **support groups**, **stress reduction**, and **physical therapy**.
  - **Pharmacologic:** Pentosan polysulfate is the only oral medication FDA-approved for PBS or IC. However, the best results may be obtained with a combination of multiple drug therapy and/or physical therapy. Oral combinations of pentosan polysulfate (Elmiron) and hydroxyzine (Vistaril) or triple therapy with pentosan, hydroxyzine, and amitriptyline have shown success but may require prolonged treatment.
  - **Bladder instillation therapy:** Dimethyl sulfoxide (DMSO) is the only intravesical therapy FDA-approved for PBS. This may need to be repeated weekly for up to 6 weeks before significant improvement is seen. Other intravesical therapies include sodium bicarbonate, lidocaine, heparin, hyaluronic acid, chondroitin sulfate, and oxybutynin.
  - **Hydrodistention:** Cystoscopy with hydrodistention should be considered in cases refractory to treatment or when the diagnosis is not clear.

- **Other treatments** that are not FDA-approved are botulinum toxin injection and sacral root neuromodulation.

## PELVIC ORGAN PROLAPSE

**POP** is defined as herniation of the pelvic organs into or out of the vaginal canal. More specifically, POP refers to loss of support of the anterior or posterior vaginal wall or the vaginal apex, which permits pelvic viscera such as the bladder (cystocele), rectum (rectocele), small bowel (enterocele), sigmoid colon, or uterus (apical or uterine prolapse) to protrude into the vagina or, in its most severe form, through the vaginal introitus. POP does not include rectal prolapse.

### Treatment of Pelvic Organ Prolapse

- The goal of treatment for POP should depend on the patient's goals. The three therapeutic categories are expectant management, nonsurgical, and surgical.
- **Expectant management** is reasonable for mildly symptomatic POP or in patients without bothersome concomitant LUTS or defecatory dysfunction. Providers can offer reassurance that treatment is available if and when prolapse becomes bothersome. Risks of expectant management include vaginal epithelial erosion and persistence of LUTS and defecatory dysfunction.
- The **nonsurgical approach** may be useful in patients with a mild degree of prolapse, who desire future childbearing, have frail health, or are unwilling to undergo surgery.
  - **Pelvic floor muscle training (PFMT) or exercises (PFME)**, also known as Kegel exercises, can alleviate the symptoms of prolapse. These treatments have also been shown in small trials to reduce the anatomic severity of mild prolapse.
  - **Pessaries:** The two basic types are supportive (most commonly a ring, with or without support) and space occupying (most commonly a Gellhorn). Pessaries can decrease symptom frequency and severity and delay or avoid surgery. Treatment with estrogen, either locally or systemically, may help the vaginal epithelium tolerate the foreign body. Because pessaries can cause vaginal wall erosion or ulceration and fistula formation, if neglected, patients should be examined routinely. Complications are minimized by avoiding excessive pressure on the vaginal epithelium and by emphasizing proper pessary care, including regular surveillance and cleansing. Serious complications are rare and more likely to occur in those who are unable to clean their pessaries regularly or who cannot come for routine cleaning visits. Risk factors for unsuccessful pessary fitting include a large genital hiatus and a short vaginal length.
- The goal of **surgery** is relief of prolapse symptoms. Overcorrection should be avoided because it can lead to new symptoms including LUTS or SUI. Although the uterus itself does not contribute to POP, most of the literature on prolapse surgery include hysterectomy concomitantly with POP repair to maximize the opportunity to correct apical support. The three categories of POP repair are obliterative, reconstructive, and compensatory.

### Surgical Procedures for Pelvic Organ Prolapse
#### Reconstructive Procedures

- **Abdominal sacral colpopexy** replaces normal vaginal support with interposition of a suspensory bridge of mesh or graft between the apical anterior and posterior vagina with the anterior sacral promontory. Success rates are 78% to 100% for the correction of apical prolapse. It has a lower rate of recurrence, dyspareunia, and is more durable than vaginal procedures such as sacrospinous ligament suspension. Its complications include rare intraoperative hemorrhage and a 3% to 4% prevalence of vaginal mesh erosion.

- **Sacrospinous ligament suspension (SSLS)** anchors the vaginal apex to the sacrospinous ligament, usually on the right side. This approach is faster, less expensive, and is associated with earlier return to daily activities than the abdominal procedures such as abdominal sacral colpopexy but has been shown to be not as effective. There is a 63% to 97% success rate. There are high rates of postoperative anterior vaginal prolapse, thought to be due to the pronounced posterior deviation of the vaginal axis (37%). Complications include hemorrhage, nerve injury, stress incontinence, dyspareunia, and buttock pain.

- **Iliococcygeus fascia suspension**, performed in patients who have suboptimal uterosacral ligaments, attaches the vaginal apex to the iliococcygeal fascia just below the ischial spine. Case-control studies report similar rates of success, complications, recurrence, and postoperative anterior vaginal prolapse as after SSLS.

- **Uterosacral ligament suspension** with fascial reconstruction suspends the apex of the vagina to the uterosacral ligaments, restoring the natural axis of the vagina. There is an 80% to 100% success rate. The most clinically relevant complication is ureteral kinking.

- **Anterior colporrhaphy** involves plicating the layers of the vaginal muscularis and pubocervical fibromuscular connective tissue to repair anterior prolapse (cystocele). The 5-year success rate is 30% to 40%. Complications include sexual dysfunction and dyspareunia.

- **Posterior colporrhaphy** is the plication of the pararectal and rectovaginal fibromuscular connective tissue over the rectum. Dyspareunia is common and occurs more frequently with posterior than anterior colporrhaphy.

- **Defect-directed repairs** isolate defects in the rectovaginal fibromuscular connective tissue and reapproximate normal anatomy.

- **Perineorrhaphy** is the reconstruction of the perineal body and attachment to the rectovaginal septum. The goal is to build up the perineum, but it has been associated with subsequent dyspareunia.

- **Enterocele**, or herniation of bowel into or through the vagina, may occur after a previous hysterectomy. Some recommend a preventative procedure concomitantly with any vaginal hysterectomy such as **McCall culdoplasty** that surgically obliterates the cul-de-sac at the time of vaginal hysterectomy and may prevent future enterocele. Once identified, an enterocele can be repaired by dissecting the bowel from the vaginal wall and endopelvic connective tissue and obliterating the cul-de-sac.

## Obliterative Procedures

- Obliterative procedures include **colpocleisis** and **colpectomy**. They may be useful for older patients who do not desire future vaginal intercourse. The benefits include decreased complications, decreased surgical time, and high success rate (86% to 100%). A **partial colpocleisis (LeFort)** involves leaving the uterus in place with lateral drainage channels for cervical secretions. In a **total colpectomy**, the vaginal epithelium is removed and the vaginal vault tissue is reduced.
  - Patients should be counseled regarding the risk of regret (5% to 10%), as the procedure precludes subsequent vaginal intercourse. If clinically indicated, preoperative evaluation can include a Pap smear, pelvic sonogram, or endometrial biopsy.

Compensatory Procedures

• When native tissue is weak or insufficient, **compensatory procedure**s with graft/ mesh placement/augmentation may be indicated. Biologic grafts can be native tissue, allografts (cadaveric tissue), and xenografts (porcine, bovine). The most commonly used synthetic mesh is type I polypropylene mesh.
  • Anterior and posterior **vaginal wall fibromuscular connective tissue replacement**. Various graft materials and synthetic meshes have been used to augment vaginal prolapse repairs. The purpose of the graft is often twofold: via replacing the weakened or absent vaginal supports and acting as an absorbable "collagen scaffold" for fibroblast infiltration and scar formation. If the repair is too tight, the loss of flexibility can lead to fecal urgency and dyspareunia.

Use of Mesh in Vaginal Prolapse Surgery

• There are many mesh/graft "kits" for anterior and posterior repairs and for apical suspension. Although some of these procedures have resulted in decreased anterior vaginal prolapse recurrence when compared with vaginal restorative procedures without mesh/graft augmentation, the FDA issued a public health notification in July 2011 regarding adverse events related to transvaginal POP repair with mesh, including mesh erosion (10% within 12 months), pain, infection, urinary complaints, bleeding, and organ perforation. Therefore, these procedures should only be performed judiciously on selected patients who are thoroughly counseled regarding the data on efficacy and complications by surgeons especially trained to perform these types of procedures.

# DISORDERS OF ANORECTAL FUNCTION

## Anal Incontinence

• **AI** includes loss of voluntary control of flatus or stool (solid or liquid). **Fecal incontinence (FI)** is the loss of control over solid or liquid stool. AI can be a psychologically devastating and socially incapacitating condition.

### Treatment of Anal Incontinence

• **Nonsurgical treatment** should be attempted with all patients before surgical reconstruction. Improvement is seen in 63% to 90% of patients. The first step is to eradicate treatable underlying causes, such as transient neurologic conditions, inflammatory bowel disease, fecal impaction, metabolic disorders, or offending diets.
  • **Environmental** adjustments are necessary to decrease social isolation and anxiety and to improve quality of life.
  • **Skin care** is important to prevent associated morbidities.
  • **Pelvic muscle–strengthening exercises and behavioral therapy:** All patients should undergo a pelvic muscle training program before contemplating surgery.
  • **Pharmacologic** agents that slow motility and reduce frequency (e.g., loperamide hydrochloride [Imodium], diphenoxylate hydrochloride [Lomotil]) may help some patients exercise more control over their stool.
  • **Dietary change:** Increasing ingestion of natural fiber or the use of bulking agents, such as psyllium preparations (Metamucil), can change the consistency of stool, making it firmer and more easily controlled. Reduced caffeine intake will decrease colonic motility. A bowel diary can assist in eliminating offending foods.

- **Surgical:** Patients with FI should try nonsurgical treatment before pursuing surgical management. The procedures performed include end-to-end or overlapping **sphincteroplasty**, **muscle transposition** (neosphincter), **artificial sphincter implantation**, and **colonic diversion**. **Sacral neuromodulation** is FDA-approved for FI.

## Constipation

- The Rome III criteria diagnoses constipation if the patient has at least 3 months of 2 or more of the following six symptoms: less than three defecations per week or 25% of defecations that involve straining, hard stools, sensation of incomplete evacuation or anorectal obstruction, or manual maneuvers to facilitate defecation.
- Constipation is not only a risk factor for pelvic floor disorders due to the chronic increase in intra-abdominal pressure, it is also a common symptom of pelvic floor disorders such as prolapse (rectocele). Some women will present with symptoms of AI due to constipation, as liquid stool escapes around impacted bowel contents.
- Management of constipation should be guided by the patient's history and physical exam. Initial options for treatment include behavior modification, changes in diet including increase in fiber intake, laxatives, or enemas. Defecatory dysfunction may respond to biofeedback or relaxation exercises, or botulinum toxin injections. If initial management is not successful, further evaluation may be necessary including imaging studies or referral to specialists.

## SUGGESTED READINGS

American College of Obstetrics and Gynecology Committee on Practice Bulletins—Gynecology. ACOG practice bulletin no. 63: urinary incontinence in woman. *Obstet Gynecol* 2005;105(6):1533–1545.

American College of Obstetrics and Gynecology Committee on Practice Bulletins—Gynecology. ACOG practice bulletin no. 85: pelvic organ prolapse. *Obstet Gynecol* 2007;110(3): 717–729.

Abrams P, Andersson KE, Birder L, et al. Fourth International Consultation on Incontinence Recommendations of the International Scientific Committee: evaluation and treatment of urinary incontinence, pelvic organ prolapse, and fecal incontinence. *Neurourol Urodyn* 2010;29(1):213–240.

Bradley CS, Zimmerman MB, Qi Y, et al. Natural history of pelvic organ prolapse in postmenopausal women. *Obstet Gynecol* 2007;109:848.

Hagen S, Stark D. Conservative prevention and management of pelvic organ prolapse in women. *Cochrane Database Syst Rev* 2011;(12):CD003882.

Handa VL, Garrett E, Hendrix S, et al. Progression and remission of pelvic organ prolapse: a longitudinal study of menopausal women. *Am J Obstet Gynecol* 2004;190:27.

Jelovsek JE, Maher C, Barber MD. Pelvic organ prolapse. *Lancet* 2007;369:1027.

Madoff RD, Parker SC, Varma MG, et al. Faecal incontinence in adults. *Lancet* 2004;364(9434):621–632.

Nygaard I, Barber MD, Burgio KL, et al. Prevalence of symptomatic pelvic floor disorders in US women. *JAMA* 2008;300:1311.

Swift S, Woodman P, O'Boyle A, et al. Pelvic Organ Support Study (POSST): the distribution, clinical definition, and epidemiologic condition of pelvic organ support defects. *Am J Obstet Gynecol* 2005;192:795.

# 32 Family Planning: Contraception, Sterilization, and Abortion

Sarah Oman and Anne E. Burke

**Family planning** is an integral part of the health care of women. By age 45 years, more than half of all American women will have had an unintended pregnancy and 3 in 10 will have had an abortion. Recognition of the potential for improved access to family planning services presents an opportunity to improve maternal mortality rates, population growth, and the status of women in society.

## CONTRACEPTION

Contraceptive use is exceedingly common among women of reproductive age, although effective and consistent contraceptive use continues to pose challenges.

- Ninety-nine percent of women of reproductive age (15 to 44 years old) in the United States have used at least one contraceptive method and 62% are currently using contraception.
- Among women affected by unintended pregnancy, 60% report contraceptive use in the month prior to the pregnancy, suggesting incorrect or inconsistent use of their chosen method(s).
- Increasing the use of long-term, highly effective methods, such as intrauterine devices and implantable contraceptives, may reduce the number of unintended pregnancies.
- Contraceptive use is associated with improved health outcomes for women and children.
- Contraceptive use prevents obstetric complications by facilitating birth spacing and preventing unintended pregnancies at the extremes of reproductive age.
- Noncontraceptive benefits of hormonal contraception include improvement in menstrual and perimenstrual symptoms, bleeding patterns, and acne and decreased risk of developing ovarian and endometrial cancer.
- Physicians can optimize consistent long-term use of contraception among their patients through counseling that takes into account medical history, ethical and religious concerns, the patient's short- and long-term childbearing plans, and prior contraceptive use history.
- Table 32-1 lists contraceptive methods available in the Unites States, along with their perfect-use and typical-use failure rates.
  - Contraceptive methods can be considered in terms of "tiers of effectiveness" based on pregnancy rates with typical use.

| TABLE 32-1 | Efficacy of Various Contraceptive Methods | |
|---|---|---|
| **Method** | **Typical Use** | **Perfect Use** |
| No method | 85 | 85 |
| Spermicides | 29 | 18 |
| Withdrawal | 27 | 4 |
| Periodic abstinence | | |
| Calendar | 25 | 9 |
| Standard days method | 12 | 5 |
| Ovulation method | 25 | 3 |
| Symptothermal | 25 | 2 |
| Postovulation | 25 | 1 |
| Diaphragm with spermicide | 16 | 6 |
| Condom | | |
| Female | 21 | 5 |
| Male | 15 | 2 |
| Pill (combined) | 8 | 0.3 |
| Mini-pill (progestin-only) | 13 | 1.1 |
| Patch (Ortho Evra) | 8 | 0.3 |
| Vaginal ring (NuvaRing) | 8 | 0.3 |
| Depo Provera | 3 | 0.3 |
| Implant (Implanon) | 0.05 | 0.05 |
| IUD | | |
| Copper T (ParaGard) | 0.8 | 0.6 |
| Levonorgestrel IUS (Mirena) | 0.2 | 0.2 |
| Female sterilization | 0.5 | 0.5 |
| Male sterilization | 0.15 | 0.10 |

IUD, intrauterine device; IUS, intrauterine system.

- An example of a visual aid that can be used for patient counseling is shown in Figure 32-1.
  - In this chapter, we will discuss methods in approximate descending order of effectiveness.
- Another useful resource is the Centers for Disease Control and Prevention's (CDC's) U.S. Medical Eligibility Criteria for Contraceptive Use (US MEC), which can be consulted to determine safe contraceptive methods for women with medical comorbidities (Table 32-2).
  - This resource, available online and as a downloadable "app," provides guidance for safe use of contraceptives; it does not address comparative risks of pregnancy in women with medical conditions.

## Most Effective Methods: Sterilization and Long-Acting Reversible Contraception

*Bilateral Tubal Ligation*

- **Bilateral tubal ligation** (BTL) is a surgical procedure in which the fallopian tubes are permanently occluded, preventing sperm from fertilizing the ovum. The proce-

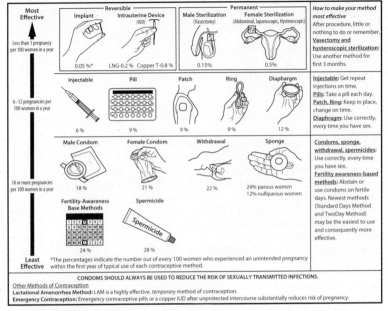

| Most Effective | Reversible | | | Permanent | | How to make your method most effective |
|---|---|---|---|---|---|---|
| | Implant | Intrauterine Device (IUD) | Male Sterilization (Vasectomy) | Female Sterilization (Abdominal, laparoscopic, Hysteroscopic) | | After procedure, little or nothing to do or remember. **Vasectomy and hysteroscopic sterilization:** Use another method for first 3 months. |
| Less than 1 pregnancy per 100 women in a year | 0.05 %* | LNG-0.2 %  Copper T-0.8 % | 0.15% | 0.5% | | |
| 6–12 pregnancies per 100 women in a year | Injectable | Pill | Patch | Ring | Diaphragm | **Injectable:** Get repeat injections on time. **Pills:** Take a pill each day. **Patch, Ring:** Keep in place, change on time. **Diaphragm:** Use correctly, every time you have sex. |
| | 6 % | 9 % | 9 % | 9 % | 12 % | |
| 18 or more pregnancies per 100 women in a year | Male Condom | Female Condom | Withdrawal | Sponge | | **Condoms, sponge, withdrawal, spermicides:** Use correctly, every time you have sex. **Fertility awareness-based methods:** Abstain or use condoms on fertile days. Newest methods (Standard Days Method and TwoDay Method) may be the easiest to use and consequently more effective. |
| | 18 % | 21 % | 22 % | 24% parous women 12% nulliparous women | | |
| | Fertility-Awareness Base Methods | Spermicide | | | | |
| Least Effective | 24 % | 28 % | | | | |

*The percentages indicate the number out of every 100 women who experienced an unintended pregnancy within the first year of typical use of each contraceptive method.

**CONDOMS SHOULD ALWAYS BE USED TO REDUCE THE RISK OF SEXUALLY TRANSMITTED INFECTIONS.**

Other Methods of Contraception
**Lactational Amenorrhea Method:** LAM is a highly effective, *temporary* method of contraception.
**Emergency Contraception:** Emergency contraceptive pills or a copper IUD after unprotected intercourse substantially reduces risk of pregnancy.

**Figure 32-1.** Contraceptive counseling tool: tiers of effectiveness.

dure can be performed postpartum (within 48 hours after vaginal delivery), at the time of cesarean delivery, or as an interval procedure (>6 weeks postpartum) via laparoscopic or transcervical hysteroscopic approach.

- The **Parkland** and **Pomeroy** salpingectomies are the most common methods used for postpartum sterilization. These involve ligating and excising portions of the tubes via an infraumbilical incision.
- **Laparoscopic tubal ligation** is performed via banding, clipping, or cauterizing the tubes.
- The Collaborative Review of Sterilization (CREST) study, a landmark analysis of tubal sterilization, compared the long-term effectiveness of numerous methods of sterilization and found a rate of 18.5 pregnancies per 1,000 procedures overall (Table 32-3).
- **Advantages** of transabdominal sterilization include the fact that these procedures offer highly effective, permanent contraception to women who desire no future childbearing. Sterilization may decrease the risk of ovarian cancer, possibly by blocking carcinogens from ascending through the fallopian tubes.
- **Disadvantages** include the need for anesthesia for sterilization via an abdominal approach, risk of surgical complications, and sterilization failure resulting in either intrauterine or ectopic pregnancy. Sterilization failure rates are higher for women younger than the age of 30 years because these women are more fertile at the time of sterilization.
- The reported 10-year cumulative probability of ectopic pregnancy for all sterilization methods in the CREST study was 7/1,000, with greater risk of ectopic

| TABLE 32-2 | Contraindications to Estrogen-Containing Hormonal Contraception |
|---|---|

Moderate or severe uncontrolled HTN
History of CVA or MI
Multiple risk factors for CAD: age, smoking, HTN, DM
History of or current DVT/PE
Migraines with aura or focal neurologic symptoms
Active hepatoma or liver cirrhosis or unexplained elevation of liver enzymes
Known or suspected breast cancer
Smoking >15 cigarettes per day and age >35 yr
Breast-feeding <6 wk postpartum (theoretic risk of growth restriction)
Diabetic neuropathy, retinopathy, neuropathy, or other vascular disease
Valvular heart disease, complicated (SBE, pulmonary HTN, or atrial fibrillation)
Known thrombogenic mutation
Migraines without aura and age >35 yr
Symptomatic gallbladder disease
Undiagnosed vaginal bleeding
Non–breast-feeding <3 wk postpartum

Category 4 (i.e., unacceptable risk) contraindications are listed.
HTN, hypertension; CVA, cerebrovascular accident; MI, myocardial infarction; CAD, coronary artery disease; DM, diabetes mellitus; DVT, deep vein thrombosis; PE, pulmonary embolism; SBE, subacute bacterial endocarditis.
From Centers for Disease Control and Prevention. U.S. medical eligibility criteria for contraceptive use, 2010. *MMWR Recomm Rep* 2010;59(RR-4):1–86.

| TABLE 32-3 | Failure Rates for Female Sterilization Methods |
|---|---|

| Method | % Pregnant in 10 years |
|---|---|
| Postpartum salpingectomy | 0.75 |
| Interval partial salpingectomy | 2.0 |
| Unipolar cautery | 0.75 |
| Bipolar cautery | 2.48 |
| Spring clip (Hulka clip) | 3.65 |
| Silastic bands (Falope ring) | 1.77 |
| Filshie clip[a] | 0.9–1.2 |

[a]Not studied in CREST.
Data from Peterson HB, Xia Z, Hughes JM, et al. The risk of pregnancy after tubal sterilization: findings from the U.S. Collaborative Review of Sterilization. U.S. Collaborative Review of Sterilization Working Group. *Am J Obstet Gynecol* 1996;174:1161–1170; Kovacs GT, Krins AJ. Female sterilizations with Filshie clips: what is the risk failure? A retrospective survey of 30,000 applications. *J Fam Plan Reprod Health Care* 2002:28:34–35.

pregnancy in younger women. However, although the relative risk of ectopic pregnancy (chance that a pregnancy, once it occurs, may be ectopic) may be higher after sterilization, the absolute risk of ectopic pregnancy is lower than in noncontracepting women due to the high efficacy of sterilization. The risk of regret of sterilization is significantly higher in women sterilized prior to age 30 years.

### Hysteroscopic Tubal Sterilization (Essure Micro-Insert)

- Essure is an irreversible method of transcervical hysteroscopic tubal occlusion that can be performed in the office or operating room. In this procedure, a 4-cm × 1-cm stainless steel and nickel-coated coil is inserted into each fallopian tube under hysteroscopic guidance. A local inflammatory response leads to tissue ingrowth around the coil and subsequent tubal occlusion. An alternative method of contraception must be used for 3 months afterward and until a hysterosalpingogram (HSG) confirms successful tubal occlusion.
  - Advantages to transcervical sterilization include the ability to perform these procedures in an office setting without risks associated with anesthesia and without the need for abdominal incisions.
    ○ This may be particularly important for women who desire permanent sterilization but are obese, have had multiple abdominal surgeries, or have serious medical comorbidities.
  - Disadvantages include a failure rate that may be higher than that seen after BTL and the need to comply with a postprocedure HSG to confirm success. Failure rate demonstrated from clinical trials was <1%, although postmarketing failure rates have been higher.
    ○ Most pregnancies result from noncompliance with the HSG protocol following an unsuccessful procedure or occur as interval pregnancies between the time of procedure and complete scarring.

### Male Sterilization: Vasectomy

- **Vasectomy** is the surgical occlusion of the vas deferens, which prevents sperm from being ejaculated.
  - Up to 20 postprocedure ejaculations are required before the procedure becomes effective (as determined by two azoospermia results on semen analysis).
  - Vasectomy is highly effective and has no long-term side effects. It is also less expensive and associated with fewer complications than tubal ligation.
  - Vasectomy requires an outpatient surgical procedure, is permanent, offers no protection against sexually transmitted diseases (STDs), and is not immediately effective.

## Long-Acting Reversible Contraception

- These may be excellent alternatives to sterilization, even in women who desire no further childbearing.
  - Long-acting methods become cost-effective after about a year of use and so can be considered for women with a wide range of fertility plans.

### Intrauterine Contraception

- Intrauterine contraception, also known as intrauterine devices (IUD) or systems (IUS), is one of the most effective methods of reversible contraception. Choice of terminology can be based on personal preference, but the term IUD is widely understood by providers and patients.

- Two types are currently commercially available in the United States: the copper-containing T380A and the levonorgestrel (LNG)-releasing IUS. Both are flexible plastic devices that are inserted into the uterus and cause a sterile inflammatory reaction in the uterus that interferes with sperm transport into and within the uterine cavity. The LNG-IUS also works through local progestin effects, such as the thickening of cervical mucus and atrophy of the endometrial lining.
  - The **Copper T380 IUD** (*ParaGard*) is effective for at least 10 years, likely 12. The copper IUD is also the most effective form of postcoital contraception (see "Postcoital Contraception" later).
  - There are now two **LNG-releasing IUD**s available in the United States: a 20-μg LNG/day device (Mirena) and a product that releases 14 μg LNG/day (Skyla) (both Bayer HealthCare Pharmaceuticals, Whippany, NJ). The 20-μg IUD is approved for 5 years in the United States and is likely effective for 7 years. A noncontraceptive benefit is the reduction of menstrual blood loss by up to 90% by suppressing growth of endometrial tissue. The 14-μg LNG IUD is effective for 3 years, after which the daily levels of LNG release decrease significantly.
- **Advantages:** IUDs provide highly effective protection against pregnancy and are easily inserted and removed. The LNG-containing IUDs may correct menstrual bleeding abnormalities and improve anemia. IUDs may also provide protection against ascending pelvic infection and even protect against endometrial cancer. Return to fertility is rapid after removal.
- **Disadvantages/side effects:** There are no hormonal side effects of the copper IUD. In some women, menstrual bleeding may be slightly heavier and longer in the initial months after insertion. This can generally be managed with nonsteroidal anti-inflammatory drugs (NSAIDs). The LNG-IUDs may have hormonally related side effects, including irregular bleeding, which generally corrects after a few months of use. Oligomenorrhea or amenorrhea may occur with the LNG-IUD, which may not be desirable to some women. Some women may experience systemic hormonal side effects, although many will not.
- **Contraindications:** There are few true contraindications to the use of IUDs. IUDs should not be used if pregnancy is suspected, if anatomic uterine abnormalities cause significant cavity distortion, if there is unexplained vaginal bleeding prior to appropriate medical workup, or if a pelvic malignancy is suspected. IUDs do not need to be removed, however, when cervical cancer or dysplasia is discovered and/or treated. Active pelvic infection is a contraindication; pelvic infection is further discussed in the following text. Although HIV infection does not contraindicate IUD placement, AIDS is considered to be a contraindication.
- **Risks:** Risks of IUD insertion include expulsion (2%), perforation (1:1,000), pregnancy (2 to 8:1,000), and infection (uncommon).
- **Other considerations: Immediate postpregnancy** (postpartum and postabortal) **IUD placement** is safe and may lead to a substantial decrease in unplanned pregnancy. Expulsion risk may be higher than when placement is not associated with pregnancy, but this risk can be balanced against other benefits and concerns.
- **Pelvic infection:** A woman's **risk of pelvic inflammatory disease (PID) is not increased** by IUD use. The progestin IUS (Mirena) may decrease risk by decreasing ascending infection due to thickening of the cervical mucus. The copper IUD does not affect risk. The historic association between IUDs and PID originated with the

*Dalkon Shield*, an IUD used in the 1970s that had a braided filament string that was associated with increased risk of PID. Modern IUDs have monofilament strings that do not share this risk.

- Placement of an IUD at the time of an active pelvic infection does increase risk of developing PID. Women with evidence of or high suspicion for active sexually transmitted infections should be screened for STDs and have these treated before having IUDs placed. Otherwise, patients with risk factors (as defined by the CDC) can be screened for chlamydia and gonorrhea at the time of placement. Women with no risk factors or symptoms need not receive additional screening prior to IUD insertion.

- History of PID or ectopic pregnancy is not a contraindication to IUD use. Diagnosis of uncomplicated chlamydia or gonorrhea infection does not necessitate IUD removal: Treatment can be offered with IUD in place. PID that is diagnosed with an IUD in place should be treated, and the IUD may be left in situ in many cases.

- **Postinsertion pregnancy:** Although the relative risk of ectopic pregnancy is higher among pregnancies occurring with an IUD in place, the overall risk of ectopic pregnancy is reduced by an IUD because pregnancy risk is markedly decreased. If a woman has a desired intrauterine pregnancy with an IUD in place, the IUD should be removed if possible.

## *Progestin-Only Implants (Nexplanon)*

- Implants are another form of highly effective, reversible contraception. The only implant currently available in the United States is Nexplanon (formerly Implanon) (Merck, New York, USA).
  - It consists of a single rod, 4 cm × 2 mm (the approximate size of a match), that releases a contraceptive dose of etonogestrel for 3 years. The dose is sufficient to suppress ovulation, as well as to prevent pregnancy through progestin-mediated cervical mucus thickening and endometrial atrophy (see the section "Progestin-Only Methods").
  - The implant is placed under the skin of the upper (usually nondominant) arm and injected from a preloaded insertion device. FDA-mandated training is required for clinicians who wish to provide or remove the implant. The implant is extremely effective and suitable for women who desire long-term reversible contraception and are comfortable with the side effect profile.

- **Advantages:** Implants provide highly effective protection against pregnancy and are relatively easy to insert and remove. Some women may experience decreased menstrual bleeding or amenorrhea. Return to fertility is rapid after removal.

- **Side effects/disadvantages:** Menstrual disturbances are common with *Nexplanon* use.
  - Bleeding patterns can be unpredictable and may vary over time in the same individual. Intolerance of bleeding may lead to discontinuation and patients should be counseled appropriately.
  - Interventions such as short-term estrogen, oral contraceptive pills, doxycycline, or scheduled NSAIDs have been studied for treatment of bothersome bleeding with the contraceptive implant, but evidence for their effectiveness is mixed at best.
  - With no intervention, about 50% of women who continue contraceptive implant use despite unacceptable bleeding will experience improvement over time.

- There may be other hormonal side effects, such as headache and acne, which may be more likely to resolve within a few months of insertion, as etonogestrel levels decrease to their steady-state following the initial period of higher hormone release.
- **Risks:** Insertion is generally quite safe, but rare complications can include infection, injury to nerves, allergic reaction, or incorrect placement leading to complications of removal.
- **Contraindications:** There are few evidence-based contraindications to progestin-only methods. These are discussed in the following text in the review of shorter acting progestin-only methods.

## Shorter Acting Methods of Hormonal Contraception

Hormonal contraceptives have been used routinely for over 50 years in the United States. These methods are extremely safe when provided appropriately. They can also be highly effective when used correctly and consistently. In addition to the long-acting reversible contraception methods, hormonal contraception refers both to progestin-only methods (mini-pill, injection) as well as combined estrogen–progesterone methods (combined oral contraceptives [COCs], transdermal patch, and vaginal ring).

### Progestin-Only Methods

- Synthetic progestin preparations prevent pregnancy without the use of estrogen.
  - Some progestin-only methods prevent ovulation, but all act on the cervical mucus to thicken it and make it unfavorable to sperm penetration.
  - Progestin-induced transformation of the endometrium creates an intrauterine environment unfavorable to fertilization and possibly implantation.
- There are few true contraindications, and these methods can be used in many women with contraindications to combined hormonal contraceptive use.
- Contraindications to progestin-only methods (implants, injections, and pills) include breast cancer, complicated diabetes, and severe active liver disease or cirrhosis.
- Most other women can safely use these methods of contraception.
- For further guidance, refer to the US MEC mentioned earlier in this chapter.

### Injectable Contraceptives

- Depo medroxyprogesterone acetate (DMPA) is a progestin-only injectable contraceptive that is injected intramuscularly (IM) (150 mg) by a medical provider every 3 months.
  - The World Health Organization recently released guidance indicating that the contraceptive effect likely persists up to 17 weeks.
  - DMPA provides highly effective contraception, although its potential effectiveness is limited by a discontinuation rate of over 40% in the first year of use.
  - There is also a subcutaneous formulation (DMPA-SC) containing 104 mg DMPA.
    - Although similar in efficacy and side effect profile to DMPA-IM, it is less widely used.
- **Advantages:** effective contraception. Noncontraceptive benefits include reduction in menstrual blood loss, improvement of anemia, protection against endometrial cancer, reduced seizure frequency in some women with epilepsy, and reduced frequency of sickle crises.

- **Side effects/disadvantages:** Side effects include irregular bleeding, delayed return to fertility, and weight gain. DMPA has also been associated with hair loss in some patients. Although irregular bleeding is common after the first injection, 50% of women become amenorrheic after the first year of use.
  - The average delay in return to ovulatory function is 6 to 10 months after the last injection but delay of up to 18 months is possible.
    - Patients should be counseled on this potential delay, as it can impact future childbearing plans.
  - There has long been concern about weight gain with DMPA.
    - In many studies, this weight gain has not proven significant and may reflect overall weight change with age and the US obesity epidemic, especially in adolescents.
    - Certain subpopulations may be more susceptible than others.
    - Although this is an ongoing area of research, indications are that obese adolescents may be more likely than nonobese adolescents to gain weight on DMPA.
    - The same link may not be true for adult women, however, women who gain weight rapidly following initiation of DMPA should be counseled that weight gain is likely to increase with continued use.
  - A "black box" FDA warning states that **DMPA may decrease bone mineral density** (BMD), especially in adolescents.
    - Studies have also shown this decrease in BMD is measurable after one injection and continues with each subsequent injection.
    - This decreased bone density is reversible after DMPA discontinuation, is generally less than one standard deviation below the mean, is comparable in magnitude to that which occurs with breast-feeding, and has not been shown to correlate with an increased risk of fracture.
    - The World Health Organization has affirmed that there need not be time re-strictions on DMPA use due to bone density concerns.
    - Nor does there appear to be a role for routine bone density screening in pre-menopausal DMPA users, and supplementation with estrogen is not advised.

## *Progestin-Only Pills (Micronor, Ovrette)*

- POP are taken daily with no hormone-free interval.
  - They contain lower doses of progestin than COCs.
  - They are probably most effective after about 6 hours of ingestion, and contra-ceptive effect diminishes significantly after 24 hours.
  - It is important for patients to take their pill at the same time each day and should be advised to use a backup method if their dose is delayed by more than 3 hours.
- POP available in the United States do not reliably suppress ovulation but rather prevent pregnancy through progestin-mediated effects on the cervical mucus and endometrium.
  - Although traditionally suspected of having a higher failure rate than COC, POP are probably about as effective: Both types of pills have a typical-use failure rate of about 9% in the first year of use.
- POP are also safe for use by the vast majority of women; it has been suggested that they would be appropriate for over-the-counter use.
  - Side effects include irregular bleeding and possible systemic hormonal effects (e.g., acne).
- Risks are few.

*Combined Hormonal Contraceptives*

- These methods contain both synthetic progestin and estrogen. Progestin contributes significantly to the contraceptive effect, whereas estrogen maintains the stability of the endometrium and contributes to ovulation inhibition.
  - This allows for monthly withdrawal bleeding and decreases irregular vaginal bleeding. Available methods include oral contraceptives, the transdermal contraceptive patch, and the vaginal contraceptive ring.
- **Advantages:** Besides providing contraception, combined methods may be used to manage dysmenorrhea, menstrual dysfunction, premenstrual symptoms, ovarian cysts, and acne. Use of COCs is associated with a 40% to 80% reduced risk of ovarian cancer (greater effect seen with longer term use) and a 50% to 70% reduced risk of endometrial cancer. The cancer prevention benefits of COCs are robust enough for some public health experts to advocate counseling women on these benefits even when the contraceptive effects of such medications are not needed. Whether these benefits extend to the other combined methods has not been reported, but it may be possible to extrapolate based on similar components and physiologic effects.
- **Side effects/disadvantages:** Combined hormonal contraceptives are highly effective and generally well-tolerated, but side effects may include:
  - *Estrogen*: bloating, headache, nausea, mastalgia, leukorrhea, hypertension, melasma, telangiectasias
  - *Progestin*: mood changes, fatigue, mild weight gain, decreased libido
- **Risks:** Systemic use of estrogen increases the risk of thromboembolism. This must be considered in context, as the overall risk of thromboembolism in most candidates for hormonal contraception is very low, and the additional risk conferred by hormonal contraception is much lower than the risk associated with pregnancy.
  - Risk of venous thromboembolism (VTE) in women per year is
    - 4/100,000 at baseline
    - 10/100,000 in women using COCs
    - 20/100,000 in women using patch
    - >100/100,000 in pregnant women
    - 550/100,000 in postpartum women
- **Contraindications:** Many contraindications to combined methods are based on concerns for elevated risk of thrombotic events, which may become unacceptably high in the setting of medical conditions that predispose to such complications. These include cigarette smoking in women age 35 years and older, hypertension, personal history of VTE, migraine with aura, the presence of multiple risk factors for cardiac disease, and the presence of antiphospholipid antibodies. Known thrombogenic mutations would also preclude use of combined methods, although routine screening for these is not recommended. Breast and uterine cancer are also contraindications to combined methods. For further guidance, providers can refer to the US MEC mentioned earlier in this chapter.

*Combined Oral Contraceptives ("The Pill")*

Current formulations of COCs contain <35 mg of ethinyl estradiol (EE) combined with variable doses of any number of synthetic progestins. One formulation, not available in the United States, contains 17β-estradiol instead of EE. Most formulations still contain 21 days of active hormones followed by 1 week of placebo. During the week of placebo pills, withdrawal bleeding will occur. Some formulations provide a longer duration of active pills (e.g., 24 or 84 days). Extended-use or continuous COCs (e.g., *Seasonale*, *Lybrel*, or standard monophasic pills used continuously) shorten or eliminate the hormone-free interval. This generally decreases or eliminates withdrawal bleeding. Extended-use preparations also improve menorrhagia, dysmenorrhea, endometriosis, chronic pelvic pain, and menstrual migraines. Spotting or breakthrough bleeding may increase with continued use. There are no medical advantages to withdrawal bleeding on any schedule nor are there risks of infrequent or absent bleeding which results from hormonal suppression of the endometrium.

COCs may be started at any time during the menstrual cycle. There are no benefits to delaying initiation until menses or a particular day of the week, and the "quick start" method of starting pills on the day of counseling is associated with improved initiation rates. A week of backup contraception is recommended following initiation after day 5 of the menstrual cycle.

Spotting, irregular menses, and nausea are common after initiation of hormonal contraception but generally resolve within the first 3 months. All brands of COCs have essentially equivalent efficacy and side effect profiles. Some women may have idiosyncratic responses to different formulations, and in these cases, it may be appropriate to switch formulations after 3 months of pill use. Monophasic pills may be associated with less breakthrough bleeding.

### Combined Transdermal Hormonal Contraceptive (Ortho Evra)

- The **contraceptive patch** releases 150 μg norgestimate (progestin) and 20 μg ethinyl estradiol daily.
  - The patch is applied weekly to any body location (other than the breast) for 3 consecutive weeks, followed by a patch-free withdrawal bleeding week.
  - Transdermal delivery avoids hepatic first-pass metabolic effects and maintains steady serum hormone levels without the peaks and troughs seen with pills.
    - Local adhesive reactions to the patch are rare (<5%), and adhesion is reliable.
    - Clinical trials suggested that the patch is less effective in women who weigh >90 kg (198 pounds).
- **Other considerations:** An FDA "black box" warning states that the patch provides approximately 60% more total estrogen than a typical birth control pill containing 35 mg EE.
  - Nonetheless, the daily peak in estrogen is approximately 25% less with the patch compared to pills.
  - The clinical significance of this finding, particularly on the risk of VTE, is unclear, especially because studies have not shown an increased risk of fatal blood clots compared to COCs.

### The Combined Hormonal Vaginal Ring (NuvaRing)

- The *NuvaRing* is a flexible plastic ring 5 cm in diameter and 4 mm in thickness that releases 15 μg/day of EE and 120 μg/day of etonogestrel (progestin).
  - It is placed in the vagina for 3 weeks and removed for 1 week, during which withdrawal bleeding occurs.
  - Alternatively, the ring can be kept in the vagina for 4 weeks followed by transition immediately to a new ring for women who desire to use this method continuously.
- Coital problems and expulsion of the device are rare.
  - If patients desire, the ring may be removed for up to 3 hours, such as during intercourse, although doing this routinely is not recommended.

- If the ring is out of the vagina for >3 hours, backup contraception should be used until the ring has been back in place for 7 days.
- The ring achieves a lower steady-state level of estrogen compared to the patch and COCs, although it is not known if this difference is clinically significant.

## Barrier Methods

*Male Condom*

- Most male condoms are made of latex, although nonlatex condoms are also available.
- They should be applied before vaginal penetration and should cover the entire length of the erect penis.
- They should not be applied too tightly or loosely and a reservoir should be left to retain the ejaculate.
- Adequate lubrication should be used on both the inside and outside of the condom, and the condom should be removed immediately after ejaculation.
  - Condoms with spermicidal lubricant are more effective at preventing pregnancy.
    ○ The CDC currently suggests that women who are at high risk for HIV infection should not use nonoxynol-9 spermicides because this ingredient may increase the risk of HIV transmission.
  - Condoms are highly effective in preventing sexual transmission of HIV and other infections (e.g., gonorrhea, chlamydia, trichomonas). However, because condoms do not cover all exposed areas, they may not be as effective in preventing infections transmitted by skin-to-skin contact (e.g., herpes simplex virus, HPV, syphilis, chancroid).

*Female Condom*

- Female condoms consist of a polyurethane sheath.
  - One type has two flexible rings at either end.
  - The closed end with the upper/inner ring is applied against the cervix and the open end with the lower/outer ring rests against the labia minora outside the introitus.
    ○ Adequate lubrication is important for function and comfort.
- Like male condoms, this method decreases sexual transmission of HIV infection and other STDs.
  - It also provides extra protection on the outside of the body that may decrease infections transmitted by skin-to-skin contact. There are other female condoms in development.

*Diaphragm*

- Diaphragms are barrier devices that are inserted into the vagina and prevent sperm from entering the upper genital tract.
  - The diaphragm consists of a rubber or latex cup with a flexible ring.
  - The edges of the diaphragm should lie just posterior to the symphysis pubis and deep into the cul-de-sac so that the cervix is completely covered behind the center of the diaphragm.
  - The largest diaphragm that comfortably fills this space should be selected during an office exam and fitting.
    ○ Diaphragms range in size from 50 to 105 mm in diameter, with the most commonly prescribed diaphragms measuring 65 to 75 mm.

- Although there is no definitive evidence to support the use of a spermicide with the diaphragm, this is a common recommendation in clinical practice.
  - If spermicide is used, it should be applied to the inside of the rubber cup before each act of coitus.
- The diaphragm should be left in place for a minimum of 6 hours after the last coital act but not >24 consecutive hours. It may be placed hours before intercourse.
- Women with uterine prolapse or structural abnormalities of the reproductive tract may not be able to use a diaphragm.
- Patients relying on a diaphragm for contraception should inspect the diaphragm regularly for holes and should replace their diaphragm at least every 2 years.
- Diaphragms may offer some protection against STD transmission but their use increases the risk of urinary tract infection.

*Cervical Cap*
- A cervical cap is a dome-shaped rubber cap with an inside rim that fits snugly against the outer cervix adjacent to the vaginal fornix.
- This method has decreased efficacy in parous women.

## Natural Family Planning
- Natural family planning (NFP) means that a couple voluntarily avoids or interrupts sexual intercourse during the fertile phase of the woman's menstrual cycle. Effectiveness varies significantly based on the individual, as this method relies on regular menses, cooperation of both partners, and abstinence at times. Methods of NFP include:
- **Symptothermal:** A woman must check her basal body temperature daily and avoid intercourse from the start of menses until 3 days after a spike occurs, indicating that ovulation has occurred and she is no longer at risk for pregnancy in that cycle.
- **Cervical mucus:** A woman must monitor the texture of her cervical mucus to detect a transition from tacky white-yellow into clear, slippery, stretchy discharge at ovulation. Intercourse is avoided from the onset of menses until 3 days after ovulation was predicted.
- **Calendar:** Menstrual cycles are charted for 6 months to detect the cycle length and this chart is used to calculate the patient's fertile days based on estimated day of ovulation.

## Lactational Amenorrhea Method
- During breast-feeding, suckling causes hormonal changes at the level of the hypothalamus that interrupt the pulsatile release of gonadotropin-releasing hormone. This, in turn, impairs LH surge and ovulation does not occur.
  - Lactation offers protection against pregnancy only if strict criteria are followed.
    - Women must be exclusively or nearly exclusively breast-feeding and feedings must occur every 3 to 4 hours during the day and every 6 hours at night.
    - Supplemental feedings should not exceed 5% to 10% of the total.
    - This method is only reliable if the infant is younger than 6 months old.
    - Once a woman has resumed menses, it can be assumed that lactation is no longer providing protection against pregnancy.

## POSTCOITAL (EMERGENCY) CONTRACEPTION

Emergency contraception (EC), or postcoital contraception, may be used after unprotected intercourse to prevent pregnancy. EC pills work mainly through ovulation prevention. EC via insertion of a copper IUD may disrupt implantation. EC does not affect a pregnancy that has already implanted and is therefore not an abortifacient.

### Emergency Contraceptive Pills

- Two types of emergency contraceptive pills (ECP) are available in the United States: LNG (e.g., Plan B) and ulipristal acetate (UPA) (Ella).
  - **LNG-ECP** includes a total of 1.5 mg LNG that may be taken in two doses (0.75 mg 12 hours apart) or one dose (1.5 mg). The single-dose regimen has better compliance with fewer side effects and increased efficacy. LNG-ECP is now available without a prescription for women of all ages. It is effective in preventing pregnancy up to 120 hours after intercourse but effectiveness is inversely related to time since intercourse; therefore, it is most effective when taken immediately after coitus. This regimen is 94% to 98% effective in preventing pregnancy with failure rates at the higher end of this spectrum observed in women who take the dose between 72 to 120 hours after unprotected intercourse. Failure rates may be increased in the obese population.
  - **Ulipristal acetate (Ella)** is a progesterone receptor antagonist taken as a single 30 mg dose within 5 days (120 hours) of unprotected intercourse. It works by directly inhibiting follicle rupture and therefore maintains high efficacy even as ovulation nears. It appears to be at least as effective as LNG, and the efficacy is more consistent over time than seen with LNG. UPA is available by prescription only. UPA is 92% to 99% effective in preventing pregnancy when taken within 5 days of unprotected intercourse. Ulipristal appears to be effective over a wide variety of weights but loses efficacy in women who are morbidly obese.
  - **IUD as EC:** The copper IUD may be inserted within 5 days of unprotected intercourse to decrease the chance of implantation. It is 99.8% to 99.9% effective if inserted within 5 days. According to a recent systematic review of all emergency contraceptive methods, the copper IUD was the most effective method; it is also the only option that addresses not only immediate but future contraception if left in place.
- There are no contraindications to use of EC. Use in pregnancy is not advised; however, the use will not cause termination of existing pregnancy and is not teratogenic. Use of EC is not an ideal method of routine contraception because it is less effective than other methods. However, repeated use is not dangerous. Irregular bleeding and delay of next menses are common after taking EC. Patients are encouraged to take a pregnancy test if menses have not resumed within 1 week after expected menstrual timing.

## ELECTIVE PREGNANCY TERMINATION

### Epidemiology and History

Forty-one million abortions occur each year worldwide. Half of these are unsafe, resulting in 67,000 maternal deaths from abortion and related complications around the world annually. This accounts for 13% of maternal mortality. Abortion is very safe in the United States, with a mortality rate of 0.6/100,000. Extensive study has shown that an abortion does not increase the risk of infertility, breast cancer, or future miscarriage. Abortion has not been shown to cause long-term negative psychological effects in the absence of risk factors.

## Evaluation, Counseling, and Follow-up

- Providers caring for women with unplanned and undesired pregnancy should be able to counsel patients on all the options available to them, including induced abortion.
- A nondirective counseling approach should be taken with the patient to ensure that she is confident in her decision. Those who do not provide this service should be able to counsel patients, make appropriate referrals, and manage postabortal complications.
- Prior to abortion, confirmation of intrauterine pregnancy and pregnancy dating should be performed. Maternal Rh status should be obtained, as Rh-negative women should receive RhoGAM at the time of induced abortion (see Chapter 21).
- Contraception should be discussed with all women, as fertility can return immediately. Women can ovulate within 10 days of abortion, and at least half of women will ovulate within 3 weeks of an abortion procedure.
- Pregnancy symptoms usually resolve within 1 week after abortion. Normal menses may take up to 6 weeks to return. Follow-up is traditionally recommended within 2 to 4 weeks to assess for complications, confirm resolution of pregnancy, and re-address contraception.

## Surgical Abortion

### Surgical Abortion in the First Trimester

Surgical abortion at <14 weeks performed surgically is referred to as dilation and curettage (D&C). This is the most common method of first-trimester abortion. Principles of care include pain management, cervical dilation, and uterine evacuation.

- A paracervical block with local anesthesia is frequently given. Intravenous sedation may also be given, as may oral anxiolytics. Choice may depend on patient preference and availability of options. First-trimester abortions generally need not be performed under general anesthesia, in the absence of other considerations.
- Adequate cervical dilation facilitates the procedure and may reduce complication rates.
  - In many cases, the cervix can be manually dilated at the time of the procedure.
    - For later first-trimester procedures, medications such as misoprostol can be used for preoperative cervical ripening.
    - The exact gestational age at which this is introduced may vary among providers and practice environments but is generally beginning at 10 to 12 weeks' gestation.
  - There may also be a role for mifepristone as a cervical ripening agent, although its expense makes this a less commonly used approach.
  - For cases performed at gestational ages approaching 14 weeks, osmotic dilators (overnight or for several hours) may be considered.
    - These are discussed further in the section on second-trimester surgical abortion.
  - Mechanical dilation uses surgical instruments that have progressively increasing diameters (e.g., Pratt, Hegar, or Denniston dilators) to open the cervix to a sufficient diameter.

- To empty the uterus of the products of conception (POCs), electric or manual vacuum aspiration (MVA) can be performed. Both use a suction curette or cannula attached to a suction device. The cannula/curette should be approximately the same diameter (in millimeters) as the weeks' gestation. The apparatus is advanced through the internal os into the uterine cavity. Uterine contents can then be aspirated by generating negative air pressure via either the syringe or suction machine, collecting the POCs.
- Electric vacuum aspiration (EVA) uses a suction curette attached to an electrically powered vacuum canister.
- MVA has been in use for >30 years. A specially designed handheld 60-mL syringe is attached to either a flexible or rigid cannula of a diameter appropriate for gestational age.
- After aspiration, the tissue should be inspected to verify that the POCs are consistent with the gestational age.
- Sharp curettage is generally not necessary. The use of sharp curettage increases the pain of the procedure. It may also contribute to bleeding and increased risk of uterine perforation.
- Antibiotics should be administered for infection prophylaxis. Doxycycline is a commonly used and cost-effective choice.

### Surgical Abortion in the Second Trimester

- The most commonly used surgical procedure for second trimester abortion is dilation and evacuation (D&E). D&E is considered the preferred method of second-trimester termination when experienced personnel are available and autopsy of an intact fetus is not required.
  - In experienced hands, D&E is the safest available method of second-trimester termination.
- The procedure for surgical termination between 14 and 22 weeks' gestation is different in several important ways from a first-trimester D&C. Instrumental removal of the POCs is usually required. It is essential to examine and account for all POCs consistent with gestational age.
  - Preoperative cervical preparation is highly recommended. This can be accomplished via medications that ripen the cervix or by osmotic dilators.
    - Choice of technique depends on provider experience, gestational age, and availability. Osmotic dilators, such as Dilapan (polyacrylonitrile) or laminaria (dried seaweed *Laminaria japonica*), absorb cervical moisture, and as they do, they enlarge and dilate the cervical canal.
    - They also cause the release of prostaglandins, which ultimately disrupt the cervical stroma and soften the cervix.
    - Osmotic dilators must be placed several hours before the procedure or overnight for maximum effect.
    - For procedures later in the second trimester, dilation is often carried out over 1 to 2 days, and sequential insertion of osmotic dilators may be used.
  - Ultrasonographic confirmation of gestational age is considered essential and has become standard in most practice environments.
    - The procedure may also be carried out under ultrasound guidance to facilitate complete and efficient evacuation.
    - Ultrasound guidance is not a substitute for competence, however, and does not eliminate risk of complications.

## Medical Abortion

*Medical Abortion in the First Trimester*

- Evidence-based medical abortion regimens are safe and effective up to 63 days of gestation, with some recent research supporting use beyond 63 days. Medical abortion can be performed using mifepristone (RU-486) and misoprostol, or methotrexate and misoprostol. The latter has fallen out of favor, as it is less effective than mifepristone/misoprostol.
  - Mifepristone is a progesterone antagonist. Its effects include alterations in the endometrial blood supply, blocking the support of pregnancy and softening the cervix.
  - Methotrexate inhibits DNA synthesis and affects rapidly dividing cells, including trophoblast.
  - Misoprostol is a prostaglandin that is used to induce uterine contractions after administration of either mifepristone or methotrexate, thus promoting expulsion of the POCs.
- Evidence-based recommendations support the use of mifepristone and misoprostol up to 63 days of gestation and with a lower mifepristone dose (200 mg vs. 600 mg) than the FDA-approved regimen, which was based on a gestational age limit of 49 days.
- Where access to other options is limited, misoprostol alone can be used in repeat 24-hour dosing intervals for medical abortion. Effectiveness may vary from 47% to 96%.
- Medical abortion is a different experience than surgical abortion, more akin to a miscarriage.
  - The abortion may take several days to complete.
  - A follow-up visit is generally required to confirm completion because surgical evacuation is advised in case of medication failure.
  - It is important for patients to be counseled accordingly and be able to follow up.
- Side effects following administration of mifepristone and misoprostol consist primarily of pain, bleeding, and gastrointestinal (GI) upset.

*Medical Abortion in the Second Trimester*

- Medical second-trimester abortion may be the best alternative in some settings. It does not require anesthesia, a skilled operator is not required, and fetal examination can be performed on an intact fetus, such as in cases of genetic termination.
- However, as compared with D&E, the procedure can take 24 hours or longer, major complications and mortality are higher, and fever and severe GI side effects are common when prostaglandins are used.
- The overall goal is to administer medications that cause uterine contractions and lead to the expulsion of the POCs. Medications include high-dose intravenous oxytocin and different preparations of vaginally administered prostaglandins (prostaglandin $E_2$ [Prostin $E_2$] and misoprostol). Less commonly, hypertonic solutions (saline or urea) may be administered intra-amniotically to induce second-trimester abortions. Antiprogestins, such as mifepristone, may also be used.

## Abortion Complications

Fortunately, legal abortion is a safe procedure. However, as with any other procedure, complications can occur. Complications with medical abortion generally stem from retained POCs, bleeding, and infection.

*Risks of Surgical Abortion*

- Perforation is a risk of surgical abortion. Management of perforation is beyond the scope of this chapter, but there are principles one can follow.
  - If perforation is suspected, the suction is stopped, suction is not applied, and the patient should be examined clinically and with ultrasound.
  - If she is stable, observation with close monitoring may be appropriate.
  - If the patient shows signs of bleeding or instability, surgical management (laparoscopy vs. laparotomy) should be performed.
- Excess uterine bleeding or hemorrhage due to atony can be managed with uterotonics, such as misoprostol, Methergine, or oxytocin. Bimanual massage is also helpful.
- Hematometra should be suspected if a patient has intense pain and an enlarged uterus immediately after surgical abortion.
  - Surgical reaspiration is the key to management, and uterotonics such as Methergine can be considered.
- Postabortal endomyometritis may present with fever and abdominal pain postabortion.
  - Oral or intravenous doxycycline and a cephalosporin, with or without metronidazole, should be administered.
  - The decision to use outpatient versus inpatient management can be made applying criteria similar to those designated for PID.
- Retained POCs after abortion can cause fever, pain, bleeding, and/or symptoms of pelvic infection. The treatment is evacuation of the uterus.
  - Oral prophylactic doxycycline administration, before or after surgical abortion, can reduce the risk of postabortion endomyometritis by 40%.

*Risks of Medical Abortion*

- Medical abortion has a low complication rate.
  - Continuing pregnancy occurs in 1% to 3% of cases.
    - Retained products may also occur.
  - These can be managed by surgical evacuation or possibly by an additional dose of misoprostol.
  - The risk of bleeding severe enough to require transfusion is far less than 1%.
- A series of case reports that appeared several years ago described a very rare risk of fatal sepsis resulting from medical abortion related to *Clostridium sordellii*.
- In response to this, some providers have come to recommend buccal administration of misoprostol over vaginal, although whether this or prophylactic antibiotics further decrease infection risk is controversial.

## SUGGESTED READINGS

Blumenthal P, Edelman A. Hormonal contraception. *Obstet Gynecol* 2008;112(3):670–684.

Chervenak FA, McCullough LB. The ethics of direct and indirect referral for termination of pregnancy. *Am J Obstet Gynecol* 2008;199(3):232–233.

Clark MK, Sowers MR, Nichols S, et al. Bone mineral density changes over two years in first-time users of depot medroxyprogesterone acetate. *Fertil Steril* 2004;82:1580–1586.

Grimes DA, Lopez LM, Manion C, et al. Cochrane systematic review of IUD trials: lessons learned. *Contraception* 2007;75(6)(suppl):S55–S59.

Jabara S, Barnhart K. Is Rh immune globulin needed in early first-trimester abortion? A review. *Am J Obstet Gynecol* 2003;188:623–627.

Morrison CS, Bright P, Wong EL, et al. Hormonal contraceptive use, cervical ectopy, and the acquisition of cervical infections. *Sex Transm Dis* 2004;31:561–567.

Mosher WD, Martinez GM, Chandra A, et al. Use of contraception and use of family planning services in the United States: 1982–2002. *Advanced Data* 2004;350:1–36.

# Intimate Partner and Sexual Violence

Maryann B. Wilbur and Abigail E. Dennis

## INTIMATE PARTNER VIOLENCE AND RELATED BEHAVIORS

### Definitions

- **Intimate partner violence (IPV):** a pattern of assaultive and/or coercive behaviors that may include physical injury, psychological abuse, sexual assault, progressive isolation, stalking, intimidation, and reproductive coercion
- **Domestic violence (DV):** an older and very similar term referring to assault-ive and/or coercive behavior within a shared household; IPV and DV strongly overlap
- **Population-specific violence:** includes different forms of population-specific violence affecting particularly vulnerable patients, such as child abuse, adolescent abuse, elder abuse, and patterns of behavior affecting vulnerable or marginalized populations

### Background

- Affects individuals of all ages, races, and educational and economic backgrounds
- Occurs in both heterosexual and homosexual relationships; however, the most common presentation is a heterosexual relationship with a female victim
- Can be thought of as part of a larger disempowerment syndrome and is seen more often in women affected by low socioeconomic status, sexually transmitted infections, and unintended pregnancy
- Long-standing abusive relationships tend to develop a cycle in which a violent episode is followed by a period of reconciliation and apology. A tension-building phase soon begins and culminates in a repeat violent attack and the cycle begins anew.
- Escape from the relationship may be difficult because of fear, shame, powerlessness, and social isolation. Over time, the degree of violence may escalate.

## Statistics

- The majority (85%) of individuals affected by IPV are women.
- In primary care practices, nearly 25% of women endorse current or previous IPV.
- Approximately 25% of women in the United States will be abused by a current or former partner sometime during their lifetime.
- IPV is the single most common cause of injury to women in the United States; more than 30% of all women's emergency room visits can be attributed to IPV.
- Fifty-four percent of IPV is reported to police; only 24% of sexual assaults are reported.
- One third of female homicides in the United States are IPV-related.
- Women are more likely to be injured, raped, or killed by a current or former male partner than by all other types of assailants combined.

## Intimate Partner Violence and Pregnancy

- According to the Centers for Disease Control and Prevention (CDC), 4% to 8% of pregnant women report abuse during pregnancy.
- One in six abused women reports her partner was first abusive in pregnancy.
- Abuse often escalates during the course of the pregnancy and postpartum.
- IPV can result in poor pregnancy outcomes, such as miscarriage, preterm labor, low birth weight, and fetal injury or death.
- Women with an unintended pregnancy have a threefold higher risk of abuse than those women whose pregnancy was planned.
- Pregnant women have a threefold higher risk of being victims of attempted or completed homicide, and IPV-related homicide is the number one cause of death in pregnancy.

## Reproductive Coercion

- Defined as "explicit male behavior to promote pregnancy unwanted by the woman and can include 'birth control sabotage' and/or 'pregnancy coercion,' such as telling a woman not to use contraception and threatening to leave her if she doesn't get pregnant."
- More broadly, clinicians will encounter a spectrum of coercive behaviors that aim to influence women's reproductive choices.
- Strongly correlated with the following demographics:
  - Ethnic and/or racial minority
  - Low educational achievement
  - Lack of employment
  - Low socioeconomic status
  - History of sexually transmitted infection (STI)
  - History of unwanted pregnancy
  - Increasing age difference between the individual and her partner
  - Current unwanted pregnancy
- Reproductive coercion represents another form of controlling behavior within a relationship displaying power differentials. Of women experiencing IPV, nearly half will also endorse reproductive coercion upon direct questioning from a clinician.

## Evaluation and Management

*Screening*

- Regular screening for IPV is the most important thing clinicians can do and routine surveillance has been recommended by the U.S. Department of Health and Human

Services, the Institute of Medicine, and the American College of Obstetricians and Gynecologists (ACOG).

- Routine IPV screening significantly increases detection. In a study of trauma victims, the institution of a screening protocol increased detection from 5.6% to 30%.
- The opinion published by ACOG supports specifically asking women about their abuse history and recommends screening at the following patient encounters:
  - New patient visits
  - Annual visits
  - Problem visits where unintended pregnancy or STI is diagnosed
  - First prenatal visit
  - Once during each trimester in pregnancy
  - Postpartum visit
- Guidelines for screening
  - Setting is very important. A patient must feel that she is in a safe and comfortable environment. Ideally, screening should be done without a partner, children, or other relatives present. Be aware that the aggressor often accompanies the woman to the appointment and wants to remain in the room to monitor what is said.
  - Ensure patient confidentiality.
  - Begin with an objective statement that demonstrates that your screening is universal and necessary to provide comprehensive health care. This type of introduction increases the detection rate and helps the patient feel that she has not been singled out.
  - Never ask what the patient did wrong or why she remains with her partner. Avoid judgment or value-laden terms, such as "abused" and "battered."
  - Choose quick screening questions that feel comfortable and make screening routine. Several useful questionnaires have been developed to address abuse:
    - Family Violence Prevention Fund questions (Table 33-1)
    - The Structured Analysis Family Evaluation questions (Table 33-2)
    - The three-question Abuse Assessment Screen (Table 33-3)
- Be patient. Patients will often fail to disclose on first questioning, but they will almost never reveal IPV if not asked. If the provider suspects abuse and the patient initially denies it, the provider should readdress the issue during a subsequent visit.
- Leave the conversation open and make sure patients are aware that they can discuss any issues at future visits. This supportive environment where information is available regarding options or resources could prompt patients to seek help in the future.

*Diagnosing Intimate Partner Violence*

- Women affected by IPV will often have numerous office or emergency room visits for injury. There may be an inconsistent explanation for the injuries or a delay in seeking treatment. The injuries classically involve multiple sites, such as three or more body parts; affect the head, back, breast, and abdomen (whereas accidental injuries are more likely to be peripheral); and are in various stages of healing.
- Patients who are abused tend to report somatic complaints, such as fatigue, headache, and abdominal pain. They are also more likely to suffer from eating disorders, gastrointestinal complaints, psychiatric disorders, and substance abuse.

| TABLE 33-1 | Screening Questions from the Family Violence Prevention Fund |
|---|---|

**Sample Intimate Partner Violence Screening Questions**

While providing privacy, screen for intimate partner violence during new patient visits, annual examinations, initial prenatal visits, each trimester of pregnancy, and the postpartum checkup.

**Framing Statement**

"We've started talking to all of our patients about safe and healthy relationships because it can have such a large impact on your health."[a]

**Confidentiality**

"Before we get started, I want you to know that everything here is confidential, meaning that I won't talk to anyone else about what is said unless you tell me that . . . (insert the laws in your state about what is necessary to disclose)."[a]

**Sample Questions**

"Has your current partner ever threatened you or made you feel afraid?"
(Threatened to hurt you or your children if you did or did not do something, controlled who you talked to or where you went, or gone into rages)[b]

"Has your partner ever hit, choked, or physically hurt you?"
("Hurt" includes being hit, slapped, kicked, bitten, pushed, or shoved.)[b]

*For women of reproductive age:*

"Has your partner ever forced you to do something sexually that you did not want to do or refused your request to use condoms?"[a]

"Does your partner support your decision about when or if you want to become pregnant?"[a]

"Has your partner ever tampered with your birth control or tried to get you pregnant when you didn't want to be?"[a]

*For women with disabilities:*

"Has your partner prevented you from using a wheelchair, cane, respirator, or other assistive device?"[c]

"Has your partner refused to help you with an important personal need such as taking your medicine, getting to the bathroom, getting out of bed, bathing, getting dressed, or getting food or drink or threatened not to help you with these personal needs?"[c]

---

[a]Modified and reprinted from Family Violence Prevention Fund. Reproductive health and partner violence guidelines: an integrated response to intimate partner violence and reproductive coercion. San Francisco, CA: Family Violence Prevention Fund, 2010. http://www.futureswith outviolence.org/userfiles/file/HealthCare/Repro_Guide.pdf. Accessed October 12, 2011, with permission.

[b]Modified and reprinted from Family Violence Prevention Fund. National consensus guidelines on identifying and responding to domestic violence victimization in health care settings. San Francisco, CA: Family Violence Prevention Fund, 2004. http://www.futureswithoutviolence.org/userfiles/file/Consensus.pdf. Accessed October 12, 2011, with permission.

[c]Modified and reprinted from Center for Research on Women with Disabilities. Development of the abuse assessment screen-disability (AAS-D). In *Violence against Women with Physical Disabilities: Final Report Submitted to the Centers for Disease Control and Prevention*. Houston, TX: Baylor College of Medicine, 2002:II-1–II-16. http://www.bcm.edu/crowd/index.cfm?pmid=2137. Accessed October 18, 2011, with permission.

| TABLE 33-2 | Structured Analysis Family Evaluation Questionnaire |
| --- | --- |

- **S**tress/safety: Do you feel safe in your relationship?
- **A**fraid/abused: Have you ever been in a relationship in which you were threatened, hurt, or afraid?
- **F**riends/family: Are your friends or family aware that you have been hurt? Could you tell them, and would they be able to give you support?
- **E**mergency plan: Do you have a safe place to go and the resources you need in an emergency?

Based on Neufeld B. SAFE questions: overcoming barriers to the detection of domestic violence. *Am Fam Physician* 1996;53:2575–2582.

- Gynecologic and obstetric clues to the presence of abuse include increased prevalence of sexually transmitted disease, chronic pelvic pain, premenstrual syndrome, unintended pregnancy, and late prenatal care (Table 33-4).

*Assessment of Risk*

- In the case that the patient reveals that she has been affected by IPV, the clinician should attempt to elicit the degree of risk to the patient. Sample questions include the following:
  - How were you hurt?
  - Has this happened before?
  - When did it first happen?
  - How badly have you been hurt in the past?
  - Have you ever needed to go to the emergency room for treatment?
  - Have you ever been threatened with a weapon, or has a weapon ever been used on you?
  - Have you ever tried to get a restraining order against a partner?
  - Have your children ever seen or heard you being threatened or hurt?
  - Do you know how you can get help for yourself if you are hurt or afraid?
  - Is the violence getting worse?
  - Are there threats of suicide or homicide?
  - Is there a weapon in the home?

| TABLE 33-3 | Abuse Assessment Screen |
| --- | --- |

- Within the last year, have you been hit, slapped, kicked, or otherwise physically hurt by someone?
- Since you've been pregnant, have you been hit, slapped, kicked, or otherwise physically hurt by someone?
- Within the last year, has anyone forced you to have sexual activities?

Based on McFarlane J, Parker B, Soeken K, et al. Assessing for abuse during pregnancy. *JAMA* 1992;267:3176–3178.

| TABLE 33-4 | Gynecologic and Obstetric Clues to Presence of Abuse |
| --- | --- |

Chronic pelvic pain
Severe premenstrual syndrome
Multiple or recurrent sexually transmitted infections or recurrent vaginitis
Medical noncompliance
Sexual dysfunction
Abdominal pain
Unintended pregnancy
Late registration for prenatal care, no prenatal care
Noncompliance and missed appointment
Fetal or maternal injury (violence is often directed toward the woman's
   abdomen during pregnancy)
Spontaneous abortion or stillbirth
Vaginal bleeding in the second or third trimester
Preterm labor
Infection
Anemia
Poor weight gain
Low-birth-weight infants

*Interventions*

- Most victims of abuse are not ready to leave their abusers. They may rely on their abuser for financial support and shelter or may have a fear of repercussions.
  - Empowerment of the patient is the first step. Provide support and do not attempt to make decisions for the patient.
  - Use resources such as social workers and violence prevention programs. Provide the patient with phone numbers of resource agencies and offer to let the patient establish first contact while she is still in your office.
  - Discuss the gravity of the situation and assess immediate safety needs.
  - Reinforce that the patient is not to blame. Emphasize that she did nothing to justify this behavior.
  - Treat the patient's injuries and screen for suicidal tendencies, depression, and substance abuse.
  - When applicable, discuss court restraining orders and laws against stalking with the help of legal and social work resources.
  - Review an exit plan or exit drill (Table 33-5). Do not force a woman to leave before she is ready; leaving is associated with increased physical aggression and resources need to be in place to minimize risk to the woman and her children during this critically vulnerable transition.
  - Abusive partners often monitor cell phone usage; therefore, offering a separate cell phone specifically to assess safety has been suggested to facilitate a woman leaving an unsafe situation.
  - Provide ongoing support, and offer referrals for counseling.
  - Provide documentation, including direct quotations and photographs.

| TABLE 33-5 | Exit Plan for Domestic Violence Intervention |
|---|---|

The following exit plan has been proposed for a woman who feels that she or her children are in danger from her partner:

1. Have a change of clothes packed for herself and her children, including toiletries, necessary medications, and an extra set of house and car keys. These can be placed in a suitcase and stored with a friend or neighbor.
2. Cash, a checkbook, and savings account information may also be kept with a friend or neighbor.
3. Have available identification papers, such as birth certificates, social security cards, voter registration card, utility bills, and a driver's license because children will need to be enrolled in school and financial assistance may be sought. If available, also take financial records, such as mortgage papers, rent receipts, or an automobile title.
4. Take something of special interest to each child, such as a book or toy.
5. Have a plan of exactly where to go, regardless of the time of day or night. This may be a friend or relative's home or a shelter for women and children.
6. Have a separate phone available to make emergency phone calls.

Modified from Helton A. Battering during pregnancy. *Am J Nurs* 1986;86:910–913.

- Report abuse in indicated situations. If the patient is a minor, an elder, or disabled, clinicians are mandated to report abuse. Most states do not require mandatory reporting of IPV in adults who do not meet these criteria.

## Special Populations

*Elder Abuse*

- A form of abuse, neglect, and/or violence, typically at the hands of adult family members or caregivers, affecting as many as 2 million Americans.
- Providers should apply the same criteria in assessing older individuals as they would in assessing a younger woman for DV.
- Elder abuse must be reported to the state elder abuse hotline.

*Disabled Women*

- Girls or women with physical, cognitive, or emotional disabilities are all at particular risk of IPV and sexual abuse and should be screened at each visit.
- Abuse of disabled persons must be reported to the Disabled Persons Protection Commission.

*Women with Undocumented Immigrant Status*

- Women with undocumented immigrant status are also particularly vulnerable and may find themselves in a situation where they are being threatened with deportation as a means of coercion. Such a woman should be reassured that this behavior is illegal under United States law. If it can be justified on humanitarian grounds, a nonimmigrant visa will allow her to remain in the United States and she should be given resources for contacting a community attorney familiar with this process.

### Sex Workers

- Women who trade sex for money and/or drugs are significantly more likely to become victims of coercive behavior and sexual abuse. Clinicians must remain cognizant of the vulnerability of this population and should screen at every encounter. Patients in this category should also be assured that illegal activity on their part should not prevent them from reporting violence to the authorities.

## SEXUAL VIOLENCE

### Definitions

- **Sexual violence:** all forms of sexual activity where consent is not given (e.g., assault, sexual harassment, threats, sex trafficking, female circumcision)
- **Sexual assault:** any sexual act performed on one person by another without consent
- **Rape:** a legal (not medical) term and should be used minimally, if at all, in medical records

### Background

- Sexual assault is the fastest growing violent crime in America.
- Nine in 10 sexual assault victims are women.
- One in 6 women will be sexually assaulted in her lifetime.
- Seventy-three percent of sexual assault victims know their offender.
- Approximately 1 in 6 sexual assaults is reported to the police. Approximately 6% of the accused spend a day in jail.

### Evaluation and Management

- A comprehensive workup should be done in a manner that is sensitive to the patient's acute mental and physical state and with an awareness that the collection of forensic evidence needs to be done in a specific, time-sensitive fashion. When possible, one should use a coordinated community response plan, with referral to a medical center that can perform a sexual assault forensic exam. This may not be possible in cases of severe trauma, and life-threatening emergencies should obviously be prioritized.
  - When evaluating a patient who has had a recent sexual assault, multiple issues should be addressed.
    - Medical: injuries, STI exposure, pregnancy
    - Emotional: crisis intervention, counseling referrals
    - Forensics: documentation, proper collection and handling of evidence, court appearances

### Coordinated Community Response Plan

- Rape crisis centers/hotlines: These centers have trained crisis counselors/advocates who provide free 24-hour counseling, referral, and victim support services.
- Sexual assault response teams (SARTs): These are multidisciplinary teams composed of law enforcement agents, medical providers, sexual assault advocates, social workers, etc. who work together to streamline care/minimize trauma to victims and to optimize collection of evidence.

- Sexual assault forensic examiner (SAFE) or sexual assault nurse examiner (SANE): These professionals have been specially trained to care for sexual assault victims.
  - They are specifically trained in forensic evaluation/precise collection of evidence, minimizing barriers to support in the legal system and providing prompt and compassionate care to patients. All efforts should be made to use these professionals and when possible, physical exams should be deferred until a forensic examiner is present so as not to interfere with evidence collection.

### Sexual Assault Evidence Collection Kit

- Walks a provider through the steps of obtaining informed consent and then performing a targeted history and physical exam with emphasis on appropriate collection of forensic evidence
- The Federal Violence Against Women Act (passed in 2005, in effect since 2009) allows for victims of sexual assault to obtain a forensic exam free of charge even if they have chosen not to report the assault to law enforcement (i.e., "Jane Doe rape kits").

### Patient History

- A chaperone of the same gender as the patient should be present at all times for the history and examination.
- Take a targeted sexual and gynecologic history, including last menstrual period (LMP), contraceptive use, and last consensual intercourse. Information about past sexual history may damage a victim's credibility in court.
- Ask about injuries; this will help tailor the examination.
- Ask specifically about the nature of the violation. Elicit specifics regarding oral, vaginal, or rectal penetration as well as condom use.
- Ask what the patient has done since the event (e.g., showering, bathing, douching, voiding, defecating, changing clothes).
- Do not impose interpretation on the description—document the patient's exact description of the event. Avoid inflammatory language. Be objective and avoid passing judgment.

### Physical Examination

- If possible, this exam should be performed by a trained examiner (e.g., SANE or SAFE).
- Obtain informed consent to proceed with the examination. This should be done for legal purposes and may help the victim regain autonomy.
- Perform the exam with a chaperone of the same gender as the patient.
- The patient should undress with a sheet beneath her to capture any debris or evidence. Collect appropriate clothing from the patient and give it to the proper personnel.
- Perform a full skin examination and evaluate all orifices for evidence of laceration, bruising, bite marks, or use of foreign objects. A Wood lamp and colposcope can be used to identify semen and subtle signs of trauma. Toluidine blue will stain underlying tissue if skin is broken. Perform an overall general examination for any other injuries, such as abdominal trauma or broken bones.
- Document the patient's emotional state. Be thorough and systematic, and record all evidence of injury; use drawings and photographs as needed.

### Laboratory Testing

- Radiographic imaging, if necessary, should be obtained.
- Gonorrhea and chlamydia tests from any sites of contact
- Wet prep to look for *Trichomonas*

- Pregnancy test
- Baseline HIV counseling and testing
- Baseline specimens for hepatitis B and C and syphilis
- Drug screening for the "date rape drugs" flunitrazepam (Rohypnol) and gamma-hydroxy butyrate (GHB) if indicated

*Treatment*

- Treat traumatic injuries as indicated.
- Treat presumptively for STIs. Recommendations, per CDC guidelines, are as follows:
  - Gonorrhea: ceftriaxone 250 mg intramuscularly
  - Chlamydia: azithromycin, 1 g orally, *or* doxycycline, 100 mg twice daily for 1 week
  - Gonorrhea and chlamydia (pregnancy/allergy): erythromycin 1.5 g orally then 500 mg 4×/day for 1 week
  - Trichomoniasis: metronidazole, 2 g orally (consider an antiemetic for side effects)
  - Provide hepatitis B vaccine if the victim has not received it already.
- In high-risk populations, consider the following additional prophylaxis:
  - Herpes: acyclovir 3 g orally
  - Syphilis: penicillin G 2.4 million units
- Offer antiretroviral therapy against HIV if <72 hours has elapsed since the assault (treatment is most effective if started within 4 hours). For help deciding whether to start HIV prophylaxis and which regimen to use, consult National Clinician's Post-Exposure Prophylaxis hotline.
  - Routine prophylaxis: Combivir
  - Resistance concerns: Combivir + nelfinavir
  - HIV resistance or assailant known to be on therapy: Combivir + Kaletra
- Offer emergency contraception. The chance of pregnancy after the assault varies according to timing of the menstrual cycle but is generally reported to be 2% to 4% in victims not protected by barrier contraception.
- Schedule visits for follow-up testing. Pregnancy testing should be repeated in 1 to 2 weeks. The CDC recommends testing for rapid plasma reagin at 6, 12, and 24 weeks; HIV at 6, 12, and 24 weeks; and hepatitis B vaccination at 1- and 6-month intervals.

*Psychosocial Sequelae and Follow-up*

- Victims may experience the *rape-trauma syndrome*, which includes feelings of anger, fear, shame, anxiety, hypervigilance, nightmares, and physical symptoms.
- Victims may develop posttraumatic stress syndrome, depression, and anxiety.
- Acute counseling should include safety planning and referral to counseling. Victims should be referred to rape crisis programs and/or should be provided with 24-hour hotline numbers. Contact hospital and clinic social workers to facilitate this process.
- Follow-up in 1 to 2 weeks for psychosocial evaluation

## Sexual Abuse in Children

*Background*

- Contact or interaction between a child and an adult in which the child is being used for sexual stimulation of that adult or another person. Abuse may also be committed by another minor either when that person is significantly older than the victim or when the abuser is in a position of power or control over the child. Sexual abuse also encompasses nonsexual contact, such as pornography or exhibitionism.

• The majority of childhood sexual abuse occurs between ages 6 and 14 years and especially between ages 12 and 14 years. The perpetrator is usually a relative or an acquaintance.

*Evaluation and Management*

• Children suspected of being victims of abuse or assault should be evaluated by professionals trained in conducting interviews, documenting questions and responses, and collecting forensic evidence. Centers designed for a multidisciplinary approach are ideal for these evaluations. The process is the same as outlined earlier, with the following considerations:

  • **History:** Take time to establish rapport with the child. Information should be recorded in the child's own words; for young children with limited verbal skills, techniques such as play interviews or drawings have been used to promote communication. Note the child's composure, behavior, and mental state, as well as interactions with parents and other people. Ask about recent changes in sleep (night terrors) and behaviors.

  • **Examination:** The examination should be complete, extending from head to toe, allowing the child to become accustomed to the touch of the evaluator and establishing trust. Physical or laboratory findings of trauma are rare. Some signs, however, can be used as diagnostic clues for childhood sexual abuse, especially if the abuse is recent or repetitive. Sexual abuse should be considered in any child with trauma or lacerations involving the posterior hymen or in cases of a vaginal foreign body. Have a low threshold for performing an exam under anesthesia.

  • **Mandatory reporting:** All suspected victims of child abuse should be referred to child protective services (CPS). Until the question of protection can be assured, providing temporary placement for the child is advisable.

  • **Psychosocial support:** A trained therapist should be available to assist both victim and family with the evaluation process, medical treatment, and encounters with CPS and law enforcement agencies.

## Sexual Abuse in Adolescents

• More than 75% of assaults are committed by an acquaintance of the victim. These include date rape, statutory rape, and incest.

• Teenagers are still learning to establish social boundaries, and they bring various expectations to dating situations. Some adolescents believe that violence is acceptable in some social situations. Furthermore, adolescents may use alcohol and illicit drugs, which alter judgment. A history of nonvoluntary sexual activity has been associated with early initiation of voluntary sexual activity, unintended pregnancy, and poor use of contraceptives.

• As part of routine screening, all teenagers should be asked direct questions regarding their sexual experiences and any incidence of coercion. This is an opportunity to identify adolescent victims and initiate discussion of contraception and STIs. The following sensitive screening question has been suggested by adolescent specialists: "Have you ever had sex when you didn't want to?"

• Providers can offer education, counseling referrals, community resource information, and prevention messages. Some teenage empowerment messages include the following:

  • You have the right to say *no* to sexual activity.

  • You have the right to set sexual limits and insist that your partner honor them.

  • Be assertive. Stay sober. Recognize and avoid situations that may put you at risk.

- Never leave a party with someone you don't know well.
- No one should ever be forced or pressured into engaging in any unwanted sexual behavior.

## Human Trafficking

- **Definition:** The recruitment, harboring, transportation, provision, or obtaining of a person for labor or services through the use of force, fraud, or coercion for the purpose of subjection to involuntary servitude, peonage, debt bondage, or slavery.
- Estimates are difficult, but approximately 15,000 individuals are trafficked into the United States annually; 80% of these individuals are female.
- The following are examples of indicators that a patient is the victim of human trafficking:
  - Lack of any official identification papers or cards
  - Vague answers about their situation
  - Inconsistencies to their stories
  - Avoiding eye contact
  - No control of their money
- Patient and clinician resources are available at the National Human Trafficking Resource Center (NHTRC) hotline: 1-888-373-7888.

## Female Genital Mutilation

- Female genital mutilation (FGM), female genital cutting (FGC), and female circumcision are terms that are often used interchangeably to describe the alteration of female genitalia for nontherapeutic reasons, usually without analgesia or aseptic technique.
- It represents a form of violence against girls and women.
- FGM is usually grouped into types I, II, III, and IV.
- Sequelae of FGM include hemorrhage, infection, menstrual abnormalities, fistulae, sexual dysfunction, and depression/anxiety.
- FGM is not an indication for a cesarean delivery.
- FGM is a cultural not a religious practice.

## SUGGESTED READINGS

American College of Obstetricians and Gynecologists. ACOG committee opinion no. 507: human trafficking. *Obstet Gynecol* 2011;118(3):767–770.

American College of Obstetricians and Gynecologists. ACOG committee opinion no. 518: intimate partner violence. *Obstet Gynecol* 2012;119(2, pt 1):412–417.

American College of Obstetricians and Gynecologists. *Female Circumcision/Female Genital Mutilation: Clinical Management of Circumcised Women.* Washington DC: American College of Obstetricians and Gynecologists, 1999.

Eisenstat SA, Bancroft L. Domestic violence. *JAMA* 1999;341(12):886–892.

Kilpatrick DG, Edmonds CN, Seymour A. *Rape in America: A Report to the Nation.* Arlington, VA: National Victim Center and Medical University of South Carolina, 1992.

Miller E, Decker MR, McCauley HL, et al. Pregnancy coercion, intimate partner violence and intended pregnancy. *Contraception* 2010;81:316–322.

Rickert VI, Wiemann CM, Harrykissoon SD, et al. The relationship among demographics, reproductive characteristics, and intimate partner violence. *Am J Obstet Gynecol* 2002; 187(4):1002–1007.

Roberts TA, Auinger P, Klein JD. Intimate partner abuse and the reproductive health of sexually active female adolescents. *J Adol Health* 2005;36:380–385.

World Health Organization. *Eliminating Female Genital Mutilation: An Interagency Statement.* Geneva, Switzerland: World Health Organization, 2008.

Zeitler MS, Paine AD, Breitbart V, et al. Attitudes about intimate partner violence screening among an ethnically diverse sample of young women. *J Adolesc Health* 2004;39(1):119.e1–119.e8.

## WEBSITES

- National Domestic Violence hotline 1-800-799-SAFE (7233)
- The National Domestic Violence: www.ndvh.org
- Rape, Abuse & Incest National Network (RAINN) hotline 1-800-656-HOPE (4673)
- The National Coalition Against Domestic Violence: www.ncadv.org
- The U.S. Department of Justice: www.usdoj.gov, www.ndvh.org
- National Human Trafficking Resources Center (NHTRC) hotline: 1-888-373-7888
- Futures Without Violence (previously known as Family Violence Prevention Fund): www.futureswithoutviolence.org
- National Coalition Against Domestic Violence: www.ncadv.org
- National Network to End Domestic Violence: www.nnedv.org
- National Resource Center on Domestic Violence: www.nrcdv.org
- Office on Violence Against Women (U.S. Department of Justice): www.usdoj.gov/ovw

# Pediatric Gynecology
Sara Seifert and Dayna Burrell

**Pediatric gynecology** presents many challenges to the general obstetrician-gynecologist unaccustomed to dealing with these young patients. Most of the obstacles may be overcome by communicating effectively and allowing the patient to feel "in control."

- The interview is the most important aspect in determining the true reason for the visit. Due to different levels of maturity in each age group of children, different approaches to communication may be used. Including parental figures in the discussion is key.
- Gynecologic problems often experienced by the pediatric patient include vulvovaginitis, trauma, foreign bodies, prepubertal vaginal bleeding, abnormal pubertal development, urogenital abnormalities, and genital tumors.

## GYNECOLOGIC EVALUATION OF A PREPUBERTAL CHILD

- The examination presents a unique set of difficulties that may be overcome by following a few key guidelines:
  - Give the patient a sense of control.
  - Display a caring and gentle attitude at all times; the initial evaluation can set the tone for all future examinations.
  - The physical exam should include an overall assessment of other organ systems. This allows the patient to feel more comfortable in the exam room and the

examiner to gain an overall appreciation of height, weight, skin disorders, hygiene, and other indicators of pubertal development.

- If the child is very young or has suffered physical abuse, she may need to be evaluated under anesthesia.
- Make it clear to the child that the examination is permitted by her caregiver and that if anyone else tries to touch her genital area, she should tell her caregiver.
- A chaperone should be present during the physical exam.

### General Pediatric Physical Exam

- The abdominal exam can be facilitated by placing the child's hand over the examiner's hand.
- Palpate the inguinal regions to identify potential hernias or gonadal masses.
- Tanner classification of the external genitalia and breast development should be used to quantify pubertal changes (Fig. 34-1).

### Pediatric Pelvic Exam: Positioning

- **Frog-leg posture:** child supine with feet together and knees bent outward. Commonly used in the younger patient.

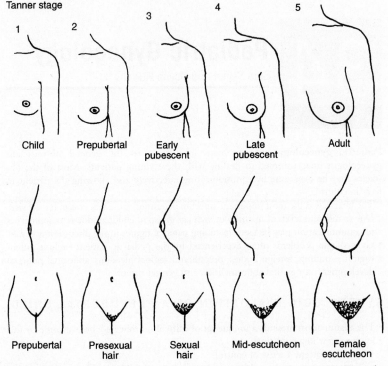

**Figure 34-1.** Tanner stages of development. (From Beckmann CR, Ling FW, Barzansky BM, et al. *Obstetrics and Gynecology*, 2nd ed. Baltimore, MD: Lippincott Williams & Wilkins, 1995:8, with permission.)

- **Knee-chest position:** when combined with a Valsalva maneuver, allows for assessment of the introital area. Using an otoscope for magnification or nasal speculum may help with visualization when the primary complaint is vaginal discharge or foreign bodies.
- **Supine lateral-spread method:** often sufficient enough to allow for visualization of the vestibular structures
- **Mother's lap positioning:** Allow the patient to sit in her mother's lap, knees bent, heels on mom's knees; combine with lateral traction of the labia for adequate exposure.
- When a child is uncooperative or evaluation of the genitalia is not optimal, an **exam under anesthesia** or a return visit may be necessary.

## Pediatric Pelvic Exam: Assessment

- Note perineal hygiene, presence of pubic hair, hymenal configuration, size of the clitoris, and the presence of vulvovaginal lesions or vaginal discharge.
- Careful inspection of the hymen must be completed before pelvic examination. A Foley catheter balloon can be placed behind the hymen and filled to visualize a redundant hymen.
- Lateral downward traction of the labia allows visualization of the hymen in prepubertal girls.
- Specimens may be collected using a small urethral Dacron swab. A second technique employs an empty butterfly catheter attached to a syringe and saline is flushed and aspirated to obtain a mix of secretions. A pediatric feeding tube attached to a 20-mL syringe also allows for vaginal irrigation.
- Use of "extinction stimuli" can greatly facilitate a first pelvic exam. Use a distracting stimulus to draw attention from a second stimulus. For example, press a nonexamining finger into the patient's perineum before touching the introitus and allow the patient to acknowledge the presence of its pressure.
- Proper instrument selection is important. Speculum exams are rarely appropriate in the prepubertal patient. Often, the hymenal ring is too tight to accommodate even a pediatric speculum. A nasal speculum can be used for an exam under anesthesia if speculum exam is necessary.
- Rectoabdominal examination may aid in examination of the uterus in a patient who cannot tolerate a vaginal exam.
- Common exam findings:
  - Newborn child: It is important to recognize that maternal estrogen influences physical development of the newborn child. Vulvar edema, whitish pink vaginal mucosa, vaginal discharge, and breast enlargement may be normal in the newborn and should regress in the first 8 weeks of life.
  - Toddler-prepubertal child: Unestrogenized vaginal mucosa appears thin, hyperemic, and atrophic. Capillary beds may appear like roadmaps and are often mistaken for inflammation, especially around the sulcus of the vestibule and in the periurethral area.

### Documentation

- A labeled sketch of the external genitalia should be included in the medical record with a diamond-shaped space used to represent the vestibule of a child in the supine position. Twelve o'clock should represent the clitoris and 6 o'clock should represent the posterior fourchette.
- Key components include assessing Tanner stage, description of labia majora; labia minora; urethral meatus; hymen; and the presence of any discolorations, hemangiomas, vulvovaginal lesions, or vaginal discharge.

# GYNECOLOGIC EVALUATION OF AN ADOLESCENT

## Adolescent Gynecologic Exam

- Given changes in Pap smear guidelines (see Chapter 45), a pelvic exam is not always necessary in the adolescent patient.
- Pelvic exams should be performed in patients younger than the age of 21 years, only if indicated by chief complaint and history.
- An evaluation of external genitalia can still be performed to confirm normal anatomy and development.
- Testing for sexually transmitted infections such as gonorrhea, chlamydia, or trichomoniasis can be performed from urine samples or vaginal swabs.
- If indicated, a Huffman (1/2 × 4 inches) or Pederson (7/8 × 4 inches) speculum is most appropriate for use in this patient population.
- Although the focus of this chapter is on the evaluation and management of prepubertal pediatric patients, several recommendations should be noted for the evaluation of adolescent patients.
- Although evaluation of Tanner stage may be appropriate at an initial visit, clinical breast exams are not necessary unless indicated by complaint or history until age 20 years.

# COMMON PEDIATRIC GYNECOLOGY COMPLAINTS

## Vulvovaginitis

- Vaginal discharge is the most common gynecologic complaint in the prepubertal girl and accounts for 40% to 50% of visits to a pediatric gynecology clinic.
- Presents as vaginal discharge that can stain the underclothing
- Vulvar burning or stinging may occur when urine comes into contact with irritated, excoriated tissues.

### History: Key Points

- Note the duration, consistency, quality, and color of the discharge.
- Symptoms may also include erythema, tenderness, pain, pruritus, dysuria, or bleeding.
- Anaerobic infections may have a foul odor.
- Bloodstains can occur if *Shigella*, group A β-hemolytic *Streptococcus*, foreign body, or trauma is present.
- Poor hygiene; back to front wiping; use of harsh soaps, bubble baths, and lotions; trauma associated with play; genital manipulation with a foreign body or contaminated hands; close fitting, poorly absorbent clothing, including prolonged exposure to a wet bathing suit; thin, unestrogenized, alkaline vaginal mucosa; and lack of labial development may predispose to vulvovaginitis.
- Ask the child to demonstrate proper front to back wiping.
- Note the type of diaper and frequency of changes in younger children.
- Ask about recent systemic infections, new medications, bed-wetting, dermatoses, and nocturnal perianal itching.

### Physical Examination

- Presentations for vulvovaginitis are extremely variable, ranging from no discharge to copious secretions. Erythema, edema, and excoriations are commonly noted. Evidence of poor perineal hygiene may be evident, with stool seen on the vulva or between the labia.
- Collect a sample of any discharge for microscopic examination and culture. Avoid contact with the hymen in prepubertal children.

- Carefully note the configuration of the hymen and evaluate for any signs of trauma. The perianal skin should also be examined.
- Vaginoscopy should be considered to exclude a foreign body, neoplasm, or abnormal connection with the gastrointestinal or urinary tract, especially in recurrent cases or those associated with bleeding.

*Etiologies of Vulvovaginitis*

Infection

- Normal prepubertal vaginal flora includes lactobacilli, α-hemolytic streptococci, *Staphylococcus epidermidis*, diphtheroid, and Gram-negative enteric organisms, especially *Escherichia coli*. Candida is present in only 3% to 4% of prepubertal girls.
- Although many cases of vulvovaginitis may be nonspecific, the most common pathogenic bacteria causing vulvovaginitis include group A *Streptococcus*, *Haemophilus influenzae*, *Staphylococcus aureus*, *Streptococcus pneumoniae*, and *E. coli*.
- Children may pass respiratory flora from the nose and oropharynx to the genitalia area, making this a possible etiology of vulvovaginitis.
- Children with chronic, nightly episodes of vulvar or perianal itching should be evaluated for *Enterobius vermicularis*.
- Shifts in flora resulting from inoculation by bacterial, viral, and yeast can result in inflammation and discharge. Several of these pathogens may be indicative of sexual activity or abuse. Sexually transmitted diseases are typically the result of sexual abuse.
- Obtain cultures if symptoms are persistent or if there is purulent discharge. Treatment with antibiotics is indicated when an infectious pathogen is identified (Table 34-1).

Vaginitis that is Nonspecific, Environmental, or Chemical

- Twenty-five percent to 75% of cases are likely caused by poor hygiene, soaps, obesity, foreign bodies, association with upper respiratory infections, and irritating clothing in the setting of unestrogenized mucosa.
- Treatment includes discontinuation of the causative agent, perineal hygiene, sitz baths, loose-fitting clothing, cotton underwear, hypoallergenic soaps, wet wipes, and emollients.
- If there is no resolution in 2 to 3 weeks, evaluate for a foreign body or infection.
- A trial of estrogen cream can be used if other etiologies are ruled out to thicken the vaginal mucosa and make it less sensitive.

Foreign Bodies

- Most common in girls aged 2 to 4 years. The foreign bodies can vary from wads of toilet paper, buttons, or coins to peanuts and crayons. Antibiotics should be started before removal.
- Presence can be an indicator of sexual abuse.
- Retained foreign bodies in the vagina often present with bloody, brown, or purulent discharge of several weeks duration. Persistent vaginal discharge in a toddler or young girl warrants an exam under anesthesia.
- Genital pruritus, abdominal pain, or fever may be present.
- If the object remains undetected, peritonitis can develop from the ascension of purulent secretions into the fallopian tubes.
- A careful examination of the vaginal wall for any defects or additional embedded foreign bodies should be performed after the object has been removed. If the rectovaginal septum is involved, a temporary colostomy with delayed repair of the vaginal and rectal tissues may be indicated.

| TABLE 34-1 | Treatment of Specific Vulvovaginal Infections in the Prepubertal Child |

| Etiology | Treatment |
|---|---|
| *Streptococcus pyogenes* | Penicillin V potassium 250 mg bid–tid × 10 d |
| *Haemophilus influenzae* | Amoxicillin 40 mg/kg/d × 7 d<br>Alternate: amoxicillin/clavulanate, cefuroxime axetil, trimethoprim-sulfamethoxazole, erythromycin-sulfamethoxazole |
| *Staphylococcus aureus* | Cephalexin 25–50 mg/kg/d × 7–10 d<br>Amoxicillin clavulanate 20–40 mg/kg/d (of the amoxicillin) × 7–10 d<br>Cefuroxime axetil suspension 30 mg/kg/d divided bid (max 1 g) × 10 d (tablets: 250 mg bid)<br>Dicloxacillin 25 mg/kg/d × 7–10 d |
| *Streptococcus pneumoniae* | Penicillin, amoxicillin, erythromycin, trimethoprim-sulfamethoxazole, clarithromycin |
| *Shigella* | Trimethoprim-sulfamethoxazole or ampicillin × 5 d<br>For resistant organisms: ceftriaxone |
| *Chlamydia trachomatis* | ≤45 kg: erythromycin 50 mg/kg/d (divide in 4 doses/d) × 14 d<br>≥45 kg, <8 yr: azithromycin 1 g once<br>≥8 yr: azithromycin 1 g once OR doxycycline 100 mg bid PO × 7 d |
| *Neisseria gonorrhoeae* | <45 kg: ceftriaxone 125 mg IM PLUS treat for *Chlamydia* as above<br>Alternate: spectinomycin 40 mg/kg (max 2 g) IM once PLUS treat for *Chlamydia* as above<br>≥ 45 kg: treated with adult regimens (see Chapter 28) |
| *Candida* | Topical nystatin, miconazole, clotrimazole, or terconazole cream; fluconazole orally |
| *Trichomonas* | Metronidazole 15 mg/kg/d given tid (max 250 mg tid) × 7 d |
| *Enterobius vermicularis* (pinworms) | Mebendazole (Vermox), 1 chewable 100-mg tablet, repeated in 2 wk |

bid, twice a day; tid, three times a day; PO, orally; IM, intramuscularly.
Modified from Emans SJ, Laufer MR, Goldstein DP, eds. *Pediatric and Adolescent Gynecology*, 5th ed. Philadelphia, PA: Lippincott Williams & Wilkins, 2005:98, with permission.
Data from Workowski KA, Berman S; Centers for Disease Control and Prevention. Sexually transmitted disease treatment guidelines, 2010. *MMWR Recomm Rep* 2010;59(RR-12):1–110.

## Anatomic Abnormalities

- **Ectopic ureter:** May result in urinary leakage. Often detected on prenatal ultrasound. After birth, an ultrasound can be used for diagnosis, followed by magnetic resonance imaging (MRI) if indicated.
- High hymenal opening: may impair vaginal drainage; hymenectomy is curative in these cases.
- Urethral prolapse (see the following text).

## Dermatologic Conditions

- Lichen sclerosis, psoriasis, atopic dermatitis, and contact dermatitis of the vulva may all present with symptoms similar to vulvovaginitis. These conditions may respond to topical corticosteroids.
- Lichen sclerosus is treated with high-potency corticosteroids, as scarring can cause permanent sexual dysfunction.
- Aphthous ulcers are typically seen in girls 10 to 15 years old and are very painful, with a purulent base and raised edges; the patient will frequently have nonspecific systemic symptoms as well. The etiology is idiopathic but thought to be viral (e.g., influenza, Epstein-Barr virus, cytomegalovirus). Oral corticosteroids are frequently prescribed. If these ulcers are recurrent, consider Behçet disease.

## Systemic Illness

- Varicella, measles, Epstein-Barr virus, Crohn disease, Stevens-Johnson syndrome, diabetes mellitus, Behçet syndrome, and Kawasaki syndrome may all result in vaginal discharge, vesicles, fistulas, ulcers, and inflammation.

### Treatment

- Treatment depends on the etiology but almost always involves improving perineal hygiene.
- Sitz or tub baths twice a day for half an hour may help eliminate the vaginal discharge.
  - Nonirritating soaps and white cotton underpants should be recommended.
  - Nylon tights, tight blue jeans, prolonged wearing of wet bathing suits, and bubble baths should be discouraged.
  - Both the caregiver and child should be instructed on proper front to back wiping.
  - The child should be instructed to urinate with her knees apart to reduce urinary reflux into the vagina.
- Persistent symptoms after therapy (>2 weeks) warrant reexamination.
- In rare idiopathic persistent cases, vaginal irrigation with a 1% solution of povidone-iodine (Betadine) may help.
- Alternate approaches to persistent cases include a 2-month course of antibiotics or 2 to 4 weeks of estrogen cream.
- Recurrence often points to continued improper hygiene. Obese girls are at higher risk for recurrence.

## Prepubertal Vaginal Bleeding

- Vaginal bleeding prior to menarche can result from a wide array of causes but must be taken seriously, as some conditions can be life-threatening.
- Etiologies may include infection, anatomic abnormalities, genital tumors, hormonal abnormalities, trauma, or sexual abuse.

### Vulvovaginitis

- Any cause of vulvovaginitis may result in vaginal bleeding. Evidence of infection, dermatoses, or retained foreign bodies should be targeted during evaluation.

### Urethral Prolapse

- Increased abdominal pressure can cause the urethral mucosa to protrude through the meatus, forming an annular, hemorrhagic mass that bleeds easily.
- Average age of onset is 5 years, and occurrence is more common in African Americans.
- Medical treatment consists of a short-term course of estrogen cream. Topical antibiotics and sitz baths may also be beneficial.

- Urinary retention or a large mass may require resection of the prolapsed tissue and insertion of an indwelling catheter.
- Differential diagnosis includes urethral polyps, caruncles, cysts, and prolapsed ureteroceles.

### Genital Tumors

- Genital tumors are uncommon in the prepubertal girl but need to be considered in a patient with a chronic genital ulcer, tissue protruding from the vagina, a malodorous or bloody discharge, or an atraumatic swelling of the external genitalia.
- Causes are outlined in Table 34-2. Masses seen can be benign polyps or cancerous. Treatment is excision.
- Sarcomas require a biopsy for diagnosis, excisional procedure, and chemotherapy.

### Abnormal Uterine Bleeding

- See Chapter 40.

### Endometrial Shedding

- Causes of endometrial shedding are outlined in Table 34-3 and often relate to a hormonal abnormality.
- Precocious puberty is often associated with endometrial shedding in this population (see the section "Disorders of Puberty").

### Trauma and Sexual Abuse

- See the following text, also Chapter 33.

## Traumatic Injuries

- The period of highest incidence is between ages 4 and 12 years, with 75% of all genital injuries occurring in young girls. Because of differences in anatomy between a child and an adult, a seemingly innocuous lesion can suggest serious injury. Common injuries include:

### Straddle Injuries

- Most present as a swollen area of painful ecchymosis or hematoma over the labia; the mons, clitoris, and urethra can be involved.
- If hematuria is present, consider a voiding cystourethrogram to rule out bladder or urethral injury.
- Periurethral injuries can result in swelling and urinary retention. Early placement of a urinary catheter is advised.
- Treat with observation and cold compresses for the first 6 hours. If the hematoma remains the same size or becomes smaller, warm sitz baths are often all that are required.
- Analgesics and prophylactic antibiotics can be used when a hematoma at the urethral orifice is causing pain and poor urination.

### Accidental Penetration

- Most frequently seen between ages 2 and 4 years, often the result of falling on a sharp object (e.g., pen or pencil).
- Presentation often includes hematuria, vaginal discharge, or bleeding. A puncture wound may be intraperitoneal with rectal pain or bleeding as the presenting complaint.
- In an unstable patient with an injury above the hymen, laparoscopy or laparotomy should be performed.

| TABLE 34-2 | Malignant Genital Tumors in Pediatric Gynecology | |
|---|---|---|
| **Tumor** | **Characteristics** | **Treatment** |
| Sarcoma botryoides (Rhabdomyosarcoma) | • Most common malignant tumor of the genital tract in girls<br>• Fast-growing, aggressive<br>• 90% before age 5 yr, peak incidence age 2 yr<br>• Arises in submucosa of vagina<br>• Hallmark polypoid mass passing from the vagina, vulva, or urethra, usually anterior<br>• Vaginal bleeding, abdominal pain | • First, stage with CXR/CT scan<br>• Chemotherapy followed by surgery (type of procedure depends on stage of disease)<br>• Possible radiotherapy<br>• Follow-up (tends to recur locally)<br>• Improved treatment regimens have led to more conservative surgical options and improved survival |
| Clear cell adenocarcinoma | • Often seen with maternal diethylstilbestrol exposure<br>• Abnormal vaginal bleeding and discharge | • In early stages, conservative approach involves wide local excision, with lymph nodes dissection followed by local radiation<br>• Advanced disease may require whole pelvic radiation |
| Germ cell tumors | • Most common ovarian neoplasm in pediatric population<br>• Arises from primitive germ cells; two types— dysgerminomas and embryonal carcinoma<br>• Presents as complex pelvic masses<br>• Tumor markers: AFP, hCG, CEA | • Management is surgical and involves at least unilateral oophorectomy and staging if needed<br>• Dysgerminomas respond to radiation, but future fertility should be taken into consideration |

CXR, chest radiograph; CT, computed tomography; AFP, alpha-fetoprotein; hCG, human chorionic gonadotropin; CEA, carcinoembryonic antigen.

| TABLE 34-3 | Causes of Endometrial Shedding in Children |
|---|---|

- Physiologic neonatal withdrawal bleed in the first 2 wk of life secondary to maternal estrogen withdrawal
- Isolated premature menarche
- Iatrogenic or factitious precocious puberty caused by medications that contain exogenous estrogens
- Idiopathic precocious puberty
- Functional ovarian cysts
- Ovarian neoplasms
- McCune-Albright syndrome
- Central nervous system lesions
- Hormone-producing neoplasms
- Hypothyroidism

- Workup involves examination with abdominal radiography, anoscopy, and sigmoidoscopy. Microscopic hematuria warrants careful urethral catheterization. Resistance to the passage of a catheter requires a voiding cystourethrogram. Catheterization should not be attempted with gross hematuria.

*Lacerations*

- Often secondary to forceful abduction of the legs, gymnastic exercise, water-skiing, bicycle accidents, or motor vehicle accidents.
- Lacerations of the vaginal orifice frequently extend into the fornix.
- Examination under anesthesia must be performed to determine the extent of the injury and rule out involvement of the rectovaginal septum or peritoneal cavity.

*Clitoral Strangulation or Ischemia*

- Difficult to diagnose; symptoms may include irritability and engorgement and cellulitis of the clitoris.
- Often results when an entrapped hair from a caretaker accidentally becomes wrapped around the base of the organ. Treatment is removal of the stricture.

**Sexual Abuse**

- Suspect with unusual injury patterns or odd behavior as well as the following associated complaints: genital trauma, bleeding, chronic genital pain, sexually transmitted infections, anal inflammation, recurrent urinary tract infections, abdominal pain, enuresis/encopresis, or anorexia.
- Behavioral changes include aggression, self-injury, conduct disorders, sleep disturbances, excessive phobias, depression, substance abuse, problems in school, or inappropriate knowledge of sexual behavior.
- History: Obtain separately from the child if possible. Avoid leading questions. A doll may provide the young child with a way to express what has happened. A multidisciplinary approach involving the child's pediatrician and social worker may also be beneficial.
- If abuse is suspected, the patient should be referred to an appropriate emergency department with individuals trained in collecting forensic evidence, preferably within 24 hours of the event.
- Sexual play involves children of the same age without coercion and is a normal part of development.

## Labial Adhesions

- In the low estrogen environment of childhood, the labia may fuse in response to any genital trauma, even diaper rash.
- Adhesive vulvitis caused by chronic irritation is common between ages 2 and 6 years.
- Asymptomatic labial adhesions do not require treatment and will resolve spontaneously with increasing estrogen levels in puberty.
- If urinary retention or urinary tract infections occur, treatment is required and involves application of estrogen cream along the white line of the adhesion, with gentle traction twice daily for 2 to 6 weeks.
- Recurrence is common after treatment. Acute urinary retention requires surgical excision.

## DISORDERS OF PUBERTY

**Puberty** is a result of pulsatile gonadotropin-releasing hormone (GnRH) secretion and activation of the hypothalamic-pituitary-gonadal axis. The onset of puberty is generally between 8 and 13 years old in girls. Tanner stages are used to describe pubertal development.

### Delayed Puberty

- Delay of puberty can be caused by anatomic abnormalities, chromosomal disorders, neoplastic growths, or nutritional deficiencies.
- Commonly presents as a physical delay in maturation combined with amenorrhea.
- Causes of delayed puberty can be classified based on the level of follicle-stimulating hormone (FSH) present, as outlined in Table 34-4.

*Hypergonadotropic Hypogonadism (High Follicle-Stimulating Hormone)*

- A sufficient amount of gonadotropins are present, but the ovaries are not responsive and therefore do not produce sex steroids.

| TABLE 34-4 | An Overview of Causes of Delayed Puberty |
|---|---|
| **FSH Level** | **Differential Diagnosis** |
| High >30 mIU/mL | • Gonadal dysgenesis syndromes: Turner syndrome, Swyer syndrome |
| | • Primary ovarian failure |
| Low <10 mIU/mL | • Constitutional delay |
| | • Intracranial neoplasms |
| | • Isolated gonadotropin deficiencies |
| | • Hormone deficiencies |
| | • Kallmann syndrome |
| | • Prader-Willi syndrome |
| | • Laurence-Moon-Biedl syndrome |
| | • Chronic disease and malnutrition |
| Normal | • *Anatomic deformities* result in normal development with primary amenorrhea. |
| | • Imperforate hymen |
| | • Transverse vaginal septum |
| | • Müllerian agenesis |

## Gonadal Dysgenesis

- Presents as a phenotypic female with persistent prepubertal development.
- May have some secondary sex characteristics and spontaneous menstruation. Most often associated with primary amenorrhea.
- **Turner syndrome** (45, X) occurs in 1 in 2,000 to 2,500 girls. Phenotype includes primary amenorrhea and short stature.
- Patients with **Swyer syndrome** (46, XY) often have a normal-to-tall stature. It is caused by a mutation or structural abnormality of the Y chromosome.

## Primary Ovarian Failure

- Ovaries develop but do not contain oocytes; may be associated with chemotherapy, radiation, galactosemia, gonadotropin resistance, autoimmune ovarian failure, or ovarian failure secondary to previous infection.
- Treatment involves administration of exogenous estrogen and progesterone to avoid osteoporosis and facilitate development of secondary sexual characteristics.

### *Hypogonadotrophic Hypogonadism (Low Follicle-Stimulating Hormone)*

- An insufficient level of gonadotropins is present to permit follicular development, and, therefore, sex steroids are not produced.
  - **Chronic disease:** Conditions including states of malnutrition (e.g., starvation, anorexia nervosa, cystic fibrosis, Crohn disease, diabetes mellitus, and hypothyroidism) may disrupt GnRH production.
  - **Constitutional delay:** A delay in the GnRH pulse generator postpones the normal physiologic events of puberty.
  - **Intracranial neoplasms:** Craniopharyngiomas and pituitary adenomas may cause delayed puberty. Visual symptoms are often associated with these tumors, as is short stature and diabetes insipidus. Diagnosis is by computed tomography (CT) or MRI of the head.
  - **Isolated gonadotropin deficiencies:** often secondary to abnormalities in genes encoding proteins related to GnRH, FSH, or luteinizing hormone (LH)
  - **Hormone deficiencies:** Aberrations of growth hormone, thyroid hormone, or prolactin can affect puberty.
  - **Kallmann syndrome:** presents with a classic triad of anosmia, hypogonadism, and color blindness. The hypothalamus cannot secrete GnRH due to dysfunction in the arcuate nucleus. Few or no secondary sexual characteristics are present.
  - **Prader-Willi syndrome:** an autosomal deletion and imprinting disorder associated with obesity, emotional instability, and delayed puberty due to hypothalamic dysfunction
  - Other uncommon causes include **Laurence-Moon** and **Bardet-Biedl syndromes**.

### *Eugonadism (Normal Follicle-Stimulating Hormone)*

- In cases of eugonadal pubertal delay, the hypothalamic-pituitary-gonadal axis remains intact, but primary amenorrhea occurs secondary to anatomic abnormalities in the genitourinary tract, androgen insensitivity, or inappropriate positive feedback mechanisms.
  - Anatomic abnormalities: See the section "Congenital Anomalies."
  - Androgen insensitivity: See the section "Ambiguous Genitalia."
  - Other causes of primary amenorrhea with eugonadism include anovulation, androgen-producing adrenal disease, and polycystic ovarian syndrome.

### *Key Points in Evaluation and Management of Delayed Puberty*

- A careful medical, surgical, and family history and exam including Tanner staging are important initial steps of evaluation.

- Initial laboratory workup should include serum FSH, prolactin, thyroid-stimulating hormone (TSH), and complete blood count (CBC).
- Further workup should be determined by initial findings with management based on etiology.

## Precocious Puberty

- **Precocious puberty** occurs in only 1 of 10,000 girls and is defined as the presence of secondary sexual characteristics at an age >2.5 standard deviations below the mean (i.e., 6 years old in African Americans and 7 years old in Caucasians).
- Accelerated growth velocity and rapid bone growth can result in short adult stature.
- Causes are divided into gonadotropin-dependent and gonadotropin-independent disorders.

*Gonadotropin-Dependent Disorders—Central Precocious Puberty*

- Related to premature development of the hypothalamic-pituitary axis
- A condition results in pulsatile secretion of GnRH from the hypothalamus, resulting in release of FSH and LH, which stimulate ovarian function.
- Most commonly **idiopathic**; secondary sexual characteristics progress in normal sequence but more rapidly than in normal puberty and may fluctuate between progression and regression.
- Characteristic signs and symptoms include breast development without pubic hair development, an increase in height, acne, oily skin or hair, and emotional changes.
- May be transmitted in an autosomal recessive fashion
- Often, ovarian follicular cysts are present due to elevated levels of LH and FSH.
- Other causes involve **central nervous system disease**, particularly mass effects near the hypothalamus. The most common neoplasm is a hamartoma in the posterior hypothalamus.
  - Disease often involves areas surrounding the hypothalamus; mass effect, radiation, or ectopic GnRH-secreting cells are thought to cause premature activation of pulsatile secretion of GnRH from the hypothalamus.
  - Diagnosis is by CT or MRI of the head; history may be significant for headache, mental status changes, mental retardation, dysmorphic syndromes, along with the premature development of secondary sexual characteristics.
  - Treatment should be directed at the underlying cause; the location of many of such tumors makes resection difficult, and, as a result, chemotherapy or radiation may be indicated.
  - Treatment with a GnRH agonist can result in a short burst of gonadotropin release, followed by downregulation and a decrease in the level of circulating gonadotropins. Follow estradiol levels to make appropriate dose adjustments.

*Gonadotropin-Independent Disorders—Pseudoprecocious Puberty*

- Exogenous hormones causing early puberty result from a peripheral source.
- Development of pubertal characteristics may be more rapid than with central causes due to a faster initial rate of hormone production.
- Differential diagnosis includes estrogen-secreting tumors, benign follicular ovarian cysts, McCune-Albright syndrome, Peutz-Jeghers syndrome, adrenal disorders, and primary hypothyroidism.

Estrogen-Secreting Ovarian Tumors

- See Chapter 48.

## Benign Ovarian Cysts

- Most common form of estrogen-secreting masses in children
- May require a diagnostic laparoscopy or possibly exploratory laparotomy to differentiate from a malignant tumor. Removal of the cyst may be therapeutic.

## McCune-Albright Syndrome

- **Triad:** café au lait spots, polyostotic fibrous dysplasia, and cysts of skull and long bones; precocious puberty is present in 40% of cases
- Associated with rapid breast development and early occurrence of menarche
- Sexual precocity results from recurrent follicular cysts. Removal of cyst is not helpful.
- Aromatase inhibitors may help control symptoms.
- Evaluate with serial pelvic sonograms to detect the presence of gonadal tumors.

## Peutz-Jeghers Syndrome

- Commonly characterized by mucocutaneous pigmentation and gastrointestinal polyposis.
- Also associated with rare sex cord tumors, including epithelial tumors of the ovary, dysgerminomas, or Sertoli-Leydig cell tumors, whose estrogen secretion may result in feminization and incomplete sexual precocity.
- Girls with Peutz-Jeghers syndrome should be screened with serial pelvic sonograms.

## Adrenal Disorders

- Some adrenal adenomas secrete estrogen and may result in sexual precocity.

## Primary Hypothyroidism

- Characterized by premature breast development and galactorrhea without an associated growth spurt. See Chapter 13.

*Key Points in Evaluation and Management of Precocious Puberty*

- Perform a detailed evaluation with Tanner staging.
- Laboratory data should include LH, FSH, prolactin, estradiol, progesterone, 17-hydroxyprogesterone, dehydroepiandrosterone, dehydroepiandrosterone sulfate, TSH, T4, human chorionic gonadotropin.
- A GnRH stimulation test can definitively diagnose central precocious puberty.
- Obtain an x-ray to determine bone age. Head CT or MRI can rule out an intracranial mass. Abdominal/pelvic ultrasound can be used to evaluate the ovaries.
- Goals for management include maximizing adult height and delaying maturation. Treat the intracranial, ovarian, or adrenal pathology if present and attempt to reduce associated emotional problems.

## Premature Thelarche

- **Premature thelarche** is defined as bilateral breast development without other signs of sexual maturation in girls before age 8 years.
- Commonly occurs by age 2 years and is rare after age 4 years.
- The etiology is unclear, but exogenous estrogen must be excluded.
- Precocious puberty must be ruled out.
  - Document the appearance of the vaginal mucosa, breast size, and presence or absence of a pelvic mass.
  - Obtain bone age. It is within normal range in premature thelarche.
  - Perform pelvic ultrasonography, which should exclude ovarian pathology.
  - Obtain plasma estrogen levels. They may be mildly elevated; significant elevations suggest another etiology.

- In idiopathic cases, regression often occurs after a few months but may persist for several years.

## AMBIGUOUS GENITALIA

### Male Feminization

- Genetic males (XY) undergo feminization related to androgen insensitivity.
- **Complete androgen insensitivity** or **"testicular feminization"**
  - Transmitted in a maternal X-linked recessive fashion
  - Pathophysiology: Androgen presence is incapable of inducing maturation of the Wolffian duct. Anti-müllerian hormone is present, and müllerian duct formation remains inhibited. The resulting phenotype is female, with a vagina derived from the urogenital sinus that ends in a blind pouch and testes that often descend through the inguinal canal.
  - Clinical presentation: primary amenorrhea, Tanner stage V breast development, and scant axillary and pubic hair
  - Management: Gonadectomy is recommended once sexual maturation is complete secondary to an increased incidence of malignancy; exogenous estrogen therapy is also recommended.
- **Incomplete androgen insensitivity**
  - Less common with presentation ranging from near complete masculinization to near complete failure of virilization
  - As minimal sensitivity to androgens is present, the Wolffian duct system develops to some extent, although spermatogenesis usually remains absent.
  - Physical exam may include a range of clitoromegaly or ambiguous genitalia.
  - Sex assignment depends on the degree of masculinization.
- **5-Alpha reductase deficiency**
  - Genotypic males (XY) who are phenotypically female in the prepubertal state and become phenotypically male at puberty. Testicular function is normal and there is no breast development.

### Female Virilization

- Genetic females (XX) are exposed to increased androgen levels that lead to inappropriate virilization, most often an indicator of organic disease in girls.
- Virilizing **congenital adrenal hyperplasia (CAH)**: most commonly associated with deficiency of 21-hydroxylase, an autosomal recessive disorder. May present in a newborn with ambiguous genitalia and possible salt wasting due to mineralocorticoid deficiency. Virilization may also be delayed until later childhood in less severe forms.
- **Cushing disease:** can manifest as growth failure, with or without virilization, obesity, striae, or moon facies
- **Ovarian tumors:** Sertoli-Leydig cell tumor (e.g., arrhenoblastoma) is the most common virilizing ovarian tumor. Others include lipoid cell tumor and gonadoblastoma.

## CONGENITAL ANOMALIES OF THE FEMALE REPRODUCTIVE TRACT

**Anatomic disorders** may present as primary amenorrhea, chronic pelvic pain, mucocolpos, hematocolpos, or hematometra.

- **Imperforate hymen:** may present as bulging, translucent mass at the introitus in the newborn or as cyclic pain, abdominal mass, hematocolpos, and/or a bluish perineal bulge after menarche. Imperforate hymen may regress as the girl enters childhood. In cases where there is no regression, surgical intervention is required to incise the hymen and allow stored debris (hematocolpos) to escape. Additional hymenal abnormalities including microperforate and septate hymen may also require surgical intervention but do not completely obstruct the vaginal introitus, and therefore, symptoms are usually absent or less severe.

- **Transverse vaginal septum:** due to failure of canalization of müllerian tubules and the sinovaginal bulb, leaving a membrane present. Presentation and examination may be similar to an imperforate hymen; however, 35% to 86% are found in the mid to upper vagina. If the membrane is thin, it can be incised and dilated. If thick, evaluation with ultrasound or MRI can guide surgical decision making.

- **Longitudinal vaginal septum:** This is often associated with uterine and/or renal anomalies. Complaints include persistent bleeding despite the use of a tampon. Surgical correction is indicated. An obstructed hemivagina is frequently seen with ipsilateral renal agenesis.

- **Müllerian agenesis:** failure of the müllerian tract to develop results in a blind vaginal pouch without uterus or fallopian tubes present. Ovaries are not of müllerian origin and puberty progresses as usual with primary amenorrhea as a presenting complaint. This must be distinguished from androgen insensitivity, as described previously. One third of these patients have associated urinary tract anomalies, and 12% have skeletal anomalies. A neovagina can be created by progressive dilation or surgery.

- **Vaginal atresia/agenesis:** This occurs in 1 in 5 to 10,000 newborns. Patients will present similarly to a transverse septum in adolescent girls. Treatment may involve progressive vaginal dilation or surgical reconstruction. Up to 50% have other congenital anomalies, so a full workup is warranted.

## SUGGESTED READINGS

American Academy of Pediatricians. Management of urinary tract infections. *Pediatrics* 1999; 103(4):843–852.

American College of Obstetricians and Gynecologists. ACOG committee opinion no. 335: the initial reproductive health visit. *Obstet Gynecol* 2006;107:745–747.

American College of Obstetricians and Gynecologists. ACOG committee opinion no. 534: well woman visit. *Obstet Gynecol* 2012;120:421–424.

Antoniazzi F, Zamboni G. Central precocious puberty: current treatment options. *Pediatr Drugs* 2004;6(4):211–231.

Carel JC, Leger J. Precocious puberty. *N Engl J Med* 2008;358:2366–2377.

Emans SJ, Laufer MR, eds. *Goldstein's Pediatric and Adolescent Gynecology*, 6th ed. Philadelphia, PA: Lippincott Williams & Wilkins, 2012.

Garden AS. Vulvovaginitis and other common childhood gynaecological conditions. *Arch Dis Child Educ Pract Ed* 2011;96(2):73.

Lara-Torre E. Physical exam of pediatric and adolescent patients. *Clin Obstet Gynecol* 2008; 51(2):205–213.

Merritt D. Genital trauma in children and adolescents. *Clin Obstet Gynecol* 2008;51(2):237–248.

Miller RJ, Breech LL. Surgical corrections of vaginal anomalies. *Clin Obstet Gynecol* 2008; 51(2):223–236.

Shulman L. Mullerian anomalies. *Clin Obstet Gynecol* 2008;51(2):214–222.

Striegel AM, Myers JB, Sorensen MD, et al. Vaginal discharge and bleeding in girls younger than 6 years. *J Urol* 2006;176(6, pt 1):2632.

# IV Reproductive Endocrinology and Infertility

# 35 Infertility and Assisted Reproductive Technologies

Cindy M. P. Duke and Mindy S. Christianson

## INFERTILITY

### Definitions

- **Infertility:** failure of a couple of reproductive age to conceive after at least 1 year of regular coitus without contraception
  - **Primary infertility:** infertility in a woman who has never been pregnant
  - **Secondary infertility:** infertility in a woman who has had one or more previous pregnancies
- **Fecundability:** probability of achieving pregnancy within one menstrual cycle. For a normal couple, this is approximately 25%.
- **Fecundity:** ability to achieve a live birth within one menstrual cycle

### Incidence

- Data from the 2002 National Survey of Family Growth (NSFG) revealed that 2% of women of reproductive age in the United States had an infertility-related medical appointment within the past year.
- Data from the 2006 to 2010 NSFG continued to show that as in the 2002 data, 11.9% of women of reproductive age reported having received infertility services at some point in their lives.
- Additionally, 6% of couples with women of reproductive age reported not becoming pregnant after not using contraception in the prior year.

| TABLE 35-1 | Differential Diagnosis of Infertility | |
|---|---|---|

| Diagnosis | Percent | Basic Evaluation |
|---|---|---|
| Male factors | 30 | Semen analysis |
| Tubal/uterine/peritoneal factors | 25 | HSG, laparoscopy, chromopertubation |
| Anovulation/ovarian factors | 25 | BBT chart, midluteal progesterone level, endometrial biopsy, luteinizing hormone testing |
| Cervical factors | 10 | Postcoital test |
| Unexplained infertility | 10 | All of the above |

HSG, hysterosalpingogram; BBT, basal body temperature.
Adapted from Fritz MA. Infertility. In Fritz MA, Speroff L, eds. *Clinical Gynecologic Endocrinology and Infertility*, 8th ed. Philadelphia, PA: Lippincott Williams & Wilkins, 2010:1137–1190.

- Demand for infertility services has increased in recent years. Reasons include the following:
  - Delayed childbearing in women due to career demands and marriage at a later age
  - An increase in variety and effectiveness of assisted reproductive technology (ART) treatments and an increased public awareness of these treatments, including in vitro fertilization (IVF)
  - An increase in tubal factor infertility as a consequence of sexually transmitted diseases
  - Relative scarcity of babies placed for adoption due to effective contraception and increased availability of abortion services.

## Differential Diagnosis

- The **differential diagnosis** of infertility encompasses five principal categories (Table 35-1):
  - Male factor
  - Ovulatory dysfunction
  - Structural (tubal/peritoneal and uterine)
  - Cervical factors
  - Unexplained causes
  - Coital factors

# EVALUATION

- Evaluation is indicated for women who fail to conceive after 1 or more years of regular, unprotected intercourse.
- Women older than the age of 35 years should be evaluated sooner (i.e., after 6 months of regular, unprotected intercourse).
- Successful reproduction requires proper structure and function of the entire reproductive axis, including hypothalamus, pituitary gland, ovaries, fallopian tube, uterus, cervix, and vagina.
- **Infertility evaluation** comprises six major elements:
  - History and physical examination
  - Semen analysis

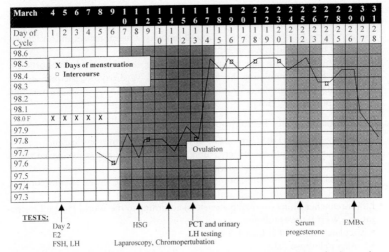

**Figure 35-1.** Sample basal body temperature (BBT) chart with complete infertility evaluation within one menstrual cycle. $E_2$, estradiol level; EMBx, endometrial biopsy; FSH, follicle-stimulating hormone level; LH, luteinizing hormone level; HSG, hysterosalpingogram; PCT, postcoital test.

- Assessment of ovarian reserve
- Tests for occurrence of ovulation
  - Tests to evaluate for structural abnormalities: These include evaluation of tubal patency, detection of uterine abnormalities, and determination of peritoneal abnormalities.
- Sperm—cervical mucus interaction (postcoital testing [PCT])—for select patients. This has fallen out of favor and is infrequently used.
- With proper coordination, the evaluation can be completed within one menstrual cycle (Fig. 35-1). No abnormality or cause of infertility is identified in 10% to 15% of couples. This group comprises a category known as "unexplained infertility."

## History and Physical Examination

- The initial assessment involves an extended and complete history from both partners and a complete physical examination.
  - Physical examination of the male partner can be deferred pending the results of the semen analysis. Abnormal results of a semen analysis warrants referral to a urologist.
- History elicited from both male and female partners should include the following:
  - Duration of infertility, methods of contraception, previous evaluation and treatment, prior reproductive history, sexual dysfunction, coital frequency and satisfaction, sexually transmitted infections, tobacco and alcohol use, caffeine use, family history of mental retardation, and birth defects
- History elicited from the female partner should include the following:
  - Complete menstrual history, dysmenorrhea or menorrhagia, pelvic or abdominal pain, dyspareunia, symptoms of thyroid disease, galactorrhea, symptoms of hirsutism, exercise habits, and indices of stress

- Components of the female physical exam should include the following:
  - Weight and body mass index, thyroid exam, breast exam, signs of hirsutism, pelvic or abdominal tenderness, uterine size and mobility, adnexal masses and/or tenderness, cul-de-sac tenderness, or nodularity
- Baseline studies and labs may include the following: thyroid-stimulating hormone, prolactin, follicle-stimulating hormone (FSH), 17-hydroxyprogesterone, serum testosterone, progesterone, dehydroepiandrosterone (DHEAS), semen analysis, and hysterosalpingogram (HSG).

## Male Factor Infertility Evaluation

- The semen analysis is the cornerstone of male factor infertility evaluation.
  - Semen sample should be collected after at least 48 to 72 hours abstinence and is best evaluated within 1 hour of ejaculation.
  - Obtained either by masturbation or by sexual intercourse with a silicone condom because latex condoms are spermicidal.
- Lower reference limits (normal parameters) according to the World Health Organization (WHO) are as follows:
  - Ejaculate volume of at least 1.5 mL
  - Semen pH above 7.2
  - Sperm concentration of at least 20 million/mL
  - Greater than 40% total motility; greater than 32% progressive motility
  - Greater than 4% normal morphology
- Semen analysis terminology:
  - **Azoospermia:** absence of sperm in the ejaculate
  - **Oligospermia:** a concentration of fewer than 20 million sperm/mL
  - **Asthenospermia:** reduced sperm motility
- Men with an abnormal semen analysis should be referred to a urologist, especially in cases of oligospermia or azoospermia. Causes of male factor infertility include the following:
  - **Klinefelter syndrome**
    - Karyotype is 47, XXY.
    - Most common genetic anomaly in azoospermic men
    - Found in 1:500 to 1:1,000 live male births
    - Incidence: 3% of infertile men, 3.5% to 14.5% of azoospermic men, 1% of couples referred to intracytoplasmic sperm injection (ICSI)
  - **Congenital absence of the vas deferens (CAVD)**
    - Associated with cystic fibrosis gene mutations in the *cystic fibrosis transmembrane conductance regulator* (CFTR) gene.
    - Partners of men with CAVD must be tested for the CFTR gene mutation before pursuing infertility treatment with retrieved sperm.
  - **Y-chromosome microdeletions**
    - May be found in up to 7% of men with male factor infertility
    - Although these men may be able to father children via IVF/ICSI, male offspring will inherit the Y-chromosome microdeletion and be infertile.

# EXCLUSION OF OVULATORY FACTOR INFERTILITY

To exclude ovulatory dysfunction, the presence of ovulation must be confirmed. In addition, ovarian reserve should be assessed to exclude oocyte depletion and premature ovarian failure.

## Confirmation of Ovulation

- The basal body temperature (BBT) chart (see Fig. 35-1) is a simple means of determining whether ovulation has occurred.
  - The woman's temperature is taken daily on awakening, before any activity, and recorded on a graph.
  - After ovulation, rising progesterone levels increase the basal temperature by approximately 0.4°F (0.22°C) through a hypothalamic thermogenic effect.
  - Because the rise in progesterone may occur anytime from 2 days before ovulation to 1 day after, the temperature elevation does not predict the exact moment of ovulation but offers retrospective confirmation of its occurrence.
  - A temperature elevation is usually sustained for 14 ± 2 days. One that persists for <11 days is suggestive of a luteal phase defect.
- Midluteal phase progesterone level is another test to assess ovulation.
  - A concentration >3.0 ng/mL in a blood sample drawn between days 19 and 23 suggests ovulation has occurred. Normal adequate luteal support usually produces a progesterone concentration >10 ng/mL.
- Daily monitoring of urinary luteinizing hormone (LH) is now widely used, given the proliferation of commercial tests for home use.
  - Using a threshold concentration of 40 mIU/mL, positive testing for urinary LH correlates well with the surge of serum LH levels that trigger ovulation.

## Assessment of Ovarian Reserve

- Depleted ovarian reserve adversely impacts fecundability given the inferior quantity and quality of remaining oocytes. The following tests help identify both a depleted reserve and the likelihood of response to controlled ovarian hyperstimulation (COH) during assisted reproduction:
  - Day 3 FSH concentration: Values below 10 to 15 mIU/mL suggest adequate ovarian reserve. The exact cutoff depends on the particular laboratory reference standards.
  - Measurement of anti-müllerian hormone (AMH) levels can also be helpful in predicting ovarian reserve. AMH is a measure of the primordial follicle pool and over a woman's reproductive lifetime steadily decreases to undetectable levels by menopause. There are kits available to assay for this hormone and the exact cutoff depends on the specific laboratory/assay reference standard.
  - Imaging of antral follicle counts by ultrasonography
  - Clomiphene citrate challenge test: The administration of clomiphene citrate 100 mg orally on menstrual cycle days 5 to 9 with measurement of day 3 and day 10 FSH. An exaggerated FSH response portends poorly for spontaneous or assisted conception.

# EXCLUSION OF STRUCTURAL FACTORS (TUBAL/PERITONEAL AND UTERINE)

- Tubal/peritoneal factors include endometriosis, pelvic adhesion disease, or previous bilateral tubal ligation. Uterine factors include leiomyomata, intrauterine synechiae (Asherman syndrome), septae, and other müllerian anomalies.
- **HSG** assesses uterine and fallopian tube contour and tubal patency (Fig. 35-2).
  - HSG shows appreciable müllerian anomalies as well as most endometrial polyps, synechiae, and submucosal fibroids. It can also determine tubal patency.
  - Performed in the early follicular phase, within 1 week of cessation of menstrual flow, to minimize chances of interrupting a pregnancy

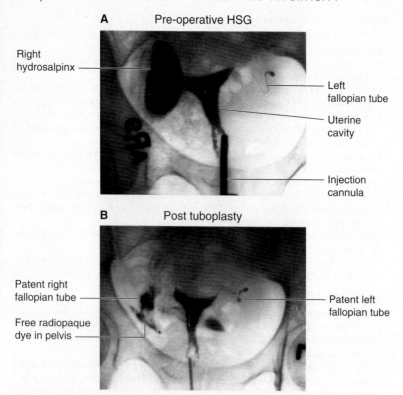

**Figure 35-2.** Hysterosalpingogram showing large right hydrosalpinx (**A**) that is resolved following successful tuboplasty (**B**). Real-time radiographs are obtained as radiopaque dye is injected through a cannula inserted in the cervical canal. Normal patent tubes demonstrate bilateral spillage from the fallopian tubes into the pelvis. (Original images courtesy of Dr. Edward Wallach, Johns Hopkins Hospital, Department of Gynecology and Obstetrics, Division of Reproductive Endocrinology and Infertility.)

- The procedure is performed by injecting a radiopaque dye through the cervix. As more dye is injected, the dye normally passes through the uterine cavity into the fallopian tubes and then spills into the peritoneal cavity.
- X-ray films are taken under fluoroscopy to evaluate tubal patency.
- Nonsteroidal anti-inflammatory drugs may be given to prevent cramping.
- HSG may have therapeutic effects. Several studies have indicated increased pregnancy rates for several months after the procedure.
- Prophylactic antibiotics (doxycycline, 100 mg orally twice daily for 5 to 7 days) are advisable when the patient has a history of pelvic inflammatory disease or when hydrosalpinges are identified during the study.
- **Saline infusion ultrasonography** (sonohysterography [SHG])
  - SHG involves transvaginal ultrasound after the introduction of sterile water or saline into the uterine cavity.

- Useful in assessment of uterine cavity abnormalities such as polyps or submucosal fibroids
- **Hysteroscopy**
  - Definitive method to evaluate the uterine cavity
  - Reserved for those patients with HSG or SHG results that merit further evaluation. It offers the possibility of minimally invasive treatment at time of the procedure
- **Diagnostic laparoscopy**
  - Assesses peritoneal and tubal factors, such as endometriosis and pelvic adhesions and can provide access for simultaneous corrective surgery
  - Laparoscopy should be scheduled in the follicular phase. This is the final and most invasive step in the patient's evaluation.
  - Findings on HSG correlate with laparoscopic findings 60% to 70% of the time.
  - Chromopertubation: dye (usually a dilute solution of indigo carmine) instilled through the fallopian tubes during laparoscopy to visually document tubal patency
  - Hysteroscopy may also be included to ensure that no intrauterine abnormalities were missed on the HSG.

## EXCLUSION OF CERVICAL FACTOR INFERTILITY

- The PCT or Huhner test allows direct analysis of sperm and cervical mucus interaction and provides a rough estimate of sperm quality.
- The test is done between days 12 and 14 of a 28- to 30-day menstrual cycle (after 48 hours of abstinence) when maximum estrogen secretion is present and the mucus is examined within 2 to 12 hours.
- Because interpretation of the PCT is subjective, the validity of the test is controversial, despite its long history of use.
- The test's use is most valuable for patients with history or physical exam findings suggestive of cervical factor, when the results will help direct treatment. However, a finding of 5 to 10 progressively motile spermatozoa per high-power field and clear acellular mucus with a spinnbarkeit (the degree to which the mucus stretches between two slides) of 8 cm generally suggests normal cervical function.
- Fecundity rates do not correlate directly with the number of motile sperm seen. The most common cause of an abnormal PCT is poor timing. Other causes include cervical stenosis, hypoplastic endocervical canal, coital dysfunction, and male factors. The sample can also be assessed for pH, mucus cellularity, white blood cell, and ferning. Clumping and flagellation of sperm without progression are often suggestive of antisperm antibodies.

## ENDOMETRIAL BIOPSY AND THE LUTEAL PHASE DEFECT

- Endometrial biopsy, historically, can document ovulation by histologic demonstration of decidualized stroma, assess for endometritis, and allows for histologic dating of the endometrium within 2 to 3 days and usually performed between days 24 and 26 of a 28-day menstrual cycle or 2 to 4 days before anticipated menstruation.
- Dates of the biopsy and subsequent menstrual cycle have been used to determine whether a luteal phase deficiency—insufficient progesterone support for the purported histologic date of the endometrium—is present. However, recent reports have

demonstrated that fertile women were at least as likely as their infertile counterparts to have an out-of-phase endometrial biopsy suggestive of a luteal phase defect.
- At present, this approach is rarely used.

## TREATMENT FOR INFERTILITY

### Anovulation

The vast majority of anovulatory women of reproductive age fall into WHO class II and, fortunately, this class proves responsive to ovulation induction. The agents most commonly used to stimulate multiple ovarian follicles are clomiphene citrate, human menopausal gonadotropins (hMG), and purified FSH. The WHO stratifies anovulatory women into three classes:
- WHO class I: hypogonadotropic hypogonadal anovulation
  - Hypothalamic amenorrhea attributable to low gonadotropin-releasing hormone (GnRH) levels or pituitary unresponsiveness to hypothalamic GnRH, with resultant low FSH and serum estradiol levels
  - Causes include excessive weight gain or loss and exercise or emotional stress.
- WHO class II: normogonadotropic normoestrogenic anovulation
  - Normal levels of estradiol and FSH; LH levels, however, are elevated. This class includes the polycystic ovarian syndrome (PCOS).
- WHO class III: hypergonadotropic hypoestrogenic anovulation
  - Main causes include premature ovarian failure (no follicles due to early menopause) or ovarian resistance.
  - These patients rarely respond to treatment for anovulation.
  - Donor eggs may be best option for these patients in achieving pregnancy.

### Clomiphene Citrate

- Mechanism of action: synthetic, nonsteroidal estrogen agonist-antagonist that increases the release of GnRH and subsequent LH and FSH release (antiestrogenic effect in hypothalamus results in increased GnRH secretion)
- Useful in women with oligomenorrhea and amenorrhea, with intact hypothalamic-pituitary-ovarian axes
- Patients who are overweight and hyperandrogenic or hypoestrogenic have decreased responsiveness to CC.
- Initiated on day 3, 4, or 5 in the menstrual cycle, usually at a starting dose of 50 mg for 5 days
- Adverse effects: vasomotor symptoms such as headache and mood change; rarely, visual symptoms such as transient blurry vision or scotomata have been reported
- Complications: cystic ovarian enlargement and multifetal gestations (5% to 10% of pregnancies)
- Another option for ovulation induction particularly in anovulatory women (e.g., PCOS) is use of aromatase inhibitors.
  - Current formulations involved are third-generation drugs letrozole (Femara) and anastrazole.
    - In particular, letrozole has been shown to be effective in PCOS women who have failed CC induction.
    - Letrozole is quickly absorbed via the gastrointestinal tract and metabolized and is generally considered safe for use.
  - However, this use of aromatase inhibitors is off-label and based on limited data from one small study, patients must be counseled regarding possible risk of congenital anomalies, specifically possible risk of cardiac and bone malformations.

- This should also be tempered by the coexisting data from another small randomized trial looking at pregnancy outcomes following treatment with letrozole, anastrazole, or CC for induction which showed no increase in congenital anomalies.

## Exogenous Gonadotropins

- GnRH, hMG, and FSH are used primarily in women who fail to respond to CC or who have hypogonadotropic amenorrhea or unexplained infertility.
  - Prescription of these expensive drugs, which are used in the more complicated protocols for IVF (see the following text), should be left to specialists trained in their use.

## Hyperprolactinemia

- Bromocriptine is used to induce ovulation in patients with hyperprolactinemia.
- Bromocriptine is a dopamine agonist that directly inhibits pituitary secretion of prolactin, which restores normal gonadotropin release.
  - The usual starting dose is 2.5 mg at bedtime to prevent dopaminergic side effects, which include nausea, diarrhea, dizziness, and headache.
  - If oral administration cannot be tolerated, vaginal administration is recommended.
- A response is usually seen in 2 to 3 months, and 80% of hyperprolactinemic patients ovulate and become pregnant.
- Cabergoline is an alternative for those who do not tolerate bromocriptine.

## Thyroid Dysfunction

- Both hypothyroidism and hyperthyroidism can lead to anovulation with subsequent infertility. These medical conditions should be corrected prior to a patient attempting pregnancy. See Chapter 13.

## Hypothalamic-Pituitary Axis Dysfunction

- Hypothalamic-pituitary axis problems including extreme weight gain or loss, excessive exercise, and emotional stress can all impact the secretion of GnRH from the hypothalamus and cause ovulatory dysfunction. These must be addressed by appropriate behavioral or psychological intervention.

## Male Factor Infertility

- Although the gynecologist does not directly treat male patients, therapies to treat male factor infertility often involve hormonal manipulation in the female partner. The evaluation is analogous to that in the woman, with examination of the hypothalamic-pituitary-testicular axis, outflow tract, and testicular function.
- Toxins, viruses, sexually transmitted diseases, varicoceles, and congenital problems can all influence infertility.
- The procedure of ICSI has revolutionized treatment of male infertility. As long as viable sperm can be retrieved by ejaculation, epididymal aspiration, or testicular biopsy, successful fertilization and pregnancy can be achieved. The fertilization rate is 95%, and the pregnancy rate is comparable to that of IVF.

## Endometriosis

- Endometriosis is the ectopic growth of hormonally responsive endometrial tissue and accounts for 15% of female infertility. Surgical treatment may be effective, although management by an infertility specialist for IVF may be necessary. See Chapter 38.

## Luteal Phase Defects

- Luteal phase defects are thought to occur in both fertile and infertile women, and the role for treatment is highly controversial. Nevertheless, in a couple with documented infertility, it is not unreasonable to treat a presumed luteal phase deficiency with intramuscular or intravaginal progesterone in the postovulatory phase of the cycle and, if pregnancy occurs, until the luteoplacental shift occurs.

## Uterine Factors

- Uterine factors, such as submucous leiomyomas, intrauterine synechiae (Asherman syndrome), and uterine deformities such as septa, cause approximately 2% of infertility. The mainstay of treatment for these conditions is surgical correction, frequently via a hysteroscopic approach.

## Infections

- Infections of the female and male genital tracts have been implicated as causes of infertility. *Chlamydia* infection and gonorrhea are the major pathogens and should be treated appropriately. *Ureaplasma urealyticum* and *Mycoplasma hominis* have also been implicated, and, if positively identified by culture, they should be treated with oral doxycycline, 100 mg twice daily for 7 days. This has been shown to increase the pregnancy rate in patients with primary infertility.

## Tubal Factor Infertility

- Tubal factor infertility has become more prevalent with the increased incidence of salpingitis. The frequency of tubal occlusion after one, two, and three episodes of salpingitis is reported to be 11%, 23%, and 54%, respectively. Appendicitis, previous abdominopelvic surgery, endometriosis, and ectopic pregnancy can also lead to adhesion formation and damaged tubes.
- Proximal tubal obstruction is identified on HSG. Tubal spasm may mimic proximal obstruction, however, and obstruction should be confirmed by laparoscopy. Treatment consists of tubal cannulation, microsurgical tubocornual reanastomosis, or IVF.
- Distal tubal disease or distortion can be seen on HSG and laparoscopy. The success of corrective surgery (neosalpingostomy) depends on the extent of disease.
- If IVF is pursued in patients with tubal factor infertility, several studies have shown that success rates of IVF are improved if hydrosalpinges are removed.
- For patients with a history of a prior bilateral tubal ligation who desire fertility, options include microsurgical sterilization reversal as well as IVF.
- Success of tubal reanastomosis depends on age, type, and location of the sterilization procedure and final lengths of repaired fallopian tubes.
- IVF may be a better option for patients who desire only a single additional child.

## ASSISTED REPRODUCTIVE TECHNOLOGIES

- Since the first successful IVF pregnancy delivered in 1978, several techniques have been developed that enhance our ability to overcome infertility.
- Among them are the capabilities for embryo cryopreservation and ovum donation.
- Of all ART cycles nationwide using fresh nondonor eggs or embryos, 36.9% resulted in pregnancy according to the 2010 National Summary Tables and Fertility Clinic data, with 81.8% of these pregnancies resulting in a live birth of one or more infant.

- The majority (57.1%) of IVF pregnancies resulted in single live births, whereas 24.8% resulted in multiple-infant births. Miscarriages occurred in 16.1%, ectopic pregnancies in 0.7%, and stillbirths in 0.6%. The following types of procedures are currently used in ART.

## Intrauterine Insemination

- May increase cycle fecundity when semen analysis contains decreased numbers of total motile sperm (<20 million).
- IUI bypasses the inability of the uterus to tolerate large amounts of unprocessed seminal plasma by washing semen to maximize the number of motile sperm.
  - Components of the ejaculate removed include seminal fluid, excess cellular debris, leukocytes, and morphologically abnormal sperm.
- Best results are achieved when the final specimen contains 10 million total motile sperm.
- Timing of IUI is critical and should optimally occur as follows:
  - The day after detection of the midcycle urinary LH surge in spontaneous or clomiphene-induced ovulatory cycles
  - Thirty-six hours after administration of exogenous human chorionic gonadotropin (hCG) in cycles stimulated with gonadotropins
- An IUI cannula is used to deliver sperm into the endometrial cavity. Following IUI, the patient remains in the recumbent position for 10 minutes.

## In Vitro Fertilization

- IVF refers to COH followed by aspiration of oocytes under ultrasound guidance, laboratory fertilization with prepared sperm, embryo culture, and transcervical transfer of the resulting embryos into the uterus. Although most IVF procedures use fresh oocytes from the patient, transfer of frozen oocytes and transfer of donor eggs are also options.
- The overall 2010 live birth/transfer rate for IVF was 36.8%. For patients undergoing IVF, the pregnancy success rate varies little by cause of infertility, with a success rate approximating the overall national rate in women with most diagnoses except for diminished ovarian reserve (Table 35-2).
- Several trends demonstrated in the 2010 data on IVF are worth noting: live birth rates declined progressively in women older than age 35 years attempting IVF using fresh nondonor eggs; there was a sharp and steady increase in the rate of miscarriages in women age older than 35 years who attempted IVF; use of ICSI increased with 74.1% of ART cycles using IVF with ICSI, whereas 25.9% used IVF without ICSI; blastocyst transfer (day 5) conferred an advantage in live birth rate over day 3, cleavage-stage embryo transfer; live birth rate per transfer was 36.8% for fresh nondonor embryos, 33.2% for frozen nondonor embryos, 55.8% for fresh donor embryos, and 34.9% for frozen donor embryos. This highlights the dependence of fertility on the age of the oocyte (donor), not on the age of the uterus (receiver or carrier).

## Intracytoplasmic Sperm Injection

- In ICSI, a single spermatozoon is injected microscopically into each oocyte, and the resulting embryos are transferred transcervically into the uterus. The advent of ICSI has revolutionized fertility treatment for couples confronting male factor infertility refractory to IUI or IVF.

**TABLE 35-2** In Vitro Fertilization Success Rates by Diagnosis

| Diagnosis of Patients Undergoing IVF | Percentage of Total Cases (%) | Live Births per Cycle (%) |
|---|---|---|
| Tubal factor | 7.3 | 33.1 |
| Ovulatory dysfunction | 6.9 | 40.4 |
| Diminished ovarian reserve | 12.1 | 15.0 |
| Endometriosis | 4.0 | 35.3 |
| Uterine factor | 1.3 | 25.7 |
| Male factor | 18.8 | 37.6 |
| Other causes | 7.0 | 28.8 |
| Unexplained cause | 13.9 | 33.6 |
| Multiple factors, female only | 10.5 | 23.7 |
| Multiple factors, female + male | 18.1 | 28.4 |

The total does not equal 100% due to rounding. Success rates are for fresh nondonor eggs or embryos.
IVF, in vitro fertilization.
Data from Centers for Disease Control and Prevention; American Society for Reproductive Medicine; Society for Assisted Reproductive Technology. 2010 Assisted reproductive technology success rates: national summary and fertility clinic reports. Atlanta, GA: U.S. Department of Health and Human Services, 2012. http://www.cdc.gov/art/Art2010. Accessed May 20, 2013.

- Success rates of ICSI for male factor infertility compare favorably to routine IVF without ICSI performed for non–male factor infertility.

## Gamete Intrafallopian Transfer and Zygote Intrafallopian Transfer

- Gamete intrafallopian transfer (GIFT) is extraction of oocytes followed by the transfer of gametes (sperm and oocyte) into a normal fallopian tube by laparoscopy.
- Zygote intrafallopian transfer (ZIFT) refers to placement of embryos into the fallopian tube via laparoscopy after oocyte retrieval and fertilization.
- Both procedures are rarely used today.

## INDICATIONS FOR IN VITRO FERTILIZATION

- **Tubal conditions:** large hydrosalpinges, absence of fimbria, severe adhesive disease, repeated ectopic pregnancies, or failed reconstructive therapy, also women with previous bilateral tubal ligation who chose IVF over reanastomosis
- **Endometriosis:** if other forms of treatment have failed
- **Unexplained infertility**
- **Male factor infertility:** low sperm count, low sperm motility, and abnormal morphology associated with reduction in fertilizing ability
- **Uterine malformations:** related to diethylstilbestrol exposure
- **HIV-positive serodiscordant couples:** Use of ICSI or sperm-washing techniques has enabled HIV-negative women to safely achieve pregnancy using the sperm of their affected male partners. Processing and handling of these specimens

require specialized facilities, protocols, training, and equipment to prevent cross contamination.

- **Men and women seeking fertility preservation:** patients about to undergo chemotherapy or irradiation of their pelvic regions can consider cryopreservation of gametes, embryos, or ovarian tissue for subsequent childbearing via ART.
- **Couples seeking preimplantation genetic diagnosis** (see later discussion).

## CONTROLLED OVARIAN HYPERSTIMULATION AND PROTOCOLS FOR IN VITRO FERTILIZATION

The agents most commonly used to stimulate multiple ovarian follicles are CC, hMG, and purified FSH. The particular products and protocols used may be tailored as the treatment progresses to boost the chances of an adequate response and increase the pregnancy rate.

### Clomiphene-Only Regimens

- These regimens are generally given on days 5 to 9 of the menstrual cycle.
- Response may be followed by BBT measurement, ultrasonography, and measurement of LH and estradiol levels.
- CC is inexpensive and has a low risk of ovarian hyperstimulation syndrome (OHSS). However, it creates a low oocyte yield (one or two per cycle), most commonly used with timed intercourse at home or IUI.
- Most treatment regimens start with 50 mg/day for 5 days beginning on cycle day 3 or day 5. If ovulation fails to occur, the dose may be increased to 100 mg/day.
- hCG, 5,000 IU to 10,000 IU, may be used to simulate an LH surge. Eighty percent of properly selected couples will conceive in the first three cycles after treatment. The most commonly used hCG formulation is choriogonadotropin alfa injection (Ovidrel).
- Potential side effects of CC are vasomotor flushes, blurring of vision, urticaria, pain, bloating, and multiple gestations (5% to 7% of cases, usually twins).

### Gonadotropin Regimens

- These regimens increase the number of recruited follicles in patients who do not achieve pregnancy with CC and in those patients with endometriosis or unexplained infertility.
- hMG, which is a combination of LH and FSH, is usually given for 2 to 7 days.
- Although gonadotropin injections prove more effective at COH than clomiphene, they are more expensive and can lead to life-threatening OHSS.
- Trade names for hMG include Humegon, Pergonal, and Repronex.
- Attempts to minimize the potentially deleterious LH component of hMG have led to the manufacture of purified urinary FSH and, more recently, recombinant FSH.
- The purity and consistency associated with recombinant FSH argue for its exclusive use, but evidence of its superior efficacy has been conflicting and inconclusive. Follicle maturation during COH is monitored using sonography and serial measurement of estradiol levels.
- To complete oocyte maturation, hCG is administered once the follicles have reached 17 to 18 mm in diameter.
- Potential disadvantages of gonadotropin use include premature luteinization, spontaneous LH surges resulting in high cancellation rates, multiple gestations, and ovarian hyperstimulation.

## Gonadotropin-Releasing Hormone Agonists

- These are used via a flare-up protocol or a luteal phase protocol in IVF cycles.
- The flare-up protocol causes an elevation of FSH in the first 4 days, which increases oocyte recruitment.
- After 5 days of administration, the GnRH agonist (GnRHa) downregulates the pituitary to prevent premature luteinization and a spontaneous LH surge.
- The luteal phase protocol involves starting GnRHa administration on the 17th to 21st menstrual day in the cycle before IVF.
- GnRHa increases the number, quality, and synchronization of the oocytes recovered per cycle and thereby improves the fertilization rate, the number of embryos, and the pregnancy rate.
- Lupron is the most commonly used GnRHa in the United States.

## Gonadotropin-Releasing Hormone Antagonists

- **Commonly used for COP in IVF cycles**
- These block LH secretion, and the premature LH surges that force cycle cancellation without causing a flare-up effect.
- They are administered in a single dose on the eight menstrual day or in smaller doses over 4 days.
- Because they block the periovulatory LH surge, less gonadotropins are required to stimulate ovulation and side effects are decreased.
- Trade names include Antagon and Cetrotide.

# OOCYTE RETRIEVAL, CULTURE FERTILIZATION, AND TRANSFER

There are two major techniques of oocyte retrieval. The most commonly used method is ultrasonographically guided follicular aspiration and the less common and rarely used method is laparoscopic oocyte retrieval.

## Ultrasonographically Guided Oocyte Retrieval

- A 17-gauge needle passed through the vaginal fornix to retrieve oocytes.
- Performed 34 to 36 hours after hCG injection under sedation
- Potential complications include risk of bowel injury and injury to pelvic vessels.

## Oocyte Fertilization

- Sperms are diluted, centrifuged, and incubated before 50,000 to 100,000 motile spermatozoa are added to each Petri dish containing an oocyte.
- Fertilization is documented by the presence of two pronuclei and extrusion of a second polar body at 24 hours.

## Embryo Transfer

- Performed 3 to 5 days after oocyte insemination
  - Day 5 blastocyst transfer is becoming more common today due to higher livebirth rates compared to cleavage-stage (day 3) embryos.
- Excess embryos not used for transfer can be cryopreserved for an unlimited period, with a survival rate of 75%.
- The actual number of embryos transferred depends on the individual's age and other risk factors for multiple pregnancy.

• The common practice is to supplement the luteal phase with progesterone given intramuscularly or by vaginal suppository, beginning the day of oocyte release and continuing into the 12th week of pregnancy.

## MATERNAL, FETAL, AND LONG-TERM EFFECTS OF ASSISTED REPRODUCTIVE TECHNOLOGY

### Ovarian Hyperstimulation Syndrome

• OHSS can be a life-threatening complication of COH characterized by ovarian enlargement and increased capillary permeability.
  • Potentiated by COH cycles using GnRH analogs for downregulation or hCG to trigger oocyte maturation
• Presentation: abdominal bloating, ascites, decreased urine output, hemoconcentration, hypercoagulability, hydrothorax, acute respiratory distress syndrome, electrolyte imbalance, and multiple organ failure
• Classified as mild, moderate, or severe according to the presenting symptoms
• Pathophysiology: thought to be mediated by vascular endothelial growth factor, produced by the ovary in response to LH or hCG
• Risk factors: young age, pregnancy, low body weight, high or rapidly climbing estradiol levels, large size and number of follicles, and the presence of PCOS
• Treatment: Moderate to severe cases of OHSS should be managed as an inpatient.
  • Includes close monitoring of fluid and renal status, frequent evaluation of electrolytes and coagulation studies, intravascular resuscitation, thrombosis prophylaxis and paracentesis, and/or thoracentesis, as indicated
• Prevention: If impending OHSS is suspected, prevention can be attempted by lowering or withholding ("coasting") the hCG triggering dose, postponing embryo transfer, or canceling the cycle.
  • OHSS is an entirely iatrogenic entity that is usually avoidable by vigilance and judicious execution and alteration of COH regimen.

### Multiple Gestation

• The 2010 data demonstrate that 30% of clinical pregnancies involved multiple gestation: 29.0% were twin pregnancies and 1% were triplet or higher order pregnancies.
• In attempting to limit the prevalence of multiple gestation, the American Society for Reproductive Medicine has issued practice recommendations governing the number of embryos transferred. These recommendations are stratified depending on whether cleavage-stage embryos or blastocysts are transferred.
  • Women younger than age 35 years: strong consideration to transfer just one embryo if a favorable prognosis; no more than two embryos (cleavage stage or blastocyst) should be transferred
  • Women aged 35 to 37 years: two cleavage-stage embryos if a favorable prognosis, otherwise three cleavage-stage embryos may be transferred; no more than two blastocysts may be transferred
  • Women aged 38 to 40 years: three cleavage-stage embryos or two blastocysts if a favorable prognosis, otherwise four cleavage-stage embryos or three blastocysts may be transferred
  • Women older than age 40 years: should receive no more than five cleavage-stage embryos or three blastocysts
• Should multiple gestation ensue, recourse to selective fetal reduction is available for patients who are comfortable with the ethics and risks of that procedure.

## Heterotopic Pregnancy

• Occurs in up to 1% of pregnancies after ART
• This incidence is dramatically higher than the corresponding ratio in the general population (1 in 30,000).
• The finding of an intrauterine pregnancy (IUP) in a woman who has undergone ART should not be automatically considered a reassuring finding, as the presence of a coexisting ectopic pregnancy is possible.
• Women, after ART who display signs or symptoms suggesting ectopic pregnancy must be closely followed despite confirmation of an IUP.

## Effects of In Vitro Fertilization

• Inconsistent and equivocal evidence links IVF to increased risks of neonatal morbidity, birth defects, developmental disabilities, or certain childhood cancers.
• Conclusive evidence, however, does link IVF to an increased risk of low-birth-weight deliveries even among full-term, singleton neonates. Most recent studies and data suggest that although fetuses resulting from ART are at higher risk of congenital abnormalities when compared to spontaneously conceived fetuses, the associated risk appears to be lower than previously believed and this is in part due to the recognition that some parental factors may play a role in this increased risk as opposed to simply the practice/inherent science of ART.

## Effects of Intracytoplasmic Sperm Injection

• ICSI has been associated with a significant increase in sex and autosomal chromosome abnormalities and, potentially, with an increased risk of imprinting disorders, such as Beckwith-Wiedemann or Angelman syndromes.
• If a male with a Y chromosome microdeletion undergoes ICSI/IVF, male offspring will inherit the same microdeletion and, thus, also have male factor infertility.

# NEW TECHNOLOGIES AND SOCIAL IMPLICATIONS

The advent of ART has raised unique ethical and social implications for couples undergoing such treatments. It has also presented an option for future childbearing with biologic offspring to individuals diagnosed with malignancies that require treatments with agents (chemotherapy, radiation, etc.) that can deplete ovarian or sperm reserve.

## Embryo Cryopreservation

• It is now common practice to cryopreserve excess embryos not used during an embryo transfer cycle.
• Although many couples will use these embryos for future cycles, the number of cryopreserved embryos in the United States is estimated to be over 400,000.
• Disposition options for supernumerary cryopreserved embryos include use, discard, donation to research (including stem cell research), donation to other couples, future embryo transfer, or continued storage.
• It is imperative that couples be aware that excess embryos could result from ART and that a plan be discussed in advance for these embryos.

## Oocyte Cryopreservation and Ovarian Tissue Preservation

• The development of more reliable and reproducible freezing and thawing protocols, namely vitrification, has resulted in egg (oocyte) cryopreservation becoming widely available and no longer considered experimental.

- Oocyte cryopreservation may be offered to any reproductive age woman who is about to undergo/initiate treatment with known gonadotoxic agents (e.g., chemotherapy) who has adequate time (2 to 3 weeks) to delay therapy for an IVF cycle.
- Oocyte freezing may also be offered to couples whose religious or ethical beliefs conflict with embryo cryopreservation or for women who plan to delay childbearing for nonmedical reasons.
- Ovarian tissue cryopreservation is a fertility preservation option for women without adequate time to freeze embryos or oocytes of prepubertal girls. It is considered highly experimental.

## Third-Party Reproduction
- Includes donor oocytes and sperm, donated embryos, and gestational carriers (surrogates)
- Ethical issues involved include the following:
  - Disclosure to children conceived by these technologies regarding their genetic origin
  - Privacy issues for donors
  - Compensation for oocyte donors and gestational carriers

## Preimplantation Genetic Testing
- Umbrella term describing all types of genetic testing of the embryo. It is further subdivided into preimplantation genetic diagnosis (PGD) and preimplantation genetic screening (PGS).
- PGD allows couples with various single-gene disorders and X-linked genetic diseases to avoid transmission of the disorder to their offspring.
- PGD proceeds by biopsy and genetic analysis of one of the following specimens:
  - One to two blastomeres of a cleavage-stage (days 2 to 3) embryo derived from IVF
  - Polar body biopsy from a metaphase II oocyte obtained after COH
  - Trophectoderm tissue from a blastocyst-stage (day 5) embryo
- Single-gene disorders
  - Using polymerase chain reaction (PCR), DNA extracted from the biopsy specimen is used to screen for a known hereditary disorder—for example, cystic fibrosis, muscular dystrophy, hemophilia, or Huntington disease.
  - Only unaffected preimplantation embryos would be transferred to the woman's uterus.
- Sibling human leukocyte antigen (HLA) matching
  - PGD was first used in 2000 to screen for Fanconi anemia and simultaneously to select for a preimplantation embryo that was HLA matched to a preexisting sibling afflicted with this disorder.
- Aneuploidy testing
  - Fluorescence in situ hybridization (FISH) is a molecular technique that uses chromosome-specific sequences that can be hybridized to complementary probes attached to differentially colored fluorochromes.
  - FISH has been used for the PGD of aneuploidy and chromosomal abnormalities, such as translocations.
  - One drawback to FISH is that it only samples some of the chromosomes (no more than 14) but not all 23. Additionally, in the event of mosaicism, selective cell sampling—further compounded by selective chromosome screening—can lead to misdiagnoses.

- PGS is a screening test for aneuploidy (numerical chromosomal abnormalities) in embryos from parents that have no known chromosomal abnormality (normal karyotype).
  - Methods to perform PGS include FISH, single nucleotide polymorphism (SNP) microarrays, and comparative genomic hybridization.
  - A role for PGS is emerging in embryo screening in women of advanced maternal age, repeated miscarriage, and repeated otherwise unexplained IVF failure.
  - PGS can screen for all 23 chromosomes and can help identify optimal (euploid) embryos for transfer before IVF. However, more data is needed to determine its effectiveness in predicting the ultimate genetic status of the fetus.
- Elective sex selection
  - Also referred to as family balancing
  - PGD, via either PCR or FISH, enables efficient and accurate gender selection by screening selectively for the Y chromosome.
- Sharp debate over the propriety of such nonmedical use of reproductive technology has limited the prevalence of this application.

## SUGGESTED READINGS

Brezina P, Brezina DS, Kearns WG. Preimplantation genetic testing. *BMJ* 2012;345:e5908.

Centers for Disease Control and Prevention, National Center for Health Statistics. 2002 National Survey of Family Growth. U.S. Department of Health and Human Services Web site. http://www.cdc.gov/nchs/nsfg.htm. Accessed May 20, 2013.

Centers for Disease Control and Prevention, National Center for Health Statistics. 2006-2010 National Survey of Family Growth. U.S. Department of Health and Human Services Web site. http://www.cdc.gov/nchs/nsfg/abc_list_i.htm#infertility. Accessed May 20, 2013.

Centers for Disease Control and Prevention, National Center for Health Statistics. 2010 Assisted Reproductive Technology Report. U.S. Department of Health and Human Services Web site. http://www.cdc.gov/art/ART2010/index.htm. Accessed May 20, 2013.

Cooper TG, Noonan E, von Eckardstein S, et al. World Health Organization reference values for human semen characteristics. *Hum Reprod Update* 2010;16(3):231–245.

Davies MJ, Moore VM, Wilson KJ, et al. Reproductive technologies and the risk of birth defects. *N Engl J Med* 2012;366:1803–1813.

Glujovsky D, Blake D, Farquhar C, et al. Cleavage stage versus blastocyst stage embryo transfer in assisted reproductive technology. *Cochrane Database Syst Rev* 2012;(7):CD002118.

Hansen M, Kurinczuk JJ, Milne E, et al. Assisted reproductive technology and birth defects: a systematic review and metaanalysis. *Hum Reprod Update* 2013;19(4):330–353.

Legro RS, Barnhart HX, Schlaff WD, et al; Cooperative Multicenter Reproductive Medicine Network. Clomiphene, metformin, or both for infertility in the polycystic ovary syndrome. *N Engl J Med* 2007;356(6):551–566.

Practice Committee of the American Society for Reproductive Medicine. Preimplantation genetic diagnosis: a practice committee opinion. *Fertil Steril* 2008;90:S136–S140.

Practice Committee of the American Society for Reproductive Medicine; Practice Committee of the Society for Assisted Reproductive Technology. Criteria for number of embryos to transfer: a committee opinion. *Fertil Steril* 2013;99(1):44–46.

Practice Committee of the American Society for Reproductive Medicine; Practice Committee of the Society for Assisted Reproductive Technology. Mature oocyte cryopreservation: a guideline. *Fertil Steril* 2013;99(1):37–43.

Savasi V, Mandia L, Laoreti A, et al. Reproductive assistance in HIV serodiscordant couples. *Hum Reprod Update* 2013;19(2):136–150.

Speroff L, Fritz MA. *Clinical Gynecologic Endocrinology and Infertility*, 7th ed. Philadelphia, PA: Lippincott Williams & Wilkins, 2010.

Twisk M, Mastenbroek S, van Wely M, et al. Preimplantation genetic screening for abnormal number of chromosomes (aneuploidies) in in vitro fertilization or intracytoplasmic sperm injection (review). *Cochrane Database Syst Rev* 2006;(1):CD005291.

# 36 Miscarriage and Recurrent Pregnancy Loss

Sara Seifert and Kristiina Altman

## FIRST-TRIMESTER MISCARRIAGE

**Miscarriage**, or spontaneous abortion, is generally defined as the spontaneous loss of a fetus weighing <500 g or at gestational age (GA) <20 weeks.

- Miscarriages are classified according to the GA at which they occur.
  - **Preclinical** or biochemical **miscarriages** happen at or before 5 weeks of gestation.
  - Clinical miscarriages must have documentation of pregnancy by an appropriate beta-human chorionic gonadotropin (β-hCG) level, ultrasound, or tissue pathology and include the following:
    - **Embryonic miscarriage** occurs at 6 to 9 weeks of gestation or crown-rump length (CRL) >5 mm without cardiac activity.
    - **Fetal miscarriage** occurs between 10 and 20 weeks of gestation or CRL >30 mm without cardiac activity.

### Incidence and Risk

- Thirty percent to 40% of all conceptions result in miscarriage.
- The risk of preclinical miscarriage is estimated as approximately 25% to 30% in women older than age 35 years.
- Ten percent to 15% percent of clinically recognized pregnancies end in first-trimester and early second-trimester losses (<20 weeks of gestation).
  - Nearly 80% of sporadic losses occur during the first trimester and typically manifest before 12 weeks' GA.
- The risk of miscarriage is 22% to 57% at <6 weeks, 15% at 6 to 10 weeks, and 2% to 3% >10 weeks.
- The risk increases significantly with advanced maternal age (AMA) from 8% to 20% in women younger than age 35 years to as high as >50% in those older than age 40 years. This increase is thought to be related to the increased risk of aneuploidic pregnancies in older women.
- Although maternal age probably has the greatest impact, several other factors carry an increased risk of sporadic first- or early second-trimester clinical miscarriage. See Table 36-1.
- Common causes of sporadic losses include the following:
  - Chromosomal abnormalities account for approximately 50% of miscarriages.
    - Incidence is inversely related to GA.
      - Ninety percent in anembryonic (gestational sac without embryonic structures) products of conception (POCs) (sometimes referred to as "blighted ovum")
      - Fifty percent in embryonic abortuses
      - Thirty percent in fetal abortuses

| TABLE 36-1 | Risk Factors for Miscarriage |
|---|---|

Increasing maternal age (>35 yr old)
History of previous miscarriage
Tobacco
Alcohol
Illicit drug use (e.g., cocaine)
NSAID use
Caffeine (high intake)
Low folate levels/intake
Maternal fever/febrile illness
Maternal obesity
Maternal medical conditions (e.g., diabetes)

NSAID, nonsteroidal anti-inflammatory drug.

- o Typically autosomal trisomies, monosomies, or polyploidies
- o Maternal conditions: uterine anomalies, endocrinopathies, autoimmune disease, hypercoagulability, infection, and teratogen exposure
- o Previous obstetric history: Risk of miscarriage increases from 20% in women with a history of one miscarriage to 43% in women with a history of three or more.
- o Tobacco: Smoking and exposure to secondhand smoke increase the risk.
- Observational and population-based studies have also implicated the following risk factors: alcohol and illicit drug use, nonsteroidal anti-inflammatory drug (NSAID) use, fever, caffeine, obesity, and low folate levels.

## Presentation

- The hallmark complaint of a pregnant woman experiencing a miscarriage is **vaginal bleeding** after a missed period, with or without pain.
- Of note, 25% of all pregnancies are complicated by bleeding before 20 weeks of gestation. Of these, 12% to 57% end in miscarriage. Several studies have found that spotting or light bleeding does not increase the risk of miscarriage.
- The types of spontaneous abortion include the following:
  - **Threatened:** often painless, cervix closed, uterine size consistent with GA
  - **Inevitable:** painful, cervix open, uterine size consistent with GA
  - **Complete** (usually *before* 12 weeks of gestation): mild pain; cervix closed; uterus small, contracted, and empty
  - **Incomplete** (usually *after* 12 weeks of gestation): painful; cervix open often with tissue in os or vagina; uterus small and not well-contracted, with POCs still in the uterus
  - **Missed** (intrauterine fetal demise at <20 weeks of gestation): retained nonviable pregnancy in which the embryo or fetus lacks heartbeat but symptoms of miscarriage have not developed. Also called delayed miscarriage. The patient typically presents due to cessation of the normal symptoms of pregnancy (i.e., nausea, vomiting, breast tenderness) or receives the diagnosis unexpectedly during ultrasound evaluation.

- **Septic:** painful, purulent discharge; cervix open; cervical motion tenderness; tender uterus; constitutional symptoms (e.g., fever, malaise); tachycardia; and/or tachypnea. The infectious source is often *Staphylococcus aureus*. Septic miscarriage is frequently a complication of unsafe induced abortion as opposed to the sequela of spontaneous loss.

## Assessment

- The **differential diagnosis** for early pregnancy bleeding includes the following:
  - Physiologic
  - Ectopic pregnancy
  - Gestational trophoblastic disease
  - Anatomic pathology of the vagina, cervix, or uterus
- The gold standard for diagnosis is imaging, usually with transvaginal ultrasound. This modality is especially useful in differentiating intrauterine and ectopic pregnancies.
  - Viability can be determined through the appearance of a gestational and/or yolk sac and with measurement of the CRL. A gestational sac should be visible at $\beta$-hCG levels of 1,000 to 2,000 mIU/mL (~5 weeks of gestation) depending on ultrasound equipment and radiologist, but the detection level may be higher in patients with difficult anatomy (e.g., morbid obesity, multiple fibroids, deeply retroflexed uterus). Newer research is elucidating the lowest discriminatory levels with modern ultrasound equipment and the 99% probability levels for visualizing a gestational sac (390 to 3,510 mIU/mL), a yolk sac (1,094 to 17,716 mIU/mL), and a fetal pole (1,394 to 47,685 mIU/mL).
  - In diagnosing a missed clinical miscarriage, the operator can use several sonographic criteria: (a) absence of fetal cardiac activity with a CRL >5 mm and/or (b) absence of a fetal pole in the presence of a mean sac diameter of >18 mm transvaginally or >25 mm transabdominally.
- The early presence of fetal cardiac activity in women of AMA is not necessarily reassuring. One series demonstrated an increased risk of miscarriage from 4% in women younger than age 35 years to 29% in women older than age 40 years.
- Evaluation also includes a complete blood, a type and screen, serum progesterone, and serial quantitative $\beta$-hCG measurements. The last is most useful in conjunction with imaging. In normal pregnancies, $\beta$-hCG levels usually rise 55% to 66% in 48 hours. The measurements should be done in the same laboratory due to intra-assay variations. Occasionally, a slower rise may be seen in normal pregnancies.

## Management and Complications

- If bleeding is minimal or symptoms have resolved, a threatened miscarriage can be managed expectantly. Bed rest or progesterone treatment does not prevent miscarriage.
- Similarly, complete abortions often require no intervention other than evaluation of passed tissue to confirm POCs. In such cases or with expectant management, patients should be advised to bring the POC to the hospital for evaluation.
- Miscarriage has a 1.5% to 2% risk of alloimmunization. Given the minimal risks of anti-D immune globulin (RhoGAM) administration compared to the potential benefits, any Rh (D)-negative woman who experiences a spontaneous loss or has a threatened miscarriage should receive it.
- Incomplete, inevitable, or missed miscarriages can be managed expectantly, medically, or surgically. These three outcomes have been extensively studied. Selecting an option is based on a combination of patient wishes, stability, and stage of miscarriage.

| TABLE 36-2 | Options for Medical Treatment of Miscarriage |
|---|---|

| Regimen | Directions |
|---|---|
| Misoprostol 800 μg vaginally or 600 μg sublingual | Give every 3 hr, may repeat twice. |
| Misoprostol 400 μg vaginally | Give every 4 hr, may give four doses. |
| Mifepristone 200 mg orally and misoprostol 800 μg vaginally | Give mifepristone followed by misoprostol 48 hr later. |
| Mifepristone 600 mg orally and misoprostol 400 μg vaginally | Give mifepristone followed by misoprostol 48 hr later. |

Adapted from Dempsey A, Davis A. Medical management of early pregnancy failure: how to treat and what to expect. *Semin Reprod Med* 2008;26:401–410.

*Expectant Management*

- **Expectant management** is an ideal option for women who present during the first trimester, are clinically stable, and would prefer no intervention.
- The success is greatest in incomplete (91%) compared to missed (76%) or preclinical (66%) miscarriages. The average time to miscarriage completion is 2 to 4 weeks.
- Surgical or medical intervention is indicated if expectant management fails.

*Medical Management*

- **Medical management** is an effective method for women who decline surgery or expectant management (Table 36-2).
- The World Health Organization recommends either 800 μg vaginal or 600 μg sublingual misoprostol, to be repeated after 3 days. This results in a completion rate of 79% by 7 days and 87% by 30 days. Cramping and bleeding typically occur within 2 to 6 hours of administration. Pretreatment with Tylenol and NSAIDs is helpful. Of note, the oral route tends to cause more undesirable side effects, such as uterine cramping and gastrointestinal symptoms.
- Several trials have included the combination of a progesterone antagonist (mifepristone) and misoprostol. The U.S. Food and Drug Administration–approved regimen includes 600 mg mifepristone and 48 hours later 400 μg misoprostol orally, with 92% efficacy. An alternative recommendation (200 mg mifepristone orally with 800 μg misoprostol per vagina) appears to have greater efficacy (95% to 99%) as well as fewer side effects and lower cost.

*Follow-Up*

- A follow-up ultrasound should show the absence of POCs, and serum β-hCG level should drop 80% 1 week following the passage of tissue. It is prudent to follow β-hCG levels to zero if an intrauterine pregnancy (IUP) was not documented.

*Surgical Management*

- **Surgical management** via dilation (or dilatation) and curettage (D&C) or dilation and evacuation (D&E) is the traditional approach in both first- and early second-trimester losses. This option is especially suitable for unstable patients, for women who would prefer not to wait for completion, or in cases of early nonviable pregnancies where the location of pregnancy is unknown. In that situation, histologic finding of chorionic villi confirms an IUP.

- Surgical management carries an increased risk of uterine perforation, cervical trauma, and anesthesia complications. Optional preoperative misoprostol treatment with 400 to 600 μg of misoprostol 4 to 6 hours before the procedure or the night before softens the cervix and makes cervical dilation easier.

- Preoperative doxycycline 100 mg PO one hour prior to the procedure or 100 mg IV thirty minutes prior to the procedure may be given. Postoperatively the patient may receive 200 mg PO once 12 hours after the procedure for prevention of infection.

- After a D&C, the serum β-hCG levels are expected to decrease by more than 20% during the following 24 hours.

- The management of septic abortions involves a combination of medical and surgical interventions. The patient must be stabilized, cultures (blood and endometrial) are obtained, and broad-spectrum antibiotics are then administered. Finally, uterine contents are removed via surgical evacuation.

## SECOND-TRIMESTER MISCARRIAGE

### Incidence and Risk

- Second-trimester losses (13 to 27 weeks of gestation) are less common and are often mistakenly grouped with early miscarriages. One percent to 5% of pregnancies result in miscarriage between 13 and 19 weeks' gestation, whereas only 0.3% spontaneously end between 20 and 27 weeks of gestation.

- "Stillbirth" is the customary term of pregnancy loss after 20 weeks of gestation.

- Compared to first- and early second-trimester losses, later second-trimester losses have similar etiologies, such as chromosomal abnormalities, maternal medical conditions, and teratogenic exposures.

- Causative factors more specific to second-trimester miscarriage include cervical insufficiency, thrombophilia, maternal infection or exposures, and placental abruption.

### Presentation, Assessment, and Management

- History should include the following: maternal symptoms of pregnancy loss, obstetric history, past medical and gynecologic history, family history, teratogenic exposures, drug use, and trauma.

- Initial assessment should also include a review of the pregnancy development, such as sequential vital signs, weight progression, sonographic data, and antenatal testing.

- There are several clinical scenarios associated with second-trimester loss:
  - **Cervical insufficiency** is the inability of the cervix to retain a pregnancy in the second trimester and presents as painless cervical dilation without contractions or labor. An ultrasound finding of a short cervix is not sufficient to make this diagnosis. See Chapter 9.
  - **Placental abruption** may present with vaginal bleeding and uterine contractions but can also be occult. Early delivery is recommended and may be performed by cesarean section. Ultrasound does not necessarily diagnose abruption, as a retroplacental clot can be obscured by the placenta itself.
  - **Preterm premature rupture of membranes** is a significant contributor to second-trimester loss. See Chapter 9.

- Discharge instructions and care after a miscarriage are vital components of the treatment. Patients should be instructed to rest the pelvis with nothing placed in the

vagina for at least 2 weeks. They should also be advised to call a doctor for heavy bleeding, fever, or persistent abdominal pain.
- There is no evidence to suggest restrictions on contraceptive use or to recommend delaying future conception following miscarriage.
- Patients should be counseled on their risk of recurrence. These risks are a function of the underlying etiology.
- Acknowledgement of parental grief with provision of emotional support and professional counseling is encouraged.

# RECURRENT PREGNANCY LOSS

**Recurrent pregnancy loss** (RPL) (Table 36-3) has traditionally been defined as three or more consecutive losses of clinically recognized pregnancies <20 weeks of gestation. The American Society for Reproductive Medicine defines RPL as two or more losses at any GA and suggests a thorough evaluation after three or more.
- Primary RPL: recurrent miscarriages (RMs) without a previous viable pregnancy
- Secondary RPL: RPL with previous delivery of a live infant (better prognosis)

## Incidence and Risk
- Five percent of all women will experience two consecutive losses; 1% will have three consecutive losses.
- Incidence of RPL significantly increases with maternal age, but risks also include genetic factors, uterine pathology, endocrine and metabolic factors, immunologic causes, antiphospholipid antibody syndrome, environmental factors, and infectious agents. At least 50% of all cases remain undiagnosed.
- A detailed history and physical examination should be the initial step followed by more specific testing.

## Etiologies and Management
### Genetic Aberration
- The incidence of chromosomal abnormalities in RPL depends on the GA of the pregnancy. It is thought that these abnormalities account for 70% of preclinical RPL and 50% of clinical RPL, similar to spontaneous miscarriages.
- The most common chromosomal abnormalities are autosomal trisomies (in descending frequency—16, 22, 21, 15, and 13), comprising 50% to 60% of clinical RPL cases. Other chromosomal abnormalities in clinical RPL cases include polyploidy (20%), monosomy (18%), and unbalanced translocations (4%).
- Parental karyotyping may be indicated in couples with RPL, particularly in those with three or more clinical miscarriages. When karyotyping is done, one partner in 3% to 5% of couples will be diagnosed with a chromosomal abnormality, usually a balanced translocation. A karyotypic abnormality is more likely with young maternal age, ≥3 losses, or a first-degree relative with RPL. A small percentage of abnormal parental karyotypes include inversions, microdeletions, and mosaicisms.
  - Balanced translocations most commonly appear in the mother. Given this increased prevalence, it is more beneficial to test the mother first followed by the father as needed.
- For evaluation of POCs, gestational tissue with the most successful cell culture growth are placenta, fascia lata, skin from nape of neck, tendons, and blood.
  - These tissues should be placed in normal saline, *not* in formalin.

| TABLE 36-3 | Evaluation for Recurrent Pregnancy Loss |
|---|---|
| *First-line tests* | • Complete medical, surgical, genetic and family history and a physical examination<br>• Sonohysterography to delineate the internal and external contours of the uterus and distinguishes between septate and bicornuate uteri. Other options to evaluate the uterine anatomy include three-dimensional ultrasound and hysterosalpingography.<br>• Anticardiolipin antibody and anti-β2 glycoprotein (IgG and IgM) titers and lupus anticoagulant performed twice, 12 wk apart<br>• Thyroid-stimulating hormone (TSH) and thyroid peroxidase antibodies<br>• Prolactin level<br>• Hemoglobin A1C and fasting glucose. Consider glucose tolerance testing in obese patients.<br>• Parental karyotype and karyotype of the abortus if the above examinations are normal. |
| *Second-line tests* | • Hysteroscopy, laparoscopy, or MRI are more invasive than sonohysterography.<br>• Ovarian reserve can be evaluated by measurement of antral follicle count (AFC), basal serum follicle-stimulating hormone (FSH), and anti-müllerian hormone (AMH). These tests predict ovarian response in assisted reproductive procedures but their usefulness in triaging patients for RPL is questionable. |
| *Evidence does **not** support these tests.* | • Routine cultures for *Chlamydia* or bacterial vaginosis<br>• ANA titers<br>• Progesterone level—Single or multiple serum progesterone levels or endometrial biopsies are not predictive of future pregnancy outcome. |

IgG, immunoglobulin G; IgM, immunoglobulin M; MRI, magnetic resonance imaging; RPL, recurrent pregnancy loss; ANA, antinuclear antibody.

## Uterine Pathology

- Uterine malformations are noted in 10% to 30% of women who experience RPL, compared to approximately 7% in the general population.
- **Congenital** anomalies include developmental defects of the müllerian duct system, such as **septate**, **arcuate**, **bicornuate**, **unicornuate**, and **didelphic uteri**. Septate and bicornuate uteri are most commonly associated with RPL and are hypothesized to interfere with uterine distention or abnormal implantation due to decreased vascularity in a septum, increased inflammation, or reduction in sensitivity to steroid hormones.
- **Acquired** conditions that cause abnormalities within the uterus and cervix include uterine synechiae, leiomyoma, polyps, and cervical laxity or shortening.

- **Leiomyomas** may be **submucosal**, **intramural**, **serosal**, or **pedunculated**. Some studies show that submucosal fibroids may be associated with RPL. Vascular supply to the placenta may be affected due to an unfavorable implantation site, whereas large fibroids may distort the uterine cavity. Fibroids may cause alterations in vascular supply of the endometrium or may interfere with gamete or embryo migration. Similarly, observational studies suggest an increased miscarriage rate in patients with large endometrial polyps but the role of small polyps is unclear.
- **Intrauterine synechiae** may occur after infections or following instrumentation of the uterus. Aggressive postpartum curettage may lead to significant synechiae formation, or Asherman syndrome, that results in insufficient endometrium to support growth.
- Published data have not established that cervical insufficiency is the result of obstetric lacerations, loop electrosurgical excision, cone biopsy, or aggressive dilation in association with D&C procedures.
  ○ According to ACOG, women with prior spontaneous preterm birth at less than 34 weeks of gestation should be offered progesterone supplementation starting between 16 and 24 weeks of gestation. A woman with this history and cervical length less than 25 mm before 24 weeks of gestation should be counseled regarding cerclage placement.

Workup for Uterine Pathology

- A variety of imaging modalities are used in the evaluation and diagnosis of uterine pathology in relation to reproductive loss. Two-dimensional abdominal or transvaginal ultrasound and hysterosalpingography (HSG) are popular screening tools although they have relatively low rates of accuracy.
- HSG aids in examination of the intrauterine cavity, but it is unable to reliably detect subtle uterine pathology.
- Sonohysterography, or saline-infused hysterography, is a more accurate diagnostic tool than plain ultrasound.
  ○ Office hysteroscopy with a flexible hysteroscope is an accurate and well-tolerated method to evaluate the uterine cavity but it does not differentiate a septate and a bicornuate uterus.
- Combined hysteroscopy and laparoscopy remain the most definitive diagnostic approach by providing examination of both internal and external abnormalities. This method is also therapeutic, as it permits septal resection if needed.
- Three-dimensional transvaginal ultrasound and magnetic resonance imaging are also promising tools to aid in displaying uterine morphology in women with RPL. Three-dimensional ultrasound seems to be the most accurate imaging modality for the exterior contour of the uterus, which can help differentiate septate and bicornuate uteri.
- Resection of uterine septa (septoplasty), hysteroscopic lysis of adhesions, myomectomy, polypectomy, and cervical cerclage placement are all treatments for congenital and acquired uterine abnormalities.

*Endocrine/Metabolic Dysfunction*

- Endocrine and metabolic factors are implicated in 15% to 60% of RM cases.
- Poorly controlled **diabetes mellitus** (A1C >8%) and **obesity** have been associated with increased risk of miscarriages. See Chapter 13. Strict glycemic control should be reinforced prior to conception to decrease fetal anomalies. Pregnancy loss is increased in obese women, possibly due to insulin resistance. Weight loss prior to pregnancy improves pregnancy outcome.

- Luteal phase deficiency:
  - Functional corpus luteum defects or abnormal endometrial progesterone receptors are thought to contribute to the RPL rate, especially embryonic losses. Currently, there is no reliable means to diagnose luteal phase deficiency using either serum progesterone measurements or serial endometrial biopsies.
  - Progestational agents are available in various preparations, including oral, vaginal, and intramuscular (IM) formulations.
    - Oral supplementation has proven to be the most convenient but less efficacious due to its rapid metabolism and inability to bolster the progestational effect at the level of the uterus.
    - There are no differences in efficacy of IM versus vaginal routes of progestational agents with regard to pregnancy or miscarriage rates.
    - However, given the side effect profile of IM progesterone agents (e.g., pain, risk of bleeding and abscess formation, oil allergy, inconvenience), trials are underway to compare several vaginal options (usually 25 to 100 μg twice daily), including gel (for instance Prometrium R or Crinone R) and micronized insert (Endometrin R).
  - Although studies have shown no statistically significant difference in the miscarriage rate between those receiving progesterone and those receiving placebo, there is a significant difference when stratified for obstetric history (i.e., three or more previous consecutive losses).

*Polycystic Ovarian Syndrome*

- A 20% risk of miscarriage has been noted in this population of women.
- Proposed mechanisms for explanation of the increased risk of miscarriage with polycystic ovarian syndrome (PCOS) include hyperandrogenism, elevated luteinizing hormone levels, obesity, hyperinsulinemia, premature or delayed ovulation, metabolic derangements of prostaglandins, growth factors, and elevated cytokines.
- Metformin has been shown to decrease miscarriage rate in women with PCOS in some studies, but randomized controlled trials offer no definitive evidence.
  - Existing prospective studies show no evidence of teratogenicity or developmental problems in the first 18 months of life in the infants of mothers who used metformin in early pregnancy. Some studies advocate using metformin 500 to 2,500 mg by mouth daily through the first trimester in affected women.

*Thyroid Dysfunction*

- Clinical and subclinical hypo- and hyperthyroidism are thought to have an association with RPL, interfering with implantation, but causation has not been demonstrated. Thyroxine therapy should be initiated in hypothyroid patients prior to conception. See Chapter 13 for thyroid disorders.
- Thyroperoxidase antibodies: if present, therapy with thyroxin decreases the risk of miscarriage.

*Hyperprolactinemia*

- In a study of 64 hyperprolactinemic women treated with bromocriptine, there was a higher rate of pregnancy (86% vs. 52%); however, research is limited on whether this intervention leads to higher rates of pregnancies without miscarriage.
- **Antiphospholipid syndrome (APS)**
  - Antiphospholipid antibodies (e.g., lupus anticoagulant, anticardiolipin or anti-β2 glycoprotein antibodies) are formed against vascular endothelium and platelets, eventually leading to vascular constriction and thrombosis. Thrombus may lead

to placental infarction and second-trimester fetal losses. Five percent to 15% of patients with RPL may have APS.

- Criteria for APS include at least one clinical and one laboratory data point.
  - Clinical criteria:
    - One or more episodes of arterial, venous, or small vessel thrombosis
    - One or more unexplained pregnancy loss of a morphologically normal fetus of greater than or equal to 10 weeks of gestation
    - One or more premature births of morphologically normal fetus at less than or equal to 34 weeks' GA due to pregnancy-induced hypertension or placental insufficiency
    - Three or more consecutive miscarriages before 10 weeks of gestation excluding anatomic, hormonal, and parental genetic factors
  - Laboratory criteria (any of the following):
    - Two positive titers of moderate to high dilution at least 12 weeks apart of anti-cardiolipin or anti-β2 glycoprotein immunoglobulin (Ig) G or IgM antibodies
    - Lupus anticoagulant (Russel viper venom test) on two occasions at least 12 weeks apart
- Studies have shown improved pregnancy outcome in women with APS who receive antithrombotic therapy.
  - Treatment with unfractionated heparin and low-dose acetylsalicylic acid (ASA) is more effective than ASA alone in increasing the live birth rate—80% compared to 40%, respectively.
  - Some studies have suggested that low-molecular-weight heparin (LMWH) may be equipotent compared to the unfractionated heparin. The benefit of LMWH is that it carries a decreased risk of heparin-induced thrombocytopenia, heparin-induced osteopenia, and maternal bleeding.

## Hereditary Thrombophilias

- Retrospective data suggests a modest association between thrombophilias and RPL. However, prospective studies have failed to give proof to this connection. Therefore, anticoagulation is not recommended for preventing RPL.
- Miscarriage risk is highest in the second and third trimesters. It is hypothesized that thrombosis in the low-flow spiral arteries leads to inadequate perfusion and precedes a cascade of events leading to late fetal loss.
- Hyperhomocysteinemia (>15 mmol/L) is associated with increased risk of RPL and placental abruption. Mutations are autosomal recessive, placing only homozygotes at increased risk; therefore, routine testing is not recommended.

## Immune Dysfunction

- Autoimmune and alloimmune factors may cause RPL similar to graft rejection or defects of the complement system.
- Celiac disease is thought to be associated with RPL and infertility and treatment appears to prevent these problems; thus women with RPL should be screened.
- Alloimmunity reflects the theory that pregnancy survival depends on maternal tolerance to foreign fetal antigens instead of maternal sensitization leading to activation of the immune response.
- Historically, attempted therapies have included leukocyte immunization, intravenous gamma immune globulin, third-party donor cell immunization, and trophoblast membrane immunization; however, these are not recommended.
- There are currently no evidence-based methods for clinical use to evaluate or treat possible immune system–related RPL.

*Infection and Environmental Exposures*

- Infectious agents (*Listeria*, *Toxoplasma*, cytomegalovirus, and primary herpes simplex virus) are known causes of miscarriage, but there is no proof of their role in RPL. Therefore, bacterial or viral cultures are not a part of the workup for RPL.
- Chemicals associated with RPL include formaldehyde, pesticides, lead, mercury, benzene, and anesthetic gases, such as nitrous oxide.
- Stress and exercise have not been found to increase the risk of RPL.

*Management*

- Stress and anxiety should be considered while caring for couples who experience RM. Consider psychosocial or spiritual support or counseling.
- Progesterone treatment empirically in patients with multiple early miscarriages of unknown etiology
- Abnormal karyotype: Referral for genetic counseling. Patient may be offered chorionic villus sampling, amniocentesis, and preimplantation genetic testing.
- Uterine abnormalities: surgical management if possible
- APS: aspirin and heparin
- Obesity: weight loss and nutrition counseling
- Correction of thyroid dysfunction
- PCOS: possibly metformin
- Hyperprolactinemia: cabergoline or bromocriptine
- Studies have shown that emotional support, close surveillance with frequent office visits, phone calls, and even serial ultrasound studies improve pregnancy outcomes.
- These strategies have been shown in controlled studies to halve the RM rate (from >50% to 25%) in the absence of any medical or surgical intervention.
- **Therapies of no proven benefit:**
  - Thrombophilias: Anticoagulation for thrombophilias other than APS does not decrease RPL.
  - Immunotherapy or steroids for allo-/autoimmunity
  - Antibiotic treatment for *Ureaplasma*- or *Mycoplasma*-positive cervical cultures

## SUGGESTED READINGS

American College of Obstetricians and Gynecologists. ACOG practice bulletin no. 24: management of recurrent early pregnancy loss. *Int J Gynaecol Obstet* 2002;78(2):179–190.

American College of Obstetricians and Gynecologists. ACOG practice bulletin no. 142: cerclage for management of cervical insufficiency. *Obstet Gynecol* 2014;123(2, pt 1):372–379.

American College of Obstetricians and Gynecologists Committee on Genetics. ACOG committee opinion no. 581: the use of chromosomal microarray analysis in prenatal diagnosis. *Obstet Gynecol* 2013;122(6):1374–1377.

Jauniaux E, Farquharson RG, Christiansen OB, et al. Evidence-based guidelines for the investigation and medical treatment of recurrent miscarriage. *Hum Reprod* 2006;21(9):2216–2222.

Michels TC, Tiu AY. Second trimester pregnancy loss. *Am Fam Phys* 2007;76(9):1341–1346.

Practice Committee of the American Society for Reproductive Medicine. Evaluation and treatment of recurrent pregnancy loss: a committee opinion. *Fertil Steril* 2012;98(5):15–28.

Robinson L, Gallos ID, Conner SJ, et al. The effect of sperm DNA fragmentation on miscarriage rates: a systematic review and meta-analysis. *Hum Reprod* 2012;27(1):2908–2012.

Trott EA, Russell JB, Plouffe L Jr. A review of the genetics of recurrent pregnancy loss. *Del Med J* 1996;68(10):495.

Zhang J, Gilles JM, Barnhart K, et al. A comparison of medical management with misoprostol and surgical management for early pregnancy failure. *N Engl J Med* 2005;353(8):761–769.

# 37 Uterine Leiomyomas

Cindy M. P. Duke, Diana Cholakian, and
Stacey A. Scheib

**Uterine leiomyomas**, also known as myomas or fibroids, represent the most common pelvic tumors in women. As benign smooth muscle neoplasms, leiomyomas only rarely undergo malignant transformation (<0.5%).

- Incidence is 30% to 70% in reproductive age women and increases with age. Lifetime risk is about 70% for whites and >80% in blacks.
- The majority of patients with fibroids are asymptomatic, only about 25% of reproductive age women have symptoms. Symptoms may include pelvic pressure, urinary or fecal complaints, reproductive dysfunction, and prolonged or heavy menstruation.
- Leiomyomas represent the single most common indication for hysterectomy and currently, there are several medical and surgical treatment options, including minimally invasive options.

## ETIOLOGY AND PATHOPHYSIOLOGY

- Leiomyomas result from monoclonal proliferation of uterine smooth muscle cells or less commonly from smooth muscle cells of uterine blood vessels. They can range in size from millimeters to large tumors reaching the costal margin. These tumors may be solitary or multiple and are classified by location within the uterus. These cells express estrogen synthetase and aromatase and are capable of converting androgens into estrogen.
- **Submucosal fibroids** develop from myometrium just deep to the endometrial lining. These can often protrude into the endometrial cavity or, if pedunculated, can even grow past the internal cervical os. The main symptoms of this subgroup of fibroids include heavy or abnormal bleeding, reduced fertility, miscarriages, and preterm labor.
- **Intramural fibroids**, located within the uterine corpus wall, may distort the uterine cavity. **Cervical fibroids** are intramural but found in the uterine cervix.
- **Subserosal fibroids** develop below the serosal layer, are often pedunculated, and occasionally extend between folds of the broad ligament. They do not cause abnormal uterine bleeding but more likely contribute to bulk symptoms.
- **Extrauterine fibroids** are leiomyomas that are found outside of the uterus. They are usually the result of hematogenous spread of neoplastic smooth muscle cells from the uterus. Extrauterine fibroids are histologically and clinically identical to the intrauterine fibroids described earlier. Extrauterine locations most commonly include the genitourinary tract, the gut mesentery, and the cardiopulmonary system. Other rarer locations include the spinal cord and blood vessels.
- A genetic basis for the presence and growth of uterine leiomyomas appears likely. Family history of leiomyomas increases an individual's risk 1.5- to 3.5-fold. It has been suggested that up to 40% of leiomyomas have associated chromosome abnormalities, including deletion of portions of 7q, trisomy 12, or rearrangements

(translocations) of chromosomes 6, 10, and 12. The Val158Met polymorphism on the catechol-O-methyltransferase (COMT) gene has been found to be a protective factor against uterine leiomyoma. The incidence of leiomyomas is estimated to be threefold greater among African American women and often occur at a younger age in this population. In addition, fibroids in African American women respond differently than those in white women. Decreased vitamin D levels may be an etiology for this increased incidence, as darker skin inhibits autologous vitamin D production.

- The growth of uterine leiomyomas is related to circulating estrogen exposure. Progesterone may exert an antiestrogen effect on the growth of leiomyomas. Fibroids are most prominent and demonstrate maximal growth during the reproductive years and tend to regress after menopause. Whenever leiomyomas grow after menopause, malignancy (e.g., leiomyosarcoma) must be considered in the differential diagnosis. Leiomyomas commonly grow during pregnancy, most likely due to the enhanced uterine blood supply that accompanies pregnancy and edematous changes in these tumors.

- As leiomyomas grow, they risk diminution of blood supply, which leads to a continuum of degenerative changes, including calcium deposition. Calcific change can be appreciated radiographically as a diffuse honeycomb pattern, a series of concentric rings, or a solid calcific mass. Necrosis, cystic changes, and fatty degeneration are manifestations of compromised blood supply secondary to growth or infarction from torsion of a pedunculated leiomyoma. Histologically, degenerative changes in myomas may also be seen with progesterone stimulation or, less frequently, malignant transformation.

- Although malignant degeneration of leiomyomas is possible, most **leiomyosarcomas** are thought to arise de novo. Leiomyosarcomas are diagnosed on the basis of counts of 10 or more mitotic figures per 10 high-power fields (HPFs). Those tumors with 5 to 10 mitotic figures per 10 HPFs are referred to as smooth muscle tumors of uncertain malignant potential. Tumors with <5 mitotic figures per 10 HPFs and little cytologic atypia are classified as cellular leiomyomas.

## COST IMPACT OF UTERINE FIBROIDS

- The management of symptomatic fibroids is expensive in both cost and disability. Costs fall under two categories: direct costs (costs of surgery, hospital admissions, outpatient visits, imaging studies, lab work, medications) and indirect costs (costs of lost work time because of absenteeism and short-term disability).

- A review of national health care databases in the United States estimated that the total direct annual cost for treatment (surgery and medications) of fibroids range between 4.1 and 9.4 billion dollars.

- A number of investigators have also looked more specifically at direct and indirect costs for treatment of symptomatic fibroids in individual patients using retrospective reviews of national health care databases and health maintenance organization reimbursement records. Costs can range anywhere from $5,900 to $20,000 per patient annually, when compared to matched controls without fibroids. A review of annual costs associated with the diagnosis of leiomyomas in women with imaging-confirmed fibroids showed a 3.1-fold increase in cost for diagnostic procedures; 10-fold increase in ultrasonic, hysteroscopic, and laparoscopic procedures; and a 35-fold greater rate of surgical procedures. Additionally, it showed that women with fibroids were 50 times more likely to get a hysterectomy than women without fibroids and were 3.1 times more likely to file disability claims.

- Symptomatic fibroids also lead to significant burden to employers, especially in the time following surgical procedures. The estimated overall lost work hour costs range from $1.55 to $17.2 billion annually.
- Overall, it is estimated that uterine fibroids cost the United States between $5.9 and $34.4 billion annually.
- Additionally, the annual cost of obstetric outcomes in the United States attributable to fibroid tumors is estimated at $238 million to $7.76 billion.

## CLINICAL MANIFESTATIONS AND DIAGNOSIS

### Signs and Symptoms

- Most patients with leiomyomas are asymptomatic. The most commonly experienced symptoms (pain, pressure, fertility dysfunction, and menorrhagia) are related to the size and location of the fibroids or to compromise of blood supply with degeneration.
- Uterine fibroids may be found on routine pelvic exam when an enlarged or irregularly shaped uterus is palpated.
- Various radiologic modalities may be useful for the diagnosis and/or characterization of uterine fibroids (Table 37-1).

| TABLE 37-1 | Diagnostic Imaging for Uterine Leiomyomas | |
|---|---|---|
| **Diagnostic Modality** | **Advantages** | **Disadvantages** |
| Hysterosalpingogram | Evaluates the contour of the uterine cavity and fallopian tube patency | Does not provide the exact location of the fibroids. Not appropriate for evaluation of subserosal fibroids. |
| Sonohysterography | Characterizes the location and amount of distortion caused by submucosal fibroids | Decreased accuracy in localizing fibroids, compared to MRI, especially in patients with a large uterus or multiple fibroids |
| Transvaginal sonogram | Useful for detection and evaluation of fibroid growth | Decreased accuracy in localizing fibroids, compared to MRI, especially in patients with a large uterus or multiple fibroids |
| Magnetic resonance imaging | Identifies the size and location of fibroids for the best surgical planning; useful before uterine artery embolization | Increased cost |

- **Excessive or prolonged menstrual bleeding** is the most frequently encountered symptom and may be due to vascular alterations in the endometrium. The obstructive effect on uterine vasculature produced by intramural tumors has been associated with the development of endometrial venule ectasia. This tends to be due to vasoactive growth factors. As a result, leiomyomas give rise to proximal congestion of the myometrium and endometrium. The engorged vessels in the thin atrophic endometrium that overlies submucosal tumors contribute to excessive bleeding during cyclic sloughing. The increased size of the uterine cavity also gives rise to the increased volume of menstrual flow.
- Patients may also present with **pressure** to adjacent organs and **increased abdominal girth**. Pressure on the bladder customarily provokes **urinary frequency**. When the leiomyoma is adjacent to the bladder neck and urethra, incontinence or acute urinary retention with overflow incontinence may occur. Ureteral obstruction is a rare complication of larger leiomyomas extending to the pelvic sidewall causing hydronephrosis. Posteriorly located fibroids may produce **constipation**, rectal pressure, or tenesmus. With especially enlarged uteri, patients can also present with back pain, lower extremity swelling, or radiating pain down one or both legs.
- **Chronic pain** symptoms may include dysmenorrhea, dyspareunia, and noncyclic pelvic pain. Acute pain may be a consequence of torsion of the stalk of a pedunculated leiomyoma, cervical dilation by a submucosal leiomyoma protruding through the lower uterine segment, or degeneration of a leiomyoma.
- Submucosal and intramural fibroids are associated with a higher rate of spontaneous miscarriage and **infertility/subfertility** due to impaired implantation, tubal function, or sperm transport. Although it has been shown that removal of submucosal fibroids significantly improves fertility outcomes, there is conflicting evidence regarding the effect of intramural myomectomy on future fertility. Subserosal fibroids are not associated with subfertility.
- **Obstetric complications** that are associated with a fibroid uterus include miscarriage, preterm labor and delivery, malpresentation, cesarean delivery, postpartum hemorrhage, and peripartum hysterectomy. Less common adverse outcomes that may be related to fibroids include intrauterine growth restriction, abnormal placentation, first-trimester bleeding, preterm premature rupture of membranes, abruption, and labor dystocia.

## TREATMENT FOR LEIOMYOMAS

### Observation

- No standard size of an asymptomatic myomatous uterus has been determined as an absolute indication for treatment. In a patient with a large asymptomatic myomatous uterus in whom dimensions have not increased and malignancy is unlikely, the patient's age, fertility status, and desire to retain the uterus or avoid surgery must be factored into the treatment plan. Physical and radiologic imaging examinations should be performed initially and may be repeated in 6 months to document the size and growth pattern of the fibroids. If growth is stable, the patient may be followed clinically with annual pelvic examination and imaging as indicated.
- Rapidly growing fibroids can raise concern for malignancy, especially in the menopausal patient. The definition of rapid growth, however, is highly variable. One commonly accepted definition is an increase of 6 weeks size over 1 year. Postmenopausal uterine growth or bleeding increases the suspicion for malignancy; however, premenopausal women with rapid growth do not necessarily require surgical excision.

## Medical Therapy

- **Nonhormonal** medical therapy is aimed at controlling the symptoms of leiomyomas, specifically excessive menstrual flow or pain. Such therapies include tranexamic acid and nonsteroidal anti-inflammatory drugs.
- **Hormonal** therapy for fibroids includes contraceptive steroids, progestins, and gonadotropin-releasing agonists or antagonists. Investigations are underway regarding treatments such as aromatase inhibitors, selective estrogen receptor modulators (SERMs), gonadotropin-releasing hormone antagonists, and selective progesterone receptor modulators. A recent study showed a reduction in the size of fibroids after treatment with SERMs.
  - Similar to the nonhormonal medical options, combinations of estrogen and progesterone may control bleeding symptoms while preventing leiomyoma growth. There is conflicting evidence regarding the effect of **progestational therapy** on changes in fibroid or uterine volume, with some small studies showing a decrease in leiomyoma size during treatment. Conversely, use of mifepristone, an **antiprogestin**, has been associated with decrease in the size of leiomyomas with slow rate of regrowth following treatment cessation.
  - The **levonorgestrel-releasing intrauterine system (LNG-IUS)**, or Mirena, slowly delivers progesterone directly to the uterus and significantly reduces menstrual bleeding. The effect of the LNG-IUS on myoma-mediated menorrhagia depends on the size of uterine cavity and patient characteristics of blood loss. A review of various studies has shown that when compared to combined oral contraceptives, the LNG-IUS significantly decreases fibroid-related menstrual bleeding. No significant decrease of fibroid or uterine volume has been demonstrated.
  - **Gonadotropin-releasing hormone analogs (GnRHa)** have been used successfully to achieve hypoestrogenism in various estrogen-dependent conditions. Maximal reduction in tumor volume of approximately 50% has been observed with the use of GnRHa over a 3-month course of treatment. The effects of hormonal treatment are transient, and within 6 months after withdrawal of hormonal therapy, leiomyomas return to their pretreatment state.
    - These agents are useful as a conservative therapy in perimenopausal women or as an adjunct to surgical treatment. Longer than 6 months of GnRHa therapy in young patients is neither practical nor desirable because of the possibility of bone loss. Common side effects of GnRHa include hot flashes, nausea, vomiting, diarrhea, constipation, rash, dizziness, acne, breast tenderness, and headaches.
    - Concomitant treatment with a low dose of steroid hormone, referred to as **add-back therapy**, can be used to minimize the adverse affects of GnRHa in patients who benefit from continued therapy after the initial 3-month course.
    - Adjunctive presurgical therapy with a 3- to 6-month course of GnRHa can reduce tumor size. Thus, use prior to scheduled hysterectomy may increase the likelihood of success of a minimally invasive approach. Additionally, by inducing amenorrhea, GnRHa therapy enables a patient to preoperatively restore her own hemoglobin levels from baseline menorrhagia-related iron deficiency anemia. There is no decrease in estimated blood loss. However, its preoperative use is associated with obscuring of surgical planes between fibroids and normal myometrium, which may make myomectomy more difficult.
  - **Aromatase inhibitors** have been shown to reduce the volume of fibroids without leading to the side effects caused by systemic hormonal therapy.

## Surgical Therapy

*Myomectomy*

- **Myomectomy**, or surgical excision of the fibroid tissue, is the only surgical option that is available when future childbearing is desired. The location and size of the myoma(s), along with surgical expertise of the operator, dictate the approach to myomectomy. Subserosal or intramural fibroids may be resected abdominally, laparoscopically, or with robotic assistance. Submucosal myomectomy should be performed hysteroscopically (preferred) or vaginally.
- Complications following myomectomy include substantial blood loss, paralytic ileus, and pain. The risk of postoperative adhesive disease following abdominal myomectomy is about 25% but may be as high as 90%. A laparoscopic approach with the use of an adhesion barrier at the time of surgery may reduce this risk by half. The recurrence risk of leiomyomas is roughly 30% following myomectomy.
- For patients who wish to conceive, a delay of 4 to 6 months after surgery before attempting pregnancy is advisable, especially if there was significant myometrial disturbance. The most common obstetric complications following myomectomy include uterine rupture, abnormal placentation, and preterm delivery. The preferred delivery method after myomectomy with extensive uterine reconstruction is cesarean section due to an increased risk of uterine rupture with labor.

*Hysterectomy*

- Removal of the uterus is the **definitive procedure** for treatment of symptomatic leiomyomas. Hysterectomy should also be considered in the event of a rapidly enlarging tumor or postmenopausal patients, in which a reasonable likelihood of malignancy exists. If malignancy is suspected, referral to a gynecologic oncologist preoperatively or at the time of surgery is advised.
- Surgical approaches to hysterectomy include abdominal, vaginal, laparoscopic, and robotic-assisted. The option of single-incision surgery may be available with laparoscopic and robotic-assisted modalities. Similar to myomectomy, the method of approach is dictated by size, location, number, patient comorbidities, and surgical expertise.
- Patient satisfaction with symptom relief from hysterectomy is very high but accompanied by the surgical morbidity of a major operation. Additionally, some patients have expressed posthysterectomy regret regarding loss of fertility; therefore, adequate preoperative counseling including discussion of desire for, timing of, and planning for future childbearing is essential.

*Uterine Artery Embolization*

- **Uterine artery embolization (UAE)** decreases the blood supply to the uterus and ultimately causes ischemic necrosis of leiomyomas. The procedure is performed by interventional radiologists and usually involves catheterization of the femoral artery to gain access to the hypogastric arteries. Under fluoroscopic guidance, the uterine arteries are occluded with substances such as Gelfoam, absolute alcohol, Ivalon particles (polyvinyl alcohol), or metal coils. This procedure is generally reserved for intramural myomas.
- The benefits of UAE include short operating and recovery time, use of local anesthesia, and minimal blood loss. Risks of the procedure include infection (4%), complications of angiography (3%), and uterine ischemia or nontarget embolization. Premature ovarian failure secondary to compromise of the ovarian circulation has

been reported. Patients typically experience cramping for the first 12 to 18 hours after the procedure. Postembolization syndrome (fever, nausea, vomiting, and severe abdominal pain) has been observed in approximately 30% of patients.

- Outcomes of UAE include a 40% to 60% reduction in uterine size and decreased menstrual bleeding with high rates of patient satisfaction. Patients have significantly less postoperative pain and return to work sooner compared to those undergoing hysterectomy but have increased rates of minor complications. Long-term outcomes may be inferior to myomectomy and hysterectomy, with the rate of reoperation in patients undergoing UAE as high as 30%. The reoperation rate is age dependent, with higher likelihood of success in women older than age 40 years.

- The impact on postprocedure fertility has not been well-studied. However, UAE is not generally recommended in patients who desire future fertility. Initial case reports and case series of pregnancy after UAE indicate an increased risk of obstetric complications such as preterm labor, miscarriage, malpresentation, and abnormal placentation (e.g., placenta accreta). Myomectomy is still the procedure of choice in patients with symptomatic fibroids who desire future fertility.

*Magnetic Resonance Imaging–Guided Focused Ultrasound Surgery*

- With magnetic resonance imaging–guided focused ultrasound surgery (MRgFUS), fibroid tissue is heated and destroyed using targeted ultrasonic energy passing through the anterior abdominal wall. This procedure is performed with magnetic resonance imaging (MRI) thermal mapping and conducted over several outpatient visits. MRgFUS is not appropriate for pedunculated myomas or those adjacent to bowel or bladder. Although the procedure is currently U.S. Food and Drug Administration approved for premenopausal women who do not desire future fertility, outcome data beyond 24 months is lacking. Potential side effects include skin or nerve burns.

- Studies are being performed to investigate similar MRI-guided radiofrequency ablation or laser photocoagulation techniques.

*Myolysis/Cryomyolysis*

- **Laparoscopic coagulation** of a leiomyoma, or myolysis, is performed with a neodymium: yttrium-aluminum-garnet (YAG) laser by causing degeneration of protein and destruction of vascularity. Dense pelvic adhesions have been found on follow-up. Bipolar coagulation and cryomyolysis affect similar results using radio-frequency energy or supercooling, respectively. There is limited long-term efficacy or safety data for these methods, and they are not recommended for women desiring future fertility.

*Laparoscopic Uterine Artery Occlusion*

- **Laparoscopic uterine artery occlusion** accesses the uterine arteries retroperitoneally and surgically occluded. Similar short-term outcomes to UAE have been shown; however, there is limited longitudinal data.

*Doppler-Guided Uterine Artery Occlusion*

- **Doppler-guided uterine artery occlusion**, currently in development, uses a transvaginal vascular clamp with Doppler guidance to occlude the uterine arteries for 6 hours after which time the clamp is removed at the bedside. This may be a future alternative to UAE.

## SUGGESTED READINGS

American College of Obstetricians and Gynecologists. ACOG practice bulletin no. 96: alternatives to hysterectomy in the management of leiomyomas. *Obstet Gynecol* 2008;112:387–400.

Breech LL, Rock JA. Leiomyomata uteri and myomectomy. In Rock JA, Jones HW, eds. *Telinde's Operative Gynecology*, 10th ed. Philadelphia, PA: Lippincott Williams & Wilkins, 2008:687–727.

Cardozo ER, Clark AD, Banks NK, et al. The estimated annual cost of uterine leiomyomata in the United States. *Am J Obstet Gynecol* 2012;206(3):211.e1–211.e9.

Carls GS, Lee DW, Ozminkowski RJ, et al. What are the total costs of surgical treatment for uterine fibroids? *J Wom Health* 2008;17(7):1119–1132.

Eltoukhi HM, Modi MN, Weston M, et al. The health disparities of uterine fibroid tumors for African American women: a public health issue. *Am J Obstet Gynecol* 2014;210(3):194–199.

Gupta JK, Sinha A, Lumsden M, et al. Uterine artery embolization for symptomatic uterine fibroids (review). *Cochrane Database Syst Rev* 2012;(5):CD005073.

Lee DW, Ozminkowski RJ, Carls GS, et al. The direct and indirect cost of burden of clinically significant and symptomatic uterine fibroids. *J Occup Environ Med* 2007;49:493–506.

Levy G, Hill MJ, Beall S, et al. Leiomyoma: genetics, assisted reproduction, pregnancy and therapeutic advances. *J Assist Reprod Genet* 2012;(29):703–712.

Pritts EA, Parker WH, Olive DL. Fibroids and infertility: an updated systematic review of the evidence. *Fertil Steril* 2009;91(4):1215–1223.

Sangkomkamhang US, Lumbiganon P, Laopaiboon M, et al. Progestogens or progestogen-releasing intrauterine systems for uterine fibroids. *Cochrane Database Syst Rev* 2013;(2):CD008994.

Van der Kooij SM, Ankum WM, Hehenkamp WJ. Review of nonsurgical/minimally invasive treatments for uterine fibroids. *Curr Opin Obstet Gynecol* 2012;24:368–375.

# 38 Menstrual Disorders: Endometriosis, Dysmenorrhea, and Premenstrual Dysphoric Disorder

Irene Woo and Melissa Yates

## ENDOMETRIOSIS

**Endometriosis** is defined as the extrauterine presence of functioning endometrial glands and stroma. It is most commonly found in the ovaries but also located in the pouch of Douglas, vesicouterine space, uterosacral ligaments, and surrounding pelvic peritoneum. It is less commonly seen in laparotomy and episiotomy scars; appendix, pleural, and pericardial cavities; and the cervix.

## Theories of the Pathogenesis of Endometriosis

- The etiology of endometriosis is unknown. Several theories involving anatomic, immunologic, hormonal, and genetic factors have been postulated.
- **Retrograde menstruation:** Sampson's original theory suggests that endometriosis is related to retrograde menstruation of endometrial tissue via the fallopian tubes into the peritoneal cavity. Support for this theory is as follows:
  - Blood flow from the fimbriated ends of fallopian tubes has been visualized during laparoscopy (seen in 90% of women with patent fallopian tubes).
  - Endometriosis is most often found in the dependent portions of the pelvis.
  - Incidence of endometriosis is higher in women with obstruction to normal outward menstrual flow (e.g., cervical stenosis).
  - Endometriosis is more common in women with shorter menstrual cycles or longer duration of flow, providing more opportunity for endometrial implantation.
- **Immunologic factors:** Increasing data suggest that specific immunologic factors at the site of endometrial implants play a major role in determining whether and to what extent a patient will develop the disease. These factors are thought to explain the attachment and proliferation of the endometriotic cells.
- **Inflammatory factors:** Elevated levels of interleukin-6 and tumor necrosis factor-$\alpha$ have been noted in the peritoneal fluid of endometriosis patients. Interleukin-8 may help in the attachment of endometrial implants in the peritoneum and is also an angiogenic agent.
- **Hormonal factors:** Unlike normal endometrial tissue, endometriotic implants can produce aromatase, leading to extraovarian estrogen production. This may explain why endometriosis can recur in women who have undergone hysterectomy and bilateral salpingo-oophorectomy. Prostaglandin $E_2$, a proinflammatory compound, has been shown to be a powerful inducer of aromatase activity in endometriotic implants.
- **Coelomic metaplasia:** This theory postulates that totipotential cells of the ovary and peritoneum are transformed into endometriotic lesions by repeated hormonal or infectious stimuli. This may explain the finding of endometriosis in mature teratomas and extraperitoneal sites.
- **Lymphatic spread:** One study showed that 29% of women with endometriosis at autopsy had positive pelvic lymph nodes for the disease. Thus, lymphatic spread may be another mechanism to explain why endometriotic implants can be found in remote anatomic areas, such as the lung.
- **Genetic factors:** Women who have a first-degree relative with endometriosis have a sevenfold greater risk of developing endometriosis. The mode of inheritance is most likely multifactorial.

## Patient Characteristics

- Mean age at diagnosis is 25 to 30 years. The greatest incidence has been observed in nulliparous women with early age at menarche and shorter menstrual cycles. Increased parity and greater cumulative lactation have been shown to be protective factors in development of endometriosis.
- Although some women with endometriosis are asymptomatic, the most common symptoms are infertility and pelvic pain.
  - **Infertility:** Incidence of endometriosis is believed to be 20% to 40% among infertile couples, with some studies showing endometriosis to be 7 to 10 times more likely in this patient group. Often, asymptomatic patients undergoing laparoscopy for infertility often will be diagnosed with mild endometriosis.

- **Pelvic pain:** Seventy-one percent to 87% of women with chronic pelvic pain have endometriosis. Endometrial lesions can lead to chronic inflammation with increase in inflammatory cytokines and subsequent overproduction of prostaglandins, both of which can be a source of pain. Furthermore, endometriotic lesions may harbor high levels of nerve growth factors. However, the severity of pelvic pain does not correlate with the amount of endometriosis present. The pain typically associated with endometriosis is central, deep, and often in the rectal area. Unilateral pain may be compatible with lesions in the ovary or pelvic sidewall. Dysuria or dyschezia can result from urinary or intestinal tract involvement, respectively, and oftentimes predict deeply infiltrating endometriosis. Forty percent to 50% of patients with deep dyspareunia have been found to have endometriosis.
- Incidence of endometriosis in patients with dysmenorrhea is believed to be 40% to 60%. One study found endometriotic implants in approximately 70% of teenagers who underwent laparoscopy for chronic pelvic pain. Dysmenorrhea often starts before the onset of menstrual bleeding and continues until bleeding abates.

## Abnormal Clinical Findings Associated with Endometriosis

- Nodularity of the uterosacral ligaments, which are often tender and enlarged
- Painful swelling of the rectovaginal septum
- Pain with motion of the uterus and adnexa
- Fixed retroverted uterus and large immobile adnexa are indicative of severe pelvic disease.

## Confirmation of Diagnosis

- **Definitive diagnosis** can be made only through **histology** and examination of lesions removed at the time of surgery. Histology reveals both endometrial glands and stroma. Hemosiderin-laden macrophages have been identified in 77% of endometriosis biopsy specimens. Pelvic ultrasonography can be useful in differentiating the presence of endometriomas from other adnexal masses.
- Experienced clinicians often presumptively diagnose endometriosis based on clinical history and timing of symptoms. First-line therapy with oral contraceptive pills can be initiated without a surgical diagnosis; however, when this fails, a thorough survey of the pelvis via **diagnostic laparoscopy** is recommended. Endometriotic lesions classically appear as blue-black powder-burn visual appearance; however, studies have reported a marked discrepancy in appearance of the lesions and the histology. Nonclassic lesions may appear vesicular, red, white, tan, or nonpigmented. The presence of defects in the peritoneum (usually scarring overlying endometrial implants) is known as Allen-Masters syndrome. Endometriomas, "chocolate cysts," appear filled with dark brown blood.

## Medical Treatment

- Estrogen stimulates the growth of endometriotic implants similar to its effect on normal endometrial tissue. Medical therapy is aimed at suppressing ovarian estrogen stimulation by interrupting the hypothalamic-pituitary-ovarian axis. Inhibition of ovulation by gonadotropin suppression removes the stimulation of endometriosis by cycling sex steroids.
- **Oral contraceptive pills (OCPs):** These pills cause anovulation and decidualization, which results in atrophy of endometrial tissue. Symptomatic relief of pelvic pain and dysmenorrhea is reported in 60% to 95% of patients. However, the

estrogenic component may potentially stimulate growth and increase pain during the first few weeks of treatment. The recommended dose is a 20- to 30-mg ethinyl estradiol pill. Continuous combined OCPs can provide significant pain relief in patients suffering mainly from dysmenorrhea.

- **Gonadotropin-releasing hormone (GnRH) agonists:** when given over the long-term suppress pituitary function by downregulating pituitary GnRH receptors. This interruption of the hypothalamic-pituitary-ovarian axis produces a "medical oophorectomy" or "pseudomenopause." Three available agents are leuprolide acetate (Lupron Depot), 3.75 mg by intramuscular injection every month for 6 months; nafarelin acetate nasal spray, 200 μg twice daily for 6 months; and goserelin acetate (Zoladex), 3.6 mg subcutaneous implants at 28-day intervals for 6 months. Side effects are related to the hypoestrogenic state. The U.S. Food and Drug Administration (FDA) has approved the use of a 12-month course to avoid the long-term consequences of the hypoestrogenic state on bone metabolism and lipid profile changes.
  - **Add-back therapy:** largely used for minimization of side effects. Numerous studies have demonstrated the efficacy of adding back combined estrogen/progesterone to patients on GnRH agonist therapy. Patients receiving add-back therapy have significantly less vasomotor side effects and bone mineral density loss over a 6-month period while still benefiting from pain improvement from their endometriosis. Vaginal bleeding is a side effect of add-back therapy and is dose dependent. A postmenopausal estrogen–progesterone add-back regimen can be used, such as daily conjugated estrogen 0.625 mg together with medroxyprogesterone acetate 2.5 mg. An alternate regimen is 2.5 mg norethindrone acetate daily.
- **Progestins:** Progestins inhibit ovulation by luteinizing hormone (LH) suppression and, eventually, may induce amenorrhea (Table 38-1). They also suppress endometriosis through decidualization and atrophy of endometrial tissue. Progesterone therapy can be continued for suppression of endometriosis symptomatology; however, health care providers should be aware of the potential for bone demineralization with long-term progesterone use.
- **Danazol (Danocrine):** a derivative of the synthetic steroid 17α-ethinyl testosterone. It suppresses the midcycle LH surge, inhibits steroidogenesis in the human corpus luteum, and produces a high-androgen and low-estrogen environment that does not support the growth of endometriosis. Approximately 80% of patients experience relief or improvement in symptoms within 2 months of beginning danazol treatment. Androgenic side effects greatly reduce compliance. Recurrence of symptoms is almost 50% within 4 to 12 months after discontinuation of therapy. Adverse side effects occur in approximately 15% of women taking danazol.
- **Aromatase inhibitors:** Recent studies have evaluated the third-generation aromatase inhibitors, letrozole and anastrozole, for treatment of endometriosis refractory to other modalities. They are used alone or combined with GnRH agonists. These medications have been shown to decrease circulating estrogen levels by 50%. The most significant side effect is decreased bone density, which is not necessarily ameliorated with the use of calcium and vitamin D; however, evidence at this point is conflicting with regard to the overall decrease in bone density, requiring further study.
- Additional side effects include vaginal spotting, hot flushes, headaches, and mood swings, which are better tolerated compared to the side effects of GnRH agonists.
- Pain control with **nonsteroidal anti-inflammatory drugs (NSAIDs)** inhibits prostaglandin production by ectopic endometrium. NSAIDs are a good first-line agent, especially when the diagnosis of endometriosis has not been firmly established.

| TABLE 38-1 | Medical Management of Endometriosis |
| --- | --- |

| Drug | Mechanism | Dosage | Side Effects |
| --- | --- | --- | --- |
| Gonadotropin-releasing hormone analogs | Downregulation of pituitary receptors, inhibition of the hypothalamic-pituitary-ovarian axis leading to ovarian suppression | Leuprolide acetate (Lupron): 3.75–7.5 mg IM qmo × 6 Nafarelin acetate (Synarel): 200–400 mg intranasally bid × 6 mo Goserelin acetate (Zoladex): 3.6 mg implant SC q12wk × 6 mo | Hot flashes, vaginal dryness, bone demineralization, insomnia, libido changes, fatigue |
| Oral contraceptives | Anovulation, atrophy, and decidualization of endometrial tissue | Monophasic pill | Weight gain, breakthrough bleeding, breast tenderness, bloating, nausea |
| Progestins | Atrophy and decidualization of endometrial tissue, suppression gonadotropins, inhibition of ovulation, amenorrhea | Medroxyprogesterone acetate: 150 mg IM q3mo × 4 or 30 mg PO qd × 90 d Megestrol acetate: 40 mg PO qd × 6 mo | Weight gain, fluid retention, breakthrough bleeding, depression Possible bone demineralization with long-term use |
| Danazol | Anovulation by decreasing the midcycle luteinizing hormone surge Inhibition of steroidogenesis, creation of high-androgen and low-estrogen environment | Danazol 400–800 mg PO qd × 6 mo | Amenorrhea, virilization, acne, hirsutism, atrophic vaginitis, decrease in breast size, hot flashes, deepening of voice |

IM, intramuscularly; bid, twice a day; SC, subcutaneously; qd, every day.
Adapted from American College of Obstetricians and Gynecologists. ACOG practice bulletin no. 114: management of endometriosis. *Obstet Gynecol* 2010;116:223–236.

## Surgical Treatment

- **Definitive surgery** entails total abdominal hysterectomy with bilateral salpingo-oophorectomy, excision of peritoneal surface lesions or endometriomas, and lysis of adhesions. A "semidefinitive" procedure that preserves an uninvolved ovary is another option because it avoids the long-term risks of surgical menopause. However, there is a sixfold increased risk of developing recurrent symptoms and an eightfold reoperation rate to remove the remaining ovary.
  - Hormone replacement therapy (HRT) after definitive surgery for the prevention of surgical menopausal symptoms is also considered safe and does not appear to increase the risk of recurrence of endometriosis.
- **Conservative surgery** is usually reserved for patients with endometriosis-related pain but who desire future fertility. Improvement in symptoms is often achieved with laparoscopic excision or destruction of endometrial implants via laser vaporization, electrocoagulation, and thermal coagulation. Although there is significant short-term improvement in pain, a few studies have shown at 3 years postoperation, approximately 30% of patients will require additional surgeries. Despite this, the American College of Obstetricians and Gynecologists does recommend, in patients with normal ovaries, removal of uterus and endometriotic lesions with ovarian conservation.

## Endometriosis and Infertility

- The exact incidence of infertility caused by endometriosis is unknown.
- Theories on the physiologic changes caused by endometriosis that affect fertility potential include abnormal folliculogenesis, elevated oxidative stress, altered immune function, alterations in peritoneal fluid cytokines, and decreased presence of integrins during the implantation phase, thus decreasing endometrial receptivity. Together, these factors decrease oocyte quality and impair fertilization and implantation.
- Fewer oocytes are retrieved when an endometrioma is present but the pregnancy rate with in vitro fertilization (IVF) is not greatly altered and the risk of removing segments of normal ovarian cortex along with the cystectomy must be weighed against the benefit.

## Endometriosis and Ovarian Malignancy

- The prevalence of endometriosis in patients with epithelial ovarian carcinoma, especially in endometrioid and clear cell types, is higher than that of the general population. Conversely, ovarian carcinoma has been documented in 0.3% to 0.8% of patients with endometriosis.
- The pathology of endometriosis exhibits many of the characteristics of neoplastic lesions: reduced cell cycle inhibitor activity, ability to resist apoptosis, angiogenic potential similar to malignant neoplasms, and ability to invade surrounding tissue.
- Endometriosis implants may represent a precancerous state. Endometriosis is related to a chronic inflammatory state involving cytokine release, which can lead to malignant mechanisms. Both atypical endometriosis and ovarian cancers associated with endometriosis have p53 overexpression; the Ki-67 index was noted to be three times higher in atypical endometriosis.
- Clear cell and endometrioid carcinoma are the most common histologies associated with ovarian endometriosis. Numerous studies reviewing the histologic slides of endometriosis demonstrate simultaneous atypical endometriosis and malignancy.

- Endometriosis-associated ovarian carcinoma is found at an earlier stage and lower grade and is associated with a better overall survival rate than sporadic ovarian cancer.
- There is a definite causal relationship between endometriosis and specific histologic types of ovarian cancer. However, the low magnitude of the conferred risk is consistent with the view that ectopic endometrium undergoes malignant transformation with a frequency similar to its eutopic counterpart.
- At present, malignant transformation of endometriotic lesions is a recognized mechanism in the development of ovarian cancer. However, definitive surgery to remove all visible evidence of endometriosis is not recommended as a prophylactic means of reducing the development of ovarian malignancy. Rather, long-term use of oral contraceptives is the preferred method of cancer risk reduction, as an 80% lower occurrence of ovarian cancer in women with endometriosis has been shown in patients using the drug for >10 years.

## DYSMENORRHEA

- Primary dysmenorrhea is painful menstruation with no evidence of hormonal or anatomic pathology. Secondary dysmenorrhea has a demonstrable cause.
- Risk factors include young age (<20 years), heavy menstrual flow, smoking, weight loss attempts, nulliparity, and psychiatric disorders such as depression and anxiety.
- It is the most commonly reported menstrual disorder, affecting up to 90% of women.
- Primary dysmenorrhea presents within 6 months of menarche. If dysmenorrhea does not appear until more than a year after menarche, secondary dysmenorrhea should be suspected. Primary dysmenorrhea, unlike secondary dysmenorrhea, tends to become less painful as patient gets older and may also improve after childbirth.
- See Chapter 30 as well.

### Pertinent Findings in History and Physical Exam

- Defined as spasmodic cramping ("labor-like" pains) beginning a few hours before or simultaneous with the onset of menses, which are often accompanied by nausea, vomiting, backache, irritability, fatigue, diarrhea, and headache.
- Symptoms with primary dysmenorrhea last only 2 to 3 days; however, pelvic pain and tenderness may persist beyond this interval with secondary dysmenorrhea. Pain is most intense during first 24 to 36 hours of menstrual flow, which is consistent with the time of maximal prostaglandin release into the menstrual fluid.
- Clinical presentation with secondary dysmenorrhea varies considerably with its cause. Endometriosis is the most common cause, but other possibilities are pelvic inflammatory disease, adenomyosis, pelvic adhesions, and uterine fibroids.
- Evaluation of dysmenorrhea includes a complete pelvic exam. The use of microbiologic cultures, ultrasound, and other imaging modalities may be required to identify the etiology of secondary dysmenorrhea. Diagnostic laparoscopy may also be indicated in particular situations, for instance, in patients that fail empiric medical therapy for presumed endometriosis related dysmenorrhea.

### Treatment of Dysmenorrhea

- Three modalities exist: pharmacologic, nonpharmacologic, and surgical. Pharmacologic is preferred for primary dysmenorrhea.

- NSAIDs are the gold standard of treatment of primary dysmenorrhea. No specific NSAID is most efficacious, but older and generically available NSAIDs are preferred. They relieve primary dysmenorrhea by reducing endometrial prostaglandin production and by exerting a central nervous system analgesic effect. They do not affect menstrual flow volume but do reduce the amount of menstrual fluid prostaglandin level to below that of normal pain-free cycles.

- Combined OCPs, contraceptive patch, single-rod contraceptive progestin implant, and levonorgestrel intrauterine devices can all reduce dysmenorrhea. Levonorgestrel intrauterine device is highly effective in reducing menstrual blood loss with concomitant clinical relief.

- Glyceryl trinitrate, magnesium, calcium channel antagonists, and vitamin $B_6$ have been shown to have varying beneficial effects on symptom reduction with primary dysmenorrhea.

- Nonpharmacologic treatment includes transcutaneous nerve stimulation (TENS), acupuncture, acupressure, and heat-wrap therapy. High-frequency TENS offers significant pain relief via raising pain threshold and increasing the release of endorphins from the spinal cord and peripheral nerves. Although acupressure only has a suggestive role in the reduction of dysmenorrhea, acupuncture has been shown to be equally beneficial to ibuprofen in pain reduction. Continuous suprapubic heat application has been shown to be more therapeutic than acetaminophen during the initial 8 hours of application.

- Surgical interventions including nerve ablation (uterosacral nerve ablation and presacral neurectomy) and spinal manipulation have shown no long-lasting therapeutic benefit according to Cochrane meta-analyses. Additionally, they carry significant risk of adverse events.

## PREMENSTRUAL DISORDER: PREMENSTRUAL DYSPHORIA AND PREMENSTRUAL DYSPHORIC DISORDER

- **Premenstrual dysphoria or more commonly premenstrual syndrome (PMS)** is a cluster of mood, cognitive, and physical disturbances with the hallmark symptom of irritability. It is distinct from depression or anxiety disorders and has a prevalence of 3% to 5% of reproductive age women.
  - Mood symptoms include irritability, mood swings, depression, and anxiety; cognitive disturbances may be confusion or poor concentration. Physical problems consist of bloating, breast tenderness, appetite changes, hot flashes, insomnia, headache, and fatigue.
- **Premenstrual dysphoric disorder (PMDD)** represents the more severe end of the spectrum. It is composed of the same blend of symptoms but involves an increased severity in perceived symptoms and a marked impairment in daily life. This diagnosis is reserved for patients who meet the *Diagnostic and Statistical Manual of Mental Disorders* criteria set by the American Psychiatric Association.
  - A woman has PMDD when she has five or more of the following symptoms:
    - Feeling depressed
    - Feeling tense, anxious, or "on edge"
    - Moodiness or frequent crying
    - Constant irritability and anger that cause conflict with other people
    - Lack of interest in things she used to enjoy

- ○ Having problems concentrating
- ○ Lack of energy
- ○ Appetite changes, overeating, or cravings
- ○ Having trouble sleeping or sleeping too much
- ○ Feeling overwhelmed
- ○ Physical symptoms such as tender or swollen breasts, headaches, joint or muscle pain, bloating, and weight gain
- Symptom onset occurs anytime in the 2 weeks prior to the onset of bleeding, continues to the start of bleeding, and resolves after a day or two of menstrual flow.
- The exact physiologic cause of premenstrual disorders is unknown. Most frequently cited theories include neuroactive progesterone metabolite, γ-aminobutyric acid receptor modulation, and critical reduction in serotonergic function during the luteal phase.

## Evaluation and Diagnosis

- Dysmenorrhea, depression and anxiety disorders, menstrual migraine, cyclic mastalgia, irritable bowel syndrome, and hypothyroidism may all present with mood or physical disturbances similar to those that manifest with PMS/PMDD. See also Chapter 30.
- There are no laboratory or physical exam findings required to make the diagnosis. Rather, these tests are used to rule out other causes of similar symptoms. Hormone levels (estrogen, progesterone, LH, follicle-stimulating hormone [FSH]) do not vary between women with and without PMS/PMDD; thus, there is no use in obtaining these values.
- For diagnosis of PMS, symptoms must begin at least 5 days before menses, persist for three menstrual cycles in a row, and end within 4 days after menses starts. It must also interfere with some of the patient's normal activities.
- Such logs are helpful for clinicians in order to determine whether the reported symptoms are limited to the luteal phase or are present throughout the cycle, suggesting a general medical condition. Additionally, they are helpful for patients for instituting self-help strategies and for anticipating symptoms.

## Treatment

- Because PMS/PMDD is a chronic problem, adverse effects, cost, and severity of symptoms should all be considered before employing a specific treatment.
- Lifestyle changes are probably most appropriate for mild to moderate PMS/PMDD. Regular aerobic exercise; relaxation therapy; stress reduction; sufficient sleep; dietary limitation of caffeine, alcohol, and salt; and increased consumption of complex carbohydrates during the luteal phase have been shown to reduce the severity of symptoms.
- Dietary supplements (especially St. John's wort but also ginkgo and kava) are somewhat effective for mild to moderate PMS but ineffective for PMDD. However, patients should be aware of their potential adverse effects (especially the affect of St. John's wort on the effectiveness of OCPs).
- In several small randomized trials, NSAIDs taken in the luteal phase have been shown to decrease all physical symptoms with the exception of breast tenderness.
- Yaz, the combined OCP containing drospirenone and 20 mg of ethinyl estradiol, was recently approved by the FDA for treatment of PMDD and has been shown effective in treating mood and physical and behavioral symptoms of PMDD.

- Selective serotonin reuptake inhibitors are the most effective pharmacologic treatment for moderate to severe PMS and PMDD. Continuous dosing exerts a greater inhibition of symptoms than intermittent dosing. Fluoxetine, sertraline, citalopram, and paroxetine all demonstrated a statistically significant improvement in symptoms.

## SUGGESTED READINGS

Allen C, Hopewell S, Prentice A. Non-steroidal anti-inflammatory drugs for pain in women with endometriosis. *Cochrane Database Syst Rev* 2005;(4):CD004753.

American College of Obstetricians and Gynecologists. ACOG practice bulletin no. 110: non-contraceptive uses of hormonal contraceptives. *Obstet Gynecol* 2010;115(1):206–218.

American College of Obstetricians and Gynecologists. ACOG practice bulletin no. 114: management of endometriosis. *Obstet Gynecol* 2010;116(1):223–236.

American Psychiatric Association. *Diagnostic and Statistical Manual of Mental Disorders.* 4th ed. Washington, DC: American Psychiatric Association, 1994:717–718.

Balasch J, Creus M, Fabregues F, et al. Visible and non-visible endometriosis at laparoscopy in fertile and infertile women and in patients with chronic pelvic pain: a prospective study. *Hum Reprod* 1996;11:387–391.

Barbieri RL, Niloff JM, Bast RC Jr, et al. Elevated serum concentrations of CA-125 in patients with advanced endometriosis. *Fertil Steril* 1986;45(5):630–634.

Brosens I, Puttemans P, Campo R, et al. Non-invasive methods of diagnosis of endometriosis. *Curr Opin Obstet Gynecol* 2003;15(6):519–522.

Diwadkar GB, Falcone T. Surgical management of pain and infertility secondary to endometriosis. *Semin Reprod Med* 2011;29(2):124–129.

Namnoum AB, Hickman TN, Goodman SB, et al. Incidence of symptom recurrence after hysterectomy for endometriosis. *Fertil Steril* 1995;64:898–902.

Sagsveen M, Farmer JE, Prentice A, et al. Gonadotrophin-releasing hormone analogues for endometriosis: bone mineral density. *Cochrane Database Syst Rev* 2003;(4):CD001297.

Sampson JA. Peritoneal endometriosis due to menstrual dissemination of endometrial tissue into the peritoneal cavity. *Am J Obstet Gynecol* 1927;71:422–469.

Shakiba K, Bena JF, McGill KM, et al. Surgical treatment of endometriosis: a 7-year follow-up on the requirement for further surgery. *Obstet Gynecol* 2008;111:1285–1292.

Somigliana E, Vigano' P, Parazzini F, et al. Association between endometriosis and cancer: a comprehensive review and a critical analysis of clinical and epidemiological evidence. *Gynecol Oncol* 2006;101(2):331–341.

Worley MJ, Welch WR, Berkowitz RS, et al. Endometriosis-associated ovarian cancer: a review of pathogenesis. *Int J Mol Sci* 2013;14:5367–5379.

Yeung P Jr, Sinervo K, Winer W, et al. Complete laparoscopic excision of endometriosis in teenagers: is postoperative hormonal suppression necessary? *Fertil Steril* 2011;95(6):1909–1912, 1912.e1.

U.S. Food and Drug Administration. Lupron and Lupron Depot (leuprolide acetate) injection. U.S. Food and Drug Administration Web site. http://www.fda.gov/safety/medwatch/safetyinformation/ucm291032.htm. Accessed May 21, 2013.

# Evaluation of Amenorrhea

Irene Woo and Kyle J. Tobler

**Amenorrhea** is the absence of menses. It is physiologic during pregnancy, lactation, and menopause. The lack of regular, spontaneous menses for any other reason after the expected age of menarche is pathologic.

- **Primary amenorrhea:** No menses by age 14 years in the absence of secondary sexual development or no menstruation by age 16 years with the presence of secondary sexual characteristics.
- **Secondary amenorrhea:** The absence of menses in a previously menstruating woman. It is also defined as the lack of menses for 6 months or for three menstrual cycles in women that have experienced menarche. Evaluation, however, need not be deferred solely to conform to these definitions.
- **World Health Organization** (WHO) amenorrhea groups
  - **WHO group I** (hypogonadotropic hypoestrogenic) has no endogenous estrogen production, normal or low follicle-stimulating hormone (FSH) levels, normal prolactin (PRL) levels, and no lesion in the hypothalamus or pituitary.
  - **WHO group II** (normogonadotropic normoestrogenic) has endogenous estrogen production and normal levels of FSH and PRL.
  - **WHO group III** (hypergonadotropic hypoestrogenic) has elevated FSH levels and low to absent estrogen, indicative of premature ovarian failure (POF).

## MENSTRUAL PHYSIOLOGY

- Spontaneous, cyclic menstruation requires an intact and functional hypothalamic-pituitary-ovarian axis (HPOA), endometrium, and genital outflow tract. Abnormalities in any of these structures may result in amenorrhea.

### Normal Physiology of the Hypothalamic-Pituitary-Ovarian Axis and Menstruation

- Hypothalamus (arcuate nucleus) secretes gonadotropin-releasing hormone (GnRH) in pulses at specific frequencies and amplitudes into the portal circulation.
- GnRH pulses stimulate gonadotrophs in the anterior pituitary to synthesize, store, and secrete gonadotropic hormones FSH and luteinizing hormone (LH) to the systemic circulation.
- FSH stimulates ovarian follicle development and estradiol ($E_2$) secretion.
- $E_2$ provides inhibitory feedback on the hypothalamus and pituitary, decreasing FSH release. $E_2$ also stimulates proliferation of the endometrium.
- Follicular growth continues until the threshold level of systemic $E_2$ is surpassed, shifting to positive feedback, which triggers the LH surge.
- LH surge causes the developing oocyte within the follicle to resume meiosis and ovulate.
- Following ovulation, the follicle becomes a corpus luteum, rapidly shifting from primarily $E_2$ production to progesterone production.

- Progesterone decidualizes the endometrium in preparation for embryo implantation.
- If pregnancy occurs, human chorionic gonadotropin (hCG) secreted from the syncytiotrophoblast supports the corpus luteum and continued progesterone release.
- If pregnancy does not occur, the corpus luteum will regress, ceasing to produce progesterone.
- Progesterone withdrawal causes the endometrium to slough, resulting in the menstrual effluent.
- The HPOA and endometrium demonstrate a finely orchestrated system that must be intact at all steps for a normal menstrual cycle to occur (Fig. 39-1).

## EVALUATION OF AMENORRHEA

### When to Evaluate for Amenorrhea

- **Rule out pregnancy**, as both primary and secondary amenorrhea require an immediate evaluation for pregnancy.

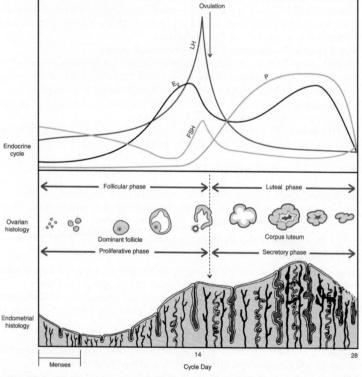

**Figure 39-1.** The normal menstrual cycle. Changes in serum hormones, ovarian follicle, and endometrial thickness during a 28-day menstrual cycle. Menses occur during the first few days of the cycle. E₂, estradiol; FSH, follicle-stimulating hormone; LH, luteinizing hormone; P, progesterone. (From Berek J, ed. *Berek and Novak's Gynecology*, 14th ed. Philadelphia, PA: Lippincott Williams & Wilkins, 2007.)

- Use clinical judgment. The aforementioned listed timeline defining amenorrhea does not need to be met prior to initiating an evaluation.
- Do not overlook gross evidence of a disease process: Turner syndrome, frank virilization, obstructed vagina, or other evidences of a disease process.
- Use a systematic approach, evaluating each critical component of menstruation: hypothalamus, pituitary, ovaries, uterus, and genital outflow tract.

## Important History for Amenorrhea

- **Present illness:** Presence of cyclic pelvic or abdominal pain, headache, visual changes, seizure, hot flushes, hot or cold temperature intolerance, vaginal dryness, urinary issues, hirsutism, virilization, galactorrhea, severe physical or emotional stress, changes in weight, diet, athletic training, or trauma
- **Past medical history:** General health; chronic illnesses (especially autoimmune and thyroid disease); birth defects; all current and recently discontinued medications or supplements; contraception history (especially the use of depot medroxyprogesterone acetate); history of pelvic infection, complications with prior pregnancies or abortions, and any instrumentation of the uterus; and abdominal or pelvic surgeries. Most recent pregnancy and delivery and lactation history can be significant, as can a personal history of cancer treatment involving radiation therapy and/or chemotherapy.
- **Development:** Age of thelarche, pubarche, and menarche, whether menarche was spontaneous or induced, and cycle regularity
- **Social:** Severe physical or emotional stress, changes in weight or diet, and athletic training
- **Family history:** History of late pubertal development, early menopause, mental retardation, or short stature

## Important Physical Examination for Amenorrhea

- Height, weight, body mass index, waist-to-hip ratio if obese, blood pressure, and pulse
- General body habitus, looking for disease stigmata of Turner syndrome, Cushing syndrome, and thyroid disease. Also gross malnutrition or obesity.
- Vision changes or peripheral loss of vision
- Mouth and teeth for tooth enamel erosion
- Skin evaluated for hyperpigmentation, acanthosis nigricans, abdominal striae, acne, hirsutism, and balding
- Thyroid gland palpated for size, shape, and nodules
- Breast development (Tanner stage), galactorrhea, or other breast discharge
- Abdominal exam for masses, fat distribution, hirsutism, and aforementioned listed skin changes
- External genitalia examined for hair distribution and virilization (clitoromegaly), imperforate hymen, or labial fusion
- Internal genitalia examined for transverse vaginal septum, lateral vaginal obstruction, estrogenized vaginal mucosa, and the presence of a cervix with visible patent external cervical os
- Rectal exam to evaluate the extent of hematocolpos and presence of uterus beyond a vaginal obstruction or absent vaginal orifice. Rectal exam can also assist in evaluating a patient with an intact hymen or infantile vaginal orifice.

## Laboratory Evaluation of Amenorrhea

- Important for laboratory evaluation to be guided by the aforementioned presenting history and physical examination
- hCG to evaluate for pregnancy

- FSH, $E_2$, thyroid-stimulating hormone (TSH), and PRL
- 17-Hydroxyprogesterone, testosterone, and dehydroepiandrosterone sulfate (DHEAS) for patients with virilization, hirsutism, or androgen excess
- Testosterone if concern for complete androgen insensitivity
- Karyotype if concern for genitourinary abnormalities, suspicion for gonadal dysgenesis, or complete androgen insensitivity. Also consider if other nonrelated physical malformations are present.

## Imaging Evaluation of Amenorrhea

- Pelvic ultrasound for both primary and secondary amenorrhea
- Hysterosalpingogram (HSG) or sonohysterography particularly for secondary amenorrhea and suspicion for Asherman syndrome

## Follow-Up Laboratory and Imaging Studies for Initial Evaluation

- Fragile X (FMR1) premutation for patients with POF
- Antiadrenal antibodies and antithyroid antibodies (antiperoxidase and antithyroglobulin) for patients with POF
- Karyotype for patients younger than 30 years with POF
- Cortisol levels (24-hour urinary free cortisol, late-night salivary cortisol, dexamethasone suppression testing) for patients with suspected Cushing syndrome, also considered in patients evaluated for polycystic ovarian syndrome (PCOS) and/or evidence of hyperandrogenism
- Insulin-like growth factor 1 (IGF-1), free T4, and morning cortisol level for patients with a pituitary lesion identified by magnetic resonance imaging (MRI)
- Adrenocorticotropic hormone (ACTH) stimulation test for patients with elevated 17-hydroxyprogesterone
- MRI of the pituitary for hyperprolactinemia or hypogonadotropic hypogonadism which has no other identifiable etiology (severe physical and emotional stress, malnutrition, medications, hypothyroidism)
- MRI of pelvis. Obtain when genitourinary abnormalities are not well characterized or for surgical planning. Particularly useful when evaluating for imperforate hymen versus transverse vaginal septum, obstructed hemivagina, and noncommunicating or hypoplastic uterine horn.
- Renal ultrasound and radiographs (computed tomography [CT] or x-ray) of spine for patients with müllerian dysgenesis
- Endometrial biopsy (suspicion of genital tuberculosis or schistosomiasis)

## Progesterone Withdrawal for Evaluation of Amenorrhea

- Progestin challenge: 5 to 10 mg of medroxyprogesterone (Provera) for 5 to 7 days. Positive response is withdrawal bleed within 2 to 7 days after discontinuation of Provera.
  - Approximately 20% of patients with POF, hypothalamic amenorrhea, and hyperprolactinemia experience withdrawal flow depending on the degree of hypoestrogenism.
  - Failure to withdraw after sequential estrogen then estrogen/progestin is supportive of Asherman syndrome or cervical stenosis, but these conditions are rarely seen in the absence of a previous surgical procedure and the amenorrhea can be temporally related to the procedure.
  - Consider use of serum $E_2$ level rather than use of progesterone withdrawal to determine status of estrogen.
  - Progesterone-induced withdrawal bleed is indicated as a treatment for amenorrhea and a thickened endometrium on ultrasound.

| TABLE 39-1 | Differential Diagnosis of Primary Amenorrhea | |
|---|---|---|
| | **Breast Development Present** | **Breast Development Absent** |
| **Uterus present** | Consider secondary amenorrhea differential<br>Hypothalamic cause<br>Pituitary cause<br>Ovarian cause<br>Uterine cause | **Gonadal dysgenesis**<br>45,X<br>46,X; abnormal X<br>Mosaic X<br>46,XX or 46,XY: pure gonadal dysgenesis<br>17-hydroxylase deficiency with 46,XX<br>Galactosemia<br><br>**Hypothalamic or pituitary failure**<br>Kallmann syndrome<br>CNS congenital defect<br>Hypothalamic-pituitary tumors<br>CNS infection<br>Physiologic delay |
| **Uterus absent** | Müllerian agenesis<br>Androgen insensitivity syndrome | 17,20-desmolase deficiency (46,XY)<br>Agonadism<br>17-hydroxylase deficiency (46,XY) |

CNS, central nervous system.

## Differential Diagnosis for Primary Amenorrhea

- History and physical examination to evaluate for genital outflow obstruction
- Keep pregnancy in differential, although less likely.
- Keep the most common causes high on differential, (gonadal dysgenesis, müllerian anomalies/dysgenesis, and complete androgen insensitivity).
- To develop a differential diagnosis, categorize the patients into four categories based on the presence or absence of a uterus and the presence or absence of breast development (indicative of estrogen) (Table 39-1).
  - Uterus present and breasts absent likely represents gonadal dysgenesis, hypothalamic failure, or pituitary failure.
  - Uterus absent and breasts present likely represents androgen insensitivity or congenital absence of the uterus.
  - Both uterus and breasts absent likely represents failure of steroidogenesis to produce sex hormones including 17- or 20-desmolase deficiency, 17α-hydroxylase deficiency, or agonadism. Frequently have 46,XY karyotype combined with gonadal failure.
  - Both uterus and breast development present likely represents pituitary etiology (hyperprolactinemia) or another subcategory that also underlies secondary amenorrhea.

## Differential Diagnosis for Secondary Amenorrhea

- Always keep pregnancy high on the differential diagnosis (Table 39-2).
- Physiologic explanations include pregnancy, menopause, and postpartum lactation.

| TABLE 39-2 | Pathologic Causes of Secondary Amenorrhea |

| Etiology | Causal Factor |
|---|---|
| **Reproductive tract** | |
| Cervical stenosis | Surgical procedure (i.e., LEEP, CKC) |
| Asherman syndrome | Endometrial scarring |
| **Ovarian** | |
| Premature ovarian failure | Idiopathic, chromosomal abnormality, auto-immune disease, infection |
| Polycystic ovary syndrome | Inappropriate gonadotropin secretion, insulin resistance |
| **Pituitary** | |
| Hyperprolactinemia | Lactotroph hyperplasia ± prolactinoma, drugs |
| Pituitary adenomas | Thyrotroph, corticotroph, or other hyperplasia |
| Sheehan syndrome | Postpartum hemorrhage |
| **CNS** | |
| Hypothalamic amenorrhea | Stress, eating disorders, weight loss, excessive exercise |
| Brain injury | Interruption of HPOA |
| Inflammatory or infiltrative process | Interruption of HPOA |
| **Other endocrinopathies** | |
| Hypothyroidism, Cushing syndrome, late-onset adrenal hyperplasia | |

LEEP, loop electrosurgical excision procedure; CKC, cold knife conization; CNS, central nervous system; HPOA, hypothalamic-pituitary-ovarian axis.

- If onset is related to previous pregnancy, abortion, or other surgical procedure, consider cervical stenosis or Asherman syndrome. Further evaluation with HSG, hysteroscopy, or sonohysterogram.
- Mildly elevated PRL: Repeat in the morning (patient needs to refrain from breast stimulation, intercourse, or exercise prior to test). Also, verify normal TSH to rule out hypothyroidism as etiology of hyperprolactinemia. MRI will confirm presence of a pituitary lesion.
- Normal $E_2$ and FSH levels: Likely anovulation, consider further evaluation for PCOS.
- Low $E_2$ and low FSH levels: Consider central nervous system (CNS) lesion or hypothalamic-pituitary failure and further evaluation with MRI.
- Low $E_2$ and elevated FSH levels: Consider POF and gonadal dysgenesis.
- Elevated TSH: occult or subclinical hypothyroidism
- Elevated DHEAS: Rule out adrenal tumor with CT scan.
- Elevated 17-hydroxyprogesterone: Consider late-onset congenital adrenal hyperplasia and confirm with ACTH stimulation test.

- Evidence of androgen excess: with a normal $E_2$, FSH, PRL, TSH, 17-hydroxy-progesterone and DHEAS, should consider PCOS. May see polycystic ovaries on pelvic sonogram; however, it is not required for diagnosis.
- Signs or symptoms of Cushing syndrome: Screen with late-night salivary cortisol (easiest), 24-hour urinary free cortisol, 1-mg overnight dexamethasone suppression, or 2-day low-dose dexamethasone suppression screening tests.

## ETIOLOGIES OF AMENORRHEA—SYSTEMATIC EVALUATION

### Genital Outflow Tract and Uterine Abnormalities Resulting in Amenorrhea

- **Imperforate hymen** and **transverse vaginal septum** are outflow tract malformations that typically present with acute cyclic pelvic or abdominal pain in a patient soon after the age of expected menarche. They will often have age-appropriate secondary development. Examination of an imperforate hymen reveals no obvious vaginal orifice and often a bulging, thin perineal membrane. In a patient with a transverse septum, physical exam will reveal a normal vaginal orifice but no visible cervix. Imperforate hymen should distend with Valsalva maneuver. In some cases, an MRI may be required to distinguish an imperforate hymen from a transverse septum.
- **Müllerian agenesis** and **hypoplasia**, also known as Mayer-Rokitansky-Küster-Hauser (MRKH) syndrome, is a relatively common cause of primary amenorrhea. The incidence ranges from 1:4,000 to 1:10,000. Subjects with MRKH commonly present in their late teens with normally developing breasts, pubic hair, and external genitalia, as the presence and function of the ovaries are normal. Depending on the location of the müllerian agenesis, the patient can present with no vagina, a portion of a vagina as well as complete uterine agenesis, or a portion of the uterus. Amenorrhea is generally the only complaint, although 2% to 7% may have rudimentary müllerian structures with functioning endometrium, resulting in cyclic pain. MRI of the pelvis can assist with classifying the anomalies and surgical planning, if required. In addition, imaging of the urinary tract should be performed in all patients with müllerian abnormalities, as approximately 30% have renal anomalies. Skeletal abnormalities are also commonly associated with MRKH. Vaginal dilator therapy or surgical construction of a neovagina can usually create a functional vagina.
- **Complete androgen insensitivity syndrome** (CAIS), previously known as testicular feminization, is an X-linked, recessive disorder that occurs in 46,XY individuals and results in phenotypic women. Testes are present and secrete normal male levels of anti-müllerian hormone (AMH) and testosterone. AMH results in regression of müllerian structures. Masculinization fails to occur because of an androgen receptor defect. Like MRKH, patients with CAIS typically present in the later teens with normal development of breasts with primary amenorrhea. Physical examination generally demonstrates normal external genitalia, a shortened or absent vagina, and no cervix or uterus. Also, physical exam can often differentiate the two conditions because pubic and axillary hair is sparse in CAIS, and testes may be palpable in the inguinal region. The diagnosis of CAIS is confirmed by documenting serum testosterone in the normal male range and a 46,XY karyotype. The incidence of gonadal neoplasia is 52%, and the incidence of gonadal malignancy is 22% in CAIS. Under these circumstances, gonadectomy must be performed. Because malignancy rarely occurs before age 20 years, deferring surgery until after pubertal maturation and epiphyseal closure have occurred is preferable. The gynecologist should refer to the removed tissue as

gonad rather than testis in initial discussions with the patient. Counseling is often indicated. Vaginal dilator therapy can usually create a functional vagina.

- **Asherman syndrome** is the most common cause of secondary amenorrhea and accounts for 7% of patients presenting with secondary amenorrhea. Asherman syndrome (i.e., intrauterine synechiae) is most commonly associated with aggressive postpartum curettage or abortion. Other risk factors include uterine or cervical surgeries, such as cesarean section, septoplasty, myomectomy, and cone biopsy procedures. Infectious causes include tuberculosis, schistosomiasis, infection associated with intrauterine devices (IUDs), and other severe pelvic infections. Diagnosis can be confirmed with HSG, sonohysterogram, or hysteroscopy. Treatment requires hysteroscopic lysis of intrauterine adhesions and placement of intrauterine stent.

- **Cervical stenosis** can be the result of congenital defects or acquired following cervical conization or loop electrosurgical excision and dilation and curettage. If cervical stenosis is the underlying etiology of secondary amenorrhea, hematometra and an enlarged uterus should be detected by physical exam and confirmed with ultrasound. Treatment includes serial dilation of the cervix.

## Ovarian Abnormalities Resulting in Amenorrhea (Hypergonadotropic Hypogonadism)

- Primary dysfunction at the level of the ovary. The ovaries no longer respond to gonadotropin stimulation limiting follicular development and production of $E_2$.

- **Gonadal dysgenesis** is the most common cause of primary amenorrhea, accounting for 43% of such cases. Peripheral blood karyotype aids in diagnosis. Although Turner syndrome is the most frequent cause of gonadal dysgenesis, any condition resulting in depletion of germ cells can cause gonadal dysgenesis and replacement of the gonads with fibrous streaks.

  - **Turner syndrome** (TS) classically results from aneuploidy involving the X chromosome. Approximately, 60% of TS patients are 45,X and the other 40% include karyotype abnormalities such as 45,X/46,XX mosaics; 46,XXqi isochromosome; and 46,XXp short arm deletion. Internal and external genitalia develop normally for females. The cohort of primordial follicles undergoes accelerated atresia so that oocytes are depleted prior to the onset of puberty. A lack of gonadal $E_2$ production results in a failure of breast development and other secondary sexual characteristics.
    - Patients with TS exhibit several cardinal features including webbed neck, shield-shaped chest, short stature, and sexual infantilism. Typically, these patients are identified in the pediatric population due to short stature, prior to noting primary amenorrhea. Some TS patients, especially those with mosaic karyotypes, can undergo spontaneous puberty and conception (16% and 3.6% of cases, respectively).

  - **Mosaicism** involving partial deletions or rearrangements of one X chromosome can cause a wide range of gonadal dysfunctions ranging from gonadal dysgenesis to POF. Determining whether a Y chromosome is present in a mosaic is important because the presence of the SRY portion of the Y chromosome predisposes to tumor formation. Presence of a Y chromosome requires gonadectomy or removal of the gonadal streaks.

  - **Pure gonadal dysgenesis** is a term used to describe 46,XX or XY individuals who experience dysgenesis of germinal tissue early in embryonic development. Such dysgenesis likely results from genetic, environmental, or infectious insults, although a specific cause is rarely identified. All subjects are phenotypic women of normal height who fail to undergo puberty. Patients with 46,XY gonadal dysgenesis, also known as **Swyer syndrome**, require removal of their gonadal streaks to prevent malignant transformation.

- **CYP17 deficiency** is a rare disorder that can affect 46,XY or XX individuals. The lack of 17α-hydroxylase and 17,20-lyase activities results in both gonadal and adrenal insufficiencies. Patients with an XY karyotype are phenotypic women (due to lack of androgen production) but also lack a uterus because AMH was secreted in early fetal life. Subjects usually present at the time of puberty with hypertension (due to excess mineralocorticoid production), hypokalemia, and hypergonadotropic hypogonadism. CYP17 deficiency is an autosomal recessive disorder.

- **LH and FSH receptor mutations** have also been identified preventing the ovaries from responding to gonadotropin stimulation and resulting in POF. They can present with varying levels of secondary sexual development and likely primary amenorrhea. However, these conditions are very rare.

- **POF** can manifest as primary or secondary amenorrhea. For patients who previously menstruated, POF is defined as amenorrhea associated with a depletion of oocytes and cessation of menses before age 40 years. In those with primary amenorrhea, approximately 50% will have an abnormal karyotype. The various possible etiologies for POF associated with secondary amenorrhea are listed in the following text; however, up to 90% of patients with POF remain unexplained following evaluation.

  - **X chromosome abnormalities**, such as short or long arm deletions or mosaicism, not severe enough to cause primary gonadal dysgenesis, may present as POF.

  - **Spontaneous POF** is not induced by chemotherapy, radiation, or surgery. The majority of cases are idiopathic; 6% have premutations in the gene responsible for **fragile X syndrome (FMR1)**; and 4% have **steroidogenic cell autoimmunity**, placing them at risk for adrenal insufficiency. Because 14% of patients with familial POF and 2% of isolated POF will have the FMR1 premutation, it is important to evaluate for the FMR1 gene premutation by obtaining a family history of POF, fragile X, unexplained mental retardation, tremor/ataxia syndrome, and/or any developmental delay in children. In addition, because up to 20% of patients with POF develop autoimmune hypothyroidism, they should undergo adrenal and thyroid antibody testing. Those younger than age 30 years with POF should also have karyotyping performed, as 13% will show some chromosomal abnormalities. Inclusion of any Y chromosomal material is an indication for gonadectomy.

  - **Iatrogenic POF** can be the result of follicular depletion by radiation, chemotherapy (especially with alkylating agents), or surgical manipulation or removal of ovarian tissue. Prior to undergoing radiation or chemotherapy, measures can be taken to decrease exposure to or mitigate damage. Prior to radiation therapy, oophoropexy can position ovaries outside the radiation field. Prior to and throughout chemotherapy treatment for malignancy or severe autoimmune diseases, GnRH agonists or antagonists can potentially provide protection, although the efficacy of these treatments is still debated. Additionally, many centers offer ovarian tissue cryopreservation; however, the optimal strategies and protocols are still under investigation.

- **Treatment of POF** involves estrogen replacement and should be initiated in essentially all patients to prevent the premature onset of osteopenia and osteoporosis. In addition, these women are at high risk for early-onset cardiovascular disease, genitourinary atrophy, vasomotor symptoms, sleep disturbance, and vaginal dryness. Often, POF patients require twice as much estrogen as compared to postmenopausal women to alleviate symptoms. This can be accomplished with use of oral contraceptive pills or higher doses of traditionally used hormone replacement therapy regimens (e.g., micronized $E_2$ 1 to 2 mg daily or conjugated equine estrogens 0.625 to 1.25 mg daily) or transdermal treatment regimens

(0.1 mg/24 hours). In patients with short stature or open epiphyseal plates, lower doses of estrogen should be used to avoid premature closure. If the uterus is intact, adjunct cyclic treatment with progestins is required to prevent endometrial hyperplasia.

- Spontaneous pregnancy following POF is possible, although unlikely (~5%). Treatment of infertility classically requires oocyte donation; however, in some cases, high doses of gonadotropins can achieve follicular development. Lastly, POF can be associated with psychological distress and appropriate counseling and emotional support should be initiated.

## Hypothalamic Dysfunction Resulting in Amenorrhea (Hypogonadotropic Hypogonadism)

- Underlying etiology is a decrease in GnRH release and stimulation of the pituitary to release gonadotropins resulting in failure of folliculogenesis and production of $E_2$.
- The term **hypothalamic amenorrhea** applies to conditions in which GnRH secretion is diminished in the absence of any organic pathology.
- Physical or **psychological stress**, **anorexia nervosa**, **exercise**, and **weight loss** can contribute to dysfunctional hypothalamic GnRH secretion. Affected women are frequently underweight, >10% below ideal body weight, and/or engage in regular strenuous exercise.
- **Kallmann syndrome** is an inherited X-linked disorder resulting from a genetic mutation that causes failure of olfactory and GnRH neuronal migration from the olfactory placode. The resultant hypogonadotropic hypogonadism is due to the absence of GnRH pulses to stimulate gonadotropin release from the pituitary. This syndrome is characterized by primary amenorrhea, absent breast development, presence of cervix and uterus, and anosmia.
- **Congenital GnRH deficiency** is a genetic condition resulting in the absence of functional hypothalamic neurons. Unlike Kallmann syndrome, it is not associated with anosmia.
- **GnRH receptor mutations** inhibit signaling of GnRH to release gonadotropins from the anterior pituitary. Patients affected have a broad range of phenotypes, depending on the particular mutation.
- **Other CNS pathologies**, such as hypothalamic neoplasms, trauma, hemorrhage, or cranial irradiation, can interrupt the function of the HPOA. **Craniopharyngioma** is the most common CNS neoplasm causing delayed puberty. An MRI should be ordered for any patient with hypogonadotropic amenorrhea when no obvious external cause is present.
- **Chronic debilitating disease** can also lead to hypogonadotropic amenorrhea as a result of alterations in GnRH pulsatility. This has been observed in renal disease, liver disease, malignancy, and HIV. However, virtually any serious chronic illness can undermine the HPOA.
- **Treatment** involves correcting the underlying causative behavior if identified. The primary treatment is estrogen/progestin replacement as described in the POF treatment section.

## Pituitary Disorders Resulting in Amenorrhea

- **Pituitary lesions** can present with amenorrhea and low or normal levels of gonadotropins. The most common pituitary lesion is a prolactinoma, but nonfunctioning adenomas, adenomas that secrete other pituitary hormones, or empty sella syndrome may also be present.

- **Hyperprolactinemia** accounts for 14% of secondary amenorrhea and a small portion of primary amenorrhea. Pregnancy and breast-feeding are physiologic causes of hyperprolactinemia. Medications that can cause hyperprolactinemia include most antipsychotics and antidepressants, $H_2$ receptor blockers, methyldopa, verapamil, reserpine, and metoclopramide. Other medical causes that must be evaluated include hypothyroidism and renal failure. However, by far the most common pathologic cause of hyperprolactinemia is a prolactinoma.
  - **Prolactinomas** are classified as either microadenomas or macroadenomas (>10 mm). Macroadenomas may be associated with bitemporal hemianopsia and therefore, visual field defects should be evaluated for during physical examination.
  - Excess PRL levels can cause negative feedback on hypothalamic GnRH secretion, thereby lowering gonadotropin release. In addition to hypogonadism, most women will experience oligo or amenorrhea and galactorrhea. Galactorrhea is secretion of a milky fluid, excluding breast-feeding. Discharge may be white/clear in color but also greenish or even bloody. Bloody discharge requires evaluation for an intraductal papilloma or cancer with mammography. In the absence of hyperprolactinemia, galactorrhea does not need further workup.
  - Laboratory evaluation of serum PRL levels between 20 and 200 ng/mL are considered elevated. A mildly elevated serum PRL should be repeated in a fasting, nonstressed environment because PRL concentration can vary with time of day, level of stress, and other factors. Occasionally, macroadenomas can produce extremely high serum PRL levels (>1,000 ng/mL), but the laboratory value could be falsely low due to the hook effect. In this phenomenon, the substrate saturates both the capture and signal antibodies used in the laboratory assays resulting in inability of the two antibodies to bind. This results in only a modestly elevated level in the sample. If clinical suspicion is high for hyperprolactinemia but the laboratory value is inconsistent, the test should be repeated with the serum diluted. Women with pituitary macroadenomas should also have additional evaluation including a serum free T4, IGF-1, and morning cortisol level.
  - A confirmed elevation in PRL prompts imaging of the pituitary gland, usually by MRI. At least 30% to 40% of women with hyperprolactinemia have a pituitary adenoma. The incidence of malignancy in prolactinomas is very rare and resection is rarely required.
  - Treatment of hyperprolactinemia is usually successful with dopamine agonist therapy (bromocriptine or cabergoline). See Chapter 13.
- **Sheehan syndrome** is a condition of pituitary necrosis and hypopituitarism following postpartum hemorrhage and hypotension. See Chapter 13.
- Infiltrative disease: most commonly caused by hemochromatosis, a disorder of excessive deposition of iron in liver, pancreas, anterior pituitary, and heart. Screen iron studies; fasting transferrin saturation >45% is indicative. Treat with phlebotomy and chelation therapy.
- **Isolated gonadotropin (FSH/LH) deficiency** is a rare condition usually associated with thalassemia major, retinitis pigmentosa, or prepubertal hypothyroidism.

## Normogonadotropic Amenorrhea

- Heterogeneous group with normal levels of gonadotropins and $E_2$. Patients have normal secondary sexual development. The underlying etiology of amenorrhea is chronic anovulation.

- **PCOS** is the most common cause of amenorrhea associated with hyperandrogenism. Patients generally have normal levels of gonadotropins and E$_2$.
  - National Institutes of Health and the Rotterdam Consensus Conference are the most commonly used diagnostic criteria for PCOS. See Chapter 41.
  - After other causes of amenorrhea and hyperandrogenism have been excluded, evidence of chronic an-/oligoovulation, androgen excess, and/or polycystic ovaries on ultrasound generally establishes the diagnosis.
  - Hyperandrogenism should be evaluated with serum testosterone and 17-hyroxyprogesterone and DHEAS levels should be assessed to exclude the late-onset congenital adrenal hyperplasia or the presence of an adrenal or other androgen-producing tumors.
  - PCOS is associated with an increased risk for type 2 diabetes, insulin resistance, hypertension, lipid abnormalities, obesity, metabolic syndrome, and endometrial hyperplasia/cancer.
  - Treatment includes weight reduction and inducing withdrawal bleed through cyclic progesterone or a combined hormonal contraceptive to decrease risk of un-opposed estrogen stimulation of uterine lining, also identification and treatment of other underlying medical comorbidities (diabetes, obesity, hyperlipidemia, hirsutism).
- **Late-onset congenital adrenal hyperplasia** generally presents similarly to PCOS with amenorrhea and hyperandrogenism. Initial screening with 17-hydroxyprogesterone followed by ACTH stimulation test establishes the diagnosis. Most patients have an autosomal recessive disorder resulting in 21-hydroxylase deficiency. Treatment of amenorrhea involves glucocorticoid replacement and/or combined contraception. See Chapter 41 for a more complete discussion.
- **Cushing syndrome** is a clinical state resulting from prolonged, inappropriate hypercortisolism. Etiology includes pituitary tumor (Cushing disease), adrenal hypersecretion of cortisol, or iatrogenic (chronic steroid use). It is characterized by loss of normal hypothalamic-pituitary-adrenal feedback mechanisms and loss of the normal circadian rhythm of cortisol secretion. Screening tests include late-night salivary cortisol (evaluated diurnal variation), 24-hour urinary free cortisol (evaluates secretion), and dexamethasone suppression testing (evaluates impaired feedback).
- **Hyperprolactinemia** frequently presents with normal gonadotropin levels and normal to mildly depressed E$_2$. See earlier discussion.
- **Thyroid disease** can present with normal levels of gonadotropins and amenorrhea. Classically, **hypothyroidism** accounts for 1% to 2% of primary and secondary amenorrhea. Hypothyroidism can lead to hyperprolactinemia. Thyrotropin-releasing hormone (TRH) stimulates the release of TSH and PRL from the anterior pituitary. Therefore, patients with poorly controlled hypothyroidism may also experience sequelae of hyperprolactinemia. Both PRL and TSH should be routinely evaluated as part of the evaluation for amenorrhea. An elevated TSH and low T4 confirm hypothyroidism. An elevated TSH and normal T4 is diagnostic for subclinical hypothyroidism. Both clinical and subclinical hypothyroidism should be treated. Treatment should be initiated with 25 to 50 μg/day of levothyroxine followed by TSH assessment every 4 to 6 weeks until TSH levels normalize.

## Menopause

- **Menopause** occurs secondary to a genetically programmed loss of ovarian follicles. The onset of menopause should be differentiated from POF based on the age of the patient. It is defined as 12 months of amenorrhea after the final menstrual period. It reflects complete, or near complete, ovarian follicular depletion and the absence of ovarian $E_2$ secretion. Mean age of menopause is 51 years with a range of 43 to 57 years in American women. It is characterized by elevated FSH and low $E_2$. See Chapter 43.

## SUGGESTED READINGS

American College of Obstetricians and Gynecologists. ACOG practice bulletin no. 108: polycystic ovary syndrome. *Obstet Gynecol* 2009;114:936–949.

Nelson LM, Covington SN, Rebar RW. An update: spontaneous premature ovarian failure is not an early menopause. *Fertil Steril* 2005;83:1327–1332.

Practice Committee of the American Society for Reproductive Medicine. Current evaluation of amenorrhea. *Fertil Steril* 2008;90:S219–S225.

Rebar RW, Connolly HV. Clinical features of young women with hypergonadotropic amenorrhea. *Fertil Steril* 1990;53:804–810.

Reindollar RH, Byrd JR, McDonough PG. Delayed sexual development: a study of 252 patients. *Am J Obstet Gynecol* 1981;140:371–380.

Reindollar RH, Novak M, Tho SP, et al. Adult-onset amenorrhea: a study of 262 patients. *Am J Obstet Gynecol* 1986;155:531–543.

Speroff L, Fritz MA. *Clinical Gynecologic Endocrinology and Infertility*, 8th ed. Philadelphia, PA: Lippincott Williams & Wilkins, 2011.

Zacur HA. Indications for surgery in the treatment of hyperprolactinemia. *J Reprod Med* 1999;44:1127–1131.

# Abnormal Uterine Bleeding

Dipa Joshi and Roxanne Marie Jamshidi

The evaluation of **abnormal uterine bleeding (AUB)** requires characterization and quantification of the bleeding, specifically the onset, duration, frequency, amount, pattern, and associated symptoms.

## MENSTRUAL DIMENSIONS

- The mean menstrual blood loss in women with normal hemoglobin and iron levels is 35 mL, with 95% of women losing <60 mL each menstrual cycle.
- **Menstrual frequency** may be characterized as:
  - Normal—21 to 35 days
  - Oligomenorrhea—menstrual intervals longer than 35 days
  - Polymenorrhea—menstrual intervals shorter than 21 days

- The **volume** of menstrual blood loss and **cycle regularity** should be determined, although this can be based on subjective patient report.
  - Normal blood loss—5 to 80 mL
  - Regular cycles—2 to 20 days cycle-to-cycle variation over 12 months
  - Light cycle—<5-mL blood loss
  - Menorrhagia—heavy, regular periods with >80-mL blood loss
  - Metrorrhagia—irregular bleeding, especially between cycles
  - Menometrorrhagia—heavy, irregular bleeding that includes intermenstrual bleeding
  - Withdrawal bleeding—a predictable pattern of bleeding that occurs after the withdrawal of progestin therapy
  - Breakthrough bleeding—unpredictable bleeding that occurs while on hormonal contraception
- **Duration** of menstrual bleeding is defined as:
  - Normal—4 to 6 days
  - Prolonged—>7 days
  - Shortened—<3 days
- **Dysmenorrhea:** pain associated with menstruation that can interfere with daily activities

## DIFFERENTIAL DIAGNOSIS OF ABNORMAL UTERINE BLEEDING

**Causes of uterine bleeding** can be organized by age groups (Table 40-1).

### Prepubertal Abnormal Uterine Bleeding

- Benign **prepubertal bleeding** may occur in the first few days of life due to the withdrawal of maternal estrogen, but all other cases of bleeding require evaluation.
- See Chapter 34.

### Reproductive Age Abnormal Uterine Bleeding

- AUB in the **reproductive years** is associated with pregnancy, anovulatory bleeding, structural causes, and coagulation disorders.

#### History and Physical Exam

- The patient's sexual history, past medical history, gynecologic and obstetric history, and contraceptive and medication regimens are pertinent. Any change in the patient's diet, weight, and exercise pattern is relevant.
- Family history should be reviewed for possible bleeding disorders.
- Adolescent girls should be screened for physical abuse.
- Notable physical exam findings include weight, evidence of hyperandrogenism (e.g., hirsutism, acne), thyroid nodules, evidence of insulin resistance (e.g., acanthosis nigricans), and evidence of bleeding disorders (e.g., petechiae, ecchymoses, skin pallor).
- Inspection of the vaginal vault may reveal discharge suggestive of infection or evidence of trauma, lesions, polyps, products of conception, or masses.
- A bimanual examination should be performed to evaluate the internal os; presence of cervical motion tenderness; size and contour of uterus and adnexa; and presence of any palpable masses, lesions, or tenderness.
- Tanner staging should be documented (see Chapter 34).

| TABLE 40-1 | Differential Diagnosis of Abnormal Uterine Bleeding by Age Group | | | |
|---|---|---|---|---|
| **Children** | **Adolescent** | **Reproductive** | **Perimenopausal** | **Menopausal** |
| • Physiologic | • Anovulatory due to im-maturity of hypothalamic-pituitary-ovarian axis | • Pregnancy related | • Anovulatory | • Atrophy |
| • Vulvovaginitis | | • Anovulatory | • Endometrial hyperplasia | • Endometrial carcinoma |
| • Trauma | | • Vaginal/pelvic infection | • Endometrial polyps | • Endometrial hyperplasia |
| • Urethral prolapse | • Coagulopathy | • Structural (leiomyo-mata, polyps) | • Leiomyomas | • Endometrial polyp |
| • Endocrinopathies | • Pregnancy | • Adenomyosis | • Adenomyosis | • Leiomyomas |
| • Precocious puberty | • Vaginal/pelvic infection | • Endocrinopathies | • Genital tract neoplasm | • Hormone replace-ment therapy |
| • Ovarian cyst | • Benign lesions | • Malignancy/hyperplasia | | |
| • Genital tract neoplasm | • Medications | • Coagulopathy | | |
| | • Mullerian anomalies | • Iatrogenic | | |
| | • Genetic abnormality | | | |

Adapted from Shwayder JM. Pathophysiology of abnormal uterine bleeding. *Obstet Gynecol Clin North Am* 2000;27:219–234, with permission.

*Diagnostic Testing*

- Order laboratory urine (or serum) human chorionic gonadotropin (β-hCG) to assess for pregnancy, thyroid-stimulating hormone (TSH), prolactin, and complete blood count.
- In patients with history or physical exam suggesting genital tract infection, cervical or vaginal swabs to assess for sexually transmitted infections such as chlamydia, gonorrhea, herpes, or trichomonas can be of use.
- In women with risk factors for neoplastic processes, a tissue diagnosis is required (i.e., endometrial biopsy).
- In women at risk for coagulopathy, targeted screening of bleeding disorders is recommended (discussed later in this chapter).
- Imaging can be ordered to look for an anatomic cause of bleeding (e.g. fibroid, endometrial polyp).

## Perimenopause Abnormal Uterine Bleeding

- **Perimenopausal AUB** is most commonly due to anovulation and structural abnormalities (e.g., fibroids, polyps), however may be attributed to hyperplasia or malignancy.

*History, Exam, and Testing*

- In addition to routine history obtained for women of other ages, menopausal symptoms (e.g., vasomotor symptoms, sleep disturbances, mood disturbances) should be explored.
- Order TSH, follicle-stimulating hormone, and prolactin.
- Imaging should evaluate for fibroids. See Chapter 37.
- Obtain tissue specimens/biopsies (e.g., cervical, endometrial) if indicated.
- Infectious workup is recommended in patients at risk.

## Postmenopause Abnormal Uterine Bleeding

- **Postmenopausal AUB** is primarily caused by endometrial and vaginal atrophy. However, as approximately 15% of these women will have some form of hyperplasia and 7% to 10% will have endometrial cancer, AUB in the age group suggests malignancy until proven otherwise.
- As with very young patients, careful attention should be paid to determine the source of bleeding, such as the rectum.
- Tissue sampling and imaging in this population are essential.
- Infectious workup is recommended in patients at risk.

# EVALUATION OF ABNORMAL UTERINE BLEEDING

## Ultrasonography

- **Transvaginal ultrasonography (TVUS)** is useful to evaluate for the presence of fibroids, polyps, intrauterine pregnancy, and ectopic pregnancy. In the workup for possible malignant processes, sonography can be used to search for a thickened endometrium and masses within the uterus, adnexa, or cervix.
  - TVUS is a better diagnostic tool in postmenopausal than premenopausal women, with a sensitivity of 94% and specificity of 78% in diagnosing an endometrial abnormality in this population using a cutoff of 5 mm for the endometrial echo.
  - On the other hand, for reproductive age women, as useful as TVUS is at assessing the myometrium, it is only 56% sensitive and 73% specific for assessment of the intrauterine cavity.

- **Saline infusion sonography**, or sonohysterography, involves distention of the uterine cavity with sterile saline to enhance visualization of the endometrial surface during TVUS. Sonohysterography is the most sensitive noninvasive method of diagnosis for endometrial polyps and submucous myomata. However, it does not distinguish between benign and malignant processes.

## Hysteroscopy

- The gold standard for evaluating the endometrial cavity is **hysteroscopy**. The advantage of this procedure is that it provides direct visualization of the endometrial cavity and can be performed in the office setting or operating room. It can be both diagnostic and operative, allowing for directed biopsies and excision of polyps and small myomas. Office hysteroscopy with targeted biopsies has a sensitivity and specificity of 98% and 95%, respectively, compared with histologic findings at the time of hysterectomy.

## Magnetic Resonance Imaging

- **Pelvic magnetic resonance imaging (MRI)** can be useful in the diagnosis of adenomyosis and can accurately localize and measure fibroids, facilitating determination of the best treatment (e.g., embolization, resection, hysterectomy).

## Endometrial Sampling

- The American College of Obstetricians and Gynecologists (ACOG) recommends **endometrial sampling** in women older than age 45 years as a first-line test. Women younger than 45 years with risk factors for unopposed estrogen (e.g., obesity, polycystic ovarian syndrome), those who have failed medical management or have persistent AUB, are also recommended by ACOG to undergo endometrial sampling.
- Endometrial sampling is a rapid, safe, and cost-effective procedure that can be performed in the office to evaluate AUB. A potential drawback is that the biopsy does not sample the entire endometrium and a localized lesion may be missed: The posttest probability of endometrial cancer from an office endometrial biopsy is approximately 80% for a positive test result and 1% for a negative test result.

## Dilation and Curettage

- **Dilation and curettage (D&C)** can be both diagnostic and therapeutic but incurs the cost of an operating room and carries the risks of anesthesia. However, D&C may be indicated in women with nondiagnostic endometrial biopsies, biopsies with insufficient tissue for analysis, or women with cervical stenosis making an office procedure unsuccessful.

# SPECIFIC CAUSES OF ABNORMAL UTERINE BLEEDING

## Pregnancy-Associated Bleeding

- **Pregnancy** should be suspected in any woman in her reproductive years.
- If urine β-hCG is positive, a pelvic examination must be performed and an ultrasonographic study obtained. The differential includes ectopic pregnancy or threatened, inevitable, incomplete, or missed abortion. A quantitative serum β-hCG test is needed if an intrauterine pregnancy is not first confirmed by ultrasound, and Rh status is needed in all of these cases.
- Any patient who is hemodynamically unstable, bleeding heavily, or septic requires surgical intervention.

- Women with missed or incomplete abortions who are stable and not bleeding heavily may be offered expectant management or treated medically with misoprostol, which has a success rate of approximately 84%.

## Dysfunctional Uterine Bleeding

- **Dysfunctional uterine bleeding (DUB)** is a diagnosis of exclusion for AUB without a demonstrable pathologic cause and is found in approximately one third of all patients evaluated. The predominant causes of DUB are anovulation or oligoovulation. Anovulation is multifactorial and related to alterations of the hypothalamic-pituitary-ovarian axis. The use of the terminology "dysfunctional uterine bleeding" is falling out of favor with major professional organizations such as ACOG and the International Federation of Gynecology and Obstetrics (FIGO).

- With long-term anovulation, estrogen production occurs without the progesterone normally produced from a corpus luteum, thus creating an unopposed estrogen state. Therefore, these women are at risk for endometrial hyperplasia. Anovulation is also associated with polycystic ovary syndrome, which also places women at risk for endometrial hyperplasia. Morbid obesity can also cause DUB. Peripheral conversion of androstenedione to estrone occurs in adipose tissue producing elevated estrogen levels. Occasionally, DUB may be associated with ovulatory cycles.

- The optimal treatment will relieve symptoms and improve quality of life with minimal side effects. It is directed toward stabilizing the endometrium and treating the underlying hormonal alterations. Treatment is usually long-term because symptoms tend to return when therapy is discontinued. Various medical therapies are available (Table 40-2).

- Administration of progestins may be especially useful in patients with contraindications to **combined oral contraceptive pills** (COCs), such as smokers older than age 35 years. Although progestin therapy does not result in ovulation, it does prevent the negative sequelae of unopposed estrogen and regulates bleeding. However, very little data are available and no consensus exists on type of progestin or dosage. Side effects of progestins include breast tenderness, weight gain, and headaches. The levonorgestrel-releasing intrauterine system (Mirena) has been shown to decrease blood loss by up to 90% in women with menorrhagia.

- **COCs** also regulate menses and often decrease flow. Extended-use regimens may be especially useful in this population.

- **Nonsteroidal anti-inflammatory drugs** (NSAIDs) may reduce menstrual volume in women with menorrhagia by at least 20% to 40% and need to be taken during menses only.

- **Danazol** has been shown to significantly reduce menstrual blood loss (~50%) and may induce amenorrhea. However, androgenic side effects limit its use.

- **Antifibrinolytic medications** (e.g., tranexamic acid) decrease menstrual blood flow by 50% and similar to NSAIDs need to be taken only during menses. Some practitioners have been reluctant to prescribe antifibrinolytics because of their prothrombotic potential; however, studies have not shown increased incidence of thrombosis in treated women versus the general population. Antifibrinolytics may be especially useful in women who cannot tolerate hormonal treatments.

- **Gonadotropin-releasing hormone** (GnRH) agonists have limited use for treating AUB long-term and have significant side effects, such as hot flashes, osteopenia, and vaginal dryness. Symptoms return shortly after discontinuation. GnRH agonists can reduce uterine volume by 30% to 50%, which may facilitate less invasive surgery (i.e., vaginal vs. abdominal hysterectomy). Add-back therapy, which typically includes a progestin or a progestin plus low-dose estrogen, alleviates menopausal symptoms.

| TABLE 40-2 | Pharmacologic Management of Abnormal Uterine Bleeding |
|---|---|

**Hormonal Management**

**Progestins**

Medroxyprogesterone (*Provera*) 10 mg 3×/d for 14 d (days 12–25) or for 5–10 d

Norethindrone acetate (*Aygestin*) 5 mg 3×/d for 14 d (days 12 and 25) for anovulatory bleeding or on days 5–25 for ovulatory bleeding

Medroxyprogesterone acetate injection (*Depo Provera*) 150 mg IM every 12 wk

Levonorgestrel-releasing intrauterine system (*Mirena*)

**Combined estrogen and progestins**

Oral contraceptives

Transdermal preparations

Vaginal ring

Hormone replacement therapy

**Androgenic steroids**

Danazol 200 mg/d

**Gonadotropin-releasing hormone (GnRH) agonists**

Leuprolide (*Lupron*) 3.75 mg IM/mo or 11.25 mg every 3 mo

Goserelin (*Zoladex*) 3.6 mg SQ every 4 wk

**Nonsteroidal Anti-inflammatory Drugs (NSAIDs)**

Mefenamic acid 500 mg 3×/d

Ibuprofen 600–800 mg every 6 hr

Meclofenamate sodium 100 mg 3×/d

Naproxen sodium 550 mg × 1, then 275 mg every 6 hr

**Antifibrinolytic Agents**

Tranexamic acid 1,300 mg tid for up to 5 d during monthly menstruation

---

IM, intramuscularly; SQ, subcutaneously; tid, three times a day.

Adapted from Singh RH, Blumenthal P. Hormonal management of abnormal uterine bleeding. *Clin Obstet Gynecol* 2005;48:337–352; Roy SN, Bhattacharya S. Benefits and risks of pharmacological agents used for the treatment of menorrhagia. *Drug Safety* 2004;27:75–90, with permission.

*Surgical Treatment for Dysfunctional Uterine Bleeding*

- Surgical treatment may be warranted in patients who fail medical management.
  - D&C may be an initial step in treating AUB but does not typically have a sustained therapeutic effect.
  - Endometrial ablation is designed to ablate the full thickness of the endometrium. A variety of modalities are available, including thermal ablation, microwave, laser, cryocautery, and radiofrequency, each with its own advantages and disadvantages.
    ○ Before performing endometrial ablation, endometrial hyperplasia or carcinoma must be ruled out. It should be used to treat AUB in women with no intra-uterine pathology, although some of the devices are approved for women with submucosal or intracavitary fibroids.

○ Across all methods, the overall success rate is approximately 80% to 90%, with 30% to 50% of women reporting amenorrhea 6 months postprocedure. Still, within 5 years, 15% will have a second ablation and 20% will have a hysterectomy. Although endometrial ablation is not recommended in women who desire future fertility, contraception should be addressed for patients undergoing ablation.

- Hysterectomy provides definitive treatment for menorrhagia and may be a reasonable option in women with severe menorrhagia, refractory to medical and less radical surgical therapy, who have completed their childbearing.

## Coagulation Disorders

- Menorrhagia during adolescence should be attributed to a **coagulation disorder** until proven otherwise. Bleeding from multiple sites (e.g., nose, gingiva, intravenous sites, gastrointestinal, and genitourinary tracts) may suggest coagulopathy. There is a higher prevalence of bleeding disorders in women with menorrhagia.

### Von Willebrand Disease

- **Von Willebrand disease (vWD)** is the most common inherited bleeding disorder, affecting 1% to 2% of the population. Low, abnormal, or absent von Willebrand factor (vWF) leads to a spectrum of disease severity with three main types of vWD: types 1, 2, and 3. In women with vWD, menorrhagia is the most common manifestation, occurring in 60% to 95% beginning at menarche.
- Women with vWD are also likely to report postpartum or postoperative bleeding or bleeding related to dental work. They may also report easy bruising, epistaxis, or family history of bleeding symptoms. The frequency of vWD in women with menorrhagia is 5% to 20%.
- Other coagulopathies may also cause AUB, including platelet abnormalities, idiopathic thrombocytopenic purpura, and hematologic malignancy (e.g., leukemia).
- Testing for vWD should be considered in women with a history of unexplained menorrhagia beginning at menarche. ACOG recommends screening for vWD in adolescents with severe menorrhagia before starting hormonal therapy and in adult women with significant unexplained menorrhagia.
  - vWF levels vary over time and are affected by various physiologic, genetic, and pharmacologic factors. Several tests are performed to diagnose vWD: factor VIIIC activity, vWF antigen, ristocetin cofactor activity (i.e., vWF activity), platelet function tests, and bleeding time. vWF multimer tests are subsequently performed to distinguish among subtypes.
  - The ristocetin cofactor assay may be the best single screening test.
- Therapy usually involves treating the underlying cause and may require administration of blood products.
- Little data are available regarding treatment of menorrhagia in women with vWD. Oral contraceptives, desmopressin, and antifibrinolytic agents are options. Nasal desmopressin appears to be an effective treatment for vWD.

## Endocrine Disorders

- **Endocrinopathies** can cause anovulation, producing an environment of unopposed estrogen. In the absence of progesterone, the endometrium eventually breaks down, which may or may not lead to the formation of hyperplasia. Hypothyroidism and hyperprolactinemia are common disorders that can lead to anovulation.
- See Chapters 13 and 41.

## Hepatic Dysfunction

- Decreased metabolism of estrogen and decreased clotting factor synthesis are common ramifications of **liver failure**. Anovulation may also ensue. Menometrorrhagia is common.
- Liver function tests are necessary to make the diagnosis. Physical examination findings of jaundice, ascites, hepatosplenomegaly, palmar erythema, pruritus, and spider angioma are suggestive of liver failure. See Chapter 17.
- If possible, the underlying cause should be treated. If the patient is coagulopathic and hemorrhaging, administration of packed red blood cells and fresh frozen plasma may be indicated. Progestin therapy may also be beneficial.

## Medication Side Effects

### Psychotropic Medications

- Certain medications used in the treatment of psychiatric patients can affect the hypothalamic-pituitary axis and interfere with ovulation.
- Antipsychotic medications (i.e., dopamine antagonists) most commonly cause hyperprolactinemia and subsequent abnormalities in menstruation.
- Phenothiazines and antidepressants, particularly tricyclics, also interfere with the normal menstrual cycle.

### Hormone Medications

- Medroxyprogesterone acetate (Depo Provera). Approximately 50% of the patients taking this medication experience amenorrhea after 1 year of use, 80% after 5 years. Irregular bleeding also may be experienced.
- Combination oral contraceptive pills. Intermenstrual (breakthrough) bleeding is a side effect associated with COCs use that often leads to discontinuation. With long-term use, AUB may result from endometrial atrophy.
- Progestational agents. High doses of progestins often are used in the treatment of AUB and endometrial hyperplasia. Prolonged use of these agents may result in endometrial atrophy, which itself can cause AUB.

### Other Medications

- Anticoagulants. If the dosage of anticoagulants is too high, the patient can experience AUB.
- Digitalis, phenytoin, and corticosteroids have been implicated as causes of AUB.
- Over-the-counter medications that may contribute to AUB include motherwort, gingko, and ginseng.

## Intrauterine Devices

- Copper-containing **intrauterine devices**, unlike the levonorgestrel-releasing Mirena intrauterine system, increase average monthly blood loss by approximately 35%.
- Such bleeding is often treated successfully with NSAIDs.

## Genital Infection

- AUB is not a common presenting symptom of either **endometritis** or **cervicitis**. If present, bleeding associated with endometritis is most commonly intermenstrual, whereas bleeding associated with cervicitis is usually postcoital.
- Endometritis is diagnosed by uterine tenderness and sometimes fever. Any recent history of instrumentation of the uterus adds to the suspicion of endometritis. Chronic endometritis may be diagnosed by endometrial biopsy as evidenced by the

presence of plasma cells. Cervicitis is diagnosed by clinical examination and results of cervical cultures. See Chapter 28.

## Benign Pathology

### Leiomyomata

- **Leiomyomata** (fibroids) are the most common uterine neoplasm and are the number one indication for hysterectomy in the United States. See Chapter 37.
- AUB is the most common presenting symptom in women with leiomyomata.
- Although submucosal fibroids, followed by intramural fibroids, are most likely to cause bleeding, fibroids of any size and in any location can cause abnormal bleeding.

### Polyps

- Generally, benign endometrial lesions tend to be asymptomatic but may be present in 10% to 33% of women with complaints of bleeding, typically metrorrhagia.
- Diagnosis can be made by saline infusion sonogram or hysteroscopy.
- Bleeding secondary to polyps may respond to hormonal therapy. When found in postmenopausal women, they should be removed via operative hysteroscopy. Cervical polyps can be removed by grasping them with forceps, twisting them off, and cauterizing the base as needed.

### Endometrial Hyperplasia

- **Endometrial hyperplasia**, a precursor to endometrial carcinoma, is classified into simple or complex, based on architectural features, and typical or atypical, based on cytologic features. Endometrial hyperplasia tends to occur during periods of long-term unopposed estrogen exposure, either secondary to anovulatory cycles or exogenous use. AUB is the most common presenting symptom.
- An endometrial tissue sample, obtained either from an endometrial biopsy or D&C, is required to diagnose endometrial hyperplasia.
- Treatment depends on age, desire for future fertility, surgical risk, and presence of atypia in the pathology specimen.
  - **Hyperplasia without atypia** may be managed by long-term follow-up with repeat endometrial sampling if abnormal bleeding recurs.
    - Cyclic medroxyprogesterone acetate is recommended (10 mg/day for 12 to 14 days/cycle for 3 to 6 months) in young anovulatory women to induce monthly withdrawal bleeding and subsequently normalize the endometrium, which occurs in approximately 86% of patients on this regimen.
    - Local progesterone administration via the levonorgestrel-releasing intrauterine system (Mirena) and combined oral contraceptives are also options.
    - Postmenopausal women with endometrial hyperplasia without atypia who are on estrogen replacement therapy should discontinue estrogen and may then be treated with medroxyprogesterone and repeat D&C.
  - **Atypical endometrial hyperplasia** is more likely to progress to carcinoma, and therefore, more aggressive treatment is needed. Atypical hyperplasia concomitantly exists with endometrial carcinoma in up to 25% to 50% of cases. Thus, a significant number of women diagnosed with atypical hyperplasia on curettage will be found to have invasive carcinoma if hysterectomy is performed.
    - For patients who wish to retain their fertility, progestational therapy is an acceptable approach. Treatment with continuous regimens of megestrol acetate (40 mg two to four times daily) is associated with a regression rate of 94%.

Treatment is continued for 6 months with endometrial biopsies performed at 3 and 6 months. Dosing is increased if regression is not observed. This approach also may be used in women who are poor surgical candidates. If regression does not occur, megestrol dose can be increased to 200 mg/day. Once regression occurs, maintenance therapy should begin with either megestrol, cyclic medroxyprogesterone acetate, or a levonorgestrel-releasing intrauterine system.

○ It must be emphasized that conservative therapy in women with complex atypical hyperplasia involves risk and close follow-up is necessary. Progesterone withdrawal regimens are not consistently effective and should not be used in the treatment of atypical hyperplasia. Also see Chapter 47.

## Malignancy

### Endometrial Cancer

* Endometrial carcinoma is rare in patients younger than age 40 years. Postmenopausal bleeding, however, should be assumed to represent endometrial cancer until proven otherwise.
* In a postmenopausal woman not receiving hormone replacement therapy, the presence of a thickened endometrial stripe (>5 mm) on ultrasonography is considered abnormal. Tissue sampling is then required. See Chapter 47 for further discussion.

### Cervical Cancer

* Cervical carcinoma is a disease of both the relatively young and the old. Almost all cervical lesions that cause abnormal bleeding are visible on examination. The most common bleeding patterns associated with cervical carcinoma are intermenstrual and postcoital bleeding. See Chapters 45 and 46 for screening and treatment.

### Ovarian Cancer

* Estrogen-producing ovarian tumors, such as a granulosa-theca cell tumor, can produce endometrial hyperplasia and AUB. See Chapter 48.

## SUGGESTED READINGS

American College of Obstetricians and Gynecologists. ACOG committee opinion no. 451: Von Willebrand disease in women. *Obstet Gynecol* 2009;114:1439–1443.

American College of Obstetricians and Gynecologists. ACOG practice bulletin no. 14: management of anovulatory bleeding. *Int J Gynaecol Obstet* 2001;72(3):263–271.

American College of Obstetricians and Gynecologists. ACOG practice bulletin no. 128: diagnosis of abnormal uterine bleeding in reproductive-aged women. *Obstet Gynecol* 2012;120(1):197–206.

Casablanca Y. Management of dysfunctional uterine bleeding. *Obstet Gynecol Clin North Am* 2008;35(2):219–234, viii.

Hashim A. Medical treatment of idiopathic heavy menstrual bleeding. What is new? An evidence based approach. *Arch Gynecol Obstet* 2013;287(2):251–260.

Lacey JV Jr, Chia VM. Endometrial hyperplasia and the risk of progression to carcinoma. *Maturitas* 2009;63(1):39–44.

# Hyperandrogenism

Katherine Ikard Stewart and Lisa Kolp

**41**

**Androgens** are necessary for normal ovarian and sexual function. They play an important role in cognition, bone health, muscle mass, body composition, mood, and energy. The obstetrician-gynecologist must have a strong knowledge base regarding the role androgens play in normal female physiology.

- Androgens are precursors for estrogen synthesis.
- Although controversial, it has been proposed that androgens may be necessary for normal sexual desire in women.
- Androgens also affect skeletal homeostasis. They affect bone metabolism directly via androgen receptors expressed by osteocytes and indirectly via conversion of androgens to estrogen. Multiple studies have shown that women with low androgen concentrations have lower bone density and increased fracture risk.

## ANDROGENS IN THE FEMALE

Androgens circulate in the body in various forms. Circulating androgens found in the blood of premenopausal women include testosterone, androstenedione, dehydroepiandrosterone (DHEA), DHEA sulfate (DHEA-S), and dihydrotestosterone (DHT). Androgens are produced by the adrenal glands and the ovary and arise from peripheral conversion.

### Testosterone

- Testosterone is the most potent androgenic hormone.
- In women, nearly 25% of testosterone is secreted from the ovaries and 25% is from the adrenal glands. The remaining one half is produced from peripheral conversion of androstenedione to testosterone in the kidneys, liver, and adipose tissue.
- Normal circulating concentrations range from 20 to 80 ng/dL.
- Approximately 65% of testosterone in the circulation is bound to sex hormone–binding globulin (SHBG). Nineteen percent to 33% of testosterone is loosely bound to albumin. The remaining 1% of testosterone circulates in the free and active form (Fig. 41-1).
- Testosterone levels decrease by 50% from ages 20 to 40 years. Less testosterone is secreted from the ovary with menopause, as the ovarian theca cells are less responsive to luteinizing hormone (LH). As menopause is entered, SHBG levels remain constant, yielding an even greater decrease in free testosterone. However, serum hormone concentrations of SHBG fall due to the lack of estrogen, finally resulting in an increase in bioavailable testosterone.

### Androstenedione

- Is a less potent androgen than testosterone but can produce significant androgenic effects when present in excess amounts
- Is produced in equal amounts by the adrenal glands (50%) and the ovaries (50%)
- Majority of androstenedione is converted to testosterone.

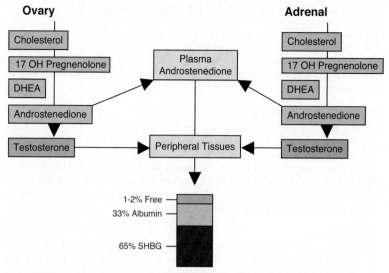

**Figure 41-1.** Endogenous production and secretion of testosterone in women. DHEA, dehydroepiandrosterone; SHBG, sex hormone–binding globulin.

- Normal serum concentration ranges from 60 to 300 ng/dL, often with a 15% increase at midcycle. Androstenedione circulates in blood, bound to both SHBG and albumin.

## Dehydroepiandrosterone and Dehydroepiandrosterone Sulfate

- Androgen precursors, much less potent than testosterone, are produced predominantly by the adrenal glands, with some component of ovarian production and peripheral conversion.
- DHEA is metabolized quickly, thus measurement of its serum concentration does not reflect adrenal gland activity. DHEA-S has a much longer half-life than DHEA, and measurement of its serum level is used to assess adrenal function.
- Serum hormone concentrations of DHEA-S in women vary widely and depend on age (normal range of approximately 35–340 $\mu$g/dL depending on the lab).

## Dihydrotestosterone

- Testosterone is converted to DHT by 5-alpha reductase, an enzyme found in many androgen-sensitive tissues.
- DHT is a very potent androgen primarily responsible for the androgenic effects on hair follicles.

## Sex Hormone–Binding Globulins

- Androgenicity is determined by free hormone concentrations. Thus, SHBG influences the hormonal state. Testosterone and insulin both decrease SHBG levels, whereas estrogen and thyroid hormone increase its levels.
- Symptoms of hyperandrogenism may be seen in patients with a normal total testosterone level if the serum hormone concentration of SHBG is reduced to a level that significantly increases the free hormone.

## CLINICAL FINDINGS IN HYPERANDROGENISM

**Hyperandrogenism** is characterized by an abnormally elevated serum concentration of androgens and/or physical findings consistent with androgen excess. Androgenic hormones in the female can stimulate abnormal terminal hair growth, voice and muscle changes, hair loss, clitoral enlargement, and reduction in breast size. Physical characteristics of hyperandrogenism are as follows.

### Androgenic Hair Changes
- During gestation, the hair follicles of the developing fetus produce fine, unpigmented hair known as **lanugo**. The total number of hair follicles is determined late in the second trimester of pregnancy. With time, some of the hair follicles produce thick, darkly pigmented **terminal hair** in response to androgen exposure. The remaining hair follicles produce **vellus hair**, which are finer and not as darkly pigmented.
- **Normal hair growth cycle** follows three stages: **anagen** (growth phase), **catagen** (involution phase), and **telogen** phase (rest phase).

*Hirsutism*
- **Hirsutism** is excessive male pattern hair growth in women. It refers to the growth of terminal hair on the face, chest, back, lower abdomen, and upper thighs caused by the overactivity or overexpression of circulating androgens. The abnormal hair growth is predominantly midline. Androgens stimulate hair growth, increase the diameter of the hair shaft, and deepen the pigmentation of the hair. In contrast, estrogens slow hair growth and decrease hair diameter and pigmentation.
  - **Idiopathic hirsutism** is the term used when a hirsute individual has normal levels of circulating androgens and has not been diagnosed with polycystic ovarian syndrome (PCOS) or another disorder.
  - **The Ferriman-Gallwey score** is an objective tool that may be used in the clinical setting to grade hair growth in women. This method evaluates nine different androgen-sensitive hair growth sites on a scale from 0 to 4. Ninety-five percent of women will have a score under 8. Scores >8 suggest an excess of androgen-mediated hair growth and this should be confirmed with a more extensive hormone evaluation.

*Hypertrichosis*
- **Hypertrichosis** is the generalized, excessive growth of vellus hair. It may be caused by genetic factors, underlying malignancy, or exposure to drugs such as phenytoin, penicillamine, diazoxide, cyclosporine, and minoxidil. It may also be seen with a number of medical conditions, including anorexia nervosa, hypothyroidism, malnutrition, porphyria, dermatomyositis, and paraneoplastic syndromes. Hypertrichosis should not be mistaken for hirsutism.

*Hair Loss*
- Recession of hair in the frontal and temporal regions of the scalp and the crown of the head (i.e., **male pattern baldness**) in response to androgens is common with aging. This is the most common pattern of hair loss and affects approximately 30% to 40% of men and women alike. However, hair loss is less evident in women because it is typically more diffuse and rarely complete. The fact that excessive androgen activity stimulates hair growth on some parts of the body while causing hair loss from others remains unexplained.

- Young men and women with **androgenic alopecia** have higher levels of 5-alpha reductase, increased androgen receptors, and lower levels of the enzyme cytochrome P-450 aromatase (which converts androgens such as testosterone and 4-androstenedione to the estrogens estradiol and estrone, respectively).

## Virilization

- This is an appearance of masculine features due to extreme excess androgenic activity. It refers to a constellation of symptoms, including deepening of the voice, male body habitus, male pattern baldness, clitoromegaly, and reduction of breast size.
- Virilization is very rare and may be associated with adrenal tumors and hyperplasia or ovarian tumors, such as theca lutein cysts, luteomas, and Sertoli-Leydig cell tumors.

## Skin Changes

- Androgens stimulate secretions from pilosebaceous glands, resulting in oily skin. Severe acne is a manifestation of excessive androgenic hormone activity.

## Voice Changes

- The vocal cords can undergo irreversible thickening, resulting in a lower tone of the voice.

## Male Body Habitus

- Hypertrophy of major muscle groups, such as arm and leg muscles, occurs in response to androgen exposure and may result in the development of a male body habitus.

## Clitoromegaly

- Enlargement of the clitoris may occur. This is a dose-dependent event and is irreversible. It is more commonly seen when the excessive androgen exposure occurs in childhood or around the time of puberty.

## Acanthosis Nigricans

- Acanthosis nigricans is a gray-brown, velvety discoloration of the skin that is associated with hyperinsulinemia and obesity. Acanthosis nigricans is typically seen in the groin, neck, axillary, and vulvar regions. These patients should undergo testing for diabetes mellitus. Acanthosis nigricans can also be a paraneoplastic syndrome and associated with an underlying malignancy, commonly an adenocarcinoma involving the gastrointestinal (GI) tract.

## DIAGNOSIS OF HYPERANDROGENISM

### History and Physical Examination

- Hyperandrogenism may be diagnosed if signs of androgen excess are present (see earlier discussion).
- A careful medical history should be taken, including a detailed menstrual history asking about age of menarche, regularity of menstrual cycles, pregnancies, oral contraceptive preparation (OCP) use, and presence of symptoms of ovulation or menstrual molimina. Patients should also be asked about a history of thyroid disease and hyperinsulinemia.
- A complete physical examination should be conducted, including evaluation for galactorrhea and acanthosis nigricans.
- Pay particular attention to medications (see earlier text) and family history.

## Laboratory Evaluation

- Measurement of serum androgen levels may be obtained to diagnose hyperandrogenism (Fig. 41-2). The clinician should check the following:
  - **Testosterone** serum hormone concentrations
  - **DHEA-S** >700 ng/dL, consistent with abnormal adrenal function
  - **17-Alpha-hydroxyprogesterone (17-OHP):** Normal level is 100 to 300 ng/dL.
  - **Prolactin** (normal range 1 to 20 ng/mL): Hyperprolactinemia can be associated with hyperandrogenism, as it is likely that prolactin receptors are located on the adrenal glands. When prolactin binds to these adrenal receptors, it stimulates the release of DHEA-S.
  - **Thyroid function tests**
- Assessment of hyperinsulinemia:
  - Normal fasting glucose <100 mg/dL
  - Impaired fasting glucose indicated by fasting glucose 100 to 125 mg/dL

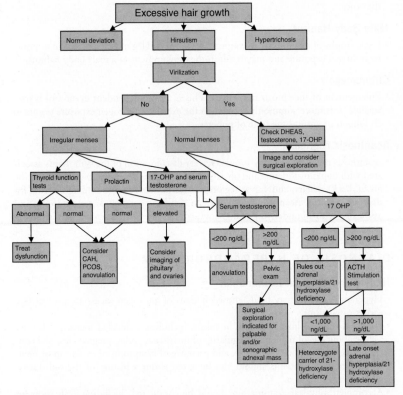

**Figure 41-2.** Algorithm for the diagnosis of hyperandrogenism. DHEAS, dehydroepiandrosterone sulfate; 17-OHP, 17-alpha-hydroxyprogesterone; CAH, congenital adrenal hyperplasia; PCOS, polycystic ovarian syndrome; ACTH, adrenocorticotropic hormone.

○ Diabetes mellitus diagnosed with fasting glucose levels >126 mg/dL, hemoglobin A1C >6.5%, 2-hour oral glucose tolerance test (75-g load) >200 mg/dL, or a random plasma glucose >200 mg/dL.

# CAUSES AND TREATMENT OF HYPERANDROGENISM

Five major causes of hyperandrogenism have been identified:
• PCOS
• Late-onset adrenal hyperplasia
• Tumors of the ovary or adrenal glands
• Cushing syndrome
• Idiopathic or drug-induced processes

## Polycystic Ovarian Syndrome

• PCOS is the most common endocrine disorder among reproductive age women. It affects approximately 4% to 12% of this population.
• In 1935, Stein and Leventhal described seven women who were amenorrheic, obese, and hirsute with cystic ovaries. From this initial description, the term **Stein-Leventhal syndrome** was originally used to identify other similarly affected women.
• Because of the cystic changes found within the ovaries of affected patients, the terms **hyperandrogenemic chronic anovulation syndrome**, **PCOS**, and **polycystic ovary disease (PCOD)** are now used to describe these patients. However, polycystic ovaries alone seen on radiologic imaging are a nonspecific finding and may be seen in normal women.
• Individuals with PCOS do not have orderly follicular development. Most cycles fail to lead to the emergence of a dominant follicle or release of an oocyte. Although follicle development occasionally proceeds to ovulation, development of the follicle to only its initial growth stage is common. The ovarian cortex becomes populated with numerous small follicles or "cysts." The hyperandrogenemic state is believed to be both a cause and effect of incomplete follicular development.
• PCOS is associated with amenorrhea, hyperandrogenism, hyperinsulinemia, and metabolic syndrome. In patients affected by this disorder, it is important to make the appropriate diagnosis early and to closely monitor these individuals, as they may be at risk for other comorbidities as a consequence of the underlying pathology.

### Diagnosis of Polycystic Ovarian Syndrome

• In May 2003, the Rotterdam European Society of Human Reproduction and Embryology/American Society for Reproductive Medicine–sponsored PCOS consensus workshop revised the diagnostic criteria to include any two of the following three manifestations:
  • Oligomenorrhea and/or anovulation
  • Hyperandrogenism (clinical and/or biochemical signs)
  • Polycystic ovaries
• In 2009, the Androgen Excess and PCOS Society also defined less inclusive criteria for PCOS which required ALL of the following criteria be met:
  • Hyperandrogenism: hirsutism and/or hyperandrogenemia **AND**
  • Ovarian dysfunction: oligo-anovulation and/or polycystic ovaries **AND**
  • Exclusion of other androgen excess or related disorders

- Of note, PCOS is always a diagnosis of exclusion in all definitions. All other etiologies of hyperandrogenism must be ruled out.
- Patients with PCOS typically present with oligomenorrhea, amenorrhea, hirsutism, obesity, and infertility. All or some of these symptoms may be present.
- Hyperandrogenism can be demonstrated by either hirsutism or elevated levels of androgens.
- Virilization is not consistent with a diagnosis of PCOS and other etiologies should be considered.
- Polycystic ovaries are defined as 12 or more follicles in each ovary measuring 2 to 9 mm and increased ovarian volume >10 mL as judged by transvaginal sonography.
- Insulin resistance and metabolic syndrome are often associated with PCOS and all obese women should be screened for comorbidities. Providers should check a cholesterol panel, blood pressure, fasting glucose, and 2-hour oral glucose tolerance test. Further studies are needed to determine the use of these tests in nonobese women with PCOS.

*Pathophysiology of Polycystic Ovarian Syndrome*

- The exact cause of PCOS remains unknown. Abnormalities of the hypothalamic-pituitary axis and the ovarian or adrenal steroidogenic pathway have been suggested as possible explanations.
  - **Pituitary and hypothalamus:** At the level of the hypothalamic-pituitary axis, increases in the frequency and amplitude of LH pulses have been recorded. A ratio of serum LH to follicle-stimulating hormone of greater than 2 is observed in PCOS patients.
  - **Ovarian androgen production:** Increased secretion of androgens from the ovaries has been observed in patients with PCOS. Elevated LH levels may lead to increased activity of ovarian theca cells, thus producing androgens. Also, elevated insulin may stimulate androgen secretion from both the ovaries and adrenals.
  - **Adrenal androgen production:** Some PCOS patients may have mild elevations of DHEA-S levels.
  - **Consequences of anovulation:** Ovulation for many women with PCOS may occur infrequently, but ovaries in these patients continue to secrete low levels of estrogen. Due to the lack of cyclic estrogen and progesterone withdrawal over time, unopposed estrogen can lead to proliferation of the endometrium that may result in abnormal bleeding and, if untreated, may progress to endometrial hyperplasia and/or endometrial carcinoma.
  - **Hyperinsulinemia and insulin resistance:** Increased resistance to insulin is often observed in patients with PCOS, whether or not they are obese. Insulin may cause or contribute to the hyperandrogenic state by activating insulin receptors within the ovary, augmenting androgen secretion, or by acting on insulin-like growth factor receptors.

*Treatment for Hyperandrogenism/Polycystic Ovarian Syndrome*

- Treatment of the patient with hirsutism, hyperandrogenism, or hyperandrogenic chronic anovulation depends on the underlying etiology and the desire for pregnancy. Hirsutism is slow to respond to hormone suppression. Results may not be seen for up to 6 months. Unfortunately, androgen suppression will not alter previous hair growth patterns. Mechanical methods of hair removal, such as shaving, waxing, depilatories, laser, and electrolysis, should also be considered.
  - **Lifestyle modifications** should be first line in the management of hyperandrogenism. For those individuals who suffer from hirsutism and obesity, weight loss of even 5% of original body weight can often improve symptoms related to

PCOS. Weight loss may result in an elevation of SHBG, a decrease in bioavailable testosterone, and an improvement in insulin sensitivity.

- **OCPs** reduce circulating gonadotropin levels and increase SHBG levels; both work to decrease circulating androgens. OCPs are the first line of treatment of oligomenorrhea caused by PCOS. Progestins decrease total androgen level by reducing the activity of 5-alpha reductase. OCP usage results in an overall decrease in the formation of new androgen-dependent hair growth and androgen-stimulated acne. All low-dose OCP preparations are believed to have similar results. If therapy with OCPs is suboptimal, addition of an antiandrogen, such as spironolactone or finasteride, is recommended.

- If combination OCPs are contraindicated or not desired, **medroxyprogesterone acetate** may be administered (5 to 10 mg for 10 to 12 days) every month or every other month to produce regular withdrawal bleeding. Patients should be cautioned that, unless contraception is used, pregnancy is possible with cyclic progestin therapy.

- **Metformin hydrochloride** is a biguanide antihyperglycemic drug, U.S. Food and Drug Administration (FDA) approved for the management of type 2 diabetes mellitus. Metformin decreases hepatic gluconeogenesis, thus reducing the need for insulin secretion. It also decreases the intestinal absorption of glucose and improves insulin sensitivity in the peripheral system, including skeletal muscle, liver, and adipose tissue. In some studies, metformin has been shown to restore menses in approximately 50% of women with PCOS. Another trial showed that metformin, compared to placebo, can improve plasma insulin and insulin sensitivity, reduce serum free testosterone, and increase serum high-density lipoprotein cholesterol.
  - **Dosing:** The optimum dose of metformin for restoration of menses in women with PCOS ranges from 500 mg by mouth three times daily to 850 mg by mouth twice daily. Patients should be titrated up to the appropriate dose of this medication, starting at the lowest dose once daily, due to the GI side effects.
  - Metformin has a limited role in the treatment of hirsutism. Other agents may be added to metformin to improve these symptoms.
  - Metformin appears to be unique among insulin-sensitizing agents in that it can improve weight loss (particularly a greater reduction in abdominal fat), hyperandrogenism, and menstrual cycles in individuals with PCOS.

- **Spironolactone** therapy is often initiated if OCP use is not an option for the treatment of hirsutism or if results from OCP therapy are not optimal. An aldosterone antagonist, spironolactone, is an antihypertensive agent that was originally found to cause gynecomastia in men. Spironolactone directly inhibits 5-alpha reductase and decreases androgen synthesis. The usual dose is 25 to 100 mg by mouth twice daily. After 6 months of therapy at 100 to 200 mg/day, there is a reduction in the diameter of terminal hair and cessation of new terminal hair growth. Doses are then tapered to a maintenance dose of 25 to 50 mg per day. Because of potential adverse effects on genitalia of male fetuses, spironolactone should be used with contraception in sexually active women. Other side effects include diuresis, orthostatic hypotension, fatigue, dysfunctional uterine bleeding, hyperkalemia, and breast enlargement.

- **Flutamide** is a nonsteroidal antiandrogen used for prostate cancer that blocks the binding of androgen to its receptor. When administered in a dosage of 250 mg/day, inhibition of new hair growth is observed. Side effects include dry skin and, rarely, hepatotoxicity. Liver function should be monitored during treatment. Due to adverse fetal effects, effective contraceptive therapy is mandatory.

- **Finasteride:** An inhibitor of mostly type II 5-alpha reductase, finasteride was developed initially as a treatment for prostate hypertrophy and cancer. By inhibiting

5-alpha reductase, the drug decreases DHT activity at the level of the hair follicle. Finasteride treatment prevents new hair growth and decreases the terminal hair shaft diameter. Finasteride is orally dosed at 5 mg daily. No major side effects have been associated with this drug. Again, due to adverse fetal effects, reliable contraception should be used.

- **Minoxidil** is the only drug approved by the FDA for treatment of androgenic alopecia in women. It promotes hair growth by increasing the duration of the anagen phase and enlarging miniaturized and suboptimal follicles. It is available over the counter as a 2% and 5% topical solution.
- **Corticosteroid therapy** is another alternative for the treatment of hirsutism and hyperandrogenism and is the primary mode of therapy for those individuals suffering from congenital adrenal hyperplasia (CAH). The steroids suppress the hypothalamic-pituitary-adrenal axis and can result in improved hirsutism and ovulatory function. Corticosteroid therapy should not be used for the long term in patients with PCOS, as it may result in debilitating osteoporosis and worsening glucose intolerance.
- **Eflornithine hydrochloride** is a cream that reduces unwanted facial hair. Eflornithine is a potent antagonist of ornithine decarboxylase, the enzyme necessary for the production of polyamines, organic compounds that stimulate and regulate the growth of hair follicles and other organs. Women who apply eflornithine hydrochloride (13.9% cream) to their faces twice daily have shown improvement after 24 weeks in some clinical trials. The benefit is usually first seen at 8 weeks.
- **Surgery:** Older women who have no desire for fertility and who do not desire continued hormonal therapy may consider bilateral oophorectomy, with or without hysterectomy.

*Fertility Treatment for Polycystic Ovarian Syndrome*

- In PCOS patients, assistance with ovulation induction frequently is required.
- **Clomiphene citrate** is usually administered orally in dosages of 50 to 100 mg/day for 5 days on a monthly basis to induce ovulation in infertile women. It is not used for cycle regulation or as a primary treatment for hirsutism. Monitoring with a basal body temperature chart, LH levels, pelvic ultrasonography, or serum progesterone 14 days after the last clomiphene citrate dose may be used to confirm ovulation. For the patient resistant to clomiphene citrate, the addition of metformin hydrochloride (500 mg three times daily) may result in ovulation.
- Direct stimulation of the ovary may be used to induce ovulation through the intramuscular or subcuticular administration of gonadotropins in the treatment of anovulatory infertility. See Chapter 32.

## Late-Onset or "Nonclassical" Adrenal Hyperplasia

- Excess androgen production is a common feature shared by most forms of **CAH**. Unlike typical CAH, symptoms of late-onset CAH are not evident until late childhood or adolescence.
- The most common adrenal enzyme defect is 21-hydroxylase (21-OH) deficiency, which is an autosomal recessive disorder.
- Enzyme deficiencies of 11-beta-hydroxylase and 3-beta-hydroxysteroid dehydrogenase are far less common.
- 21-OH converts progesterone to 11-deoxycorticosterone or 17-OHP to 11-deoxycortisol (Table 41-1). A decrease in the activity of this enzyme causes diminished cortisol production by the adrenal gland, resulting in increased pituitary secretion of adrenocorticotropic hormone (ACTH). ACTH stimulates the adrenal gland to

| TABLE 41-1 | Enzymes and Their Characteristics | | |
|---|---|---|---|
| Deficient Enzyme | Androgen Levels | Mineralocorticoid Levels | Female Virilization at Birth |
| 21-Hydroxylase | Excess | Deficiency | Yes |
| 11-β-Hydroxylase | Excess | Excess | Yes |
| 17-α-Hydroxylase | Deficiency | Excess | No |

produce increased precursor 17-OHP. Higher 17-OHP levels lead to secretion of androstenedione, which is then converted to testosterone.

*Diagnosis*

- Measure the basal levels of 17-OHP in the morning. Levels of 17-OHP should be <200 ng/dL.
  - Levels that exceed 200 ng/dL but are <800 ng/dL require ACTH stimulation testing (see Fig. 41-2).
  - Levels over 800 ng/dL are virtually diagnostic of CAH.
  - Patients with late-onset hyperplasia have 17-OHP levels >1,500 ng/dL in response to a 250-μg ACTH stimulation challenge.
- Patients should be tested for 21-hydroxylase deficiency (CYP21A2 deficiency) especially when they present with symptoms of hyperandrogenism at a young age or if they have a known family history of CAH. Women of Hispanic or Eastern European Jewish descent should also be tested, as the prevalence of this disorder among these populations is greater than in the general population.

*Treatment*

- Individuals diagnosed with late-onset adrenal hyperplasia may be treated by the administration of glucocorticoid agents to restore ovulation. This treatment also reduces circulating androgen levels. Glucocorticoid administration is therefore appropriate therapy for infertility or hirsutism in individuals with late-onset adrenal hyperplasia. In patients with 21-OH deficiency, prednisone 5 mg before bedtime is used to suppress endogenous ACTH.
- Alternatively, OCPs or antiandrogens may be used successfully to treat hirsutism, alone or in combination with dexamethasone. Ovulation-inducing drugs may also be used to treat infertility.

## Androgen-Producing Ovarian or Adrenal Tumors

- Tumors of the ovary or adrenal gland that secrete androgens are rare.
- The presence of an **androgen-producing tumor** is suspected on the basis of clinical findings.
- Palpation of an adnexal mass in a patient with symptoms of hyperandrogenism or rapid onset of virilization even in the presence of normal testosterone levels should prompt a workup for a pelvic tumor. These tumors may often be small and difficult to detect on physical examination alone.
- Testosterone levels exceeding 200 ng/dL and DHEA-S levels >1,000 mg/dL are concerning for the presence of an ovarian or adrenal androgen-producing tumor.
- Surgical removal with or without adjuvant therapy is the treatment of choice.

## Cushing Syndrome

- Patients with **Cushing syndrome** often exhibit specific physical findings. See Chapter 13.

## Idiopathic and Drug-Induced Hirsutism

- **Idiopathic hirsutism** is diagnosed in hirsute individuals who have a negative workup for other causes of hirsutism. Studies show that 5% to 15% of hirsute patients may have idiopathic hirsutism. An alternative explanation is based on the hypothesis that patients with idiopathic hirsutism demonstrate increased skin sensitivity to androgens. One theory is that patients with idiopathic hirsutism convert testosterone to DHT in greater quantities than normal due to increased activity of 5-alpha reductase.
- Occasionally, drugs may be causative. Danazol and methyltestosterone are two drugs that may cause iatrogenic hirsutism.
- The same medications used to treat hirsute PCOS patients may be used to treat patients with idiopathic hirsutism.

## SUGGESTED READINGS

American College of Obstetricians and Gynecologists. ACOG practice bulletin no. 108: polycystic ovary syndrome. *Obstet Gynecol* 2009;114:936–949.

Brodell LA, Mercurio MG. Hirsutism: diagnosis and management. *Gend Med* 2010;7(2):79–87.

Ferriman D, Gallwey JD. Clinical assessment of body hair growth in women. *J Clin Endocrinol Metab* 1961;21:1440–1447.

Hock DL, Seifer DB. New treatments of hyperandrogenism and hirsutism. *Obstet Gynecol Clin North Am* 2000;27(3):567–581, vi–vii.

# 42

# Female Sexual Response and Sexual Dysfunction

Nina Resetkova and Linda Rogers

## EPIDEMIOLOGY

- In the 1999 National Health and Social Life Survey, 1,410 men and 1,749 women aged 18 to 59 years were surveyed and 43% of these women reported sexual concerns. A British national survey found that 54% of women reported at least one sexual problem lasting at least 1 month but only 21% sought help.
- The most common female sexual problem in both studies was a lack of interest. Difficulty with orgasm was reported by 24%, difficulty with arousal by 19%, and pain

with sex by 14%. Accurate assessments of female sexual dysfunction are hampered by the fact that many patients have more than one type of dysfunction. Additionally, many patients complaining of lack of interest actually have a problem with another phase of the sexual response cycle, in part because they lack familiarity with the terms.

- Multiple studies have found that female sexual dysfunction is associated with a decreased sense of physical and emotional satisfaction and a decreased sense of overall well-being.

## DIAGNOSIS OF SEXUAL DISORDERS

### Screening

- Many physicians infrequently discuss sexual dysfunction due to limited time and training, embarrassment, or the perceived notion that there is an absence of effective treatment options. A few simple questions can initiate the discussion:
  - Are you currently involved in a sexual relationship?
  - Do you have sex with men, women, or both?
  - Do you have any concerns about or pain with sex?
  - Do you have any concerns you would like to discuss?
- Once a dialogue has been initiated, a complete history can be obtained. This should include the nature and frequency of the problem, the degree of distress, whether the problem is lifelong versus newly acquired, situational, or generalized. Additionally, the partner's sexual problems or concerns, partner reaction, and history of prior treatment or intervention should be discussed.
- It is important to elicit the patient's thoughts concerning the cause of the problems and their expectations from treatment. The physician must also get a medical history, a psychological/psychiatric history (e.g., mood disorders, body image disorders), sexual history including sexual abuse or violence, and a psychosocial history (e.g., relationship difficulties, cultural and religious beliefs that may affect function, work/finance/children, and other life stressors). It is also important to inquire about the use of medications that may cause sexual side effects and about the use of personal hygiene products such as soaps, laundry products, douches, or other possible skin irritants.

### Physical Exam

- A thorough physical exam can help identify causes, address concerns, and educate the patient about her anatomy.
- During visual inspection of the external female genitalia and perineum, it is important to note any atrophy, lack of estrogenization, loss of architecture, scarring, hypopigmentation or hyperpigmentation, or possible infection. The exam should include the urethral meatus and anus. Wet prep and pH should be performed to evaluate signs of infection. Fungal cultures or polymerase chain reaction (PCR) testing should be sent if there is any doubt about the presence of yeast, as wet prep has a sensitivity of only 50%. Suspicious skin changes on the vulva warrant biopsy.
- A moistened cotton swab is used to systematically examine the vulva and map any areas of pain. If present, tenderness is most commonly found adjacent to the hymenal ring, but it is important to check the rest of the vulva for more generalized tenderness.
- A speculum exam and gentle digital exam are then performed. Attention should be paid to tenderness, adnexal masses or nodularity, pelvic floor muscle tone, prolapse, and the anal reflex.
- Laboratory tests are rarely useful, as they are poorly predictive of function and perception of function.

## PHYSIOLOGY OF FEMALE SEXUAL FUNCTION

Female sexual function is a complex interplay of the central nervous system (CNS), peripheral nervous system, and end organs.

- The medial preoptic, anterior hypothalamic, and limbohippocampal areas are involved in sexual arousal.
- Estrogens, androgens, oxytocin, and dopamine are believed to promote female sexual response. In contrast, progesterone, prolactin, and serotonin are inhibitory.
- The vasculature and musculature changes involved in arousal are mediated by dopaminergic stimulation of the peripheral nervous system. Autonomic nerves release nitric oxide and vasointestinal polypeptide that modulate vasodilatation.
- Increased blood flow causes labial engorgement, increased vaginal lubrication, vaginal lengthening and dilation, and increased clitoral size.
- The pelvic floor muscles and the smooth muscle of the vagina spasm during orgasm. Contraction of the pelvic floor muscles involves adrenergic and cholinergic mechanisms from the efferent pudendal nerve.
- Estrogen primarily maintains the integrity of the tissues. Androgen levels are associated with libido and arousal.
- The arousal response in women involves increased heart rate, muscle tension, changes in breast sensations, and a subjective state of arousal.

## THEORIES OF SEXUAL FUNCTION

For many years, female sexual function was described with a model more characteristic of men than of women. In 1966, Masters and Johnson defined the human sexual response as a sequential model including excitement (desire and arousal), plateau, orgasm, and resolution (Table 42-1). Recent research has found that the female sexual response is much more complex and is usually not linear.

- The Study of Women's Health Across the Nation (SWAN) surveyed 2,400 women of various ethnicities (Hispanic, White non-Hispanic, African American, Chinese, and Japanese) in six US cities. The study found that 40% of these women never or infrequently felt desire, although the majority reported being capable of arousal. Only 13% expressed discontent.
- In 2011, Rosemary Basson developed a model of sexual arousal that incorporated psychological and social aspects of women's lives. In her model, desire does not always precede sexual arousal. Instead, women often begin at a state of "sexual neutrality" and respond to or seek sexual stimuli based on many possible psychological motivations. The response to this stimulus is usually arousal, which leads to desire and improved arousal. This model can be explained to patients concerned about lack of desire and can normalize what women commonly experience (a lack of spontaneous desire but the presence of reactive desire) (Figure 42-1).
- The *Diagnostic and Statistical Manual of Mental Disorders,* fifth edition (*DSM-V*), recently published in 2013, made some significant changes compared to the prior edition. Importantly, the diagnosis of sexual dysfunction requires a minimum duration of 6 months. The new edition combines female sexual desire disorder and female sexual arousal disorder into female sexual interest/arousal disorder, reflecting the research showing that most women experience both of these disorders and have difficulty distinguishing between them. A new diagnosis, genitopelvic pain/penetration disorder, merged vaginismus and dyspareunia, reflecting the difficulty women have in distinguishing the cause of penetration pain and the inadequacy of vaginal muscle spasm.

| TABLE 42-1 | Physiologic Female Sexual Response | |
|---|---|---|
| **Phase** | **Sex Organ Response** | **General Sexual Response** |
| **Excitement** | Vaginal lubrication<br>Thickening of vaginal walls and labia<br>Expansion of inner vagina<br>Elevation of cervix and corpus<br>Tumescence of clitoris | Nipple erection<br>Sex-tension flush |
| **Plateau** | Orgasmic platform in outer vagina<br>Full expansion of inner vagina<br>Secretion of mucus by Bartholin gland<br>Withdrawal of clitoris | Sex-tension flush<br>Carpopedal spasm<br>Generalized skeletal muscle tension<br>Hyperventilation<br>Tachycardia |
| **Orgasm** | Contractions of uterus from fundus toward lower uterine segment<br>Contractions of orgasmic platform at 0.8-s intervals<br>External rectal sphincter contractions at 0.8-s intervals<br>External urethral sphincter contractions at irregular intervals | Specific skeletal muscle contractions<br>Hyperventilation<br>Tachycardia |
| **Resolution** | Ready return to orgasm with retarded loss of pelvic vasocongestion<br>Return of normal color and orgasmic platform in primary (rapid) stage<br>Loss of clitoral tumescence and return to position | Diaphoresis<br>Hyperventilation<br>Tachycardia |

From Beckman CR, Ling F, Barzansky BM, et al. *Obstetrics and Gynecology*, 4th ed. Philadelphia, PA: Lippincott Williams & Wilkins, 2002:610, with permission.

## SEXUAL DYSFUNCTION DISORDERS

- **Hypoactive sexual desire disorder**—persistent or recurrent deficient or absent sexual fantasies or desire for sexual activity that causes marked distress or interpersonal difficulty
- **Sexual aversion disorder**—persistent or recurrent aversive response to any genital contact with a sexual partner, emphasizing the role of avoidance
- **Female sexual interest/arousal disorder** in *DSM-V* is a combination of the *DSM-IV* female sexual arousal disorder and female orgasmic disorder—persistent or recurrent deficient or absent sexual fantasies or desire for sexual activity and/or inability to attain or to maintain until completion of sexual activity an adequate genital lubrication–swelling response of sexual excitement and/or delay in or absence of orgasm following a normal sexual excitement phase that causes marked distress or interpersonal difficulty.

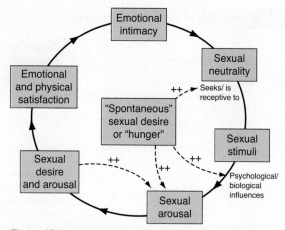

**Figure 42-1.** Basson's model of female sexual response. (From Basson R. Female sexual response: the role of drugs in the management of sexual dysfunction. *Obstet Gynecol* 2001;98:350–353, with permission.)

- **Sexual pain disorders**
  - **Genitopelvic pain/penetration disorder** combines vaginismus and dyspareunia. **Vaginismus** was defined as persistent or recurrent involuntary spasm of the outer third of the vagina that interferes with sexual intercourse. Although this has been eliminated in the *DSM-V*, many providers continue to use this terminology. **Dyspareunia** was defined as genital pain associated with sexual activity that causes distress or interpersonal difficulty.
  - Vulvodynia and vaginismus—these disorders typically present with introital dyspareunia. The International Society for the Study of Vulvovaginal Disease (ISSVD) defines vulvodynia as "vulvar discomfort, most often described as burning pain, occurring in the absence of relevant visible findings or a specific clinically identifiable, neurologic disorder." Vulvodynia is then further divided into generalized and localized.
    - Generalized
      - Provoked (sexual, nonsexual, or both)
      - Unprovoked
      - Mixed (provoked and unprovoked)
    - Localized (vestibulodynia—previously known as vulvar vestibulitis, clitorodynia, hemivulvodynia, etc.)
      - Provoked (sexual, nonsexual, or both)
      - Unprovoked
      - Mixed (provoked and unprovoked)
    - Although there may be no visible physical findings or microbiologic abnormalities, vulvodynia is now understood to involve changes in the nervous system, including an increase in nerve density and sensitivity in the vulva (peripheral sensitization), and changes in the CNS, which amplify the pain rather than diminish it (central sensitization).

○ Localized vulvodynia in the vestibule is the most common subset of vulvodynia. According to a 2003 population-based study, the lifetime incidence of localized vulvodynia in women is about 12%, compared to 3% for generalized vulvodynia.

## Assessment of Vulvodynia and Vaginismus

- The highest incidence of vulvodynia is in women ages 18 to 32 years. When perimenopausal or menopausal women present with these symptoms, it is important to first evaluate for and treat vaginal atrophy if indicated. Breast-feeding mothers and oral contraceptive pill users can also present with atrophic vaginitis and pain. This may be in part because of their progestogenic effect, which can block estrogenic effects. Additionally, there may be estrogen-related elevation in sex hormone–binding globulin, which binds preferentially to androgens, preventing their binding to androgen receptors in vaginal and vulvar tissue.
- Patients with vulvodynia are more likely to have other pain disorders such as migraine headaches, fibromyalgia, irritable bowel syndrome (IBS), and interstitial cystitis. Allergies and endometriosis may also be more prevalent. Reed et al. demonstrated that the presence of vulvodynia was associated with the presence of fibromyalgia, interstitial cystitis, and IBS with 27% of patients surveyed screening positive for multiple conditions.
- Many patients with vaginismus have a significant phobia regarding penetration and have never experienced penetration. Their physical exam may be indistinguishable from the vulvodynia patient. Introital hypersensitivity and muscle hypertonicity are commonly identified.
- Question carefully about hygiene practices. Patients may attribute their symptoms to uncleanliness and overwash with harsh soaps or use over-the-counter products with potential irritants, such as benzocaine (Vagisil).

## Treatment for Vulvodynia and Vaginismus

- Nearly all patients with these disorders benefit from **pelvic floor physical therapy** performed by a physical therapist with specialized training.
- **Mental health counseling** is helpful for patients or couples to cope with the disorder.
- **Vaginal dilator therapy** can be initiated for those patients who are willing and exhibit identifiable introital muscle tightness. Begin by teaching Kegel exercises and relaxation, then helping patient to insert the smallest dilator while in the office. Patients may use a mirror. Daily use is preferable.
  - Dilators can be purchased online, or other cylindrically shaped objects can be used, including culturette tubes, syringes (with the Luer-lock tips removed), and candles.
  - Patients can be encouraged to use their own fingers and later their partner's fingers as dilators.

### Medical Treatments

- Many of the same **oral medications** that are used for other types of neuropathic pain are used. These patients tend to be anxious, hypervigilant, and sensitive to side effects, so start with a low dose and increase gradually.
  - Tricyclic antidepressants (e.g., amitriptyline, desipramine): 25 to 150 mg/day
  - Gabapentin 900 to 3,600 mg/day
  - Topiramate 25 to 200 mg/day
  - Venlafaxine 37.5 to 150 mg/day
  - Duloxetine 60 mg/day

- **Topical medications** are often preferred by patients. No randomized controlled trials exist, and medications must usually be compounded in a specialized pharmacy. The vehicle is important because many patients are prone to irritant reactions. In general, gels and ointments are tolerated better than creams. Cellulose gel, acid-mantle cream, and stearin-lanolin are examples of vehicles that tend to be well tolerated. Patients should be shown where to apply the product, as they may lack knowledge of their own anatomy.
  - Lidocaine 2% to 5%, applied three times daily. This may cause stinging in some patients.
  - Gabapentin 6%, applied three times daily
  - Amitriptyline 2%/baclofen 2%
  - Estradiol 0.01% is often tolerated better in a noncream base such as cellulose gel
  - Topical steroids are generally not recommended, especially for long-term therapy, because of the potential for tissue thinning and steroid rebound dermatitis.

*Surgical Treatment*

- Surgical management with **vestibulectomy** has an approximately 85% success rate.
- Success rates are lower for women with vulvodynia or vaginismus who decline sexual counseling, those who have untreated hypertonicity, and those with a longer duration of symptoms.

## Follow-Up for Vaginismus/Vulvodynia Patients

- Patients should be reevaluated periodically during treatment (e.g., every 4 to 8 weeks) to track their response to treatment and to check for emergence of other disorders, such as vulvovaginal candidiasis or other infections, dermatologic problems, worsening pelvic floor muscle function, or relationship issues. Compliance with and tolerance of medications need to be reassessed periodically.

## Vulvovaginal Atrophy

- Atrophy has become an increasingly common cause of sexual pain in the years since the Women's Health Initiative Study was published due to the decrease in use of systemic estrogen. Very tiny amounts of topical estrogen (a low-dose vaginal ring, 10-µg pills, or 0.5 g of estrogen cream twice weekly) are extremely effective and have little systemic absorption. When there is introital discomfort, it is critical that estrogen also be applied topically to the introitus; vaginal application will not affect this area. Topical estrogen is thought to be superior to systemic estrogen for the treatment of vulvovaginal atrophy and has shown benefit for overactive bladder symptoms and recurrent urinary tract infections. Symptom relief may occur within 3 to 4 weeks but may last up to 6 to 12 weeks. Women who do not wish to use topical estrogen can be counseled that regular sexual activity can be very effective at maintaining tissue integrity and elasticity.
- Ospemifene was approved by the U.S. Food and Drug Administration (FDA) in February of 2013 for the treatment of moderate to severe dyspareunia when the symptoms are related to vulvar and vaginal atrophy. This is a once-daily oral selective estrogen receptor modulator. It has a positive effect on the vaginal epithelium with lower rates of adverse effects of estrogen, such as stimulation of the endometrium and thrombosis.

## Treatments for Sexual Interest and Arousal Disorder in Women

- Given that there is so much overlap among these disorders and that the female sexual response is a complex interaction, treatment must often be multifaceted.

- Pharmacology
  - Androgens—there are currently no FDA-approved androgen treatments available for women, although there are several under development. Of women who have undergone oophorectomy and hysterectomy, those with a 300-mg transdermal testosterone patch had significantly increased numbers of sexual fantasies, amount of masturbation, and number of episodes of sexual intercourse. The feeling of positive well-being increased and depressed mood decreased at 300 mg versus 150 mg or placebo. There are concerns about the lack of safety data and the risks of clitoromegaly, hirsutism, acne, hepatotoxicity, and worsening lipid profile with prolonged use. Androgens can masculinize a female fetus. The risk of breast cancer with androgen use is unknown, and results from studies are contradictory.
  - Estrogen—improves vaginal atrophy. The Women's Health Initiative trial did not show a significant difference in satisfaction with estrogen use.
  - Sildenafil—a randomized trial of 781 women with arousal disorder showed no conclusive impact of sildenafil. It does appear to be beneficial for patients taking selective serotonin reuptake inhibitors (SSRIs) or those with spinal cord injury. The phosphodiesterase inhibitor *tadalafil* (*Cialis*) is longer acting.
- Counseling
  - Cognitive behavioral therapy—identifies and modifies factors such as maladaptive thoughts, unreasonable expectations, behaviors that reduce trust, and insufficient stimuli and works to increase communication among partners. Orgasmic function can be treated as a learned skill, and cognitive behavioral treatments (e.g. directed masturbation) are highly effective.
  - Sex therapy—includes sensate therapy that initially starts with nonsexual intimacy and focuses on feedback on what is pleasurable. This technique is effective in reducing sexual anxiety and helps both partners avoid "spectating" or monitoring their own response during the encounter.
  - Bupropion—as a non-SSRI antidepressant with dopaminergic activity, it may help with mood disorders, and can be used instead of SSRIs, or may be used to counteract SSRIs' effects on sexual function. There is some evidence that bupropion has prosexual effects in nondepressed women.
- Other treatments
  - The suction vacuum device—the clitoral suction vacuum increases clitoral engorgement when the vacuum is applied and may lead to improved vascularization and sensation.
  - Several over-the-counter, topically applied, arousal-enhancing products are available in the form of personal lubricants. There is limited research showing improvement in arousal or orgasm. These products can cause irritation of mucous membranes and should be applied to the labia majora or clitoris. Some herbal products also have limited research showing improvement in desire and satisfaction.
  - Self-treatment books such as *For Yourself* by Lonnie Barbach, or *Becoming Orgasmic* by Julia Heiman and Ray Lopiccolo, are useful.

## Persistent Genital Arousal Disorder

- First described in 2001, this disorder is characterized by persistent sensations of genital arousal even without sexual or emotional stimuli, causing the patient at least moderate distress. There are many proposed etiologies of PGAD, which may involve a range of psychological, pharmacologic, neurologic, and vascular causes. It has been associated with other conditions including overactive bladder and restless leg syndrome and may often indicate a pudendal neuropathy. Treatment requires a multidisciplinary approach as well as cognitive therapy. Physical therapy, topical lidocaine, pudendal nerve blocks, transcutaneous electrical nerve stimulation units, or medications for chronic pain such as gabapentin may be helpful.

## SEXUAL FUNCTION AND SPECIAL POPULATIONS

- **Postpartum**—sexual activity postpartum is affected by many things including fatigue, breast-feeding, adjustment to the new baby, hormonal changes, pain, and healing. In one study of 796 women, 32% resumed intercourse within 6 months and 89% after 6 months. Additionally, fewer women with anal sphincter tears reported sexual activity compared to those without these lacerations.
- **Menopause and premature ovarian failure**—postmenopausal women or those with premature ovarian failure are significantly affected by dysfunction and dyspareunia. One contributing factor in this population is vulvovaginal atrophy.
- **Nonheterosexual relationships**—regardless of a patient's sexual orientation, providers should address sexual concerns such as pain, risk for sexually transmitted diseases, and screening for domestic violence.
- **Medical disorders and medications** can affect sexual arousal and function. For example, diabetes and peripheral vascular disease may affect vasocongestion. Depression, substance abuse, and tobacco use can affect sexual function. Medications such as SSRIs, antipsychotics, antihypertensives, oral contraceptive pills, and medroxyprogesterone acetate are also known to affect sexual function.
- **Pelvic floor disorders** are associated with decreased arousal, infrequent orgasm, and increased dyspareunia. Patients may have loss of self-esteem, embarrassment, and decreased desire. Urinary or fecal incontinence may additionally cause fear of odor. Surgical management for pelvic floor disorders may increase sexual function, although patients should be counseled about operative risks such as dyspareunia or damage to nerves such as the dorsal nerve of the clitoris.
- **Posthysterectomy**—there are theoretical concerns that total or supracervical hysterectomy can disrupt the complex neurologic and vascular anatomy involved in sexual response. However, sexual function has not been shown to be compromised for most women and may actually be improved once issues such as menorrhagia are resolved. Additionally, studies have shown no difference for patients who preserved their cervix or not.
- **Breast cancer and gynecologic oncology patients**—disease and treatment can cause decreased desire, arousal, opinion of self, and overall decreased quality of life. Patients may have pain or bleeding. Radiotherapy, in particular, has sexual side effects. Symptoms such as vaginal atrophy or dyspareunia can be specifically addressed. Women can be encouraged to use vaginal moisturizers (applied two or three times weekly) and engage in regular sexual activity or masturbation to maintain blood flow to the genitals. The use of topical estrogens may be contraindicated or at least controversial in some patients, for instance those on aromatase inhibitors or with a history of estrogen receptor–positive breast cancer. However, it is sometimes done after consultation of the patient's oncologist. Estradiol levels can be followed to reassure the patient of minimal absorption. Options in the future may include ospemifene, topical testosterone, topical estriol, or topical oxytocin.
- **Infertility**—many infertile couples think of sexual intercourse as goal-oriented and may have trouble finding pleasure in sexual activity.

## SUGGESTED READINGS

American College of Obstetricians and Gynecologists Committee on Practice Bulletins—Gynecology. ACOG practice bulletin no. 119: female sexual dysfunction. 2011;117(4): 996–1007.

Basson R. Sexual desire and arousal disorders in women. *N Engl J Med* 2006;354(14):1497–1506.

Carey JC. Pharmacological effects on sexual function. *Obstet Gynecol Clin North Am* 2006;33: 599–620.

Facelle TM, Sadeghi-Nejad H, Goldmeier D. Persistent genital arousal disorder: characterization, etiology, and management. *J Sex Med* 2012;10(2):439–450.

Haefner HK, Collins ME, Davis GD, et al. The vulvodynia guideline. *J Low Genit Tract Dis* 2005;9(1):40–51.

Kammerer-Doak D, Rogers R. Female sexual function and dysfunction. *Obstet Gynecol Clin North Am* 2008;35:169–183.

Reed BD, Harlow SD, Sen A, et al. Relationship between vulvodynia and chronic comorbid pain conditions. *Obstet Gynecol* 2012;120(1):145–151.

Rosen RC, Barsky JL. Normal sexual response in women. *Obstet Gynecol Clin North Am* 2006;33: 515–526.

Shifren JL, Braunstein GD, Simon JA, et al. Transdermal testosterone treatment in women with impaired sexual function after oophorectomy. *N Engl J Med* 2000;343(10):682–688.

Srivastava R, Thakar R, Sultan A. Female sexual dysfunction in obstetrics and gynecology. *Obstet Gynecol Surv* 2008;63(8):527–537.

# 43

# Menopause
Chantel Washington and Howard A. Zacur

## DEFINITIONS AND EPIDEMIOLOGY OF MENOPAUSE

Menopause is the permanent cessation of menses, dated by the last menstrual period followed by 12 months of amenorrhea.

- The average age of menopause is 51 years, with a normal range of 43 to 57 years.
  - Can also be induced by oophorectomy or iatrogenic ablation of ovarian function.
- In 2001, the Stages of Reproductive Aging Workshop divided normal female reproductive aging into stages, with the goal of clarifying terminology relating to menopause (Fig. 43-1).
  - The transition from reproductive to postreproductive life is divided into several stages, with the final menstrual period (FMP) serving as an anchor.
    - Five stages (−5 to −1) precede the FMP and two stages follow (+1 and +2).
- **Menopausal transition**, traditionally termed **perimenopause** or the **climacteric**, is the transition period from regular menstruation until menopause.
  - May last for 5 years or more, highly variable in duration
  - Characterized by menstrual cycle changes that include variable cycle length, with skipped periods and increasingly longer intervals of amenorrhea

|  |  |  |  |  |  | Final Menstrual Period (FMP) |  |  |
|---|---|---|---|---|---|---|---|---|
| Stages: | −5 | −4 | −3 | −2 | −1 | 0 | +1 | +2 |
| Terminology: | Reproductive | | | Menopausal Transition | | | Postmenopause | |
|  | Early | Peak | Late | Early | Late* | | Early* | Late |
|  |  |  | | Perimenopause | | | | |
| Duration of Stage | variable | | | variable | | | (a) 1 yr / (b) 4 yrs | until demise |
| Menstrual Cycles | variable to regular | regular | | variable cycle length (>7 days different from normal) | ≥2 skipped cycles and an interval of amenorrhea (≥60 days) | Amenorrhea | none | |
| Endocrine: | normal FSH | | ↑ FSH | ↑ FSH | | | ↑ FSH | |

*Stages most likely to be characterized by vasomotor symptoms   ↑ = elevated

**Figure 43-1.** Stages/nomenclature of normal reproductive aging in women. (From Soules MR, Sherman S, Parrott E, et al. Executive summary: stages of reproductive aging workshop [STRAW]. *Fertil Steril* 2001;76:874, with permission.)

- Associated with the cessation of ovulation, a marked decline in estradiol production, and a modest decline in androgen production
- Early menopausal transition (−2) is depicted by variable cycle length (>7 days different from the norm) and increased follicle-stimulating hormone (FSH).
- Late menopausal transition (−1) is characterized by two skipped cycles and an interval of amenorrhea >60 days.
- Diagnosis of menopause is clinical, without reliance on hormonal measurements.
  - When any doubt exists about menopause, other causes of secondary amenorrhea must be ruled out. See Chapter 39.

## PHYSIOLOGY OF MENOPAUSE

- Oocytes undergo atresia throughout a woman's life, with follicular quantity and quality undergoing a critical decline approximately 20 to 25 years after menarche. This follicular decline results in loss of ovarian sensitivity to gonadotropin stimulation.
- During perimenopause, follicular dysfunction can lead to variable menstrual cycle length. The follicular phase of the cycle is usually shortened due to the decreased number of functional follicles.
- The early menopause transition is typified by increased levels of FSH leading to overall higher estrogen levels.
- As follicular depletion continues, decreased inhibin produced by follicles leads to continued increased FSH. Follicular depletion also leads to recurrent anovulation and subsequent increase in FSH and luteinizing hormone levels.

## MENOPAUSAL SYMPTOMS AND TREATMENT

### Vasomotor Symptoms

- Seventy-five percent of menopausal women experience vasomotor symptoms such as hot flashes and night sweats.
  - Symptoms begin an average of 2 years before the FMP.
  - Eighty percent of women who have hot flashes endure them for longer than 1 year and 50% for longer than 5 years.

- **Pathophysiology:** due to vasomotor instability thought to be secondary to dysfunction of the thermoregulatory nucleus which is responsible for maintaining body temperature within a set range known as the thermoregulatory zone
  - Characterized by a sudden reddening of the skin over the head, neck, and chest, accompanied by a feeling of intense body heat, palpitations and anxiety, sleep disturbance, and irritability. Concludes with profuse perspiration.
- **Risk factors:** surgical menopause (up to 90% of women will have vasomotor symptoms), early menopause, low circulating levels of estradiol, smoking, and possibly low body mass index (BMI)
- **Treatment:** Hormone therapy (HT) is first-line treatment. Current recommendations are that HT use should be limited to the lowest effective dose for the shortest treatment duration and that ongoing use should be reevaluated periodically.
  - **Estrogen** administration: the most effective treatment for hot flashes, given orally, transdermally, or vaginally (Table 43-1)
    - Oral dosing: results in plasma level fluctuations and an estradiol to estrone ratio of <1
    - Oral estrogen plus androgen combinations are available and may help with decreased postmenopausal libido, but this is somewhat controversial.
    - Transdermal estrogen: Delivers estrogen at a relatively constant rate of 50 to 100 µg/dL, comparable to premenopausal endogenous estrogen production. Maintains the 1:1 ratio of estradiol to estrone that approximates the natural, premenopausal ratio.
      - Avoids first-pass liver metabolism effect, which prevents an effect on synthesis of clotting factors and decreases the effect on lipid metabolism
  - Dosing of HT for vasomotor symptoms is listed in Table 43-1.
  - In women with a uterus, **progestins** must be added to any estrogen regimen to prevent the increased risk of endometrial cancer associated with unopposed estrogen use.
    - The progestin is administered either continuously with daily dosing or cyclically with daily dosing only during the last half of each cycle.
  - **Contraindications for HT:** history of venous thromboembolism or stroke or those at high risk for developing these conditions, history of breast cancer, or coronary heart disease (CHD)
  - **Alternatives** to HT for vasomotor symptoms are for patients who feel estrogen produces unacceptable side effects or who have contraindications.
    - **Selective serotonin and norepinephrine reuptake inhibitors (SSRI, SNRI):**
      - **Venlafaxine** 150 mg daily reduces hot flashes by 61% over a 4-week treatment course, and **paroxetine** at either 12.5 mg or 25 mg/day also reduces hot flashes by approximately 60%.
    - **Clonidine** is a centrally acting alpha-adrenergic agonist. In a meta-analysis of 10 trials, clonidine was effective in less than half of the trials at treating vasomotor symptoms compared to placebo.
    - **Gabapentin** (900 mg/day) is also used to treat side effect symptoms. Clinical trials have shown that gabapentin reduces symptoms by 35% to 38% compared to placebo.
    - **Progestins:**
      - Oral and intramuscular progestins have shown good efficacy in randomized trials. There is conflicting evidence regarding the effectiveness of transdermal preparations.
      - Medroxyprogesterone acetate, 150 mg intramuscularly per month, has been shown to be 90% effective in the treatment of hot flashes.
      - These agents are not recommended for patients with a history of breast cancer.

| TABLE 43-1 | Hormone Replacement Therapies |

| Drug | Dosage |
| --- | --- |
| **Oral estrogens** | |
| Conjugated equine estrogens (Premarin) | 0.3–2.5 mg daily |
| Synthetic conjugated estrogens (Cenestin, Enjuvia) | 0.3–1.25 mg daily |
| Micronized estradiol (Estrace) | 0.5–2 mg daily |
| Esterified estrogens (Menest) | 0.3–2.5 mg daily |
| Estropipate (Ogen, Ortho-Est) | 0.625–2.5 mg daily |
| Estradiol (Femtrace) | 0.45–1.8 mg daily |
| **Oral progestins** | |
| Micronized progesterone (Prometrium) | 200 mg for 12 d each mo or 100 mg daily |
| Medroxyprogesterone acetate (Provera) | 10 mg daily for 12 d each mo |
| Norethindrone acetate (Aygestin) | 2.5–10 mg for 12 d each mo |
| **Oral estrogen/progestin combinations (continuous)** | |
| Conjugated estrogens/medroxyprogesterone acetate (Prempro) | 0.3/1.5 mg/daily, 0.45/1.5 mg/daily, 0.625/2.5 mg or 0.625/5 mg/daily |
| Estradiol/norethindrone acetate (Activella) | 1.0/0.5 mg daily |
| Estinyl estradiol/norethindrone acetate (FemHRT) | 5 μg/1 mg daily, 2.5 μg/0.5 g daily |
| Estradiol + drospirenone (Angeliq) | 1 mg/0.5 mg daily |
| **Cyclical oral** | |
| Estradiol/norgestimate (Prefest) | 1 mg estradiol for 15 d and then 1 mg estradiol/0.09 mg norgestimate for 15 d |
| Conjugated estrogens/medroxyprogesterone acetate (Premphase) | 0.625 mg conjugated estrogens for 14 d, then 0.625 mg conjugated estrogens/5 mg medroxyprogesterone for 14 d |
| **Transdermal estrogen preparations** | |
| Transdermal estradiol patch (Alora, Climara, Esclim, Estraderm, Menostar, Vivelle, Vivelle-Dot) | Variable dosing; apply twice weekly or weekly, depending on brand |
| Topical estradiol gel (Divigel, Elestrin, Estragel) | Variable dosing; apply once daily |
| Topical estradiol emulsion (Estrasorb) | 1.74 g/pouch; two pouches applied daily |
| Topical estradiol spray (Evamist) | 1.53 mg/spray; two or three sprays daily |

| TABLE 43-1 | Hormone Replacement Therapies *(Continued)* |
|---|---|

| Drug | Dosage |
|---|---|
| **Vaginal estrogen preparations** | |
| Vaginal conjugated estrogens (Premarin) | 0.625 mg/g; apply daily |
| Vaginal estradiol cream (Estrace) | 0.01% cream; daily then one to three times/wk |
| Vaginal estradiol ring (Estring, Femring) | 50–100 μg/d (Femring), 7.5 μg/d (Estring); replace every 90 d |
| Vaginal estradiol tablets (Vagifem) | 10 μg daily for 2 wk, then twice weekly |
| **Transdermal estrogen and progestin preparations** | |
| Estradiol + levonorgestrel (Climara Pro) | 0.45 mg/0.015 mg; apply weekly |
| Estradiol + norethindrone acetate (Combipatch) | 0.05 mg/0.14 mg; 0.05 mg/0.25 mg; apply twice weekly |
| **Oral estrogen and androgen combinations** | |
| Esterified estrogens + methyltestosterone (Estratest H.S.) | 0.625 mg/1.25 mg daily |
| Esterified estrogens + methyltestosterone (Estratest) | 1.25 mg/2.5 mg daily |

- Alternative therapies such as soy, black cohosh, red clover, dong quai, and acupuncture have been used to treat hot flashes. However, the limited trials in this area have not shown a benefit compared to placebo. Further investigation is needed to clarify their role in the alleviation of hot flashes and their side effects.
- **Behavior modification:**
  o The North American Menopause Society recommends maintaining a low core body temperature by using a fan and drinking cool beverages to manage mild hot flashes.
  o Relaxation techniques, such as slow breathing and yoga, can reduce the frequency of menopausal symptoms and alleviate hot flashes.
  o Exercise may increase the severity of symptoms by raising core body temperature.

## Urogenital Atrophy

- **Pathophysiology:** The vagina, urethra, and bladder trigone have high estrogen receptor concentrations. Loss of estrogen that accompanies menopause thus leads to urogenital atrophy.
- Atrophic vulva loses most of its collagen, adipose tissue, and water-retaining ability and becomes flattened and thin. Sebaceous glands remain intact, but secretions decrease, leading to vaginal dryness.
- Vaginal shortening and narrowing occur, and the vaginal walls become thin, lose elasticity, and become pale in color.

- Dyspareunia is the most common complaint related to vaginal atrophy.
- Estrogen deficiency within the urethra and bladder is associated with urethral syndrome, which is characterized by recurrent episodes of urinary frequency and urgency with dysuria.
- **Treatment:**
  - **Moisturizers and lubricants** are used to relieve symptoms related to vaginal dryness and dyspareunia.
    - Astroglide and K-Y jelly are used at the time of coitus to alleviate dyspareunia, whereas Replens is used on a sustained basis.
  - Local **estrogen therapy** improves vaginal atrophy and associated symptoms.
    - Can also relieve dysuria and may protect against recurrent lower urinary tract infections
    - Estrogen therapy does not improve urinary stress or urge incontinence.
    - Different forms of estrogen therapy are available.
    - Low-dose estrogen creams are applied intravaginally from daily to two times a week at doses of 0.3 mg of conjugated estrogens or 0.5 g of estradiol per application.
    - Estring is a silicone ring embedded with estrogen that releases 6 to 9 mg of estradiol daily and is kept in place for 3 months. It has minimal systemic absorption.
    - Vagifem tablets are given vaginally as one per day for 14 days followed by twice per week. They have also been shown to estrogenize the vaginal mucosa without resulting in significant systemic absorption.

## Menstrual Cycle Disturbances

- Because of the changing hormonal milieu, complaints of irregular bleeding are very common during the menopausal transition.
- If episodes of bleeding occur more often than every 21 days, last longer than 8 days, are very heavy, or occur after a 6-month interval of amenorrhea, evaluation of the endometrium must be undertaken to rule out neoplasm. This includes pelvic ultrasound, endometrial biopsy, and possible dilation and curettage with hysteroscopy.
- **Oral contraceptive pills** can be used during the menopausal transition until the onset of menopause.
  - Benefits of this therapy, in addition to relief of vasomotor symptoms, include contraception, decreased risk of endometrial and ovarian cancers, establishment of regular menses, and increased bone density.

# SPECIAL CONCERNS FOR MENOPAUSAL WOMEN

## Osteoporosis

- **Osteoporosis** is the condition of decreased bone mass and bone microarchitectural deterioration with resulting increased risk of skeletal fractures.
- In the United States, 4 to 6 million women (13% to 18% of those older than 50 years old) have osteoporosis, resulting in 1.5 million fractures per year.
- Ninety percent of all hip and spine fractures in Caucasian women aged 65 to 84 years are secondary to osteoporosis.
- **Pathophysiology**
  - Estrogen deficiency causes an imbalance of skeletal remodeling, with an increase in resorption that is greater than bone formation.
  - Results from a dominance of osteoclasts, which break down bone, and a decrease in osteoblastic activity. Estrogen binds to receptors on osteoclasts and inhibits their activity.

- Decreased serum calcium levels lead to an increase in parathyroid hormone (PTH), which stimulates osteoclastic activity. Estrogen deficiency also leads to increased bone sensitivity to PTH.
- Bone resorption matches bone formation until approximately age 25 to 35 years old. Bone mass decreases after that at a rate of 0.4% per year.
- After menopause, bone mass decreases 2% to 5% annually for 10 years and then the rate stabilizes to 1% per year.
- Most common fracture sites include the lumbar vertebrae, wrist (distal radius), and hip (femoral neck).
- Known **risk factors** account for 30% of osteoporosis incidence (Table 43-2).
- **Prevention and treatment** guidelines are in Table 43-3.
- **Diagnosis** is determined by bone mineral density (BMD) with dual-energy x-ray absorptiometry (DEXA) being the preferred technique.
  - BMD is best measured at the hip and is predictive of hip fracture and fracture at other sites.
    - $T$-scores are standard deviations above or below the comparison mean BMD of young women aged 20 to 29 years.
    - $Z$-scores correspond to the same measurements using women of the same age as the reference.
    - Normal bone $T$-scores are above $-1.0$.
    - Osteopenia $T$-scores are between $-1.0$ and $-2.5$.

| TABLE 43-2 | Risk Factors for Osteoporosis |
| --- | --- |

Family history of osteoporosis
Current cigarette smoking
Low body weight: <127 pounds for average height or BMI <22
Estrogen deficiency due to menopause, especially early menopause (younger than 45 yr)
Anorexia nervosa and other eating disorders
Insufficient vitamin D intake
Prolonged premenopausal amenorrhea (older than 1 yr)
Lifelong low calcium intake
Excessive alcohol intake
Current low bone mass
Inadequate physical activity
Medications, including glucocorticoids, gonadotropin-releasing hormone analogs, anticonvulsants, long-term heparin, excessive thyroid hormones, cholestyramine
Personal history of fracture as an adult
History of a fracture in a first-degree relative
Caucasian/Asian women
Advanced age
Numerous medical conditions (e.g., HIV/AIDS, Cushing syndrome, hyperthyroidism, diabetes, rheumatoid arthritis)

BMI, body mass index.
Adapted from National Osteoporosis Foundation. Risk factors for osteoporosis. National Osteoporosis Foundation Web site. www.nof.org/prevention/risk.htm. Accessed April 15, 2013.

| TABLE 43-3 | Prevention and Treatment of Osteoporosis in Women after Age 50 years |
|---|---|

**Prevention**

Calcium, 1,200 mg/d
Vitamin D, 800–1,000 IU/d
Regular weight-bearing, muscle-strengthening exercise
Smoking cessation
Moderate alcohol consumption

**Treatment**

Treatment for all women 50 yr or older with the following:
• Vertebral or hip fracture
• T-score ≤2.5 at the femoral neck or spine
• T-score between 1.0 and 2.5 at the femoral neck or spine and 10-yr hip fracture risk[a] ≥3%
• Ten-year major osteoporosis-related fracture probability[a] ≥20%

---

[a]Ten-year fracture risk based on the US-adapted World Health Organization absolute fracture risk model, FRAX (found at www.sheffield.ac.uk/FRAX).
Adapted from National Osteoporosis Foundation. Clinician's guide to prevention and treatment of osteoporosis. Washington, DC: National Osteoporosis Foundation, 2008.

○ Osteoporosis T-scores are at or below −2.5.
○ For each reduction in bone mass of one standard deviation, the risk of fracture doubles.
• **Screening** should be offered to all women aged 65 years or older, regardless of clinical risk factors. Other candidates for BMD determination are postmenopausal women older than age 50 years with clinical risk factors including medical risk factors or a history of a fragility fracture. (A fragility fracture is defined as fracture from a fall from standing height.)
• The Fracture Risk Assessment Tool (FRAX) is a World Health Organization (WHO) funded, web-based program that calculates a patient's 10-year probability of osteoporotic fracture based on T-score and other variables.
○ Can help in determining when a patient should be screened for osteoporosis and when treatment should be initiated
○ The U.S. Preventive Services Task Force (USPSTF) uses the FRAX algorithm to determine who should be screened. The USPSTF recommends screening before age 65 years for women who have risk for fracture that is equal to or greater than that of a 65-year-old Caucasian woman.
○ The strongest risks for osteoporosis identified were low body weight, older age, weight under 57.7 kg (127 pounds) or BMI <22 kg/m², and not taking estrogen.
• Repeat DEXA screening:
○ Every 15 years for women with normal bone density or mild osteopenia
○ Every 5 years for women with moderate osteopenia
○ Every year for women with advanced osteopenia
○ Every 1 to 2 years for women undergoing therapy for osteoporosis

- **Treatment:** should be initiated in the following groups of women:
- Any postmenopausal woman with a history of an osteoporotic vertebral or hip fracture
- Any postmenopausal woman with a BMD score consistent with osteoporosis
- Any postmenopausal woman with a *T*-score of −1.0 to −2.5 and a 10-year FRAX risk of a spine, hip, or shoulder fracture of 20% or a hip fracture risk of at least 3%.
- **Oral bisphosphonates:** A class of drug analogous to physiologically occurring inorganic pyrophosphates, inhibitors of bone resorption. They are generally considered first-line treatment for osteoporosis.
    - **Alendronate** sodium (Fosamax)
        - Mechanism: oral bisphosphonate
        - Dosing: 5 mg daily or 35 mg weekly for prevention of osteoporosis and 10 mg daily or 70 mg weekly for treatment
        - Treatment not only prevents bone loss but also progressively increases bone mass of the spine, hip, and total body.
        - Also reduces risk of vertebral fractures, progression of vertebral deformities, and height loss in postmenopausal women with osteoporosis
    - **Risedronate** sodium (Actonel)
        - Mechanism: oral bisphosphonate
        - Dosing: 5 mg daily or 35 mg weekly, 75 mg on 2 consecutive days per month, or 150 mg once monthly for prevention and treatment of osteoporosis
        - Prospective studies of postmenopausal women with normal lumbar spine BMD values found that patients who received 5 mg daily had increased spine and femoral trochanter BMD, whereas patients in the placebo group experienced decreased BMD at both sites.
        - Benefits of treatment are sustained—1 year after cessation of therapy, lumbar spine BMD was 2.3% lower than baseline in patients given risedronate but 5.6% lower in patients who received placebo.
        - In women with osteoporosis, risedronate has been shown to reduce vertebral fractures.
    - **Ibandronate** (Boniva)
        - Mechanism: oral bisphosphonate
        - Dosing: 2.5 mg daily or 150 mg monthly
        - Demonstrated to be effective at decreasing bone turnover in postmenopausal women but has not been shown to reduce hip fracture risk
    - **Bisphosphonate side effects:**
        - Heartburn, esophageal irritation, esophagitis, abdominal pain, and diarrhea
        - Oral calcium supplementation may interfere with the absorption of bisphosphonates.
        - Patient should take each dose after an overnight fast, while sitting in the upright position, and should follow by drinking a glass of water.
        - The patient must remain upright and not eat for 30 minutes after administration.
        - Long-term side effects are unknown.
- **Intravenous (IV) bisphosphonates** are an alternative for patients unable to tolerate the oral forms.
    - **Zoledronic acid** (Reclast) is given annually (5 mg IV) for treatment and every 2 years for prevention.

- **Ibandronate** (Boniva) may be given 3 mg IV every 3 months.
- IV bisphosphonate side effects include flu-like symptoms and hypocalcemia (more common in those with vitamin D deficiency). Check 25-hydroxy vitamin D level and treat as needed before infusion.

- **Selective estrogen receptor modulator**
  - **Raloxifene hydrochloride** (Evista)
    - Estrogen-like effects on bone and the cardiovascular system and antiestrogen effects on breast and uterus. It is U.S. Food and Drug Administration (FDA) approved for the prevention and treatment of osteoporosis.
    - Dosing: 60 mg daily
    - A study involving postmenopausal women, both with and without osteoporosis, found that patients treated with raloxifene daily for 2 years had statistically significant increases in lumbar spine and hip BMD compared to patients who received placebo. It has not been shown to decrease risk of hip fracture.
    - Also has been shown to reduce vertebral fractures
    - Side effects: hot flashes and leg cramps
    - An increased risk of thromboembolic events is found with raloxifene use.
    - A trial involving postmenopausal women with osteoporosis found a decreased risk of breast cancer in these patients.

- **Peptide hormone**
  - Salmon **calcitonin**
    - Mechanism: inhibits bone resorption by decreasing osteoclast activity; may also have an analgesic effect
    - Dosing: nasal form, Miacalcin 200 IU daily, used effectively in the treatment of postmenopausal osteoporosis; can also be administered subcutaneously or intramuscularly in a 100-IU dose every other day
    - Calcitonin, in both injectable and nasal spray preparations, is effective in preventing early postmenopausal bone loss.
    - Side effects: Nausea and flushing. Rhinitis and epistaxis may occur with intranasal dosing. No long-term adverse effects are found.
  - **Synthetic PTH: teriparatide** (Forteo)
    - Mechanism: a synthetic human PTH that stimulates bone formation during short-term use
    - Shown to reduce spine fractures by 65% and nonspine fractures by 54%
    - A daily dose of 20 mg is injected subcutaneously.
    - Side effects: nausea, leg cramps, and dizziness
    - Use for longer than 24 months is not recommended because long-term side effects are unknown.
    - Usually given to patients who have a history of osteoporotic fracture and inability to take bisphosphonates
  - **Hormone therapy**
    - Has been demonstrated to increase spine and hip BMD and decrease hip and vertebral fractures in women with osteoporosis and in those without osteopenia or osteoporosis
    - Recent studies have suggested that lower doses of oral HT than previously used can also prevent bone loss.
    - FDA has approved a lower dose transdermal estrogen patch with 0.014 mg of estradiol (Menostar) for the prevention of osteoporosis.

○ HT combined with bisphosphonate treatment has been shown to result in a greater increase in bone density than either treatment alone.
- **Immunologic agents**
  ○ **Denosumab** (Prolia [R])
  ○ Mechanism: Denosumab is a receptor activator of nuclear factor kappa-B ligand (RANKL) inhibitor on the surface of osteoclasts, preventing activation.
  ○ Dosing: 60 mg subcutaneously once every 6 months
  ○ Side effects: aseptic necrosis of the bone or jaw, cancer, cellulitis, dermatitis, dyspnea, endocarditis, erysipelas, hypocalcemia, hypophosphatemia, pancreatitis, and rash
  ○ A meta-analysis of four randomized controlled trials comparing denosumab to alendronate found no significant difference in fracture risk reduction between groups; however, denosumab was associated with greater increases in BMD.

## Cognition and Dementia

- There is an accelerated deterioration of cognitive function once menopause begins.
- Alzheimer disease is three times more common in women than in men.
- In cultured cells and animal models, estrogen has a protective effect on neurons.
- Limited evidence exists, however, regarding beneficial effects of estrogen on cognition.
  - The Baltimore Longitudinal Study of Aging showed women taking estrogen performed better on a short-term visual memory test.
  - The Women's Health Initiative Memory Study noted a slightly increased risk of cognitive decline and dementia in women 65 years and older taking estrogen alone or with progestin.
  - Studies to date have lacked consistency in testing outcomes and specific aspects of memory function.

## Cardiovascular Health

- Coronary artery disease (CAD) is the leading cause of death among postmenopausal women.
- Women lag 10 years behind men in terms of CAD risk prior to menopause.
- By age 70 years, a woman has the same risk of CAD as a male of the same age.
- Estrogen has a protective effect on reducing cardiovascular disease (CVD) risk in premenopausal women.
- Estrogen aids in vascular smooth muscle relaxation, decreases inflammation, decreases low-density lipoprotein levels, and increases high-density lipoprotein levels.
  - The Framingham study showed a two- to sixfold increased incidence of CAD in postmenopausal women compared to premenopausal women in the same age group.

## Hormone Replacement Therapy

*Hormone Therapy and Coronary Heart Disease*

- This is an area that is currently undergoing extensive review and debate.
- Observational studies
  - Nurses' Health Study was the largest cohort study of US women, following 121,700 premenopausal women aged 30 to 55 years. A 10-year follow-up study found a reduced risk of major coronary disease and mortality from CVD for women taking estrogen compared to women who never used estrogen.

(The primary indication for HT in users was for primary prevention or treatment of vasomotor symptoms.)

- Prospective randomized clinical trials
  - The **Postmenopausal Estrogen/Progestin Interventions** or PEPI trial found that women on HT had greater high-density lipoprotein cholesterol levels than women taking placebo. However, the **Heart and Estrogen/progestin Replacement Study (HERS)** concluded that the use of estrogen plus progestin did not prevent further heart attacks or death from CHD. There were significantly more thromboembolic events in the HT users.
  - The **Women's Health Initiative (WHI)** enrolled postmenopausal women aged 50 to 79 years (mean age 63 years; however, approximately one fourth of women were older than 70 years). In the estrogen plus progestin arm, approximately one third of women were receiving treatment for hypertension and 13% had high cholesterol. Women with severe menopausal symptoms were discouraged from participating.
    - Participants received either estrogen plus progestin, estrogen alone if they had a hysterectomy, or placebo.
    - The primary outcome was CHD, with fractures being a secondary outcome.
    - Adverse events monitored were breast cancer and venous thromboembolism.
    - After 5 years, the estrogen plus progestin arm of the study was stopped early because the number of cases of breast cancer in the treatment group exceeded the predetermined threshold for increased risk.
      - In 1 year, of 10,000 postmenopausal women who took estrogen plus progestin, 38 were diagnosed with breast cancer compared to 30 of 10,000 women who took placebo.
      - Women in the estrogen alone group have not shown increased rates of breast cancer.
    - Regarding CHD and other vascular events, results showed that per 10,000 women annually, the number of heart attacks, strokes, and blood clots were 37, 29, and 34 in the estrogen plus progestin arm compared to 30, 21, and 16 per 10,000 women taking placebo.
      - Women taking estrogen alone also showed increased risk of these events relative to placebo.
    - There were fewer bone fractures and diagnoses of colon cancer in both hormone groups.
    - A secondary analysis showed that women who initiated HT closer to menopause (within 10 years) had reduced CHD risk compared to women more distant from menopause.
      - Lower risk was found for young women and higher risk for older patients.
  - The "timing hypothesis": Given the findings of the Nurses Health Study and the secondary analyses of the WHI, it has been theorized that there could be a "window of opportunity" in the early postmenopause stage, when HT can have a protective effect on CVD risk. Further prospective, randomized controlled trials are necessary to evaluate this theory.

*Hormone Therapy Conclusions*

- HT remains the most effective treatment for menopausal signs and symptoms. It should not be used for the prevention of chronic diseases.
- Further study is required to determine the role and cardiovascular effects of estrogen in women less than 10 years post menopause.

## SUGGESTED READINGS

American College of Obstetrics and Gynecologists Committee on Practice Bulletins—Gynecology. ACOG practice bulletin no. 129: osteoporosis. *Obstet Gynecol* 2012;120(3):718–734.

American College of Obstetricians and Gynecologists Women's Health Care Physicians. Executive summary. Hormone therapy. *Obstet Gynecol* 2004;104(4)(suppl):1S–4S.

American College of Obstetricians and Gynecologists Women's Health Care Physicians. Vasomotor symptoms. *Obstet Gynecol* 2004;104(4)(suppl):106S–117S.

Anderson GL, Limacher M, Assag AR, et al. Effects of conjugated equine estrogen in postmenopausal women with hysterectomy: the Women's Health Initiative randomized control trial. *JAMA* 2004;291:1701.

Archer DF, Sturdee DW, Barber R, et al. Menopausal hot flushes and night sweats: where are we now? *Climacteric* 2011;14:515–528.

Barrett-Connor E, Grady D, Sashegyi A, et al. Raloxifene and cardiovascular events in osteoporotic postmenopausal women: four-year results from the MORE (Multiple Outcomes of Raloxifene Evaluation) randomized trial. *JAMA* 2002;287:847.

Bone HG, Hosking D, Devogelaer JP, et al. Ten years' experience with alendronate for osteoporosis in postmenopausal women. *N Engl J Med* 2004;350:1189.

Grady D. Management of menopausal symptoms. *N Engl J Med* 2006;355:2338.

Grady D, Herrington D, Bittner V, et al. Cardiovascular disease outcomes during 6.8 years of hormone therapy: Heart and Estrogen/progestin Replacement Study follow-up (HERS II). *JAMA* 2002;288:49.

Gourlay ML, Fine JP, Preisser JS, et al. Bone-density testing interval and transition to osteoporosis in older women. *N Engl J Med* 2012; 366(3):225–233.

Harlow SD, Gass M, Hall JE, et al. Executive summary: stages of reproductive aging workshop +10: addressing the unfinished agenda of staging reproductive aging. *Menopause* 2012;4:387–395.

Management of osteoporosis in postmenopausal women: 2010 position statement of the North American Menopause Society. *Menopause* 2010;17(1):25–54; quiz 55–56.

Nelson HD. Commonly used types of postmenopausal estrogen for treatment of hot flashes: scientific review. *JAMA* 2004;291:1610.

Rossouw JE, Anderson GL, Prentice RL, et al. Risks and benefits of estrogen plus progestin in healthy postmenopausal women: principal results from the Women's Health Initiative randomized controlled trial. *JAMA* 2002;288:321.

Rossouw JE, Prentice RL, Manson JE, et al. Postmenopausal hormone therapy and risk of cardiovascular disease by age and years since menopause. *JAMA* 2007;297:1465.

The Writing Group for the PEPI Trial. Effects of estrogen or estrogen/progestin regimens on heart disease risk factors in postmenopausal women: the Postmenopausal Estrogen/Progestin Interventions (PEPI) Trial. *JAMA* 1995;273:199.

# V Gynecologic Oncology

# 44 Diseases of the Vulva and Vagina

Amelia M. Jernigan and Robert L. Giuntoli II

**Vulvar and vaginal disease** should be understood by its presentation, etiology, location, and associated systemic and laboratory findings. Clinicians should have a low threshold to biopsy any suspicious vulvar abnormalities because the appearance of malignant lesions is often similar to that of benign processes. The majority of patients with vulvar cancer experience symptoms for at least months prior to diagnosis. Early biopsy of suspicious lesions is preferable in order to make a diagnosis of vulvar and vaginal malignancies, if present, and to potentially avoid progression to advanced disease.

## ANATOMY OF THE VULVA AND VAGINA

- The **vulva** is that area of skin encompassing the labia majora to the hymen. See Chapter 26.
- The vulva is bordered laterally by the genitocrural folds, anteriorly by the mons pubis, and posteriorly by the perineal body. The medial side of the labia minora to the hymen is known as the vulvar vestibule or introitus.
  - Hart line is the thin zone of color and texture change between the labia minora and the vestibule, marking the transition from the skin of the external genitalia to the mucosa of the vestibule.
  - Within the vestibule lie the urethral meatus, vaginal introitus, ostia of Bartholin glands (major vestibular glands), minor vestibular glands, and Skene ducts.
- Branches of the external and internal pudendal arteries provide the vascular supply to the vulva (Fig. 44-1).
- Sensory innervation of the anterior vulva is via the genitofemoral nerve and the cutaneous branch of the ilioinguinal nerve, whereas the posterior vulva and the clitoris are innervated by the pudendal nerve.
- The medial group of superficial inguinal nodes collects the lymphatic drainage of the vulva (Fig. 44-2).

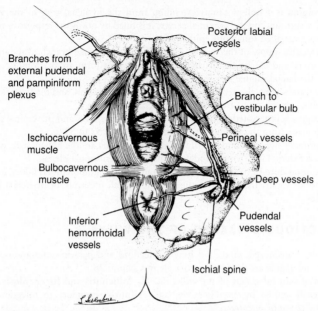

**Figure 44-1.** Superficial vulvar musculature and vascular supply of the vulva. (From Rock JA, Jones HW, TeLinde RW. *Te Linde's Operative Gynecology*, 10th ed. Philadelphia, PA: Lippincott Williams & Wilkins, 2008:505, with permission.)

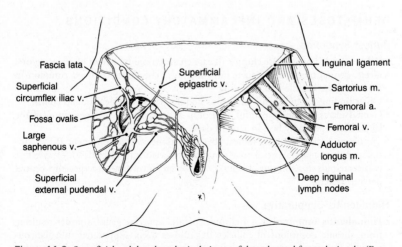

**Figure 44-2.** Superficial and deep lymphatic drainage of the vulva and femoral triangle. (From Rock JA, Jones HW, TeLinde RW. *Te Linde's Operative Gynecology*, 10th ed. Philadelphia, PA: Lippincott Williams & Wilkins, 2008:85.)

- The **vagina** is a hollow viscus extending from the hymenal ring to the vaginal fornices surrounding the proximal cervix; it is lined by hormone-responsive nonkeratinized stratified squamous epithelium.
- The vascular supply of the vagina is provided by the vaginal branch of the internal iliac artery and extensions of the uterine artery that form an anastomotic plexus along the lateral vaginal sulci.
  - The distal vagina also receives blood from pudendal vessels, and the posterior wall receives contributions from the middle rectal artery.
- The vagina is innervated by fibers from the pudendal nerves and the vaginal plexus, which arises from the hypogastric plexus (sacral rami S2 to S4).
- The primary sites of lymphatic drainage for the vagina are the hypogastric, obturator, and external iliac lymph nodes via the lateral perivaginal plexus.
  - The distal third of the vagina may also drain to the inguinofemoral nodes, and the posterior vagina may drain to the inferior gluteal, presacral, or perirectal lymph nodes.

## INFECTIOUS DISEASES OF THE VULVA

- Sexually transmitted, viral, and fungal infections and parasite infestations of the vulva and vagina are discussed separately in Chapter 28.
- Bacterial skin infections of the vulva include **folliculitis** and **furunculosis**, most frequently caused by *Staphylococcus*, and **cellulitis** secondary to infection with *Staphylococcus* or *Streptococcus*.
- Treatment of initial infection: warm compresses three times a day (tid) and cephalexin 500 mg orally (PO) four times a day (qid) or dicloxacillin 500 mg PO qid or clindamycin 300 to 450 mg PO tid
- For recurrent infections: Add to previous regimen Hibiclens washes + 2% mupirocin ointment tid × 10 days.

## DERMATOSES AND INFLAMMATORY CONDITIONS

### Behçet Syndrome

- **Behçet syndrome** is a rare chronic disease characterized by a triad of relapsing oral ulcers, genital ulcers, and ocular inflammation. The disease is most common in Japan and the Middle East.
- Other findings include acne, cutaneous nodules, thrombophlebitis, and colitis.
- Genital ulcers are small, painful, and deep and may result in fenestration of the labia. Ulcers generally heal in 7 to 10 days.
- Treatment options include topical (betamethasone valerate ointment 0.1%), intralesional (triamcinolone, 3 to 10 mg/mL, injected into ulcer base), or systemic corticosteroids (prednisone 1 mg/kg for severe involvement, especially central nervous system).

### Hidradenitis Suppurativa

- **Hidradenitis suppurativa** is a chronic, painful apocrine gland disorder resulting from chronic occlusions of follicles that causes deep, suppurated subcutaneous nodules that form sinus tracts and confluent masses. The axillae and anogenital region are most frequently involved. The lesions wax and wane; flares are common with menstruation. The lesions ulcerate, resulting in draining sinuses and extensive scarring.

- The severity of this disease varies, and it can be graded by the Hurley clinical staging system:
  - **Stage I:** single or multiple abscesses but no sinus tracts or scarring
  - **Stage II:** recurrent abscesses, tract formation and scarring, widely separated lesions
  - **Stage III:** diffuse or near diffuse involvement or multiple interconnected sinus tracts and abscesses across the entire area
- Superinfection of hidradenitis suppurativa is polymicrobial and cultures help guide treatment. The effectiveness of medical therapy wanes as deeper tissues become involved.
- Treatment options are extensive and are approached in stepwise fashion.
  - Advise patients to wear loose, light clothing; avoid manipulation of lesions or trauma to the area (e.g., with loofah sponges); keep the area dry; and use gentle, nonirritating cleansers.
  - Stage I disease: Topical therapy with clindamycin 1% twice a day (bid) with or without intralesional corticosteroids may be a useful initial approach to stage I (mild) disease. After this, 7 to 10 days of doxycycline, minocycline, clindamycin, or amoxicillin clavulanate are sometimes recommended.
  - Stage II disease: Oral tetracyclines (tetracycline, doxycycline, or minocycline) for several weeks are often used for 8 to 12 weeks or until lesions resolve. If disease persists, clindamycin (300 mg PO bid) with rifampin (600 mg PO daily) has shown promising results. For its antiandrogenic properties, some suggest that an oral contraceptive containing drospirenone or norgestimate with spironolactone may be helpful. Surgery is reserved for cases resistant to medical management.
  - Stage III or refractory disease of any stage sometimes requires surgical debridement. This must be extensive; simple incision and drainage is not adequate. Postoperative recurrences at previously affected and new sites can occur and close surveillance is indicated. Medical therapies that are potentially helpful in severe or refractory disease include tumor necrosis factor-$\alpha$ inhibitors, interleukin-12/23 inhibitors, oral retinoid, or systemic immunosuppressants or glucocorticoids.

## Fox-Fordyce Disease

- **Fox-Fordyce disease** is a rare disease characterized by papular eruption caused by the occlusion of apocrine sweat glands in the axilla and anogenital region. Patients present with flesh-colored or dark dome-shaped papules in clusters that are intensely pruritic, often leading to lichenification. It predominantly affects African Americans. Exacerbations tend to occur before and during menses. Symptoms regress during pregnancy.
- Treatment is with oral contraceptives (high estrogen content), topical estrogen ointment (1 mg estrone in peanut oil [Theelin] per ounce of petrolatum), or antiacne topical agents.

## Atrophic Vulvovaginitis

- The hypoestrogenic state of menopause produces atrophy of the vulvar and vaginal epithelium leading to dryness, pain, burning, pruritus, dyspareunia, and dysuria. The mucosa becomes friable and easily irritated and is more prone to infection. The diagnosis is clinical.
- On physical examination, the labia majora appear lax, whereas the labia minora are significantly atrophied. The mucosa is thin, pale, and smooth with loss of the normal rugae of the vagina. Fissures may be present.
- Avoid use of harsh soaps and hygiene products. Treatment with estrogen replacement therapy, either topical or oral, helps relieve symptoms.

## Contact Dermatitis

- Soaps, detergents, hygiene products, vaginal creams, and clothing can all produce a local reaction on the vulva, which may last days to weeks.
- On physical examination, symmetric eczematous lesions are seen at the area of contact.
- Identify and remove the offending agent. Oatmeal soaks and sitz baths can be used to help control symptoms, and for severe reactions, a mild steroid ointment may be used sparingly.

## Psoriasis

- **Psoriasis** typically appears as erythematous plaques with silvery, thick scales. However, the scales are often more difficult to identify on the vulva.

## Lichen Simplex Chronicus

- **Lichen Simplex Chronicus** is characterized by intense and persistent pruritus. The rash often involves the perineum.
  - Continual scratching of the vulva leads to lichenification, producing a thickened, leathery appearance with prominent skin markings and scaling (hyperkeratosis).
- Foci of atypical hyperplasia or cancer can develop, with a 3% chance of developing invasive squamous cell carcinoma.
  - Evaluation should include colposcopy and full-thickness biopsy.
- Initial treatment with topical tricyclic/antipruritic ointments (doxepin 5% ointment), antihistamines (hydroxyzine 25 to 50 mg nightly), or an anxiolytic/sedative may relieve pruritus. For more difficult cases, topical corticosteroid preparations covered by continuous dry occlusive gauze dressings (betamethasone valerate ointment 0.1%) or intralesional corticosteroids (triamcinolone 3 mg/mL) are effective.

## Lichen Planus

- **Lichen planus** is an uncommon, papulosquamous eruption that can affect the genitalia and oral mucosa. The pathophysiology is thought to involve T-cell autoimmunity to basal keratinocytes.
- Patients present with complaints of itching, pain, and burning of the vulva.
- White papules in a linear or reticular pattern are often seen on the vulva (Wickham striae).
- A wide range of morphologies are seen, the most common and most difficult to treat is the erosive form. When the erosive disease progresses, the vulva and vagina become denuded and scarred with loss of the clitoris and labia minora. Introital stenosis is present in severe disease.
- Lichen planus is a chronic recurrent disease; hence, complete control is not typical and spontaneous remission is unlikely. The use of ultrapotent topical steroids is first-line treatment. Surgery is not curative and is reserved for treatment of postinflammatory sequelae, such as labial adhesions and introital stenosis.

## Lichen Sclerosus

- **Lichen sclerosus** is of unknown etiology and is characterized by white, wrinkled, atrophic lesions associated with severe vulvar pruritus, atrophy, and scarring, with gradual loss of the labia minora and prepuce of the clitoris. The perirectal area is often involved.
- This chronic disease occurs at any age but most commonly affects postmenopausal white women.
- Women with lichen sclerosus have a 20% risk of having other autoimmune disease, most frequently alopecia areata, vitiligo, or thyroid disease.

- Patients have a 5% chance of developing vulvar squamous cell carcinoma, although lichen sclerosus is usually not considered a premalignant lesion.
- Vulvar punch biopsies should be performed to confirm the diagnosis.
- Treatment includes chronic use of ultrapotent topical corticosteroid (0.05% clobetasol propionate ointment). Topical estrogen (0.01% estradiol cream) is indicated for atrophic symptoms. Periodic clinical examinations should be performed and patients should return for biopsy if ulcerations persist or new lesions appear. Surgery is reserved for management of malignancy and postinflammatory sequelae, such as labial adhesions and introital stenosis.

## VULVAR PAIN SYNDROMES

- See also Chapters 30 and 42.

### Vulvodynia

- **Vulvodynia** is defined as chronic vulvar discomfort, occurring in the absence of relevant visible findings or a specific identifiable neurologic disorder. The pain is often described as burning, stinging, or throbbing. These symptoms interfere with the ability of women to have vaginal intercourse, wear tight clothing, exercise, or even sit down. Vulvodynia affects roughly 15% of the female population.
- Symptoms may be generalized, localized, provoked, unprovoked, or mixed.
  - The cotton swab test has been described to systematically map affected areas of the vestibule, perineum, and inner thigh for initial evaluation, to differentiate localized from generalized vulvodynia, and to gauge treatment success.
- Vulvodynia is a diagnosis of exclusion and thorough evaluation is needed to rule out other pathologies.
- Often, a combination of multiple treatments may be required to improve symptoms of vulvodynia.
  - These include general vulvar care, topical local anesthetics and estrogen creams, oral medications (e.g., tricyclic antidepressants, gabapentin, carbamazepine), trigger point injections with combined steroids and local anesthetics, dietary changes, cognitive behavioral therapy, biofeedback and physical therapy, and surgery for resistant localized pain.

### Vulvar Vestibulitis Syndrome

- **Vulvar vestibulitis syndrome (VVS)** is chronic inflammation of the vestibular glands and is characterized by erythema and severe pain elicited by touch only. The main presenting symptoms are dyspareunia and terminal dysuria.
- Patients with VVS usually benefit from pelvic rest, anti-inflammatory/antiallergenic therapy (e.g., Burow soak baths/sitz baths, antihistamine therapy, stearin-lanolin cream application), and pelvic relaxation exercises. Infectious etiologies, if present, should be treated. Medical therapies as described earlier for vulvodynia may be appropriate.
- Surgical repair of the vulva and perineum is usually performed for patients who fail to respond to conservative therapy or those who suffer from scars or recurrent perineal tears.

### Levator Ani Myalgia

- **Pelvic floor myalgia** is often the result of trauma or inflammation of the perineal branch of the pudendal nerve causing painful spasms of the affected muscles and fascia.

- Treatment of pelvic muscle myalgia may require pudendal block (triamcinolone + local anesthetic) and pelvic physiotherapy/biofeedback.

## Vulvar Neuropathy

- The pudendal, genitofemoral, and ilioinguinal nerves are the main nerves serving the vulvovaginal area. Trauma to these nerves may result in continuous dull, aching, or burning neuropathic pain.
- Gabapentin 300 to 1,200 mg PO tid or amitriptyline 0.5 to 2 mg/kg PO every night at bedtime have been shown to be effective treatments.

# BENIGN VULVAR LESIONS

## Urethral Caruncle

- **Urethral caruncle** is a benign, generally asymptomatic exophytic papule at the urethral meatus that may cause bleeding. It must be differentiated from malignancy. No treatment is required unless symptomatic, in which case topical estrogen therapy (0.01% Estrace cream, 2 to 4 g daily for 1 to 2 weeks), cryosurgery, or laser vaporization will control bleeding.

## Acrochordon

- **Acrochordons** (i.e., skin tags) are common, frequently pedunculated fibroepithelial polyps that have a rubbery consistency. They often arise in areas of chronic irritation. Acrochordons do not need to be removed unless they are symptomatic.

## Seborrheic Keratoses

- **Seborrheic keratoses** are flat to slightly raised pigmented lesions that have a characteristic waxy, "stuck-on" appearance. Although benign, providers should have a low threshold to perform excisional biopsy to rule out carcinoma.

## Lipoma

- **Lipomas** are benign tumors composed of adipose tissue. They are soft and sometimes pedunculated. They commonly appear on the mons pubis and labia majora. No treatment is necessary unless the lipoma is bothersome, in which case it can be excised.

## Ectopic (Extramammary) Breast

- Supernumerary ectopic breast tissue may be found anywhere along the milk line, which extends from the groin to the axillae. The tissue may undergo cyclical changes with the menstrual cycle like normal breast tissue and is subject to similar pathologies. Evaluation for associated renal system anomalies should be considered.

# BENIGN VULVAR CYSTS

## Bartholin Cyst

- Bartholin glands (greater vestibular glands) produce a clear, mucoid secretion that provides continuous lubrication for the vestibular surface. They are lined by transitional epithelium and are prone to obstruction, which results in **Bartholin cyst** formation. Superinfection results in an abscess. Usually polymicrobial, approximately 10% of **Bartholin abscesses** may be caused by *Neisseria gonorrhoeae*.

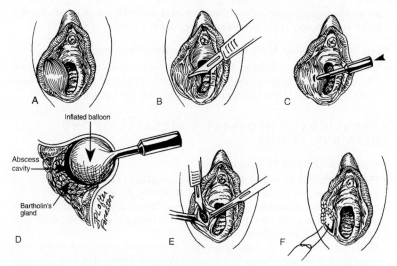

**Figure 44-3.** Surgical management of Bartholin abscess. (**A**) Typical presentation of a Bartholin cyst or abscess; (**B**) small stab incision of the cyst near the hymenal ring; (**C**) insertion of a Word catheter which is inflated in (**D**) to allow fistula drainage tract formation; (**E**) opening of the cyst wall for marsupialization seen in (**F**). (From Beckmann CR, Ling F, Barzansky BM, et al. *Obstetrics and Gynecology*, 4th ed. Philadelphia, PA: Lippincott Williams & Wilkins, 2002:372.)

- Treatment of Bartholin gland abscesses may include incision and drainage, marsupialization, or in case of recurrence, resection of the gland (Fig. 44-3). Attempts at incision and drainage are therapeutic only when the lesion becomes fluctuant. The incision is made near the hymenal ring (i.e., at the vaginal introitus near the duct orifice), and a Word catheter is inserted.
- In women aged 40 years or older, biopsy is recommended because of the risk of Bartholin adenocarcinoma.
- Antibiotic therapy, even after incision and drainage, is not usually necessary unless cellulitis is also present. Simple Bartholin cysts that are not infected and not causing symptoms may not need treatment.

## Epidermal Cysts

- **Epidermal inclusion cysts** are seen frequently on the labia majora, containing a white or yellow material made up of keratin and lipid-rich debris. They arise from blockage of pilosebaceous ducts. If traumatized, they can become erythematous and tender. If symptomatic, cysts can be surgically excised.

## Mucus Cysts

- **Mucus cysts** are found within the vestibule and develop from vestigial embryonic structures or from obstruction of the minor vestibular glands. They are lined by mucus-secreting simple columnar epithelium without myoepithelial cells.

## Gartner Cysts

- **Gartner duct cysts** arise from remnants of the mesonephric ducts. They most often appear as multiple small cysts along the lateral vagina and hymenal ring. These cysts are usually asymptomatic and are discovered incidentally. Treatment is not necessary unless cysts are very large, in which case they can be excised.

## Cysts of the Canal of Nuck (Processus Vaginalis Peritonei)

- These peritoneal-lined cysts are found in the superior aspect of the labia majora. They arise from inclusions of the peritoneum at the insertion of the round ligament to the labia majora. These cysts must be distinguished from an inguinal hernia.

# PREMALIGNANT NEOPLASTIC DISEASES OF THE VULVA AND VAGINA

## Vulvar Intraepithelial Neoplasia

- Histologic criteria for **vulvar intraepithelial neoplasia (VIN)** include disordered maturation and nuclear abnormalities, loss of polarity, pleomorphism, mitotic figures, and coarsened nuclear chromatin. Cytologic atypia is present throughout the epithelium. Historically, the degree of maturation present in the surface epithelium defined the grade of dysplasia.
  - VIN 1 (mild dysplasia) demonstrates loss of squamous maturation in the lower one third of the epithelium. This usually reflects self-limited disease.
  - VIN 2 (moderate dysplasia) shows loss of maturation in the lower two thirds of the epithelium. Surface maturation is present.
  - VIN 3 (severe dysplasia, carcinoma in situ) presents with full-thickness loss of squamous maturation. Stromal invasion does not occur. Cytologic atypia may be severe.
- In a newer system of classification, VIN 1 is eliminated and only high-grade disease (VIN 2 or 3) is categorized. There are three subcategories that reflect the malignant potential of the lesion:
  - VIN usual type (basaloid, warty, or mixed variants): associated with human papillomavirus (HPV) infection (especially 16 and 18), seen in younger women, tends to be multifocal lesions, 5% to 6% progress to invasive cancer
  - VIN differentiated: not associated with HPV and generally seen in older women, associated with atrophy and dermatoses (lichen sclerosus, lichen simplex chronicus, etc.), often unifocal, aggressive with one third progressing to invasive cancer
  - VIN unclassified: rare cases that cannot be classified as discussed earlier
- One third of VIN cases will recur, regardless of how they are treated.

## Vaginal Intraepithelial Neoplasia

- This rare condition affects 0.2 to 2 per 100,000 women.
- Vaginal intraepithelial neoplasia (VaIN) is **usually asymptomatic**, although patients can present with postcoital spotting or vaginal discharge. It is diagnosed by persistently abnormal Pap smears with no evidence of cervical neoplasia. After VaIN is diagnosed, invasive disease must be excluded by colposcopy and biopsy, especially before undertaking nonexcisional therapy. VaIN progresses to invasive cancer in 3% to 7% of patients.
- Risk factors include HPV infection, current or prior lower genital preinvasive or invasive lesions, immunosuppression, history of radiation exposure, pessary use, and prolapse.
- **VaIN** is a preinvasive lesion defined by the presence of squamous cell atypia without invasion. Lesions are classified according to the depth of epithelial involvement.

- VaIN 1: Cytologic atypia is present throughout the lower one third of the epithelium.
- VaIN 2: Cytologic atypia is present throughout the lower two thirds of epithelium.
- VaIN 3: Cytologic atypia involves more than two thirds of the epithelium.

### Treatment of Vulvar Intraepithelial Neoplasia and Vaginal Intraepithelial Neoplasia

- **Surgical resection** is the mainstay of treatment and should be performed if invasion cannot be excluded.
  - Wide local incision: 5-mm margin, ideal for localized lesions
  - Skinning vulvectomy: large, extensive, or multifocal lesions
  - Total vulvectomy or vaginectomy
- Topical agents (5% imiquimod and 5-fluorouracil cream): useful for persistent low-grade, multifocal lesions or women who are poor surgical candidates
- Intracavitary radiation therapy: effective for VAIN; associated with morbidity; and should be reserved for women who are poor surgical candidates, have multifocal disease, and/or have failed other treatments
- $CO_2$ laser ablation: Must rule out invasion with pretreatment biopsies; useful with multifocal disease, minimal scarring, and sexual dysfunction. VIN lesions should be ablated to 3 mm in hair-bearing areas and 1 mm on nonhairy surfaces.

## MALIGNANT NEOPLASTIC DISEASES OF THE VULVA

**Vulvar neoplasms** are relatively rare and represent 3% to 5% of all primary malignancies of the female genital tract. The American Cancer Society estimates that 4,850 women will be diagnosed with and 1,030 women will die from cancer of the vulva in 2014. Squamous cell carcinoma is the most common histopathology found in vulvar cancer, followed by melanoma, basal cell carcinoma, and sarcoma. These lesions most commonly present as pruritus and are often misdiagnosed by health care providers.

### Squamous Cell Vulvar Neoplasia

- Squamous cell lesions account for 85% to 90% of vulvar malignancies.
- As with VIN, two subtypes of **invasive squamous cell carcinomas** exist.
  - The classic, warty, or Bowenoid type is identified in younger patients and is related to HPV. These lesions may be multifocal.
  - The keratinizing, differentiated, or simplex types occur in older women and is not associated with HPV. These lesions tend to be unifocal, and a significant number are associated with atrophic lesions, such as lichen sclerosus.
- Accurate **surgical staging** predicts prognosis, as nodal status has the most prognostic significance, and directs treatment for squamous cell carcinoma of the vulva. The International Federation of Gynecology and Obstetrics (FIGO) staging system was recently revised to reflect the risk of nodal metastases on survival (Table 44-1).
- **Treatment.** Vulvar carcinomas, especially early-stage lesions, are treated surgically. Good margins and reliable assessment of lymph nodes are essential, as recurrences are often fatal.
  - Stage IA (microinvasive) vulvar cancer: Radical local excision with a 1-cm margin at the time of resection. Inguinofemoral lymphadenectomy is not recommended because the risk of metastasis to the lymph nodes is extremely low.

| TABLE 44-1 | International Federation of Gynecology and Obstetrics Staging for Carcinoma of the Vulva (2009) and 5-Year Survival | |
|---|---|---|

| Stage | Description | 5-Year Survival[a] |
|---|---|---|
| 0 | **Carcinoma in situ, intraepithelial neoplasia** | |
| I | **Tumor confined to vulva or perineum** | **98%** |
| IA | Tumor confined to vulva or perineum; lesion ≤2 cm with stromal invasion ≤1 mm, no nodal metastasis | |
| IB | Tumor confined to vulva or perineum; lesion >2 cm or stromal invasion >1 mm, with negative nodes | |
| II | **Tumor of any size with extension to adjacent perineal structures (lower one third of urethra, lower one third of vagina, anus) with negative nodes** | **85%** |
| III | **Tumor of any size with or without extension to adjacent perineal structures with positive inguinofemoral lymph nodes** | **74%** |
| IIIA | (i) With one lymph node metastasis (≥5 mm) or (ii) One or two lymph node metastasis(es) (<5 mm) | |
| IIIB | (i) With two or more lymph node metastases (≥5 mm) or (ii) Three or more lymph node metastases (<5 mm) | |
| IIIC | With positive nodes with extracapsular spread | |
| IV | **Tumor invading other regional (upper two third of urethra, upper two third of vagina) or distant structures** | **31%** |
| IVA | Tumor invading any of the following: (i) upper urethra and/or vaginal mucosa, bladder mucosa, rectal mucosa, or fixed to pelvic bone (ii) fixed or ulcerated inguinofemoral lymph nodes | |
| IVB | Distant metastasis to any site including pelvic lymph nodes | |

[a]Five-year survival data according to previous FIGO staging system.
Adapted from Pecorelli S. Revised FIGO staging for carcinoma of the vulva, cervix, and endometrium. *Int J Gynecol Obstet* 2009;105:103–104.

- Early-stage disease: Treat surgically with a radical procedure and lymph node assessment. More aggressive traditional surgeries are making way for less invasive approaches.
  o Historically, this was accomplished with a butterfly-shaped en block excision of the vulva, inguinal and femoral lymph nodes, and the skin and lymphatics in between. A modified three-incision technique has fewer complications and similar survival.

○ A radical excisional procedure (total radical vulvectomy, partial radical vulvectomy, radical local excision) obtains 1- to 2-cm clinical margins and dissects down to the perineal membrane.
- Inguinofemoral lymphadenectomy: removal of nodal tissue from the lateral border of the adductor longus to medial border of the sartorius muscle, the mons pubis and pubic tubercle medially and cephalad, and the external oblique laterally.
  ○ This inguinofemoral lymphadenectomy may be ipsilateral only if the tumor is >2 cm lateral to the midline and <2 cm in diameter with both groins clinically negative for metastasis. However, if the ipsilateral side is positive for tumor, the bilateral node dissections should be performed.
- Sentinel lymph node biopsy (SLNB) uses the principle that tumor will metastasize to the first lymph node in its path, the sentinel node. Therefore, a negative sentinel node excludes metastasis beyond it. Candidates should have clinically negative lymph nodes.
  ○ The Groningen International Sentinel Node for Vulvar Cancer trial showed an overall survival of 97% and a 3% relapse rate 2 years after excision with a negative SLNB in women with vulvar cancer <4 cm.
  ○ SLNB is more successful when radiocolloid and blue dye are used for identification of the sentinel node.
  ○ If tumor involves midline structures, SLNB should be performed bilaterally.
  ○ All nodes that take up blue dye and/or radiotracer should be excised (even if it is more than one node). If no nodes are identified, a lymphadenectomy should be performed.

## Verrucous Carcinoma

- **Verrucous carcinoma** is a variant of squamous carcinoma that occurs in postmenopausal women. These tumors are large, fungating masses that may be mistakenly diagnosed as condyloma acuminata resistant to treatment. Because the histologic appearance of verrucous carcinoma closely resembles normal squamous epithelium, a sufficiently deep biopsy must be obtained for diagnosis. Although lymph node metastasis is exceedingly rare, local destruction and tumor recurrence are common.
- **Treatment** consists of radical local excision.
- Radiation therapy is contraindicated because it may induce increased aggression in malignant activity.

## Basal Cell Carcinoma

- In contrast to other locations where **basal cell carcinoma** is the most common skin cancer, this malignancy constitutes only 2% to 3% of all vulvar carcinomas. They occur most commonly in postmenopausal white women. In contrast to other areas of skin, ultraviolet light exposure plays no role in the etiology of vulvar basal cell carcinoma.
- Grossly, these lesions appear as flesh colored to whitish nodules or plaques that are often ulcerated. The prognosis is good, despite a 20% risk of local recurrence. Metastases to the inguinal lymph nodes are rare.
- **Treatment** is with wide local excision.

## Melanoma

- **Melanomas** constitute the second most common primary malignancy of the vulva, comprising 5% to 10% of vulvar neoplasms. Anogenital lesions account for 3% of all melanomas. Vulvar melanoma most commonly occurs in the sixth to seventh decades of life.

- Melanomas are typically raised lesions, with irregular pigmentation and borders. They are found with equal frequency on the labia majora and on mucosal surfaces. Prognosis depends primarily on tumor thickness and on the presence or absence of lymph node involvement.
- They may be staged via the American Joint Committee on Cancer (AJCC), FIGO, Clark, Breslow, or Chung system.
- **Treatment:** Radical local excision (1-cm margins for lesions ≤1 mm thick and 2-cm margins for lesions >1 mm thick) is recommended for the primary lesion. Although nodal status has prognostic significance, the therapeutic role of regional lymphadenectomy is not well defined. Five-year survival rate is 35%. High-dose alpha-interferon may improve survival in cases at high risk for recurrence.

## Paget Disease of the Vulva

- **Paget disease of the vulva** is rare. Most affected patients are in their seventh or eighth decade of life and experience local irritation, pruritus, and bleeding.
- The lesion has slightly raised edges and is erythematous, with islands of white epithelium. Lesions are multifocal and are sharply demarcated and often have foci of excoriation and induration.
- Adenocarcinoma of the underlying sweat glands is found in 10% to 15% of patients who have intraepithelial Paget disease.
  - Ten percent of patients with vulvar Paget disease are found to have associated breast, colon, or genitourinary cancer; thus, the workup should include colonoscopy, cystoscopy, mammogram, and colposcopy.
  - If the disease is limited to the epithelium, its clinical course is usually prolonged and indolent.
- **Treatment:** Although radical surgery was formerly the mainstay of therapy, newer evidence suggests that local excision with 2- to 3-cm borders of all involved tissue carries similar prognosis. Local recurrence is common and can be treated with laser ablation. Five-year survival rates are high, and, because of the late age of onset of disease, patients usually die of illness other than Paget disease. If an underlying adenocarcinoma is identified, the patient should undergo radical excision and inguinal lymphadenectomy. The prognosis in patients with lymph node involvement is poor.

## Bartholin Gland Carcinoma

- Although primary vulvar adenocarcinomas are rare, the majority arise from the Bartholin gland.
- Primary cancers of the Bartholin gland include **adenocarcinomas and squamous cell carcinomas**. The latter may be associated with HPV. Bartholin gland malignancies typically occur in the sixth decade of life, and biopsy of suspicious lesions is recommended in women age 40 years and older.
- **Treatment:** Radical excision is recommended for the management of the primary lesion. Unfortunately, given an extensive vascular and lymphatic supply, metastatic disease is common. Inguinofemoral lymphadenectomy is recommended.

## Vulvar Sarcoma

- **Sarcomas** of the vulva are rare and account for 1% to 2% of vulvar malignancies. The age range is broader than for squamous cell carcinoma of the vulva. Lymphatic metastasis is uncommon.
- **Treatment:** Wide local excision is recommended, followed by adjuvant radiation, chemotherapy, or both.

# MALIGNANT NEOPLASTIC DISEASES OF THE VAGINA

Most malignancies identified in the vagina are secondary (i.e. recurrent or metastatic cervical cancer). Primary **vaginal cancer** is very rare, accounting for <2% of all primary malignancies of the female genital tract. Squamous cell carcinoma is the most common histopathology (80%), followed by adenocarcinoma (10%), melanoma (3%), sarcoma (3%), and other rare histologies. The American Cancer Society estimates that in 2014 there will be 3,170 new cases of and 880 deaths from vaginal cancer.

## Squamous Cell Vaginal Cancer

- Patients may present with painless vaginal bleeding and discharge or an abnormal Pap smear.
- Most are associated with HPV infection.
- Visual inspection of the vagina as the speculum is being inserted or removed may reveal a gross lesion. Often, vaginal tumors are detected incidentally as a result of cytologic screening for cervical cancer. The posterior wall of the upper one third of the vagina is the most commonly affected site. Colposcopy is helpful for visualization. Definitive diagnosis is accomplished by biopsy.
- **Staging** is performed clinically based on findings from physical and pelvic examination, cystourethroscopy, proctosigmoidoscopy, and chest radiography. The prognosis of squamous cell carcinoma of the vagina depends on FIGO staging (Table 44-2). Lymphatic dissemination from lesions in the upper third of the vagina spreads to pelvic and para-aortic lymph nodes, whereas tumors in the distal third of the vagina spread to inguinofemoral and then pelvic nodes.

| TABLE 44-2 | International Federation of Gynecology and Obstetrics Staging Classification of Vaginal Cancer and 5-Year Survival | |
|---|---|---|
| Stage | Description | 5-Year Survival |
| 0 | Carcinoma in situ, intraepithelial neoplasia | |
| I | The carcinoma is confined to the vaginal wall. | 95% |
| II | The carcinoma involves subvaginal tissue but has not extended to the pelvic sidewall. | 67% |
| III | The carcinoma extends to the pelvic sidewall. | 32% |
| IV | The carcinoma extends beyond the true pelvis or involves the bladder or rectum; bullous edema as such does not permit a case to be allotted to stage IV. | |
| IVA | Tumor invades bladder or rectal mucosa or there is direct extension beyond the true pelvis. | 18% |
| IVB | Spread to distant organs | Almost 0% |

Adapted from FIGO Committee on Gynecologic Oncology. Current FIGO staging for cancer of the vagina, fallopian tube, ovary and gestational trophoblastic neoplasia. *Int J Gynecol Obstet* 2009;105:3–4.

- **Treatment:** Treatment depends on the location, size, and clinical stage of the tumor. Invasive disease can be treated with surgery and radiation. Cisplatin is often used for chemosensitization in the setting of radiation therapy.
  - In stage I disease:
    - Surgery is preferred if negative surgical margins can be achieved and low risk for needing radiation. Disease limited to the vaginal fornix can be treated with radical hysterectomy and/or partial vaginectomy with parametrectomy and pelvic lymphadenectomy. If the distal third of the vagina is involved, dissection of groin nodes should be performed. Lymph nodes are not accounted for in the FIGO staging system, but positive lymph nodes are poor prognosticators. SLNB is still experimental.
    - Radiotherapy can be delivered by external beam radiation or brachytherapy. Proximity of the bladder, urethra, and rectum to the vagina precludes the administration of high-dose radiation.
  - Stage II and III disease is treated with external beam radiation with or without brachytherapy and/or chemotherapy.
  - Stage IV disease:
    - If pelvic nodes are involved, external beam radiation with or without brachytherapy and/or chemotherapy
    - IVA disease: Consider pelvic exenteration versus external beam radiation. Both can be used with or without radiotherapy and or chemotherapy.
    - Patients with distant metastases should receive supportive care with chemotherapy or radiation for palliative purposes.
    - Recurrent disease may require pelvic exenteration or diverting surgeries.

## Adenocarcinoma of the Vagina

- **Vaginal adenocarcinoma** is rare, accounting for <10% of vaginal cancers. Clear cell adenocarcinoma may arise from areas of adenosis in women exposed to diethylstilbestrol in utero. Screening in these patients should begin at menarche or 14 years of age. Prognosis of clear cell adenocarcinoma is good and the overall survival is 78%. However, primary non–clear cell adenocarcinoma of the vagina carries a worse prognosis than squamous cell carcinoma.
- **Treatment:** In general, adenocarcinoma is treated similarly to squamous cell carcinoma.

## Melanoma

- Primary malignant **melanoma of the vagina** is rare. It usually presents with vaginal bleeding and is typically described as blue-black or black-brown masses, plaques, or ulcerations, commonly in the distal one third of the anterior vaginal wall. Symptoms include vaginal bleeding, mass, or discharge. Staging should be based on tumor thickness (Breslow or AJCC, not FIGO or other melanoma staging systems).
- Historically, the **treatment** has been radical surgery and more recently has included wide local excision. Although generally thought to be radioresistant, radiotherapy may help with local control. Primary malignant melanomas of the urogenital mucous membranes may be aggressive. The 5-year survival rate for vaginal melanomas is usually <20%. Groin SLNB may be reasonable for prognostic reasons in women with lower vaginal lesions.

## Sarcoma

- These rare vaginal malignancies often follow a history of pelvic radiation therapy.
- Treatment is preferably surgery.

*Embryonal Rhabdomyosarcoma (Sarcoma Botryoides)*

- **Sarcoma botryoides** is a highly malignant tumor that occurs during infancy and early childhood. It usually presents as soft nodules that resembles a bunch of grapes. The polypoid mass may fill or protrude from the vagina. See also Chapter 34.
- **Treatment:** Treated with multimodality chemotherapy with vincristine, dactinomycin, and cyclophosphamide (VAC) and limited surgery in order to preserve reproductive function

## SUGGESTED READINGS

Apgar B, Cook JT. Differentiating normal and abnormal findings of the vulva. *Am Fam Physician* 1996;53:1171–1180.

Barhan S, Ezenagu L. Vulvar problems in elderly women. *Postgrad Med* 1997;102:121–132.

Boardman L, Kennedy C. ACOG practice bulletin no. 93: diagnosis and management of vulvar skin disorders. *Obstet Gynecol* 2008;111(5):1243–1253.

Duong TH, Flowers LC. Vulvo-vaginal cancers: risks, evaluation, prevention, and early detection. *Obstet Gynecol Clin North Am* 2007;34:783–802.

Foster D. Vulvar disease. *Obstet Gynecol* 2002;100:145–163.

Haefner HK, Collins ME, Davis GD, et al. The vulvodynia guideline. *J Low Genit Tract Dis* 2005;9:40–51.

Larrabee R, Kylander D. Benign vulvar disorders. *Postgrad Med* 2001;109:151–164.

Van der Zee AG, Oonk MH, De Hullu JA, et al. Sentinel node dissection is safe in the treatment of early-stage vulvar cancer. *J Clin Oncol* 2008;26:884.

# 45 Cervical Intraepithelial Neoplasia

Reinou S. Groen and Cornelia Liu Trimble

## EPIDEMIOLOGY OF CERVICAL NEOPLASIA

- In the United States, **cervical cancer** is diagnosed in approximately 12,000 women annually and fatal for approximately 4,000. It is the second leading cause of death in women aged 20 to 39 years. Approximately 50% of cervical cancer diagnoses can be attributed to inadequate screening.
- Persistent infection with the oncogenic (high-risk) **human papillomavirus (HPV)** types 16, 18, 31, 33, 35, 39, 45, 52, 56, 58, 59, and 68 is required but not sufficient to develop cervical cancer and its precursor lesions. HPV 16 is the most common carcinogenic genotype, followed by HPV 18. Together, they are responsible for 70% of HPV-related cervical cancers. Although approximately 80% of women will be infected through sexual intercourse by an HPV type at some point in their lives, 90% of these infections are transient and will be cleared immunologically within

1 to 2 years. Risks for persistent infection include tobacco exposure and immune compromise, including coinfection with HIV. HPV infection in women older than 30 years is more likely to indicate a persistent infection than detectable HPV in younger women. Cervical cancer is thought to occur after a median of 20 to 25 years following the initiation of a persistent HPV infection.

- The conventional cervical cytology smear or the liquid-based cytology (both referred to as **Pap smear**) is used as a screening test to identify the presence of visually abnormal cervical epithelial cells. Both techniques are equally sensitive and specific. Oncogenic HPV infection can be detected with the Digene hybrid capture test, which can be performed either on cytology specimens or using the Digene sampling brush.
- Annually, 4.8 million women have an abnormal Pap smear in the United States. Cytologic abnormalities are categorized using the Bethesda system (see the following text).
- Histologic abnormalities are classified in a two-tiered system of low-grade and high-grade squamous intraepithelial lesions. Low-grade squamous intraepithelial lesions (LSILs) include mild dysplasia and cervical intraepithelial neoplasia (CIN 1). High-grade squamous intraepithelial lesions (HSILs) include moderate and severe dysplasia, carcinoma in situ, and CIN 2/3.
- CIN 1 is associated with a high rate of spontaneous regression, whereas untreated CIN 3 has a reported cumulative incidence of invasive cancer of 30.1% at 30 years.

## PRIMARY PREVENTION

- **Smoking cessation:** Women who smoke have an increased risk of developing cervical cancer compared to nonsmokers. This is thought to be related to the fact that smoking triples the likelihood of persistent HPV infection and doubles the risk of progression to CIN 3.
- All women with abnormal Pap smears should be offered testing for HIV and other sexually transmitted infections.
- A quadrivalent HPV vaccine directed against HPV types 6, 11, 16, and 18 (Gardasil, Merck, Whitehouse Station, NJ) was approved for use in 9- to 26-year-old females by the U.S. Food and Drug Administration (FDA) in 2006. The vaccine is very effective in HPV 16/18 naïve women, preventing essentially 100% of HSILs. However, the **preventive vaccine does not have therapeutic effect against existing infection**. Both the Advisory Committee on Immunization Practices (ACIP) and American College of Obstetricians and Gynecologists (ACOG) recommend administration of the vaccine to females aged 9 to 26 years.
- The vaccine is administered in three doses at 0, 2, and 6 months. See Chapter 1. Currently, HPV vaccination does not change screening recommendations. However, looking forward, HPV vaccination is likely to influence positive and negative predictive values of the Pap smear by decreasing cervical abnormalities in the population.

## SCREENING

- Cytologic changes associated with HPV infection and neoplasia can be identified using Pap smears, which are the basis of cervical cancer screening programs. Abnormal Pap smears are followed by colposcopic evaluation of the cervix, as indicated in the flow diagrams later.
- **Screening guidelines** are formulated by the American Society for Colposcopy and Cervical Pathology (ASCCP) and used in the 2013 ACOG practice bulletin. The guidelines were issued in 2001, 2006, and 2012, adapting new scientific insights and epidemiologic changes.

- HPV vaccination may change the HPV genotype distribution as well as the positive and negative predictive value of Pap smears. Furthermore, vaccination may influence adherence to screening. Therefore, new guidelines will be needed to accommodate to those changes.
- Based on the ASCCP guidelines from 2012:
  - Regular screening should begin at 21 years of age, regardless of the age of first sexual intercourse. Women aged 21 to 29 years should be screened every 3 years with cytology only. In this age cohort, HPV infections are likely to be transient.
  - In women aged 30 to 65 years, screening can be performed every 3 years with cytology alone. However, preferably, screening can be performed every 5 years with HPV cotesting (cytology and high-risk HPV testing).
  - Screening can be stopped at age 65 years if a woman does not have risk factors and has 10 years of negative screening that includes at least three negative test results. Screening should not be reinstituted, even in the case of a new sexual partner after the age of 65 years. Annual well-woman exams are still recommended for all adult women.
  - Women who have had a total hysterectomy for benign indications and who do not have a history of high-grade lesion do not require further screening.
  - Women with a history of CIN 2/3 should undergo screening every 3 years for at least 20 years after an initial adequate posttreatment surveillance period, regardless of their age. The same period of vaginal screening is advised for those who underwent a hysterectomy as part of treatment for recurrent CIN 2/3.
  - HIV-positive women should be screened at 6-month intervals for 1 year after the diagnosis of HIV and then may resume an annual screening schedule. Immunocompromised and women who were exposed to diethylstilbestrol (DES) in utero should also be screened annually.
- Visual inspection with acetic acid and direct treatment with cryotherapy is currently the most effective cervical cancer prevention in low-resource settings where pathology laboratories and personnel are scarce and monetary and/or logistical constraints prohibit follow-up.

## PAP SMEAR

- Pap smear reports include specimen type, specimen adequacy, results, and any ancillary testing performed (i.e., high-risk HPV probe).
- Specimen type indicates whether the test is a vaginal or cervical sample.
- Adequacy is reported as satisfactory, unsatisfactory, or endocervical cells not present/lack of transformation zone.
  - Unsatisfactory Pap smears should be repeated in 2 to 4 months.
  - Pap smears that lack an endocervical component can be repeated in 1 year or postpartum unless any of the following risk factors are present, all of which necessitate repeat screening in 6 months:
    - History of atypical squamous cells of undetermined significance or greater abnormalities in the past, without three-interval normal Pap smears
    - High-risk HPV positivity in the previous 12 months
    - Previous glandular abnormality
    - Immunosuppression
    - Inability to visualize the endocervical canal
  - Patient noncompliance
- The results section relays any cytologic abnormality.

## DIAGNOSTIC CATEGORIES: CYTOLOGY

The 2001 revision of the Bethesda system is used to describe abnormal cervical cytology employing the following categories:
- Atypical squamous cells (**ASC**)
  - Of undetermined significance (**ASC-US**)
  - Cannot exclude high grade (**ASC-H**)
- Low-grade squamous intraepithelial lesion
- High-grade squamous intraepithelial lesion
- Atypical glandular cells (**AGC**) (endocervical or endometrial)
  - Not otherwise specified (**AGC-NOS**)
  - Favor neoplasia (**AGC-favor neoplasia**)
  - Adenocarcinoma in situ (**AIS**)

### Atypical Squamous Cells

- Approximately 2 million ASC Pap smears a year are recorded in the United States.
- ASC-US is present in 4.7% of samples and is associated with a 7% to 12% prevalence of CIN 2/3.
- ASC-H is present in 0.4% of samples and CIN 2/3 is present in 26% to 68% of women with this result.
- The risk of invasive cancer associated with an ASC Pap is 0.1% to 0.2%.

### Atypical Glandular Cells

- AGC are found in 0.4% of Pap smears.
- AGC are associated with significant neoplasia in 9% to 38% (CIN 2/3, AIS) and in 3% to 17% associated with cancer.
  - One study found that the malignancies of the women with AGC were found in women older than 35 years, are mainly of endometrial origin, and therefore suggested endometrial biopsy for every woman with AGC after the age of 35 years.
- AGC-favor neoplasia has a higher risk of neoplasia (27% to 96%) than AGC-NOS (9% to 41%).

### Low-Grade Squamous Intraepithelial Lesions

- LSIL is reported in 2.1% of Pap smears and is strongly correlated with HPV infection.
- High-grade dysplasia or neoplasia is found in 12% to 17% of women who undergo colposcopy for LSIL.

### High-Grade Squamous Intraepithelial Lesions

- HSIL is reported in 0.7% of Pap smears.
- CIN 2/3 is found in 53% to 97% of women with HSIL cytology. Invasive cancer is identified in 2.0% of women with HSIL cytology.

## TREATMENT OPTIONS

- Treatment options can be classified as ablative or excisional.
- Ablative procedures do not obtain a sample for pathologic examination.
- Excisional procedures should be performed when invasive cancer cannot be ruled out, microinvasive cancer is suspected on a biopsy, a two-level discrepancy between cytology and histology exists, and whenever concern is raised for endocervical disease.

## Ablative Methods

- **Cryotherapy** is performed with a supercooled probe applied directly to the lesion. Not appropriate for endocervical disease.
- **Carbon dioxide laser** is used to vaporize the tissue to 7-mm depth. Special equipment is necessary, but more irregular areas can be treated.
- Ablative methods are not acceptable for AIS or for unsatisfactory colposcopy.

## Excisional Methods

- Excisional procedures may increase a woman's risk of future preterm delivery or premature rupture of the membranes.
- **Loop electrosurgical excision procedure (LEEP)** is an excisional procedure employing a wire with an electrical current. The shape and size of the loop can be altered, and a second "hat" can be done to obtain further endocervical tissue.
  - Cautery artifact can make interpretation of margins difficult.
- **Cold** knife cone **(CKC)** employs a scalpel to excise a cone-shaped wedge of the cervix. The size and shape of the cone can be tailored to the lesion, and this method allows for pathologic determination of margin status.
  - CKC should be considered over LEEP for cases with AIS, suspected microinvasion, unsatisfactory colposcopy, or a lesion extending into the endocervical canal.

# MANAGEMENT STRATEGIES: CYTOLOGIC ABNORMALITIES

## Atypical Squamous Cells of Undetermined Significance

- **Reflex testing for high-risk HPV:** A positive result should be followed by colposcopy. A negative result allows for resumption of standard screening. With this strategy, the sensitivity for detection of CIN 2/3 is 92% (Fig. 45-1).

### *Special Populations*

- Adolescents (between 13 and 20 years old) have a higher prevalence of HPV but are likely to clear the infection. Therefore, they should not be tested for HPV.
- Delaying first testing until age 21 years is designed to reduce unnecessary diagnostic procedures or interventions and potential iatrogenic morbidity in young women.

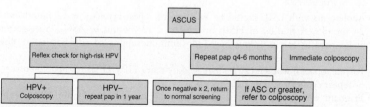

**Figure 45-1.** Triage strategy for ASC-US. ASC-US, atypical squamous cell of undetermined significance; HPV, human papillomavirus; ASC, atypical squamous cell. (Adapted from Massad LS, Einstein MH, Huh WK, et al. 2012 consensus guidelines for the management of women with abnormal cervical cancer screening tests and cancer precursors. *J Low Genit Tract Dis* 2013;17:S1–S27.)

- Pregnant women are tested according to their age group, with the exception that colposcopy can be deferred to 6 weeks postpartum. Endocervical curettage is never acceptable in pregnancy.
- Immunosuppressed and postmenopausal women are managed in a manner identical to the general population.

## Atypical Squamous Cells, Cannot Exclude High Grade

- These patients require colposcopic examination. Negative colposcopy should be followed by cytology in 6 and 12 months or cotesting at 12 months.

## Atypical Glandular Cells

- All women with AGC should undergo colposcopy with endocervical biopsy; HPV DNA testing is preferred.
- Endometrial sampling should be performed routinely for the finding of atypical endometrial cells.
- Endometrial sampling should be performed in women aged 35 years and older and in those with risk factors for endometrial cancer.
- Follow-up for AGC-NOS after negative findings is repeat cytology/HPV DNA testing at 6 months if they are initially HPV DNA positive and 12 months if negative.
- Follow-up for AGC-favor neoplasia after a negative evaluation is a diagnostic excisional procedure, preferably CKC.
- AIS is managed by a diagnostic excisional procedure, preferably CKC.

*Special Populations*

- Pregnant women should be managed in an identical fashion to the general population with the exception that endometrial and endocervical biopsies are unacceptable.
- Benign-appearing endometrial cells on a Pap smear in postmenopausal women should be evaluated with endometrial biopsy.

## Low-Grade Squamous Intraepithelial Lesion

- LSIL carries the same risk of high-grade dysplasia as ASC-US + HPV and is therefore managed identically (colposcopy).
- Endocervical curettage is preferred in those with an unsatisfactory or negative colposcopic examination.
- A finding of less than CIN 2/3 can be followed by cytology at 6 and 12 months or HPV DNA testing at 12 months.

*Special Populations*

- Adolescents with LSIL should be followed by repeat cytology at 12 months and 24 months. A finding of HSIL or greater at 12 months or ASC-US or greater at 24 months merits colposcopy. Only immunosuppressed adolescents are now screened.
- Postmenopausal women can be managed by reflex HPV DNA testing, colposcopy, or repeat cytology at 6 and 12 months.
- Pregnant women with LSIL should have a colposcopic examination. Postpartum follow-up is also acceptable.

## High-Grade Squamous Intraepithelial Lesion

- Due to the high risk of significant cervical disease, one approach is to "see and treat" with immediate LEEP.

- Colposcopy with endocervical curettage is also acceptable. An unsatisfactory colposcopy should be managed by a diagnostic excisional procedure.
- A satisfactory colposcopy that results in a diagnosis of less than CIN 2/3 can be followed by colposcopy/cytology at 6 and 12 months, excisional diagnostic procedure, or review of the original pathologic material to verify the diagnosis.

*Special Populations*

- A satisfactory colposcopy detecting less than CIN 2/3 should be followed by colposcopy/cytology every 6 months for up to 2 years.
- Persistent HSIL for 24 months should be evaluated with an excisional diagnostic procedure.
- Two consecutive negative Pap smears and no high-grade lesions on colposcopy allow for resumption of a normal screening schedule.
- Pregnant women with HSIL should be evaluated by colposcopy. Lesions suspicious for CIN 2/3 or cancer should be biopsied; it is unacceptable to biopsy other lesions.
- Evaluation no sooner than 6 weeks postpartum should be performed for women with a diagnosis of less than CIN 2/3.

## DIAGNOSTIC CATEGORIES VIA COLPOSCOPY: HISTOLOGY

- Colposcopy is used for the evaluation of abnormal cervical cytology. The average sensitivity of cytology is only 48%. Therefore, colposcopic examination should include a biopsy of a visible lesion, with the exception of pregnant women, or those who will undergo a diagnostic excision.
- A colposcope is used to examine the cervix after the application of a dilute, 3% acetic acid wash. The dilute acid dehydrates epithelial cells with a high nuclear-to-cytoplasmic ratio, resulting in acetowhite changes.
- Colposcopy is considered satisfactory if the entire squamocolumnar junction is visualized circumferentially and if all lesions are completely visualized.

### Cervical Intraepithelial Neoplasia 1

- CIN 1 is the histologic diagnosis applied to low-grade lesions. However, it is not equivalent to LSIL.
- An estimated 1 million women are diagnosed with CIN 1 annually in the United States, and the annual incidence of CIN 1 is estimated to be 1.2 per 1,000 women.
- CIN 1 progresses in approximately 11% to CIN 2/3 (Table 45-1).

### Cervical Intraepithelial Neoplasia 2/3

- CIN 2/3 is the histologic diagnosis applied to high-grade lesions; it is not equivalent to HSIL.
- An estimated 500,000 women are diagnosed with CIN 2/3 annually in the United States, and the annual incidence of CIN 2/3 is estimated to be 1.5 per 1,000 women.

### Adenocarcinoma In Situ

- Unlike squamous lesions, AIS lesions are often multifocal. Therefore, negative margins do not reliably predict excision of all disease.

| TABLE 45-1 | Natural History of Untreated Cervical Intraepithelial Neoplasia | | | |
|---|---|---|---|---|
| | Regression to Normal (%) | Persistent Dysplasia (%) | Progression to CIN 2/3 (%) | Progression to CIS (%) |
| CIN 1 | 57 | 30 | 11 | 0.3 |
| CIN 2 | 43 | 35 | — | 14–22 |
| CIN 3 | 32 | 48–56 | — | 12 |

CIN, cervical intraepithelial neoplasia; CIS, carcinoma in situ.
Adapted from Mitchell MF, Tortolero-Luna G, Wright T, et al. Cervical human papillomavirus infection and intraepithelial neoplasia: a review. *J Natl Cancer Inst Monogr* 1996;(21):17–25.

## MANAGEMENT STRATEGIES: HISTOLOGIC ABNORMALITIES

### Cervical Intraepithelial Neoplasia 1

- The management of CIN 1 depends on the cytology, as the risk of an occult high-grade lesion is greater when the referral cytology is HSIL or AGC (Fig. 45-2).
- CIN 1 preceded by ASC-US, ASC-H, or LSIL
  - Follow-up with repeat cytology at 6 and 12 months or HPV DNA testing at 12 months. A positive HPV DNA or cytology equal to or greater than ASC-US necessitates repeat colposcopy.
  - Two negative Pap smears or a single negative HPV DNA allows for resumption of standard screening.
  - Persistent (>2 years) CIN 1 can be followed as mentioned earlier or treated. Ablative and excisional procedures are acceptable given a satisfactory colposcopy. Ablation is unacceptable after unsatisfactory colposcopy.

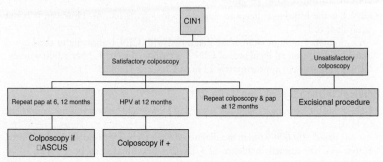

Figure 45-2. Triage strategy for CIN 1. CIN, cervical intraepithelial neoplasia; HPV, human papillomavirus; ASC-US, atypical squamous cell of undetermined significance. (Adapted from Massad LS, Einstein MH, Huh WK, et al. 2012 consensus guidelines for the management of women with abnormal cervical cancer screening tests and cancer precursors. *J Low Genit Tract Dis* 2013;17:S1–S27.)

- CIN 1 preceded by HSIL or AGC-NOS
  - Diagnostic excisional procedure or colposcopy/cytology at 6-month intervals is acceptable. Endocervical curettage should be performed if colposcopy is selected.
  - Unsatisfactory colposcopy or persistence of HSIL or AGC-NOS cytology requires a diagnostic excisional procedure.
  - Negative cytology/colposcopy for 1 year allows for resumption of routine screening.

*Special Populations*
- Adolescents with CIN 1 should be followed with yearly cytology. HSIL or greater at 1 year should be evaluated with colposcopy, as should ASC-US or greater after 24 months.
- Pregnant women with CIN 1 should be followed without treatment.

## Cervical Intraepithelial Neoplasia 2 and 3
- CIN 2/3 requires excision or ablation after a satisfactory colposcopy.
- Recurrent CIN 2/3 should be excised. Ablation is unacceptable for CIN 2/3 and an unsatisfactory colposcopy.
- Hysterectomy is not an acceptable management for CIN 2/3.
- After treatment, CIN 2/3 can be followed by HPV DNA testing at 6 to 12 months, cytology every 6 months, or cytology/colposcopy at 6-month intervals.
- Either HPV DNA positivity or ASC-US or greater on cytology require colposcopy with endocervical sampling.
- If testing is negative after posttreatment evaluation for 1 year, routine screening should be employed for at least 20 years.
- Hysterectomy is acceptable for persistent or recurrent CIN 2/3.
- Positive margins can be followed with Pap smear, colposcopy, and endocervical curettage every 4 to 6 months, or a further excisional procedure can be performed.

*Special Populations*
- In younger women, future fertility should be taken into account; because CIN 2/3 can regress spontaneously, colposcopy evaluation with endocervical assessment is therefore an appropriate initial evaluation.
- The main goal for pregnant women is to exclude invasive cancer. Biopsy is important if the colposcopy impression is high grade and a biopsy during pregnancy is not jeopardizing the pregnancy. Reassessment not earlier than 6 weeks postpartum is warranted for follow-up and further management.

## Adenocarcinoma In Situ
- Cold knife conization is the first-line treatment for AIS.
- Diagnostic excisional procedure can be considered for women who want to maintain fertility. An endocervical curettage should be performed at the time of the resection.

## SUGGESTED READINGS

American College of Obstetricians and Gynecologists. ACOG practice bulletin no. 99: management of abnormal cervical cytology and histology. *Obstet Gynecol* 2008;112(6):1419–1444.
American College of Obstetricians and Gynecologists. ACOG practice bulletin no. 140: management of abnormal cervical cancer screening test results and cervical cancer precursors. *Obstet Gynecol* 2013;122(6):1338–1367.

American College of Obstetricians and Gynecologists Committee on Practice Bulletins—Gynecology. ACOG practice bulletin no. 131: screening for cervical cancer. *Obstet Gynecol* 2012;120(5):1222–1238.

Saslow D, Solomon D, Lawson HW, et al. American Cancer Society, American Society for Colposcopy and Cervical Pathology, and American Society for Clinical Pathology screening guidelines for the prevention and early detection of cervical cancer. *Am J Clin Pathol* 2012;137(4):516–542.

Siegel R, Naishadham D, Jemal A. Cancer statistics, 2012. *CA Cancer J Clin* 2012;62:10–29.

World Health Organization. *Cervical Cancer, Human Papillomavirus (HPV), and HPV vaccines: Key Points for Policy-Makers and Health Professionals.* Geneva, Switzerland: World Health Organization, 2008.

World Health Organization. *Prevention of Cervical Cancer through Screening Using VIA and Treatment with Cryotherapy.* Geneva, Switzerland: World Health Organization, 2012. http://apps.who.int/iris/bitstream/10665/75250/1/9789241503860_eng.pdf. Accessed February 2, 2013.

# Cervical Cancer

Amy H. Gueye and Teresa P. Díaz-Montes

**Cervical cancer** is the most common gynecologic malignancy in the world and the second most frequently diagnosed cancer in women worldwide after breast cancer. Eighty percent of cases occur in developing countries. In the United States, cervical cancer is the third most common gynecologic malignancy and the second most common cause of gynecologic cancer death. Mortality and incidence rates for cervical cancer have declined in most developed countries due to the introduction of national standardized screening protocols using routine Papanicolaou smear (Pap test) and, more recently, human papillomavirus (HPV) screening.

## EPIDEMIOLOGY OF CERVICAL CANCER

Approximately 60% of women diagnosed with cervical cancer in developed countries have either never been screened or have not been screened in the preceding 5 years. The mean age for cervical cancer is 52.2 years, and the distribution of cases is bimodal, with peaks at 35 to 39 years and 60 to 64 years.

## RISK FACTORS FOR CERVICAL CANCER

- The main **risk factors** for cervical cancer include exposure to HPV, smoking, parity, and immunosuppression; other factors that have been linked with cervical cancer are race/socioeconomic status and sexually transmitted infections.
  - **HPV infection** is present in 99.7% of all cervical cancers. HPV is a nonenveloped, double-stranded DNA virus. The DNA is enclosed in a capsid shell with

major L1 and minor L2 structural proteins. The virus is spread through sexual contact. Thus, traditional risk factors for cervical cancer include early age at first coitus, multiple sexual partners, multiparity, lack of barrier contraception, and history of sexually transmitted infections.

o High-risk HPV types 16, 18, 31, 33, 35, 45, 52, and 58 are associated with 95% of squamous cell carcinomas of the cervix. HPV 16 is most commonly linked with squamous cell cervical cancer. HPV 18 is most commonly present in adenocarcinoma.

o Most HPV infections are transient, resulting in either no change in the cervical epithelium or low-grade intraepithelial lesions that are often spontaneously cleared. The progression from high-grade lesion to invasive cancer takes approximately 8 to 12 years, yielding a long preinvasive state with multiple opportunities for detection through screening.

• **Cigarette smoking** is an independent risk factor in the development of cervical disease. Smokers have a 4.5-fold increased risk of carcinoma in situ (CIS) compared with matched controls. Additionally, an increased risk of cervical cancer has been noted in women exposed passively to tobacco smoke. The potential effect of smoking appears to be limited to squamous cell carcinoma of the cervix.

• **Immunosuppression** may increase the risk of developing cervical cancer, with more rapid progression from preinvasive to invasive lesions. Patients with HIV infection present earlier and with more advanced disease than noninfected patients. The Centers for Disease Control and Prevention has described cervical cancer as an AIDS-defining illness.

• **Race and socioeconomic status**
  o The incidence per 100,000 women per year of cervical cancer in the United States varies by ethnicity/race.
    o African Americans, 11; Caucasians, 8; Native Americans, 12; Hispanics, 6; and Asians, 7
  o These differences are partially accounted for by the increased risk of cervical cancer among women of low socioeconomic status. When access to care is made equal, the excessive risk of cervical cancer precursor lesions among African American women decreases.
  o Racial differences are also apparent in survival; 58% of all African Americans with cervical cancer survive 5 years, compared with 72% of all whites.

## SCREENING, PRESENTATION, AND DIAGNOSIS

Cervical neoplasia is presumed to be a continuum from dysplasia to CIS to invasive carcinoma. **Screening** for cervical cancer with the use of an exfoliative cytologic study (i.e., Pap smear) has significant effects on the incidence, morbidity, and mortality of invasive disease by facilitating the discovery and early treatment of precursor lesions. See Chapter 45.

### Clinical Presentation

• **Early symptoms:**
  • Abnormal vaginal bleeding may take the form of postcoital, intermenstrual, or postmenopausal bleeding.
  • Serosanguineous or yellowish vaginal discharge, at times foul-smelling
  • Dyspareunia

- **Late symptoms:**
  - Hematometra due to occlusion of the endocervical canal
  - Symptomatic anemia
  - Pelvic pain
  - Sciatic and back pain can be related to sidewall extension, hydronephrosis, or metastasis.
  - Bladder or rectal invasion by advanced-stage disease may produce urinary or rectal symptoms (e.g., vaginal passage of stool or urine, hematuria, urinary frequency, hematochezia).
  - Lower extremity swelling from occlusion of pelvic lymphatics or thrombosis of the external iliac vein.

## Diagnosis of Cervical Cancer

- Most women with cervical cancer have a visible cervical lesion.
  - On **speculum examination**, cervical cancer may appear as an exophytic cervical mass (Fig. 46-1) that characteristically bleeds on contact. Endophytic tumors develop entirely within the endocervical canal, and the external cervix may appear normal. In these cases, bimanual examination may reveal a firm, indurated, and often barrel-shaped cervix. The vagina should be inspected for extension of disease. Rectal exam provides information regarding the nodularity of the utero-sacral ligaments and helps determine extension of disease into the parametrium.
  - On **general physical examination**, advanced cervical cancer may present with pleural effusions, ascites, and/or lower extremity edema. Unilateral lower extremity edema may indicate involvement of the pelvic sidewall. Groin and supraclavicular lymph nodes may be indurated or enlarged, indicating spread of disease.

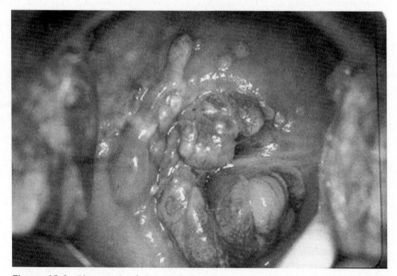

**Figure 46-1.** Photograph of the cervix demonstrating an exophytic cervical carcinoma. (Courtesy of Dr. Robert Giuntoli, The Johns Hopkins Hospital, Department of Gynecology and Obstetrics, Division of Gynecologic Oncology.)

- With obvious exophytic lesions, cervical biopsy is usually all that is needed for histologic confirmation.
- In patients with a grossly normal cervix and abnormal cytology on Pap smear, colposcopic examination with directed biopsies and endocervical curettage (ECC) is necessary. See Chapter 45.
- If a definite diagnosis of cervical cancer cannot be made on the basis of office biopsies, diagnostic cervical conization may be necessary.

## DISEASE PROGRESSION, STAGING, AND PROGNOSIS

### Routes of Cervical Cancer Spread

- Cervical cancer usually spreads by **direct extension**.
  - **Parametrial extension:** The lateral spread of cervical cancer occurs through the cardinal ligament lymphatics and vessels, and significant involvement of the medial portion of this ligament may result in ureteral obstruction.
  - **Vaginal extension:** The upper vagina is frequently involved (50% of cases) when the primary tumor has extended beyond the confines of the cervix.
  - **Bladder and rectal involvement:** Anterior and posterior spread of cervical cancer to the bladder and rectum is uncommon in the absence of lateral parametrial disease.
- Cervical cancer may also progress via **lymphatic spread** (Fig. 46-2). The cervix is drained by preureteral, postureteral, and uterosacral lymphatic channels.
  - The following are considered first station nodes: obturator, external iliac, hypogastric, parametrial, presacral, and common iliac.
  - Para-aortic nodes are second station, are rarely involved in the absence of primary nodal disease, and are considered metastases.
  - The percentage of involved lymph nodes increases directly with primary tumor volume and stage of disease.
- **Hematologic spread metastases** from cervical carcinomas occur but are less frequent and are usually seen late in the course of the disease.

### Staging of Cervical Cancer

- **Staging of cervical cancer** is based on clinical rather than surgical evaluation (Tables 46-1 and 46-2).
  - Routine laboratory studies should include a complete blood count, complete metabolic profile, and urinalysis. No tumor marker has achieved widespread acceptance.
  - Inspection and palpation should begin with the cervix, vagina, and pelvis and continue with examination of extrapelvic areas, including the abdomen and supraclavicular lymph nodes.
  - Lymphangiograms, arteriograms, computed tomography (CT), magnetic resonance imaging (MRI), positron emission tomography, laparoscopy, or laparotomy findings are not used for clinical staging, but their results may be valuable for planning treatment. Imaging studies beyond chest x-ray should be obtained only when the findings will have an impact on treatment.
- Cervical cancer is staged according to the **International Federation of Gynecology and Obstetrics (FIGO) system** (see Table 46-1; Fig. 46-3). Lymph–vascular involvement does not alter the classification.
  - When doubt exists concerning the stage to which a tumor should be assigned, the earlier stage is chosen. Once a clinical stage has been determined and treatment

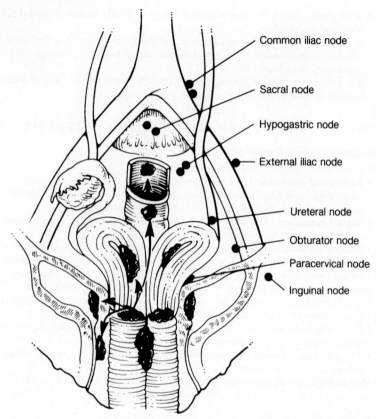

**Figure 46-2.** Possible sites of direct extension of cervical cancer to adjoining organs or metastases to regional lymph nodes. The uterus, cervix, and vagina are depicted bisected and opened to reveal the possible sites of tumor implantation. (From Scott JR, DiSaia PJ, Hammond CB, et al. *Danforth's Obstetrics and Gynecology*, 7th ed. Philadelphia: Lippincott-Raven Publishers, 1997:909, with permission.)

has begun, subsequent findings do not alter the assigned stage. Overstaging and understaging of the parametria are problematic and may affect therapeutic decisions. FIGO stage correlates with prognosis, and strict adherence to the rules of clinical staging is necessary for comparison of results between institutions.

- The distribution of patients by clinical stage is as follows: 38% stage I, 32% stage II, 25% stage III, 4% stage IV. Clinical stage of disease at the time of presentation is the most important determinant of survival regardless of treatment modality.
- Five-year survival declines as FIGO stage at diagnosis increases from stage IA (95%) to stage IV (14%).
- Only the subclassifications of stage I (IA1, IA2) require pathologic assessment.
- Vast discrepancies can exist between clinical staging and surgicopathologic findings, such that clinical staging fails to identify extension of disease to the para-aortic

**TABLE 46-1** International Federation of Gynecology and Obstetrics Staging System for Carcinoma of the Cervix (2009)

| Stage | Description | Comments |
|---|---|---|
| I | **The carcinoma is strictly confined to the cervix (extension to the corpus would be disregarded).** | The diagnosis of both stage IA1 and IA2 cases should be based on microscopic examination of removed tissue, preferably a cone, which must include the entire lesion. The depth of invasion should not be more than 5 mm taken from the base of the epithelium, either surface or glandular, from which it originates. The depth of invasion should always be reported in millimeters, even in those cases with "early (minimal) stromal invasion" ~1 mm. The second dimension, the horizontal spread, must not exceed 7 mm. Vascular space involvement, either venous or lymphatic, should not alter the staging but should be specifically recorded because it may affect treatment decisions. |
| IA | Invasive carcinoma, which can be diagnosed only by microscopy, with deepest invasion ≤5 mm and largest extension ≤7 mm | |
| IA1 | Measured stromal invasion of ≤3 mm in depth and extension of ≤7 mm | |
| IA2 | Measured stromal invasion of >3 mm and not >5 mm in depth with an extension of not >7 mm | |
| IB | Clinically visible lesions limited to the cervix uteri or preclinical cancers greater than stage IA. All gross lesions, even with superficial invasion, are stage IB cancers. | As a rule, estimating clinically whether a cancer of the cervix has extended to the corpus or not in preclinical lesions higher than stage IA is impossible. Extension to the corpus should therefore be disregarded. |
| IB1 | Clinically visible lesion ≤4 cm in greatest dimension | |
| IB2 | Clinically visible lesion >4 cm in greatest dimension | |

*(Continued)*

**TABLE 46-1** International Federation of Gynecology and Obstetrics Staging System for Carcinoma of the Cervix (2009) *(Continued)*

| Stage | Description | Comments |
|---|---|---|
| II | **Cervical carcinoma extends beyond the uterus but not to the pelvic wall or to the lower third of the vagina.** | |
| IIA | Without parametrial invasion | |
| IIA1 | Clinically visible lesion ≤4.0 cm in greatest dimension | |
| IIA2 | Clinically visible lesion >4.0 cm in greatest dimension | |
| IIB | With obvious parametrial invasion | |
| III | **The tumor extends to the pelvic wall and/or involves the lower one third of the vagina and/or causes hydronephrosis or nonfunctioning kidney.** | On rectal examination, no cancer-free space is found between the tumor and the pelvic wall. Hydronephrosis or nonfunctioning kidney due to stenosis of the ureter by cancer and no other known cause permits a case to be allotted to stage III even if, according to the other findings, the case should be assigned to stage I or stage II. |
| IIIA | Tumor involves lower third of vagina, with no extension to the pelvic wall. | |
| IIIB | Extension to the pelvic wall and/or hydronephrosis or nonfunctioning kidney | |
| IV | **The carcinoma has extended beyond the true pelvis or has involved (biopsy proven) the mucosa of the bladder or rectum.** | The presence of bullous edema, as such, should not permit a case to be assigned to stage IV. Ridges and furrows in the bladder wall should be interpreted as signs of submucous involvement of the bladder if they remain fixed to the growth during palpation (i.e., examination from the vagina or the rectum during cystoscopy). A finding of malignant cells in cytologic washings from the urinary bladder requires further examination and biopsy of the wall of the bladder. |
| IVA | Spread of the growth to adjacent organs | |
| IVB | Spread to distant organs | |

Adapted from Pecorelli S. Revised FIGO staging for carcinoma of the vulva, cervix, and endometrium. *Int J Gynaecol Obstet* 2009;105:103–104.

| TABLE 46-2 | Staging Procedures for Cervical Cancer |
|---|---|
| Physical examination[a] | Palpation of lymph nodes |
| | Examination of vagina |
| | Bimanual rectovaginal examination (under anesthesia recommended) |
| Radiologic studies[a] | Intravenous pyelogram (IVP) |
| | Barium enema |
| | Chest radiograph |
| | Skeletal radiograph |
| Procedures[a] | Biopsy |
| | Conization |
| | Hysteroscopy |
| | Colposcopy |
| | Endocervical curettage |
| | Cystoscopy |
| | Proctoscopy |
| Optional studies[b] | CT scan |
| | Lymphangiography |
| | Ultrasonography |
| | Magnetic resonance imaging (MRI) |
| | Radionuclide scanning |
| | Laparoscopy |

[a]Allowed for cervical cancer staging by International Federation of Gynecology and Obstetrics (FIGO).
[b]Information that is not allowed by FIGO to change the clinical stage but may be useful for treatment and planning.
Adapted from Berek JS, Hacker NF, eds. *Practical Gynecologic Oncology*, 4th ed. Baltimore, MD: Lippincott Williams & Wilkins, 2004.

nodes in 7% of patients with stage IB disease, 18% with stage IIB, and 28% with stage III. Thus, some clinicians emphasize surgical staging in women with locally advanced cervical carcinoma to identify occult tumor spread and allow treatment of metastatic disease beyond the traditional pelvic radiation field.

## Prognostic Factors for Cervical Cancer

- **Prognosis** is directly related to tumor characteristics including histologic subtype, histologic grade, FIGO stage, lymph node status, tumor volume, depth of invasion, and lymph–vascular space involvement (Table 46-3). Other prognostic variables include age, race, socioeconomic status, and immune status.

### Histologic Subtype

- Conflicting data exist on the influence of histologic subtype on tumor behavior, prognosis, and survival.
  - **Invasive squamous cell carcinoma** is the most common histologic type of cervical cancer, comprising about 80% of cases. Squamous cell carcinomas are also subclassified according to cell type: **large cell keratinizing**, **large cell nonkeratinizing**, and **small cell** types. Rarer types include **verrucous carcinoma** and **papillary squamous cell carcinoma**.

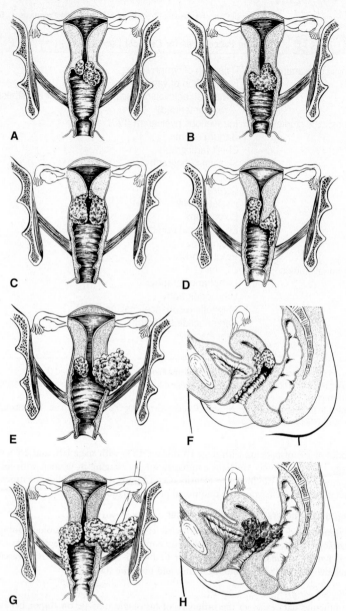

**Figure 46-3.** FIGO classification of carcinoma of the cervix. In stage I (**A,B**), only the cervix is involved. In stage II (**C,D,E**), the parametrium or upper two thirds of the vagina is involved. In stage III (**F,G**), the tumor involves the lower one third of the vagina or extends to the pelvic sidewall. In stage IV (**H**), areas beyond the true pelvis are involved or the bladder or rectal mucosa. (Adapted from Chi DS, Abu-Rustum NR, Hoskins WJ. Cancer of the cervix. In Rock JA, Jones HW III, eds. *TeLinde's Operative Gynecology*, 9th ed. Philadelphia, PA: Lippincott Williams & Wilkins, 2003:1378–1379, with permission.)

| TABLE 46-3 | Cervical Cancer Survival by International Federation of Gynecology and Obstetrics Stage[a] |
|---|---|

| Stage | 5-Year Survival (%) |
|---|---|
| IA | 97.0 |
| IB | 78.9 |
| IIA | 54.9 |
| IIB | 51.6 |
| IIIA | 40.5 |
| IIIB | 27.0 |
| IV | 12.4 |

[a]Based on 1994 FIGO staging of carcinoma of the cervix uteri.
From Kosary CL. FIGO stage, histology, histologic grade, age and race as prognostic factors in determining survival for cancers of the female gynecological system: an analysis of 1973–87 SEER cases of cancers of the endometrium, cervix, ovary, vulva, and vagina. *Semin Surg Oncol* 1994;10:31–46.

- **Adenocarcinomas** comprise 15% of invasive cervical carcinomas. Grossly, cervical adenocarcinoma may appear as a polypoid or papillary exophytic mass. However, in nearly 15% of adenocarcinomas, the lesion is located entirely within the endocervical canal and escapes visual inspection.
  - **Mucinous adenocarcinoma** is the most common type and is well differentiated with plentiful mucin production.
  - **Endometrioid carcinoma**, 30% of cervical adenocarcinomas, resembles those typical of the uterine corpus.
  - **Clear cell carcinomas**, approximately 4% of adenocarcinomas, are nodular, reddish lesions with punctate ulcers and cells with abundant, clear cytoplasm. Diethylstilbestrol exposure is a risk factor.
  - **Minimal deviation adenocarcinoma**, or adenoma malignum, is reported to represent 1% of cervical adenocarcinomas.
- Primary cervical carcinoma with both malignant-appearing glandular and squamous elements is referred to as **adenosquamous carcinoma**. The clinical behavior of these tumors is controversial, with some studies suggesting lower survival rates and others higher survival rates than with the more common squamous tumors.
- **Small cell carcinomas** of the uterine cervix are similar to small cell neuroendocrine tumors of the lung and other anatomic locations. These tumors are clinically aggressive, with a marked propensity to metastasize. At diagnosis, disease is often disseminated, with bone, brain, and liver being the most common sites. Because of high metastatic potential, local therapy alone (surgery, radiation, or both) rarely results in long-term survival. Multiagent chemotherapy, in combination with external beam and intracavitary radiation therapy, is the standard therapeutic approach.

*Histologic Grade*
- Histologic differentiation of cervical carcinomas includes three grades.
  - Grade 1 tumors are **well differentiated** with mature squamous cells, often forming keratinized pearls of epithelial cells. Mitotic activity is low.

- Grade 2 tumors are **moderately well-differentiated** carcinomas having higher mitotic activity and less cellular maturation accompanied by more nuclear pleomorphism.
- Grade 3 tumors are composed of **poorly differentiated** smaller cells with less cytoplasm and often bizarre nuclei. Mitotic activity is high. Poorly differentiated tumors have lower 5-year survival rates.

*Other Prognostic Factors*

- The most important factor in the prognosis for cervical cancer is **clinical stage**.
- **Node status:** Among surgically treated patients, survival is related to the number and location of involved lymph nodes.
  - When pelvic nodes alone are involved, the 5-year survival rate is about 65%. Five-year survival drops to 25% when common iliac lymph nodes are positive, and involvement of para-aortic nodes further lowers survival. Bilateral pelvic lymph node involvement has a worse prognosis than unilateral disease.
- **Tumor volume:** Lesion size is an important predictor of survival, independent of other factors. Five-year survival rates for lesions <2 cm, 2 to 4 cm, and >4 cm are approximately 90%, 60%, and 40%, respectively.
- **Depth of invasion:** Survival rates are inversely correlated with depth of stromal invasion.
- **Lymph–vascular space invasion:** No clear relationship exists between lymph–vascular space involvement and survival.

## MANAGEMENT OF CERVICAL CANCER

Surgery and radiation therapy are the two modalities most commonly used to treat invasive cervical carcinoma.

### Surgical Management

- In general, **primary surgical management** is limited to stages I through IIA.
- Advantages of surgical therapy:
  - Allows for thorough pelvic and abdominal exploration, which can identify patients with a disparity between the clinical and surgicopathologic stages. These patients can be offered an individualized treatment plan based on their disease status.
  - Permits conservation of the ovaries with their transposition out of radiation treatment fields
  - Avoids the use of radiation therapy and its complications
- Disadvantages to surgical therapy:
  - Risks of surgery, including bleeding; infection; and damage to organs, vessels, and nerves
  - Radical hysterectomy results in vaginal shortening; however, with sexual activity, gradual lengthening may occur.
  - Fistula formation (urinary or bowel) and incisional complications related to surgical treatment. These tend to occur early in the postoperative period and are usually amenable to surgical repair.
- Other indications for the selection of radical surgery over radiation:
  - Concomitant inflammatory bowel disease
  - Previous radiation for other disease
  - Presence of a simultaneous adnexal neoplasm

- The abdomen is opened through either a low transverse incision using the Maylard or Cherney method or through a vertical midline incision. Once inside the peritoneal cavity, a thorough abdominal exploration should be performed to evaluate for visual or palpable metastases. Particular attention should be paid to the vesicouterine peritoneum for signs of tumor extension or implantation and palpation of the cardinal ligaments and the cervix. The para-aortic nodes should be palpated transperitoneally.
- Five distinct **classes of hysterectomy** are used in the treatment of cervical cancer (Table 46-4 and Fig. 46-4 for a brief comparison).
  - **Class I** hysterectomy refers to the standard **extrafascial total abdominal hysterectomy**. This procedure ensures complete removal of the cervix with minimal disruption to surrounding structures (e.g., bladder, ureters). This procedure may be performed in patients with stage IA1 cervical cancer.
  - **Class II** hysterectomy is also referred to as a **modified radical hysterectomy** or **Wertheim hysterectomy** and is well suited for patients with stage IA2 and small lesions that do not distort the anatomy.
  - **Class III** hysterectomy, also known as **radical abdominal** or **Meigs hysterectomy**, is recommended for stages IB and IIA.
  - **Class IV** or **extended radical hysterectomy** includes removal of the superior vesical artery, periureteral tissue, and up to three fourths of the vagina.
  - In a **class V** or **partial exenteration** operation, the distal ureters and a portion of the bladder are resected. Class IV and class V procedures are rarely performed today because patients with disease extensive enough to require these operations can be more adequately treated using primary radiation therapy.
- In the past 15 years, surgeons have begun to investigate **minimally invasive methods** of treating early cervical cancers. These include laparoscopic procedures and, more recently, robotic-assisted laparoscopic procedures. Several small studies have compared laparoscopic and robotic radical hysterectomy with the open laparotomy approach. Findings include no significant differences in postoperative complications among the three groups, with longer mean operating times, shorter length of hospital stay, and smaller estimated blood loss for laparoscopic procedures compared with laparotomy.

### Fertility-Preserving Surgical Options

- Fertility-preserving surgeries are used for younger women who have not completed childbearing and require treatment for early-stage cervical cancer. These methods include **cervical conization** and **radical trachelectomy** (i.e., Dargent operation) and appear to have similar recurrence rates to radical hysterectomy if candidates are selected appropriately.
  - Cervical conization is generally reserved for stage IA cervical cancers but has also been performed with lymphadenectomy for IB1 cancers. Of the few published studies, no recurrences were noted with a minimum of 14 months follow-up.
  - Radical trachelectomy can be performed for up to stage IB1 cancer with negative nodes in patients with tumors <2 cm in diameter. The obstetric consequences for radical trachelectomy appear to be similar to those for loop electrosurgical excision procedure and conization, which include risk of preterm delivery and low birth weight.

## Primary Radiation Therapy

- **Radiation therapy** can be used for all stages of disease and for most patients, regardless of age, body habitus, or coexistent medical conditions. Radiation therapy

**TABLE 46-4**  Types of Abdominal Hysterectomy

<table>
<tr><th></th><th colspan="4">Type of Surgery</th></tr>
<tr><th></th><th>Intrafascial</th><th>Extrafascial Class I</th><th>Modified Radical Class II</th><th>Radical Class III</th></tr>
<tr><td>Cervical fascia</td><td>Partially removed</td><td>Completely removed</td><td>Completely removed</td><td>Completely removed</td></tr>
<tr><td>Vaginal cuff</td><td>None removed</td><td>Small rim removed</td><td>Proximal 1–2 cm removed</td><td>Upper one third to one half removed</td></tr>
<tr><td>Bladder</td><td>Partially mobilized</td><td>Partially mobilized</td><td>Mobilized</td><td>Mobilized</td></tr>
<tr><td>Rectum</td><td>Not mobilized</td><td>Rectovaginal septum partially mobilized</td><td>Mobilized</td><td>Mobilized</td></tr>
<tr><td>Ureters</td><td>Not mobilized</td><td>Not mobilized</td><td>Unroofed in ureteral tunnel</td><td>Completely dissected to bladder entry</td></tr>
<tr><td>Cardinal ligaments</td><td>Resected medial to ureters</td><td>Resected medial to ureters</td><td>Resected at level of ureter</td><td>Resected at pelvic side wall</td></tr>
<tr><td>Uterosacral ligaments</td><td>Resected at level of cervix</td><td>Resected at level of cervix</td><td>Partially resected</td><td>Resected at post pelvic insertion</td></tr>
<tr><td>Uterus</td><td>Removed</td><td>Removed</td><td>Removed</td><td>Removed</td></tr>
<tr><td>Cervix</td><td>Partially removed</td><td>Completely removed</td><td>Completely removed</td><td>Completely removed</td></tr>
</table>

From Perez CA. Uterine cervix. In Perez CA, Brady LW, eds. *Principles and Practice of Radiation Oncology*, 2nd ed. Philadelphia, PA: JB Lippincott, 1992, with permission.

should *not* be used in patients with diverticulosis, tubo-ovarian abscess, or pelvic kidney. Radiation therapy has evolved to include concurrent chemotherapy as a radiosensitizer, which results in improved disease-free and overall survival compared with radiation therapy alone.

- Preservation of sexual function is significantly related to the mode of primary therapy. Pelvic radiation produces persistent vaginal fibrosis and atrophy, with loss of both vaginal length and caliber. In addition, ovarian function is lost in virtually all patients who undergo tolerance-dose radiation therapy to the pelvis. Fistulous complications associated with radiation therapy tend to occur late and are more difficult to repair because of radiation fibrosis, vasculitis, and poorly vascularized tissues.
- The two main methods for delivering radiation therapy are external photon beam radiation and brachytherapy.

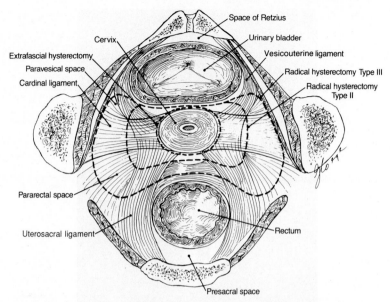

**Figure 46-4.** Diagram of pelvic anatomy and types of hysterectomy. (From Berek JS, Hacker NF. *Practical Gynecologic Oncology*, 4th ed. Philadelphia, PA: Lippincott Williams & Wilkins, 2005:356, with permission.)

- **External photon beam radiation** is usually delivered from a linear accelerator. Microscopic or occult tumor deposits from epithelial cancers require 4,000 to 5,000 cGy for local control. A clinically obvious tumor requires in excess of 6,000 cGy.
- Once external therapy has been completed, **brachytherapy** can be delivered using various intracavitary techniques, including intrauterine tandem and vaginal colpostats, vaginal cylinders, or interstitial needle implants. The tandem is placed through the cervix into the uterus, and the ovoids are placed in the lateral vaginal fornices (Fig. 46-5). Brachytherapy can be delivered as low-dose rates (LDR) or high-dose treatments. LDR treatments are inpatient over 3 to 4 days and receive 40 to 70 cGy/hr. High-dose rate treatments may be delivered on an outpatient basis over five visits.
  - Two **reference points** are commonly used to describe the dose prescription for cervical cancer:
    - **Point A** is 2 cm lateral and 2 cm superior to the external cervical os and theoretically represents the area where the uterine artery crosses the ureter.
    - **Point B** is 3 cm lateral to point A and corresponds to the pelvic sidewall and to the location of the obturator lymph nodes.
  - The cumulative dose to point A, regardless of method, adequate for central control is usually between 7,500 and 8,500 cGy. The prescribed dose to point B is 4,500 to 6,500 cGy, depending on the bulk of parametrial and sidewall disease.

## Chemotherapy

- **Single-agent chemotherapy** is used to treat patients with extrapelvic metastases as well as those with recurrent tumor who have been previously treated with surgery or radiation and are not candidates for exenteration procedures.

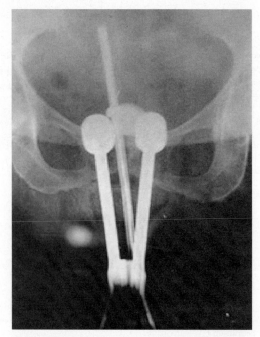

**Figure 46-5.** Brachytherapy: pelvic radiograph showing tandems and ovoids. (Image courtesy of Dr. Robert Giuntoli, The Johns Hopkins Hospital, Department of Gynecology and Obstetrics, Division of Gynecologic Oncology.)

- The best candidates for chemotherapy are those with an excellent performance status and disease that is both outside of the field of radiation and not amenable to surgical resection.
  - Cisplatin has been the most extensively studied agent and has demonstrated the most consistent clinical response rates (20% to 25%).
- The most active **combination chemotherapy** regimens for cervical cancer contain cisplatin.
- The agents most commonly used in combination with cisplatin are bleomycin, 5-fluorouracil, mitomycin C, methotrexate, cyclophosphamide, and doxorubicin.
- A limited number of randomized trials comparing dual-agent regimens with either triple-agent regimens or single-agent regimens have demonstrated that combination therapy leads to a slightly higher response rate and a longer progression-free survival; however, no difference was found among the regimens in terms of overall survival.

## Combined Modalities

- **Postoperative adjuvant radiation** therapy has been advocated for patients with microscopic parametrial invasion, pelvic lymph node metastases, deep cervical invasion, and positive or close surgical margins. Postoperative radiation therapy reduces the rate of pelvic recurrence after radical hysterectomy in high-risk patients.

- **Neoadjuvant chemotherapy:** Trials testing the efficacy of preoperative chemotherapy suggest improved outcomes, but results have not been consistent.
- **Chemoradiation** confers significant survival benefit over radiation alone in the treatment of cervical cancer. When combined with radiation, weekly cisplatin administration reduces the risk of progression for stage IIB through stage IVA cervical cancer.
  - Cisplatin acts as a radiosensitizer, yielding a large reduction in the rate of local recurrence and a more modest reduction in the rate of distant metastases.

## Management by Stage of Disease

- **Stage IA1** without lymph–vascular invasion is managed with conservative surgery, such as excisional conization or extrafascial hysterectomy. Conization may be used selectively if preservation of fertility is desired, provided that the surgical margins are free of disease. Patients treated with conization should be followed closely with Pap smear, colposcopy, and ECC every 3 months for the first year. For medically inoperable patients, stage IA carcinoma can be effectively treated with chemoradiation.
- **Stage IA2** is associated with positive pelvic lymph nodes in 5% of cases. The preferred treatment of these lesions is modified radical (class II) hysterectomy with pelvic lymphadenectomy. In patients who desire preservation of fertility, radical trachelectomy with laparoscopic or extraperitoneal lymphadenectomy may be performed.
  - In a **radical trachelectomy,** cervical and vaginal branches of the uterine artery are ligated, whereas the main trunk of the uterine artery is preserved. Once the blood supply has been controlled, the cervix is amputated at a point approximately 5 mm caudal to the uterine isthmus. The uterus is then suspended from the lateral stumps of the transected paracervical ligaments. Once the uterus has been suspended, isthmic cerclage is performed, using a technique similar to that used as prophylaxis against miscarriage. Subsequently, the vaginal and isthmic mucosa are reapproximated.
- **Stages IB1, IB2, and IIA:** Radical hysterectomy (class III hysterectomy) and radiation are equally effective in treating stages IB and IIA carcinoma of the cervix (studies based on 1994 FIGO staging).
  - Management of patients with bulky stage I disease (IB2) is controversial. The two options are a class III hysterectomy or radiation. Often, surgery is first performed with postoperative radiation. Alternatively, a gynecologic oncology group study showed that weekly cisplatin 40 mg/m$^2$ (six doses) with external radiation and a single implant to give 55 Gy at point B, followed by extrafascial hysterectomy, gave the best outcome.
- **Stages IIB, III, IVA, and IVB:** Radiation therapy is the treatment of choice for patients with stage IIB and more advanced disease. Long-term survival rates with radiation therapy alone are approximately 70% for stage I disease, 60% for stage II disease, 45% for stage III disease, and 18% for stage IV disease. With the routine use of chemoradiation, long-term survival and disease-free progression are expected to increase for all stages of disease. Patients with stage IVB disease are usually treated with chemotherapy alone or chemotherapy in combination with local radiation. These patients have a uniformly poor prognosis regardless of treatment modality.

## Treatment-Related Complications

- Modern surgical techniques and anesthesia have reduced the operative mortality rate.

- Febrile morbidity is common after radical hysterectomy due to typical postoperative reasons.
- Major causes of morbidity include lower extremity venous thrombosis, vesicovaginal fistulas (<1%), ureteral fistulas, permanent ureteral stenosis, voiding dysfunction, and pelvic lymphocyst formation.
- Acute complications of radiation therapy that occur during or immediately after therapy include uterine perforation, proctosigmoiditis, and acute hemorrhagic cystitis.
- Chronic complications that occur months to years after completing therapy include vaginal stenosis, rectovaginal and vesicovaginal fistulas, small bowel obstruction, and radiation-induced second cancers.

### Posttreatment Surveillance

- Abdominal exam, leg and groin exam, speculum exam, bimanual rectovaginal examination, and evaluation of lymph nodes should be performed every 3 months for 3 years following treatment for cervical cancer.
  - After the first 3 years, examinations should be done every 6 months for an additional 2 years and every 6 months to 1 year thereafter.
  - More frequent examinations are warranted if abnormal signs or symptoms develop.
  - Pap smears should be obtained at every visit, with consideration for annual chest x-ray and intravenous pyelogram or abdominal pelvic CT.
- Cervical cancer detected within *the first 6 months after therapy* is termed **persistent cancer**. Disease *diagnosed >6 months later* is referred to as **recurrent disease**.
  - Treatment of recurrent cervical cancer is dictated by the site of recurrence and by the mode of initial therapy.
    o Only patients with central recurrence and no evidence of disease outside the pelvis are candidates for pelvic exenteration.

### Special Management Issues
*Cervical Cancer in Pregnancy*

- Cervical cancer is the most common malignancy in pregnancy, ranging from 1 in 1,200 to 1 in 2,200 pregnancies. Cervical cancer coincident with pregnancy requires complex diagnostic and therapeutic decisions that may jeopardize both mother and fetus.
- The symptoms of cervical cancer are the same in pregnant patients and nonpregnant patients. Pregnant women are at risk of delay of diagnosis of cervical cancer.
  - Directed cervical punch biopsies can be performed safely during pregnancy when high-grade intraepithelial lesions or microinvasion is suspected.
  - ECC should be avoided due to the risk of rupturing the amniotic membranes.
  - Cervical conization should be performed only if it is strictly indicated and between **12 and 20 weeks of gestation**.
- Pregnant women with cervical cancer should undergo the same evaluation as nonpregnant women.
  - Because the bimanual examination may be difficult in pregnancy, MRI may be useful to identify extracervical disease.
- In patients with intraepithelial lesions or microinvasive disease stages IA1 and IA2, there appears to be no harm in delaying definitive therapy until after fetal lung maturity has been attained.

- Patients with less than 3 mm of invasion and no lymph–vascular space involvement may be followed to term and delivered vaginally.
- The major risk during delivery is hemorrhage due to tearing of the tumor.
- Recurrences of cervical cancer have been reported at the episiotomy site in women who deliver vaginally.
- Following vaginal delivery, these women should be reevaluated and treated at 6 weeks postpartum.
- If delivery is by cesarean section, extrafascial hysterectomy can be performed at the time of delivery or after a delay of 4 to 6 weeks if further childbearing is not desired.
- Patients with 3 to 5 mm of invasion or lymph–vascular invasion can also be safely followed until term.
  - In these cases, however, surgical treatment should include a modified radical hysterectomy with pelvic lymph node dissection, performed either at the time of cesarean delivery or at 4 to 6 weeks postpartum.
  - Radiation therapy is associated with survival rates comparable to those after surgical treatment.
- In patients with stages IB1, IB2, and IIA (studies based on 1994 FIGO staging), a delay in therapy *in excess of 6 weeks* may impact survival. If the diagnosis is made after 20 weeks of gestation, consideration may be given to postponing therapy until fetal viability.
  - Standard treatment consists of classical cesarean delivery followed by radical hysterectomy with pelvic and para-aortic lymph node dissection; however, this procedure is associated with longer operative time and greater blood loss than in nonpregnant patients.
  - Lower segment transverse cesarean section is not recommended because of the increased risk of cervical extension with this procedure that may increase intraoperative bleeding.
  - Radiation therapy results in equivalent survival rates and may be preferable for patients who are poor surgical candidates.

### Cervical Hemorrhage

- Profuse vaginal bleeding from cervical malignancies is a challenging therapeutic situation. Generally, conservative measures to control cervical hemorrhage are preferable to emergency laparotomy and vascular (i.e., hypogastric artery) ligation. Attention must first be directed toward the stabilization of the patient with appropriate intravenous fluid and blood product replacement.
  - Immediate control of cervical hemorrhage can usually be accomplished with a vaginal pack soaked in **Monsel solution** (ferric subsulfate). Topical acetone (dimethyl ketone) applied with a vaginal pack placed firmly against the bleeding tumor bed has also been used successfully to control vaginal hemorrhage from cervical malignancy.
  - Definitive control of cervical hemorrhage can be accomplished with external radiation therapy of 180 to 200 cGy/day if the patient has not previously received tolerance doses of pelvic irradiation.
  - Alternatively, arteriography can be used to identify the bleeding vessel(s), and Gelfoam or steel coil embolization can then be performed.
    - Vascular embolization has the disadvantage of producing a hypoxic local tumor environment and potentially compromising the efficacy of subsequent radiation therapy.

## CERVICAL CANCER AND GLOBAL HEALTH

- Cervical cancer is the leading cause of cancer death in women of developing countries where over 85% of worldwide deaths from cervical cancer are clustered in low-income countries.
  - The World Health Organization estimates that over half a million women will be newly diagnosed with cervical cancer every year, and the majority of these women are between the ages of 15 and 45 years, living in developing nations. Regions at highest risk include East and West Africa, South Africa, Central Asia, and Middle Africa. It is estimated that by 2030, the majority (98%) of cervical cancer deaths will occur in developing countries.
- The disparity can be explained by the lack of widespread screening for cervical cancer. The Papanicolaou screening tool is neither feasible nor practical in most low-resource settings, as cytology requires infrastructure, expertise, and resources.
  - Much research has been conducted on the "see and treat" method that makes use of the visual inspection with acetic acid (VIA) test as an alternative to the Pap smear in low-resource settings. This tool uses application of acetic acid directly to the cervix followed by visualization and immediate treatment of acetowhite lesions with cryotherapy or cervical conization. Women thus do not need to make several trips for screening and treatment.
    - A large screening study performed in Bangladesh showed that among the 100,000 women screened with VIA, only half of the 5% who were screened positive returned for a colposcopy, and of those, only half returned for treatment.
    - Across several large studies, VIA has shown varying sensitivities and specificities; one meta-analysis showed a sensitivity of 82% and a specificity of 60%.
- More recently, HPV screening has emerged as a good alternative or addition to VIA in low-resource settings. Minimal training is required for sample collection or may even be performed by the patient.
  - A cost analysis in South Africa found that HPV DNA testing followed by treatment could decrease cervical cancer incidence by 27% for only $39 of years of life saved (YLS) compared to 26% for VIA followed by treatment. Cytology would decrease incidence by 19% in low-resource settings and would be more costly per YLS.
- Finally, an important debate in the global fight against cervical cancer will be the introduction of vaccines in low-income settings.
  - Studies have shown that for the vaccine to be cost-effective, the three shots must cost between US $10 and $25. Although it will take several decades to see an impact on mortality, this will be an important milestone in overcoming the global cervical cancer burden.

## SUGGESTED READINGS

Amant F, Van Calsteren K, Halaska MJ, et al. Gynecologic cancers in pregnancy: guidelines of an international consensus meeting. *Int J Gynecol Cancer* 2009;19(suppl 1):S1–S12.

Green JA, Kirwan JM, Tierney JF, et al. Survival and recurrence after concomitant chemotherapy and radiotherapy for cancer of the uterine cervix: a systematic review and meta-analysis. *Lancet* 2001;358:781–786.

Hacker NF, Friedlander ML. Cervical cancer. In Berek JS, Hacker NF, eds. *Practical Gynecologic Oncology*, 4th ed. Baltimore, MD: Lippincott Williams & Wilkins, 2005.

Schiffman M, Castle PE, Jeronimo J, et al. Human papillomavirus and cervical cancer. *Lancet* 2007;370:890–907.

# 47 Cancer of the Uterine Corpus

Amelia M. Jernigan and Amanda Nickles Fader

**Endometrial cancer** is the fourth most common cancer in women and the most common gynecologic malignancy, accounting for 6% of all female cancers.

## EPIDEMIOLOGY OF UTERINE CANCER

In the United States and other developed countries, 1 in 38 women will develop uterine cancer, making it the most common gynecologic malignancy in these settings. The American Cancer Society estimates that there will be 49,560 new cases and 8,190 deaths from uterine cancer in 2013. The incidence has increased 0.8% each year since 1998. Most commonly, these are endometrial cancers; only 2% of uterine cancers are sarcomas. Seventy-two percent of cases will be localized at the time of diagnosis because endometrial cancer often presents with postmenopausal or irregular bleeding.

### Risk Factors for Uterine Cancer

- A woman's risk of endometrial cancer increases with **age**. The median age at diagnosis is 61 years, and the peak incidence occurs from ages 55 to 70 years. Women older than 50 years old account for 90% of the diagnoses of endometrial cancer and 5% develop disease before age 40 years.
- Other risk factors are based on **increased estrogen exposure**.
  - **Estrogen replacement** without concomitant progesterone carries a relative risk of 4.5 to 8.0 and persists for 10 years after treatment is stopped (Table 47-1).
  - **Chronic anovulation** states, such as seen in polycystic ovarian syndrome (PCOS), lead to constant estrogen stimulation of the endometrium and increase the risk of cancer due to the lack of a corpus luteum to produce progesterone.
  - **Obesity** increases endogenous estrogen by peripheral conversion of androstenedione to estrogen by aromatase in adipose tissues. Nearly 70% of early-stage endometrial cancer patients are obese. The relative risk of death increases with increasing body mass index (BMI), and a BMI $>30$ kg/m$^2$ will triple the risk of endometrial cancer.
  - **Nulliparity** (related to infertility) and **diabetes mellitus** are independent risk factors and have a relative risk of two or three for endometrial cancer, whereas the association of **hypertension** seems related to obesity.
- A woman taking **tamoxifen** has an annual risk of 2 in 1,000 of developing endometrial cancer and 40% of women will develop cancer more than 12 months after stopping therapy.
- Women with **hereditary nonpolyposis colon cancer (HNPCC)** syndrome have a 39% risk of developing endometrial cancer by age 70 years.
- Some factors can decrease the risk of endometrial cancer.
  - Factors that decrease circulating estrogen, such as cigarette smoking and oral contraceptive pill (OCP) use, may be protective.

| TABLE 47-1 | Risk Factors for Endometrial Cancer |
|---|---|

| Risk Factor | Relative Risk |
|---|---|
| Nulliparity | 2.0 |
| Estrogen replacement without progesterone | 4–8 |
| Obesity | |
| 30–49 pounds | 3.0 |
| >50 pounds | 10.0 |
| Type 2 diabetes mellitus | 2.8 |
| Tamoxifen | 2.2 |

From Barakat RR, Markman M, Randall ME, et al. Corpus: epithelial tumors. In Hoskins WJ, Perez CA, Young RC, eds. *Principles and Practice of Gynecologic Oncology*, 2nd ed. Philadelphia, PA: Lippincott-Raven Publishers, 1997:884.

- OCPs decrease endometrial cancer risk by 40%, even up to 15 years after discontinuation, and this protection increases with length of use. Four years of use reduces risk by 56%, 8 years decreases risk by 67%, and 12 years of use decreases risk by 72%.
- **Hyperplasia** appears to be the precursor lesion for most endometrial cancer. A study that followed women for 10 years after a diagnosis of hyperplasia showed that the risk of progression to cancer increased from simple hyperplasia to complex, and the presence of atypia further increased the risk.
- A recent study revealed that 43% of hysterectomies performed in community hospitals for complex atypical hyperplasia will have endometrial cancer on final pathology.

## PRESENTATION, EVALUATION, AND DIAGNOSIS

### Clinical Presentation

- Seventy-five percent to 90% of endometrial cancer cases present with **postmenopausal bleeding**. In one study of women with postmenopausal bleeding, 7% had cancer, 56% had atrophy, and 15% had endometrial hyperplasia.
  - The likelihood that postmenopausal bleeding is due to cancer significantly increases with a woman's age. One study showed that 9% of women in their 50s with postmenopausal bleeding had endometrial cancer, whereas the rate was 16% for women in their 60s, 28% for women in their 70s, and 60% for women in their 80s.
- Although endometrial cancer is mostly a disease of postmenopausal women, 20% of cases are diagnosed before menopause. **Perimenopausal menometrorrhagia**, especially in women at high risk for endometrial cancer, should be investigated with endometrial biopsy.
- **Abnormal cervical cytology** can prompt the workup for and diagnosis of endometrial cancer. However, routine Pap smear screening will only detect half of endometrial cancer cases and is not a screening test. Workup should be considered with the following Pap smear results:
  - Endometrial cells (remote from menstrual bleeding) in a woman older than 40 years

- Atypical glandular cells of undetermined significance (the risk of endometrial cancer in women older than 35 years with this Pap result is 23%)
- Adenocarcinoma (consider endometrial and cervical sampling)
- Some cases of endometrial cancer are discovered **incidentally at the time of hysterectomy**. If this is the case, a surgeon skilled on endometrial cancer staging procedures should be involved if available. To avoid this, it is recommended that all women with abnormal uterine bleeding have endometrial sampling prior to their hysterectomy.
- With a few exceptions, there are no guidelines or recommendations to screen for endometrial cancer.

### Tamoxifen

- Women who are on **tamoxifen** have an increased risk of developing endometrial cancer.
- Routine screening with ultrasound or endometrial biopsies is not recommended in this setting.
  - Use of ultrasound for screening is of limited use because tamoxifen causes subepithelial stromal hypertrophy and therefore increases the thickness of the endometrial stripe and may result in unnecessary surgical procedures.
- Women on tamoxifen should be counseled on warning signs and followed with yearly pelvic exams. Any episode of vaginal bleeding should trigger an evaluation.

### Hereditary Nonpolyposis Colon Cancer

- HNPCC, or Lynch syndrome, is inherited in an autosomal dominant fashion, resulting from a germline mutation in one of the mismatch repair genes (MMR genes MLH1, MSH2, MSH6) and comprises the majority of inherited cases of endometrial cancer. It also increases risk of cancer of the colorectum, small intestine, ureter, renal pelvis, and ovary.
- Genetic assessment for HNPCC is strongly recommended in women with a 20% to 25% risk of HNPCC.
  - This includes women with a family pedigree meeting Amsterdam criteria, patients with metachronous or synchronous colorectal and endometrial or ovarian cancers before age 50 years, or those with a first- or second-degree relative with a known germline mutation in an MMR gene.
- Women with HNPCC have a high risk of endometrial cancer (as high as 50% lifetime). A prophylactic hysterectomy should be considered.
- There is limited evidence regarding endometrial cancer screening in this population, but current recommendations advise women to undergo endometrial biopsies annually starting at the age of 30 to 35 years or 10 years before the age that first case appeared in the family and to undergo hysterectomy and bilateral salpingo-oophorectomy once childbearing is completed.

## Evaluation and Diagnosis of Postmenopausal Bleeding

- The appropriate evaluation for postmenopausal bleeding is widely debated. Ultrasound and endometrial biopsy are the two main tools available.

### Ultrasound

- **Pelvic ultrasound** measurement of the endometrial stripe can be used with a minimum cutoff of 5 mm in thickness based on the Postmenopausal Estrogen/Progestins

Intervention (PEPI) trial. This trial showed that with a 5-mm cutoff, postmenopausal ultrasound has a positive predictive value of 9%, a negative predictive value of 99%, a sensitivity of 90%, and a specificity of 48% for endometrial cancer.

- Meta-analysis shows that the posttest probability of cancer following a pelvic ultrasound with a stripe <5 mm is 2.5%. Conversely, a stripe >5 mm conveys a 32% posttest probability of cancer.
- Even with a thin stripe, if a woman persistently bleeds, sampling should be performed.

*Biopsy*

- **Endometrial biopsy** provides a cancer detection rate of 99.6% in premenopausal women and 91% in postmenopausal women. Specificity is 98%, and sensitivity is 99%. The false-negative rate is between 5% and 15%.
- The posttest probability of endometrial cancer is 82% if the biopsy is positive and 0.9% if it is negative.
  - However, a biopsy read as "insufficient sample" should trigger further evaluation because on further investigation, 20% of these women will have pathology and 3% will have cancer.

*Further Workup*

- No matter which method is used for initial evaluation, if bleeding persists or clinical suspicion is high, further evaluation with a **dilation and curettage (D&C)** should be pursued. The false-negative rate of a D&C is 2% to 6%.
- **Hysteroscopy** with D&C has a positive predictive value of 96%, a negative predictive value of 98%, a sensitivity of 98%, and a specificity of 95%.
- A recent Gynecology Oncology Group (GOG) prospective study demonstrated the difficulty in diagnosing complex atypical hyperplasia (CAH). One third of cases of CAH were deemed to be "less than" CAH by study pathologists, one third were deemed to be "greater than" CAH (i.e., endometrial cancer), and another third of the diagnoses were consistent with the original diagnosis of CAH.

## STAGING AND PROGNOSIS

### Pretreatment Evaluation

- Complete history, assessing for hereditary cancer syndromes
- Complete physical exam including comprehensive pelvic exam assessing the size and mobility of the uterus and assessment for metastasis (i.e., supraclavicular lymphadenopathy)
- Consider cancer antigen 125 (CA-125). Elevated CA-125 levels are associated with metastatic disease and can be used to follow the patient if it was elevated at diagnosis.
- Imaging: Chest imaging should be ordered. A plain film is reasonable. A computed tomography (CT) or magnetic resonance imaging (MRI) is not necessary if surgical staging is planned. If no surgery is planned, an MRI is the best modality to assess myometrial or cervical and lymph node involvement.

### Surgical Staging Procedures

- Staging for endometrial cancer is performed surgically, and because many patients have early-stage disease at the time of diagnosis, this is often the only intervention necessary.
  - **Surgical staging** most commonly involves a minimally invasive surgical approach for apparent early-stage disease. The procedure includes total extrafascial

hysterectomy, bilateral salpingo-oophorectomy, a pelvic and periaortic lymph node assessment/dissection, as well as cytoreduction of all visible disease.

- o Peritoneal washings are not part of surgical staging, but if performed, they should be obtained as the first step once abdominal access has been achieved.
- o Omentectomy should be performed if serous or clear cell histology is suspected.
- Current standard of care is minimally invasive surgery when possible. The Gynecologic Oncology Group Study LAP 2 (GOG LAP-2) randomized trial demonstrated that a laparoscopic approach to endometrial cancer staging was feasible and safe with similar intraoperative complications but fewer postoperative adverse events and a shorter hospital stay.
  - Long-term follow-up data suggest similar recurrence rates and 5-year overall survival in the open and laparoscopic groups.
- The lymphatics of the uterine fundus drain to the aortic nodes; the lower uterine segment drains to the internal and external iliac lymph nodes; and the round ligaments can drain to the superficial inguinal lymph nodes.
- **Pelvic and para-aortic lymph node dissection** is required for complete surgical staging of endometrial cancer. Pelvic lymph node dissection involves the removal of nodal tissue from the distal half of each common iliac artery, the anterior and medial proximal of each external iliac artery, and vein and the distal half of the obturator fat pad anterior to the obturator nerve.
  - Para-aortic lymph node dissection involves the removal of nodal tissue over the distal vena cava from the inferior mesenteric artery to the mid common iliac artery and between the aorta and ureter from the inferior mesenteric artery to the left mid common iliac artery.
  - Morbid obesity may render a lymph node dissection more challenging, but it is still a required component of the procedure if indicated based on histologic and pathologic risk factors (see the following text).
- One pitfall of lymph node dissection is the occurrence of lymphedema (5% to 20%). The incidence increases with the removal of more nodes and administration of adjuvant radiation.
- Furthermore, the performance of lymph node dissection is not clearly associated with improved survival. Retrospective data supports improved survival with more extensive lymph node resection, especially in patients with high-risk features. However, Consolidated Standards of Reporting Trials (CONSORT) and Adjuvant External Beam Radiotherapy in the Treatment of Endometrial Cancer (ASTEC) are two prospective randomized trials which demonstrated no difference in survival when lymph node dissection was performed.
  - Importantly, ASTEC did not require para-aortic lymphadenectomy and is criticized for including many patients who were low risk and would not have benefited from lymph node dissection in the first place as well as a low median number of lymph nodes resected. In the CONSORT trial, more nodes were removed (median = 30) but only 26% of patients in the lymphadenectomy group underwent para-aortic dissection. Therefore, it is difficult to generalize and state that a full lymph node dissection conveys no survival benefit. Furthermore, many would argue that it is the information gained from the dissection that helps guide adjuvant therapy and may convey a survival benefit, which was not adequately tested in these trials.
- The decision as to whether or not to proceed to lymph node dissection is often made in the operating room based on frozen section evaluation of the uterus for histologic cell type, tumor differentiation (grade), and depth of myometrial invasion.

| TABLE 47-2 | Lymph Node Metastasis by Grade and Depth of Invasion of Endometrial Cancer | | | |
|---|---|---|---|---|

| | Pelvic Lymph Nodes (%) | | | |
|---|---|---|---|---|
| Grade | No Invasion | Inner 1/3 | Mid 1/3 | Outer 1/3 |
| 1 | 0 | 3 | 0 | 11 |
| 2 | 3 | 5 | 9 | 19 |
| 3 | 0 | 9 | 4 | 34 |

| | Para-aortic Lymph Nodes (%) | | | |
|---|---|---|---|---|
| 1 | 0 | 1 | 5 | 6 |
| 2 | 3 | 4 | 0 | 14 |
| 3 | 0 | 4 | 0 | 23 |

From Creasman WT, Morrow CP, Bundy BN, et al. Surgical pathologic spread patterns of endometrial cancer. A Gynecologic Oncology Group Study. *Cancer* 1987;60:2035–2041.

- Lymph node dissection, if deemed surgically possible, should be pursued in the following instances: the presence of invasion to the outer one half of the myometrium (any grade), high-grade differentiation with any myometrial invasion, clear cell histology, papillary serous histology, tumor size >2 cm in maximal diameter, lymph–vascular space invasion, cervical or lower uterine segment invasion, adnexal involvement, clinically bulky lymph nodes, or disease outside of the uterus.
- Women without any of these risk factors have <5% risk of positive lymph nodes and >90% 5-year survival rate with a total abdominal hysterectomy bilateral salpingo-oophorectomy (TAH-BSO).
  - However, with the presence of any of these risk factors, the risk of positive lymph nodes increases to >10% and 5-year survival rate decreases to 70% to 85% without further treatment (Table 47-2).
- More than half of patients with a preoperative diagnosis of CAH are found to have some myometrial invasion.
- Routine CT scan rarely alters management and is a poor predictor of nodal disease, and MRI has not been shown to have sufficient accuracy to predict myometrial invasion. Neither modality should be used to determine which patient should undergo lymphadenectomy.
- Approximately 50% of positive lymph nodes will be <1 cm. Palpation and visual evaluation of retroperitoneal lymph nodes should not be considered diagnostic.
  - Gross examination of myometrial invasion is less accurate than frozen section and should not be used to determine who should undergo lymphadenectomy.
- Sentinel lymph node biopsy remains investigational but is gaining considerable traction. A meta-analysis demonstrated 93% sensitivity for detecting lymph node metastases. Pericervical injection is associated with an increased detection rate compared to hysteroscopic injection.
  - A recent study demonstrated that the incorporation of a modified staging approach using an algorithm for sentinel lymph node mapping decreases the need to perform a full lymphadenectomy but does not decrease the rate of detection of IIIC disease.

- If visible disease is noted elsewhere in the abdomen, principles of surgical cytoreduction to a point at which there is no visible disease should be employed. Complete cytoreduction is associated with a longer median survival.
- Multiple recent series from different institutions have shown the feasibility and accuracy of **laparoscopic and robotic staging** for endometrial cancer. Minimally invasive surgical staging is generally well tolerated and results in equivalent overall survival and recurrence rates.
  - A meta-analysis including 331 patients demonstrated fewer postoperative complications, less blood loss, longer operating time, shorter hospital stay, and no significant difference between overall survival and recurrence when minimally invasive surgical techniques were used versus open surgery for endometrial cancer.
  - In the **LAP-2 trial**, the GOG randomized 2,600 women to laparoscopy or laparotomy for endometrial cancer staging. Of those randomized to the laparoscopy group, 76% were successfully staged laparoscopically. No difference was noted in peritoneal cytology, lymph node metastases, or stage. Laparoscopy resulted in longer operating times but shorter hospital stays, fewer postoperative adverse events, and improved quality of life. Five-year overall survival was essentially identical (89%) in the laparotomy and laparoscopy arms, and therefore, minimally invasive surgery via conventional laparoscopy or robotics is considered a standard of care in the management of apparent early-stage endometrial cancer.

## Staging of Uterine Cancer

- Staging of endometrial cancer is demonstrated in Table 47-3 and is based on surgical findings, as described in the International Federation of Gynecology and Obstetrics (FIGO) 2009 staging criteria. In this new staging system, positive cytology no longer changes the stage but is still reported.

## Histopathologic Factors for Endometrial Cancer

- **Type I** endometrial cancers (endometrioid adenocarcinomas) are estrogen dependent, arise in a background of hyperplasia, and account for 80% of endometrial cancers.
- **Type II** tumors are not estrogen dependent, arise in a background of endometrial atrophy, are poorly differentiated, and are often of uterine serous, mucinous, or clear cell histology. They account for 10% to 20% of histologies but as much as 40% of the mortality.
- The PTEN tumor suppressor gene, K-ras oncogene, and microsatellite instability resulting from mutations in DNA mismatch repair proteins (e.g., MLH1, MSH2, or MSH6) are associated with endometrioid cancer pathogenesis and CAH.
- Uterine serous carcinoma (USC) histologically resembles and behaves like ovarian serous cancer. It tends to metastasize early (72% have extrauterine spread at the time of diagnosis) and spreads throughout the peritoneal cavity. Therefore, omentectomy along with upper abdominal and peritoneal biopsies should be performed as part of surgical staging for a known USC.
- Carcinosarcoma, leiomyosarcoma (LMS), and endometrial stromal sarcoma, make up the remaining 2% to 5% of uterine cancers.
- **Tumor grade** affects the risk of spread and recurrence and is therefore important in determining the need for adjuvant therapy.
  - **Grade 1** tumors have <5% solid, nonsquamous, or morular component.
  - **Grade 2** tumors are 6% to 50% composed of these features.
  - **Grade 3** tumors have these features in >50% of the tumor.

| TABLE 47-3 | Staging of and National Comprehensive Cancer Network Management Recommendations for Endometrial Carcinoma by Stage and Grade | | | |
|---|---|---|---|---|
| Stage[a] | Description | Grade 1 | Grade 2 | Grade 3 |
| IA | Confined to uterine corpus but <50% myometrial invasion | –RF: observe<br>+RF: observe or VBT ± pelvic RT | –RF: observe or VBT<br>+RF: observe or VBT ± pelvic RT | –RF: observe or VBT<br>+RF: observe or VBT ± pelvic RT |
| IB | Confined to uterine corpus but ≥50% myometrial invasion (not to serosa) | –RF: observe or VBT<br>+RF: observe or VBT ± pelvic RT | –RF: observe or VBT<br>+RF: observe or VBT ± pelvic RT | –RF: observe or VBT ± pelvic RT<br>+RF: observe or pelvic RT ± VBT ± chemotherapy |
| II | Invasion of cervical stroma but confined to uterus[b] | VBT ± pelvic RT | Pelvic RT + VBT | Pelvic RT + VBT ± chemotherapy |
| IIIA | Invasion of uterine serosa or adnexae | Chemotherapy ± pelvic or tumor-directed RT ± chemotherapy or pelvic RT ± VBT | | |
| IIIB | Involvement of vagina and/or parametrium | Chemotherapy ± tumor-directed RT | | |
| IIIC | Metastasis to pelvic (IIIC1) and/or para-aortic (IIIC2) lymph nodes | Chemotherapy ± tumor-directed RT | | |
| IVA | Tumor invasion of bladder and/or bowel mucosa | Chemotherapy ± RT (optimally debulked) | | |
| IVB | Distant metastases including intra-abdominal metastasis and/or positive inguinal lymph nodes | Chemotherapy ± RT (optimally debulked) | | |

[a]Staging based on the 2009 FIGO guidelines as presented in the National Comprehensive Cancer Network guidelines and recommendations are based on National Comprehensive Cancer Network guidelines. http://www.nccn.org/professionals/physician_gls/f_guidelines.asp. Accessed July 21, 2013.

[b]Endocervical glandular involvement without stromal involvement is stage I. Endocervical stromal involvement is required for a stage II designation.

RF, risk factors (age, positive lymph–vascular space invasion, tumor size, lower uterine or cervical involvement); VBT, vaginal brachytherapy; RT, radiation therapy.

## Prognostic Factors for Endometrial Cancer

- The most significant prognostic factors for recurrence and survival are stage, grade, and depth of myometrial invasion. Age, histologic type, lymph–vascular space invasion (LVSI), and progesterone receptor activity also have prognostic significance. LVSI is associated with a 35% rate of recurrence.
- Positive peritoneal cytology is controversial as a prognostic factor. Multiple large studies show conflicting results. Altering therapy for this finding as an isolated result does not improve survival.
- Prognosis for the more aggressive histologic types is less favorable. Even without myometrial invasion, 36% of uterine papillary serous carcinoma cancers will have positive lymph nodes.
  - Five-year survival for disease stages I to II is 36% and is unusual for more advanced disease.
  - Clear cell cancer portends a 72% 5-year survival for stage I disease and a 60% 5-year survival for stage II disease.
  - Overall 5-year survival for the aggressive histologic subtypes is 40%.
- Relapses tend to occur distally, often in the lungs, liver, or bones.

## MANAGEMENT OF ENDOMETRIAL CANCER

Appropriate treatment is determined by stage, grade, histologic type, and the patient's ability to tolerate therapies (Table 47-3).
- Patients with **low-risk endometrial cancer** of endometrioid type require no further therapy beyond surgery, particularly patients with grade 1, stage 1 endometrial cancer and no risk factors.

### Management of High-Risk Endometrial Cancer

- Treatment for women with higher risk disease is more controversial. Multiple studies have sought to define the appropriate role for adjuvant therapy.

*Radiation Therapy*
- The Post Operative Radiation Therapy in Endometrial Carcinoma (PORTEC) study randomized women with stage IC grade 1, stage IB and stage IC grade 2, or stage IA grade 3 (under 1988 FIGO staging). All women were treated with TAH-BSO without a lymph node dissection. These women were then randomized to receive or not receive **pelvic radiation** with 4,600 cGy.
  - Local recurrence occurred in 4.2% of radiated women versus 13.7% of those not radiated. However, the rate of death from cancer was not statistically different between the two groups (9.2% vs. 6.0%, respectively).
  - Additionally, radiation therapy for vaginal recurrence in the nonradiated group was successful in inducing a complete response in 89%, and 5-year survival of this salvage radiation group was 65%. Therefore, postoperative radiation can significantly increase local control but does not appear to impact survival. The authors concluded that postoperative radiation should be limited to women with two out of three risk factors: older than age 60 years, stage IC, or grade 3.
  - One problem with the PORTEC data was the lack of full surgical staging. The GOG addressed this in a phase III trial of 392 intermediate-risk patients who underwent TAH-BSO and lymph node surgery followed by observation (12% recurrence and 86% 4-year survival) versus radiation therapy (3% recurrence and 92% 4-year survival) and found similar results to the PORTEC data.

- GOG-99 randomized 448 women with stage IB to II disease (1988 FIGO staging) to postoperative radiation (50.4 Gy) versus no adjuvant treatment after hysterectomy, bilateral salpingo-oophorectomy, and pelvic and para-aortic lymphadenectomy. Again, they showed a decreased recurrence rate but no improved overall survival with radiation. The lower recurrence rate with radiation was especially notable (2-year recurrence rate of 26% vs. 6%) in the "high intermediate risk" subgroup: (1) any age with poorly differentiated tumor, LVSI, or outer one third myometrial invasion; (2) 50 years or older with any two of the preceding risk factors; and (3) 70 years or older with any one of the preceding risk factors.
- A multicenter retrospective trial demonstrated an 81% response rate to salvage radiation for isolated vaginal recurrences in surgical stage I patients who did not initially receive adjuvant radiation.
- In PORTEC-2, women with stage I or IIA endometrial cancer were randomized to postoperative external beam radiation therapy (46 Gy) or vaginal brachytherapy (21 Gy) after hysterectomy and bilateral salpingo-oophorectomy with pelvic and para-aortic lymph node sampling of suspicious nodes. There were no differences in 5-year vaginal or locoregional recurrence rates, distant metastases, and disease-free or overall survival. Patients in the vaginal brachytherapy group reported better social functioning and fewer gastrointestinal complaints.

### Cytoreductive Surgery

- Stage II uterine cancer significantly increases the risk for vaginal recurrence. If cervical involvement is known preoperatively, a **radical hysterectomy** should be considered, which has been shown to result in a 75% 5-year survival rate. A combination of extrafascial hysterectomy followed by radiation is associated with a 5-year survival rate of 70%.
  - If the diagnosis is made postoperatively, vaginal brachytherapy should be offered.
- These data may need to be updated in light of the new staging system.
- For stages III and IV cancers, **optimal cytoreductive surgery** has been shown to improve survival. Adjuvant therapy after cytoreduction is advised; however, the optimal mode of adjuvant therapy is unclear.
- Complete **salvage cytoreduction** for recurrent disease has been associated with a prolonged postrecurrence survival (39 months) versus patients with gross residual disease (13.5 months).

### Chemotherapy

- Chemotherapy can also be used; however, the optimal chemotherapy regimen for endometrial cancer is unknown. Single-agent response rates are low. Multiple trials have been conducted with various regimens.
- Cisplatin and doxorubicin together have a 43% response rate. The addition of paclitaxel to the cisplatin and doxorubicin regimen (TAP) in a randomized trial (GOG-177) resulted in an increase in response rate and survival. There was a significantly higher rate of peripheral neuropathy in the group treated with paclitaxel. Preliminary data from GOG 209 suggest that carboplatin and paclitaxel may be noninferior and less toxic compared to TAP.
- Hormonal therapies (progesterones like Megace, selective estrogen receptor modulators like tamoxifen, and aromatase inhibitors) are largely more useful in the palliative setting and are not used with an intention to cure.
- Targeted therapies that act on the PI3K/AKT/mTOR pathway, angiogenesis, and epidermal growth factor receptors are experimental but promising.

- Patients who fail first-line chemotherapy generally have a very poor prognosis, with a response rate to second- and third-line agents of <10% and overall survival of <9 months.

## Posttreatment Surveillance

- After treatment, surveillance for recurrence should include an examination every 3 to 6 months for 2 years and then every 6 months or annually.
  - Vaginal cytology should be performed every 6 months for 2 years and then each year.
  - If serum CA-125 was elevated at the time of diagnosis, it can be followed at each visit. Most recurrences are diagnosed by symptoms. Chest x-ray may be performed annually, but CT/MRI should be ordered as needed based on exam or symptoms.
- Continue to assess for high-risk features or family diagnoses that might prompt a genetic evaluation.

## Special Problems

*Clear Cell and Uterine Serous Carcinoma*

- These are often treated with adjuvant therapy regardless of stage. Adjuvant chemotherapy and pelvic radiation are appropriate. Despite therapy, these tumors are often very aggressive.
- The overall 5-year disease-free survival for clear cell endometrial cancers is only 40%. Relapses are often distant and tend to occur in the lungs, liver, and bone.
- As opposed to type I endometrial cancers, the precursor lesion to USC is endometrial intraepithelial carcinoma not endometrial hyperplasia. USC usually shows evidence of LVSI, and 36% of women with no myometrial invasion will have positive lymph nodes. Five-year survival is only 30% to 50% for stage I disease.
- As in ovarian cancer, chemotherapy regimens with carboplatin and Taxol have been the most successful.
- Multiple recent reports have suggested that stage IA patients, after undergoing complete surgical staging, may not require adjuvant therapy. Three-year overall survival rates range from 95% to 100%. These data may need to be updated in light of the new staging system.

*Carcinosarcoma*

- **Carcinosarcoma (mixed müllerian mesodermal tumors)** are very aggressive and are associated with previous pelvic radiation. They are often large and necrotic. Carcinosarcoma is an independent predictor of survival with a hazard ratio of 3:2 for recurrence compared to the other histologies. Thus, carcinosarcoma should be studied separately from high-risk endometrial cancers given the difference in behavior.
  - These are **no longer considered a sarcoma but are poorly differentiated endometrial cancer.**
- The 5-year survival rate is 50% for stage I tumors and 20% for stage IV.
- Lymph node dissection has not been shown to be therapeutic for these tumors. Stage and mitotic grade are the most predictive of disease course.
- Chemotherapy regimens, including cisplatin, doxorubicin, ifosfamide, and paclitaxel, have been used for malignant mixed müllerian tumors. Chemotherapy with ifosfamide and paclitaxel resulted in an improved response rate, overall survival, and progression-free survival but also more neuropathy compared to ifosfamide alone.
- Pelvic radiation improves local control but not overall survival.

*Fertility Preservation*

- Women with very early endometrial cancer who wish to preserve their fertility have been treated with progesterone rather than surgery. A review of 81 patients with stage IA1 endometrial cancer treated with progesterone revealed the following:
  - Two thirds responded with median time to response of 12 weeks, and median duration of treatment was 24 weeks. Of those who responded, 24% recurred and median time to recurrence was 19 months.
  - Forty-seven percent of the women who recurred were retreated, and 72% had a second complete response.
- A multicenter prospective study examined 28 women with endometrial carcinoma and 17 women with atypical hyperplasia who were treated with progesterone.
  - Complete response was noted in 55% of the patients with carcinoma and 82% of those with atypical hyperplasia. The patients were followed for 3 years during which there were 12 pregnancies and a 47% recurrence rate.
- A recent prospective trial followed 105 women with endometrial hyperplasia treated with a levonorgestrel-releasing intrauterine device and showed a 90% regression rate after 2 years.
- Women who wish to retain their fertility should be counseled that risks are associated with such an approach, and a TAH-BSO is recommended after childbearing is completed.
- D&C should be done to confirm pathology. An MRI is recommended to assess for myometrial invasion. D&C should be repeated every 3 months to assess response.

*Incomplete Surgical Staging*

- Treatment depends on risk factors.
- Grade 1 or 2 tumors with <50% myometrial invasion have a <10% risk of having positive lymph nodes and >90% 5-year survival without any further treatment.
- However, any grade 3 cancer or grade 1 and 2 cancers with more than 50% invasion pose a >10% risk of positive pelvic lymph nodes, and 5-year survival is decreased to 70% to 85% without further treatment. Therefore, restaging or use of adjuvant radiation is appropriate. Laparoscopic node dissection can be used for patients who were incompletely staged at their initial surgery. Additionally, fluorodeoxyglucose positron emission tomography scanning may hold promise for evaluating lymphadenopathy but further study is needed.

*Medical Contraindications to Surgery*

- Women who are medically unable to undergo surgery can be treated with pelvic radiation alone. However, 5-year survival for clinical stage I disease is decreased to 69% with this approach versus 87% for surgery alone.
- It has been shown that for stage I disease with a preoperative CA-125 of <20 U/mL, the risk of extrauterine spread was only 3%. In these cases, vaginal hysterectomy is a therapeutic option for those women unable to undergo a more extensive operation.
- In a small series of patients with a well-differentiated endometrial adenocarcinoma, a progestin-secreting intrauterine device has been shown to be effective therapy.

## UTERINE SARCOMA

**Sarcomas** represent 5% of uterine cancers. They usually present with postmenopausal bleeding, and often on exam, the woman will be found to have a fungating mass protruding from her cervix. They are divided based on their sarcomatous elements.

| TABLE 47-4 | Staging of Endometrial Stromal Sarcoma and Leiomyosarcoma[a] |
|---|---|

| Stage[b] | Description |
|---|---|
| IA | Tumor limited to the uterus and ≤5 cm |
| IB | Tumor limited to the uterus and >5 cm |
| IIA | Tumor involves the adnexae. |
| IIB | Tumor involves other pelvic tissues. |
| IIIA | Tumor infiltrates abdominal tissues at one site. |
| IIIB | Tumor infiltrates abdominal tissues at more than one site. |
| IIIC | Metastasis to pelvic and/or para-aortic lymph nodes |
| IVA | Tumor invades bladder and/or rectum. |
| IVB | Distant metastases (beyond the adnexa, pelvic, and abdominal tissues) |

[a]Carcinosarcomas should be staged as endometrial carcinomas, not as a sarcoma.
[b]Staging based on the 2009 FIGO guidelines as presented in the National Comprehensive Cancer Network Guidelines. http://www.nccn.org/professionals/physician_gls/f_guidelines.asp Accessed July 21, 2013.

## Staging of Uterine Sarcoma

- In 2009, a **staging system for uterine sarcomas** was defined (Table 47-4).

### Leiomyosarcoma

- **Uterine LMS** are an aggressive and rare subtype of uterine sarcoma. They usually arise in the myometrium and rarely in fibroids. Vaginal bleeding is the most common presenting symptom. Ten percent of patients will have lung metastases at the time of diagnosis. The typical picture is a postmenopausal woman with a rapidly enlarging fibroid.
- In a series of 1,432 patients who underwent a hysterectomy for a fibroid uterus, only 0.49% were found to have LMS. Another series of 1,332 patients who underwent hysterectomy for fibroids had a subset of patients with "rapidly growing fibroids" and only 0.2% were found to have LMS.
- These tumors appear like leiomyomas but have **>10 mitoses per 10 high-power fields** and **diffuse nuclear atypia**. Additionally, the presence of **coagulative necrosis** is suggestive of LMS.
- No benefit of adjuvant radiation has been noted.
- Fixed-dose-rate gemcitabine plus docetaxel have had promising response rates as first-line therapy for metastatic uterine LMS.

### Endometrial Stromal Sarcoma

- **Endometrial stromal sarcoma (ESS)** arises from the endometrium and can be separated into low and high grade. They represent 10% of sarcomas. They are the least aggressive uterine sarcomas. However, even in low-grade ESS, 36% of patients will relapse and 10% will die from the disease.
- Low-grade ESS often responds to progestins and aromatase inhibitors. Higher grade ESS should be treated with surgery and pelvic radiation. Chemotherapy has not been shown to be beneficial; however, with metastatic disease, doxorubicin and ifosfamide have been used.

## Prognosis for Uterine Sarcoma

- A retrospective study including women with all forms of sarcoma showed a 3-year survival rate of 82%, 60%, and 20% for sarcomas with low-, medium-, and high-grade histology, respectively.
- Three-year survival was 56%, 45%, 33%, and 5% for stages I, II, III, and IV sarcomas. These data may need to be updated in light of the revised staging criteria.
- Survival rates of 77%, 60%, and 30% were seen for sarcomas treated with surgery and then pelvic radiation with vaginal brachytherapy, surgery with just pelvic radiation, and no adjuvant therapy, respectively.

## SUGGESTED READINGS

Benedetti PP, Basile S, Maneschi F, et al. Systematic pelvic lymphadenectomy vs. no lymphadenectomy in early-stage endometrial carcinoma: randomized clinical trial. *J Natl Cancer Inst* 2008;100:1707–1716.

Ben-Shachar I, Pavelka J, Cohn DE, et al. Surgical staging for patients presenting with grade 1 endometrial carcinoma. *Obstet Gynecol* 2005;105:487–493.

Bristow RE, Santillan A, Zahurak ML, et al. Salvage cytoreductive surgery for recurrent endometrial cancer. *Gynecol Oncol* 2006;103:281–287.

Chan JK, Cheung MK, Huh WK, et al. Therapeutic role of lymph node resection in endometrioid corpus cancer: a study of 12,333 patients. *Cancer* 2006;107:1823–1830.

Chung HH, Kang SB, Cho JY, et al. Accuracy of MR imaging for the prediction of myometrial invasion of endometrial carcinoma. *Gynecol Oncol* 2007;104:654–659.

Kitchener H, Swart AM, Quian Q, et al; ASTEC Study Group. Efficacy of systematic pelvic lymphadenectomy in endometrial cancer (MRC ASTEC trial): a randomized study. *Lancet* 2009;373:125–136.

Leitao MM Jr, Khoury-Collado F, Gardner G, et al. Impact of incorporating an algorithm that utilizes sentinel lymph node mapping during minimally invasive procedures on the detection of stage IIIC endometrial cancer. *Gynecol Oncol* 2013;129:38–41.

Lin F, Zhang QJ, Zheng FY, et al. Laparoscopically assisted versus open surgery for endometrial cancer—a meta analysis of randomized controlled trials. *Int J Gynecol Cancer* 2008;18(135):1315–1325.

Mutch DG. The new FIGO staging system for cancers of the vulva, cervix, endometrium and sarcomas. *Gynecol Oncol* 2009;115:325–328.

Nout RA, Smit VT, Putter H, et al. Vaginal brachytherapy versus pelvic external beam radiotherapy for patients with endometrial cancer of high-intermediate risk (PORTEC-2): an open-label, noninferiority, randomized trial. *Lancet* 2010;375:816–823.

Schmeler KM, Lynch HT, Chen LM, et al. Prophylactic surgery to reduce the risk of gynecologic cancers in the Lynch Syndrome. *N Engl J Med* 2006;354(3):261–269.

Thomas MB, Mariani A, Cliby WA, et al. Role of systematic lymphadenectomy and adjuvant therapy in stage I uterine papillary serous carcinoma. *Gynecol Oncol* 2007;107:186–189.

Trimble CL, Kauderer J, Zaino R, et al. Concurrent endometrial carcinoma in women with a biopsy diagnosis of atypical endometrial hyperplasia: a Gynecologic Oncology Group study. *Cancer* 2006;106:812–819.

von Gruenigen VE, Tian C, Frasure H, et al. Treatment effects, disease recurrence, and survival in obese women with early endometrial carcinoma: a Gynecologic Oncology Group study. *Cancer* 2006;107:2786–2791.

Walker JL, Piedmonte MR, Spirtos NM, et al. Laparoscopy compared with laparotomy for comprehensive surgical staging of uterine cancer: Gynecologic Oncology Group Study LAP2. *J Clin Oncol* 2009;27:5331–5336.

Walker JL, Piedemonte MR, Spirtos NM, et al. Recurrence and survival after random assignment to laparoscopy versus laparotomy for comprehensive surgical staging of uterine cancer: Gynecologic Oncology Group LAP2 Study. *J Clin Oncol* 2012;30:695–700.

Zaino RJ, Kauderer J, Trimble CL, et al. Reproducibility of the diagnosis of atypical endometrial hyperplasia: a Gynecologic Oncology Group study. *Cancer* 2006;106:804–811.

# 48 Ovarian Cancer

Jill H. Tseng and Edward J. Tanner III

**Ovarian cancer** is the 10th most common cancer and the fifth leading cause of cancer-related death in American women. Ovarian cancer is the second most common gynecologic cancer following cancer of the uterine corpus and has the highest mortality of all female reproductive system malignancies.

## EPIDEMIOLOGY OF OVARIAN CANCER

* For women in the United States, the lifetime risk of developing ovarian cancer is estimated to be 1 in 72 (1.4%). This likelihood increases with age, with a median age at diagnosis of 63 years.
* The risk of malignancy in a solid adnexal mass is 7% in a premenopausal woman and increases to 30% in a postmenopausal woman. Each year, an estimated 22,240 women will be diagnosed with ovarian cancer and 14,030 will die from their disease.
* Ovarian neoplasms, of which 80% are benign, are divided into three major groups: epithelial, germ cell, and sex cord–stromal tumors (Table 48-1). The ovary can also be a site of metastatic cancer from other sites, particularly from the breast or the gastrointestinal tract (e.g., Krukenberg tumors).

## EPITHELIAL OVARIAN TUMORS

* Tumors derived from the coelomic epithelium are the most common ovarian neoplasms, accounting for 65% of ovarian neoplasms and 90% of ovarian cancers.
  * Histologic types include serous, mucinous, endometrioid, clear cell, and transitional (Brenner).

### Risk Factors
* Age older than 40 years, white race, nulliparity, infertility, history of endometrial or breast cancer, and family history of ovarian cancer have been consistently found to increase the risk of invasive epithelial cancer. Increased parity, use of oral contraceptive pills (OCPs), history of breast-feeding, tubal ligation, and hysterectomy have been associated with a decreased risk of ovarian cancer.
* Patients with a **family history** of ovarian, breast, endometrial, or colon cancer are at increased risk of developing ovarian carcinoma.
  * Hereditary familial ovarian cancer accounts for approximately 10% of all newly diagnosed cases. Women with one first-degree relative with ovarian cancer have a 5% lifetime risk of developing the disease and those with two first-degree relatives with ovarian cancer have a 7% risk.
  * There are three distinct autosomal dominant syndromes that have been termed familial ovarian cancer: site-specific ovarian cancer, breast–ovarian cancer (BRCA1 and BRCA2), and hereditary nonpolyposis colorectal cancer (HNPCC or Lynch syndrome II).

| TABLE 48-1 | Classification of Ovarian Neoplasms |
| --- | --- |

**Epithelial Tumors**

Serous (histology resembles the lining of the fallopian tube)
Mucinous (histology resembles endocervical epithelium)
Endometrioid (histology resembles endometrial lining)
Clear cell (histology resembles vaginal mucosa)
Transitional cell (Brenner; histology resembles bladder)

**Germ Cell Tumors**

Dysgerminoma
Endodermal sinus tumor
Embryonal carcinoma
Polyembryoma
Choriocarcinoma
Teratoma:
• Immature
• Mature

**Sex Cord–Stromal Tumors**

Granulosa–stromal cell
• Granulosa cell
• Thecoma-fibromas
Sertoli-Leydig cell
Sex cord tumor
Sex cord tumor with annular tubules
Gynandroblastoma

**Unclassified and Metastatic**

• **HNPCC**, also known as Lynch syndrome II, is an autosomal dominant cancer susceptibility syndrome that describes a familial predisposition to multiple cancers (primarily colon and also endometrial, ovarian, and genitourinary tract).
  • Women with HNPCC have a 40% to 60% lifetime risk for endometrial cancer and a 12% lifetime risk for ovarian cancer. Mutations in three DNA mismatch repair genes, MLH1, MSH2, and MSH6, account for over 95% of mutations found with Lynch syndrome.
• **BRCA:** Two breast and ovarian cancer susceptibility genes (BRCA1, located on chromosome 17q, and BRCA2, located on chromosome 13q) have been identified. These genes, which are involved in DNA repair, have been linked to familial breast cancer, breast-ovary, and site-specific ovarian cancer syndromes.
  • Women with BRCA gene mutations have a lifetime breast cancer risk of 82%. The lifetime ovarian cancer risks of BRCA1 and BRCA2 carriers are 25% to 60% and 15% to 25%, respectively. These women also develop the disease at an earlier age than women without mutations. Genetic screening tests are available.
• **Environmental factors** may play a role in ovarian cancer. A recent meta-analysis does not support a causal relationship between talc exposure and ovarian cancer.

- Reproductive factors play an important role in ovarian cancer risk. Increasing **parity** is associated with a decreased relative risk of developing ovarian cancer, whereas **nulliparity** is associated with an increased risk.
- The use of **OCPs** also has been associated with a decreased relative risk.
- Women with a history of **breast-feeding** have a lower risk of ovarian cancer than nulliparous women and parous women who have not breast-fed.
- Women with **infertility** have an elevated risk of ovarian cancer, independent of nulliparity.
  - Although fertility drugs have been implicated in the development of ovarian cancer, their association has not been clearly separated from the risk that nulliparity and infertility confer.
- **Tubal ligation** and **hysterectomy** with ovarian preservation both appear to lower the risk of ovarian cancer, although the mechanisms remain unclear.

## Screening and Prevention

- Early ovarian cancer is often asymptomatic. No available screening test has sufficient positive predictive value for early-stage ovarian cancer.
- **Routine yearly pelvic examination** is currently recommended for the general population as a screening tool, but it has poor sensitivity for detecting early disease.
- **Cancer antigen 125 (CA-125)** is a biomarker for ovarian cancer. A level >35 U/mL in postmenopausal women is usually considered abnormal. Approximately 50% of ovarian cancer cases confined to the ovary, and >85% of advanced ovarian cancer cases have elevated CA-125 levels. However, this biomarker alone is neither sufficiently sensitive nor specific enough to be diagnostic for ovarian cancer.
  - CA-125 levels may be elevated in several benign conditions (including pelvic inflammatory disease, endometriosis, fibroids, pregnancy, hemorrhagic ovarian cysts, liver disease, and any other lesion that causes peritoneal irritation) as well as in other malignant conditions (including breast, lung, pancreatic, gastric, and colon cancer). In addition, CA-125 is normal in approximately half of women with stage I ovarian cancer. The most important use is following serial CA-125 levels to monitor response to treatment and to detecting recurrence in women with known ovarian cancer.
- Human epididymis protein 4 (HE4) has similar sensitivity to CA-125 when ovarian cancer patients are compared to healthy controls; however, it has greater sensitivity when compared to those with benign gynecologic disease. Although not yet used for screening, HE4 is currently approved in the United States for monitoring disease progression or recurrence.
- **Other biomarkers:** CA 19-9, CA 15-3, CA 72-4, carcinoembryonic antigen, lysophosphatidic acid, sFas, mesothelin, haptoglobin-alpha, bikunin, HE4, and OVX1 are and have been investigated with combined biomarker tests commercially available for use in high-risk patients.
- **Transvaginal ultrasonography** has been evaluated as a potential screening tool. Characteristics suggestive of malignancy include complex ovarian cysts with solid components, the presence of septations, papillary projections into the cyst, thick cyst walls, surface excrescences, ascites, and neovascularization. When used to screen the general population, transvaginal ultrasonography has a poor positive predictive value. However, when limited to postmenopausal women with pelvic masses, a sensitivity of 84% and specificity of 78% has been reported.
- **Multimodal screening** using CA-125 measurement with transvaginal ultrasonography yields a higher specificity and positive predictive value than either modality alone. In postmenopausal women, the combination of transvaginal ultrasound

and a CA-125 >65 U/mL increased sensitivity to 92% and specificity to 96%. However, the role of multimodal screening remains unclear.

- A large prospective screening study, the Prostate, Lung, Colorectal, and Ovarian Cancer Screening Trial, found that concurrent multimodal screening did not reduce ovarian cancer mortality. Another ongoing large randomized trial, the United Kingdom Collaborative Trial of Ovarian Cancer Screening, demonstrated sequential multimodal screening (abnormal CA-125 followed by transvaginal ultrasound) to have a much greater sensitivity for primary ovarian and tubal cancers compared to transvaginal ultrasound alone in the initial years of screening. Final results are not expected until 2015. For this reason, additional studies are needed to determine the appropriateness of multimodal screening for ovarian cancer at this time.
- **Current recommendations for screening:** According to the U.S. Preventive Services Task Force, no existing evidence suggests that any screening test, including CA-125, ultrasound, or pelvic examination, reduces mortality from ovarian cancer; therefore, **routine screening is not recommended**. The American College of Obstetricians and Gynecologists (ACOG) agrees that routine screening tests are not beneficial for low-risk, asymptomatic women. ACOG advises the obstetrician-gynecologist to remain vigilant for the early signs and symptoms of ovarian cancer. The American Cancer Society does not recommend routine screening but states that women at high risk of ovarian cancer should be offered the combination of a pelvic exam, transvaginal ultrasound, and CA-125.
- **Prophylactic bilateral salpingo-oophorectomy:** Women older than age 45 years who are undergoing any pelvic surgery may consider prophylactic removal of the ovaries and fallopian tubes. A bilateral salpingo-oophorectomy will essentially eliminate the risk for developing ovarian cancer, although a small risk of developing primary peritoneal cancer still remains. The sequelae of surgical menopause must be weighed against the potential benefit of averting ovarian malignancy.
  - For this reason, there is no commonly agreed upon age at which bilateral salpingo-oophorectomy is recommended for normal-risk women, although studies have shown that prophylactic oophorectomy prior to age 45 years may decrease life span and risk of all-cause mortality.
  - Women at high risk of ovarian cancer (e.g., Lynch syndrome, BRCA mutations) should consider prophylactic bilateral salpingo-oophorectomy when childbearing is complete.
- **OCP prophylaxis** is the only documented method of chemoprevention for ovarian cancer, and the effect is substantial. The overall estimate of protection with OCPs is approximately 40%. Increased duration of use appears to be associated with further decreased risk, and the protective effect persists for 10 or more years after discontinuation. The use of OCPs in BRCA mutation carriers also confers a decreased risk of ovarian cancer without increasing the risk of breast cancer.

## Presentation and Diagnosis

- **Presentation:** Only 19% of ovarian cancer cases are diagnosed while the cancer is localized (stage I), and approximately 68% of patients with epithelial ovarian cancer have advanced disease (stage III or greater) at time of diagnosis. Although some women with early disease experience symptoms, the majority are asymptomatic.
  - When symptoms develop, they are nonspecific and can include abdominal bloating, early satiety, weight loss, constipation, anorexia, urinary frequency, dyspareunia, fatigue, and irregular menstrual bleeding.

| TABLE 48-2 | Risks of Specific Types of Cancers Associated with Autosomal Dominant Genetic Risk Syndromes | | |
|---|---|---|---|
| **Genetic Syndrome** | **BRCA1** | **BRCA2** | **HNPCC** |
| **Type of Cancer** | | | |
| **Ovarian cancer** | 25%–60% | 15%–25% | 12% |
| **Breast cancer** | 82% | 82% | Not associated |
| **Endometrial cancer** | Not associated | Not associated | 40%–60% |
| **Colon cancer** | Possibly increased risk | Not associated | 70%–80% |
| **Stomach cancer** | Not associated | Possibly increased risk | 20% |

HNPCC, hereditary nonpolyposis colorectal cancer.

- On physical examination, a pelvic mass is an important sign of disease. In more advanced stages, abdominal distention may develop, and chest examination may reveal evidence of pleural effusion.
- **Workup:** Evaluation of a pelvic mass varies depending on the patient's age, significant medical and family history, and the sonographic characteristics of the mass. Women with pelvic masses that are suspicious for malignancy should be referred to a gynecologic oncologist (Table 48-2). In premenopausal women, an adnexal mass <8 to 10 cm in diameter with no other concerning features is typically monitored with serial sonograms. If the decision is made to proceed with surgical evaluation, the preoperative evaluation should include a full history and physical examination, including a pelvic examination and a Pap smear.
- Additional tests should be performed on the basis of a patient's risk factors and underlying medical status. Consideration should be given to performing a computed tomography (CT) scan of the chest, abdomen, and pelvis to evaluate for metastatic disease. If surgery is necessary, a surgeon capable of performing an adequate staging procedure should be available, preferably a gynecologic oncologist, to optimize outcomes in cases of malignancy.

## Staging and Prognosis

- Epithelial ovarian tumors are classified by cell type and behavior as benign, atypically proliferating, or malignant. Atypically proliferating tumors are also referred to as tumors of low malignant potential (LMPs) or "borderline" tumors.
- Ovarian cancer is **surgically staged** (Table 48-3). The importance of complete surgical staging in treatment planning and prognosis cannot be overemphasized. The standard surgical approach involves a vertical midline incision to allow for adequate exposure, although more recent advances in laparoscopic surgery have made minimally invasive options available (Table 48-4).
- Ovarian cancer can spread by direct extension, by exfoliation of cells into the peritoneal cavity (transcoelomic spread), via the bloodstream, or via the lymphatic system. The most common pathway of spread is transcoelomic. Cells from the tumor are shed into the peritoneal cavity and circulate following the clockwise path of the

| TABLE 48-3 | Pelvic Gynecologic Oncology Referral Mass Evaluation: Criteria for Gynecologic Oncology Referral |
|---|---|

| Premenopausal Women | Postmenopausal Women |
|---|---|
| Very elevated CA-125 | Elevated CA-125 (>35 U/mL) |
| Ascites | Ascites |
| Evidence of abdominal or distant metastasis (by examination or imaging) | Evidence of abdominal or distant metastasis (by examination or imaging) |
| | Nodular or fixed pelvic mass |

From American College of Obstetricians and Gynecologists. ACOG committee opinion no. 477: the role of the generalist obstetrician-gynecologist in the early detection of ovarian cancer. *Obstet Gynecol* 2011;117:742–746.

peritoneal fluid. All peritoneal surfaces are at risk. Lymphatic spread to the pelvic and para-aortic lymph nodes can occur. Hematogenous spread to the liver or lungs can occur in advanced disease.

*Prognostic Factors*

• The most important prognostic factors are stage, grade, histology of the tumor, the amount of residual disease remaining after initial debulking surgery, and the age of the patient.
• The 5-year survival rate of patients with epithelial ovarian cancer correlates directly with **tumor stage** (Table 48-5).
• Within each **histologic subtype**, tumors may be described as benign, of LMP, or malignant.
    • The **serous** subtype is the most common, accounting for over 50% of all malignant ovarian tumors. Approximately one third are malignant, one half are benign, and one sixth are LMP. Serous carcinoma of the ovary closely resembles fallopian tube and peritoneal cancer in histology as well as in clinical behavior, and thus, they are often referred to as one entity. The mean age of patients at diagnosis is 57 years. Psammoma bodies are present in 25% of serous tumors.
    • **Mucinous** tumors are lined by cells that resemble endocervical glands or intestinal epithelium. Primary ovarian mucinous tumors account for 3% to 4% of epithelial tumors. Sixty percent of mucinous tumors are stage I, and most are unilateral. They are typically large, often filling the abdominal cavity, cystic, and multiloculated. The mean age of patients diagnosed with malignant mucinous tumors is 54 years. CA-125 levels may not be markedly elevated.
        ◦ **Pseudomyxoma peritonei** is a condition associated with mucinous neoplasms, usually of gastrointestinal origin, and is characterized by gelatinous mucus or ascites in the abdomen.
        ◦ Primary ovarian mucinous tumors may be difficult to differentiate from metastatic neoplasms of the gastrointestinal tract (colon, appendix, pancreas). Prior studies have shown that in general, primary ovarian mucinous tumors are unilateral and measure $10 cm, whereas metastatic tumors are bilateral and measure <10 cm in diameter. Using these criteria, approximately 84% of all mucinous tumors are correctly classified, including 100% of primary ovarian tumors.

| TABLE 48-4 | International Federation of Gynecology and Obstetrics Staging System for Carcinoma of the Ovary (1988) |
|---|---|

| Stage | Tumor Characteristics |
|---|---|
| **I** | **Growth limited to the ovaries** |
| IA | Growth limited to one ovary; no ascites; no tumor on the external surface; capsule intact |
| IB | Growth limited to both ovaries; no ascites; no tumor on the external surfaces; capsule intact |
| IC | Tumor either stage IA or IB but with tumor on surface of one or both ovaries; or with capsule ruptured; or with ascites present containing malignant cells; or with positive peritoneal washings |
| **II** | **Growth involving one or both ovaries with pelvic extension** |
| IIA | Extension or metastases to the uterus or tubes |
| IIB | Extension to other pelvic tissues |
| IIC | Tumor either stage IIA or IIB but with tumor on surface of one or both ovaries; or with capsule ruptured; or with ascites present containing malignant cells; or with positive peritoneal washings |
| **III** | **Tumor involving one or both ovaries with peritoneal implants outside the pelvis and/or positive retroperitoneal or inguinal nodes. Superficial liver metastasis equals stage III. Tumor is limited to the true pelvis but with histologically proven malignant extension to small bowel or omentum.** |
| IIIA | Tumor grossly limited to the true pelvis with negative nodes but with histologically confirmed microscopic seeding of abdominal peritoneal surfaces |
| IIIB | Tumor of one or both ovaries with histologically confirmed implants of abdominal peritoneal surfaces, none exceeding 2 cm in diameter; nodes are negative |
| IIIC | Abdominal implants >2 cm in diameter or positive retroperitoneal or inguinal nodes |
| **IV** | **Growth involving one or both ovaries, with distant metastases. If pleural effusion is present, cytologic findings must be positive to allot a case to stage IV. Parenchymal liver metastasis equals stage IV.** |

From Current FIGO staging for cancer of the vagina, fallopian tube, ovary, and gestational trophoblastic neoplasia. FIGO Committee on Gynecologic Oncology. *Int J Gynecol Obstet* 2009;105:3–4.

- **Endometrioid** tumors resemble the histology of the endometrium and account for 6% of epithelial tumors. Most are malignant; 20% may be tumors of LMP. The mean age of patients diagnosed with malignant tumors is 56 years. About 14% of women will also have endometrial cancer, and 15% to 20% or more will have endometriosis. Endometrioid tumors appear to have a better prognosis than serous tumors, most likely because of their early stage at diagnosis.
- **Clear cell** carcinomas account for 3% of epithelial ovarian cancers. These are the most chemoresistant type of ovarian cancer and overall are associated with a poor prognosis among subtypes. Endometriotic implants are present in 30% to 35%

| TABLE 48-5 | Surgical Staging Procedures for Ovarian Cancer |
|---|---|

Obtain ascites for cytologic evaluation
Washings from the pelvis, gutters, and diaphragm
Systematic exploration of all organs and surfaces
Hysterectomy[a]
Bilateral salpingo-oophorectomy[a]
Infracolic omentectomy
Sampling pelvic and para-aortic lymph nodes
Multiple biopsy specimens from peritoneal sites
   Pelvic side walls
   Surfaces of the rectum and bladder
   Cul-de-sac
   Lateral abdominal gutters
   Diaphragm

[a]May be preserved in select patients, particularly if future fertility is desired.
From Young RC, Decker DG, Wharton JT, et al. Staging laparotomy in early ovarian cancer. *JAMA* 1983;250(22):3072–3076; Trimbos JB, Schueler JA, van Lent M, et al. Reasons for incomplete surgical staging in early ovarian carcinoma. *Gynecol Oncol* 1990;37:374–377.

of cases, and although an uncommon occurrence, clear cell carcinomas may be associated with paraneoplastic syndromes such as hypercalcemia. About 50% of patients present with stage I disease. Tumors are large, with a mean diameter of 15 cm. Histologically, **hobnail-shaped cells** are characteristic of these tumors. The mean age at diagnosis is 57 years.

- **Transitional cell** tumors histologically resemble the bladder. The two types of malignant transitional cell tumors are Brenner tumors and transitional cell carcinomas. Approximately 10% to 20% of advanced-stage ovarian carcinomas contain a transitional cell carcinoma component. The mean age for malignant Brenner tumors is 63 years.

- **Grade** is an important independent prognostic factor, particularly in patients with early-stage disease.
  - Based on a combination of architecture (glandular, papillary, or solid), degree of nuclear atypia, and mitotic index.
  - Grade 1 is well differentiated, grade 2 is moderately differentiated, and grade 3 is poorly differentiated.
  - More recently, a two-tiered grading system has been proposed. Low-grade tumors exhibit a low degree of atypia with infrequent mitotic figures and are thought to develop from adenofibromas or borderline tumors in a slow, stepwise process. High-grade tumors demonstrate atypical nuclei and numerous mitotic figures. These tumors are thought to develop rapidly de novo.

- **Tumor ploidy** has been demonstrated to be an independent prognostic variable. Diploid tumors are often stage IA, whereas aneuploid tumors are seen in more advanced cancer.

- Debulking, also called **cytoreduction**, is defined as removal of as much tumor as possible during surgical exploration. Optimal cytoreduction implies that any remaining tumor nodules are less than 1 cm in diameter. Cytoreduction of all visible disease is associated with the greatest survival advantage, reinforcing the importance of a gynecologic oncologist involvement of primary diagnostic and cytoreductive surgery.

## Management of Epithelial Ovarian Cancer

- Treatment of epithelial ovarian cancer depends on the stage and grade of the disease, type of disease (i.e., primary or recurrent), previous treatment, and the patient's performance status.

### Tumors of Low Malignant Potential

- These tumors show a different pattern of behavior than do malignant ovarian disease. Approximately 15% of all epithelial ovarian tumors are classified as LMP and are often found in younger patients. They are most commonly of serous histology (85%) followed by mucinous.
- Serous LMP tumors with invasive implants tend to behave as low-grade carcinomas with a mortality rate of 34%.
- Mucinous LMP tumors confined to the ovary have a survival rate approaching 100%, whereas those with advanced-stage disease have a survival rate of 40% to 50%. They may be associated with a concurrent appendiceal primary tumor, and affected patients should also undergo appendectomy. Mucinous LMPs that display aggressive behavior are associated with pseudomyxoma peritonei, which is indicative of appendiceal origin.
- Surgical staging of LMPs is advocated because of the possibility of identifying an invasive cancer on final pathology. Because of their indolent growth, adjuvant therapy is not recommended even in patients with advanced disease.
  - If disease recurs, it does so an average of 10 years after initial diagnosis, and resection can be performed again at the time of recurrence. Most patients die *with* the disease rather than *from* the disease.
- In addition, early-stage disease in women who desire future fertility may be treated with unilateral salpingo-oophorectomy, or even with unilateral cystectomy, with good outcomes.

### Early Invasive Disease (Stage I or II)

- **Initial surgical resection** is necessary for establishing a histologic diagnosis and appropriate staging. Options exist for young patients who wish to preserve fertility. If intraoperative findings are consistent with stage I disease and the contralateral ovary is normal in appearance, unilateral salpingo-oophorectomy with thorough surgical staging may be performed. The uterus and normal-appearing contralateral ovary may remain in situ. The patient should be counseled about the potential for a second primary in the preserved ovary, and a total abdominal hysterectomy with removal of the remaining tube and ovary should be considered after childbearing is completed.
- **Chemotherapy:** For patients with stage IA, grade 1 or 2 disease, chemotherapy is not required. For patients with early-stage disease with prognostic factors placing them at higher risk for recurrence (stage IC or II, grade 3 disease, or clear cell histology of any stage), postoperative chemotherapy is recommended. Although platinum-based regimens are most commonly used, the optimal chemotherapy regimen for patients with early-stage disease is still being evaluated.

- **Radiation:** With relatively effective chemotherapeutic options available as well as frequency of widespread metastasis, radiation therapy is used infrequently in the treatment of ovarian cancer.

### Advanced Invasive Disease

- **Advanced disease** requires surgical staging, debulking, and a course of platinum-based chemotherapy.
- Primary **cytoreductive surgery**, or debulking, is central in the treatment of advanced disease because optimal cytoreduction is one of the most powerful predictors of survival in patients with advanced ovarian cancer.
  - The determination of residual disease upon completion of the procedure does not include the total volume of tumor cells left behind but rather the diameter of the largest single residual nodule. For example, a patient with one unresected nodule measuring 2.5 cm has not undergone optimal debulking, whereas debulking is considered to be optimal in a patient with residual miliary studding of the entire peritoneal cavity.
- **Neoadjuvant therapy**, treatment prior to surgery, has been associated with a lower overall survival compared to initial surgery. However, it may be an appropriate alternative for patients whose performance status prohibits initial surgery. In addition, for patients in whom suboptimal debulking is likely, neoadjuvant chemotherapy has been used as an alternate strategy prior to surgery in an attempt to increase the likelihood of optimal tumor debulking.
- **Combination chemotherapy** is most often used as postoperative (adjuvant) treatment for advanced epithelial ovarian cancer. Combination chemotherapy with six cycles of carboplatin plus paclitaxel is the treatment of choice for patients with advanced disease. One cycle is given every 3 weeks, with monitoring of tumor status by physical examination, CA-125 levels, and CT imaging.
- **Intraperitoneal chemotherapy:** Data suggest a substantial improvement in overall survival and progression-free survival in patients with newly diagnosed, optimally debulked stage III ovarian cancer by the administration of cisplatin and paclitaxel via an intraperitoneal (IP) port rather than the conventional intravenous (IV) administration. Studies have demonstrated an approximately 1-year increased survival with IP administration as compared to IV administration, although an increase in toxic events and catheter-related complications is a disadvantage of this therapeutic approach and may prevent completion of all six cycles.
- **Alternative therapies** including dose-dense (weekly) chemotherapy and biologic therapies are under investigation.
- **Consolidation treatment:** Eighty percent of patients who complete optimal tumor debulking followed by six cycles of carboplatin and paclitaxel will achieve a clinical remission. Consolidation treatment strategies to lengthen time to recurrence are currently being investigated. Prior studies using platinum and taxane agents for maintenance chemotherapy have not shown significant improvements in overall survival. Recent studies have demonstrated an improvement in progression-free survival when bevacizumab was administered along with IV carboplatin and paclitaxel and continued as a single agent for 10 months, although there was significantly no improvement in overall survival. Consideration of its use must reflect on its significantly increased cost without an improvement in overall survival. In patients with estrogen-positive primary tumors, hormonal therapies such as tamoxifen or aromatase inhibitors can also be considered.

## Posttreatment Surveillance in Asymptomatic Patients

- Appropriate follow-up for asymptomatic patients after primary surgery and chemotherapy should include a physical examination with rectovaginal examination, CA-125 testing, and CT scan if clinically indicated. Patients should be seen every 3 months for the first 2 years, then every 6 months for the next 3 years.
- In patients whose CA-125 level was elevated preoperatively, CA-125 is a reliable marker of disease recurrence with a sensitivity of 62% to 94% and specificity of 91% to 100%. Levels are often elevated 2 to 5 months prior to clinical detection of recurrence. However, a recent prospective randomized trial showed no difference in survival outcome for patients who were treated for recurrent ovarian cancer based on CA-125 level alone versus waiting for the development of symptomatic disease.
- CT scans have a sensitivity and specificity of 40% to 93% and 50% to 98% respectively for recurrent disease. One limitation is the poor sensitivity of detecting small volume disease. In a retrospective study, asymptomatic patients with recurrence detected by CT scan had a higher rate of optimal secondary cytoreductive surgery and improved overall survival compared to patients with symptomatic recurrence.
- Combined positron emission tomography imaging and CT may have clinical use in detecting disease recurrence in select patients and is often recommended prior to secondary cytoreduction.
- **Second-look surgery** by laparotomy or laparoscopy can be performed on patients with advanced epithelial ovarian cancer who have no clinical evidence of disease after undergoing primary debulking and adjuvant chemotherapy. The use of second-look surgery remains controversial and should be performed only in the setting of a clinical trial or on an individualized basis, as there are no data demonstrating improved survival with this approach. Patients need to be counseled that the procedure is not therapeutic but may provide prognostic information.

## Recurrent or Persistent Disease

- **Secondary debulking:** Patients with recurrent or persistent disease may be candidates for further surgical therapy or secondary cytoreduction. Surgery should be reserved for patients in whom additional therapy has a good chance of prolonging life or palliating symptoms. The best candidates for secondary cytoreduction are those with longer disease-free intervals (at least 6 to 12 months) and fewer sites of recurrence.
- **Second-line chemotherapy:** Response rates for second-line chemotherapy are in the range of 20% to 40%. A host of chemotherapy options are available for recurrent ovarian cancer.
- **Hormone therapy** has been used as salvage treatment. Both megestrol acetate (Megace) and tamoxifen have been used to treat recurrent disease. Response rates are low.
- **Radiation therapy** is generally not used except for palliation of distant metastases.
- **Experimental studies:** Many investigators are currently studying the underlying molecular biology of epithelial ovarian cancer. Microarray analysis and proteomics provide insight into the differential expression of mRNA and proteins, respectively. Translational studies to further characterize these molecular changes, as they relate to the clinical disease state, provide an opportunity for novel therapeutic agents. Clinical trials are also currently investigating antiangiogenic drugs.

*Complications of Advanced Ovarian Cancer*

- **Intestinal obstruction:** Many women with ovarian cancer develop intestinal obstruction, either at initial diagnosis or with recurrent disease. Obstruction may be related to mechanical blockage or carcinomatous ileus. Correction of intestinal obstruction at initial treatment is usually possible; obstruction associated with recurrent disease, however, is a more complex problem. Some of these obstructions may be treated conservatively with IV hydration, total parenteral nutrition, and gastric decompression. The decision to proceed with palliative surgery must be based on the physical condition of the patient and her expected survival. If patients are unable to undergo surgery or are judged to be poor operative candidates, placement of a percutaneous gastric tube may offer some symptomatic relief. In cases of large bowel obstruction, the use of colorectal stents may be an option in order to avoid the significant morbidity and mortality associated with surgical management.

- **Ascites:** Initial ascites on presentation with ovarian cancer is almost always improved by debulking surgery and several courses of chemotherapy. Persistent ascites is difficult to manage and is a very poor prognostic sign. Ascites is best managed by serial paracenteses with fluid removal and chemotherapy.

*Survival*

- **Age:** Overall survival rate 5 years after diagnosis in women younger than age 65 years is nearly twice that of women older than age 65 years (57% and 28%, respectively).

- **Stage:** Patients with stage I disease have up to a 94% 5-year survival rate. In contrast, overall survival for women with distant disease on presentation is 29% (see Table 48-5).

- **Performance status:** The Karnofsky Performance Scale Index (Table 48-6) classifies patients according to their functional impairment and can be used to assess prognosis in individual patients. Lower scores are associated with worse survival for most serious illnesses.

*Primary Peritoneal Carcinoma*

- Primary malignant transformation of the peritoneum is termed **primary peritoneal carcinoma**, which clinically and pathologically resembles serous epithelial ovarian

| TABLE 48-6 | 5-Year Survival for Epithelial Ovarian Cancer by Stage (2010) | | |
|---|---|---|---|
| Stage | 5-Year Survival (%) | Stage | 5-Year Survival (%) |
| IA | 94 | IIC | 57 |
| IB | 91 | IIIA | 45 |
| IC | 80 | IIIB | 39 |
| IIA | 76 | IIIC | 35 |
| IIB | 67 | IV | 18 |

From American Cancer Society. Survival rates for ovarian cancer. American Cancer Society Web site. http://www.cancer.org/cancer/ovariancancer/overviewguide/ovarian-cancer-overview-survival. Accessed September 20, 2010.

cancer. Primary peritoneal carcinoma can therefore appear with a clinical presentation similar to ovarian cancer in patients with a history of oophorectomy or with pathologically normal-appearing or minimally involved ovaries. Extensive upper abdominal disease is common, and clinical course, management, and prognosis are similar to those for epithelial ovarian cancer.

## FALLOPIAN TUBE CANCER

- **Epidemiology:** Carcinoma of the fallopian tube is very rare, accounting for <1% of cases of gynecologic cancer in women. Carcinoma of the fallopian tube is seen most often in the fifth and sixth decades of life.
  - Recent evidence suggests a common precursor lesion for both ovarian and fallopian tube cancers arising in the fallopian tube. In support of this theory, patients with ovarian and peritoneal high-grade serous carcinomas were found to have concurrent serous tubal intraepithelial carcinomas (STICs), usually in the mucosa of the fimbria. Furthermore, almost all STICs demonstrated overexpression of p53 similar to high-grade serous carcinoma.
- **Histology:** To confirm a histologic diagnosis of fallopian tube cancer, most of the tumor must be present in the fallopian tube, the mucosa of the tube must be involved, and a demonstrable transition from benign to malignant tubal epithelium must exist. Over 90% of tumors are papillary serous adenocarcinomas, resembling ovarian serous carcinomas.
- **Clinical presentation and diagnosis:** The triad of symptoms of fallopian tube carcinoma is watery vaginal discharge (hydrops tubae profluens), pelvic pain, and a pelvic mass. However, only 15% of patients present with this triad. Vaginal discharge or bleeding is the most common presenting symptom (50% to 60%), followed by abdominal pain and an abdominal mass. As in ovarian cancer, presentation may be nonspecific. Ascites may be present if the disease is advanced.
  - Unlike ovarian cancer, fallopian tube carcinoma more often presents at an early stage. A preoperative diagnosis of fallopian tube cancer is made in only a minority of patients; the usual clinical diagnosis is ovarian tumor or pelvic inflammatory disease. The majority of patients will have elevated CA-125 levels.
- **Natural history and patterns of spread:** Tubal cancers spread in a similar fashion to ovarian cancers.
- **Staging:** Fallopian tube cancer is staged using the ovarian cancer staging system.
- **Treatment** is similar to that of ovarian cancer, with surgical debulking as the mainstay of treatment, followed by combination platinum-based chemotherapy. Chemotherapy for early-stage disease is the subject of controversy.
- **Prognosis and survival** are related to the stage of disease. Data on 5-year survival rates are as follows from stage I to IV: 95%, 75%, 69%, and 45%.

## GERM CELL OVARIAN TUMORS

### Epidemiology

- Approximately 20% of all ovarian tumors are of germ cell origin, with only 2% to 3% of these being malignant. Types include the following: dysgerminoma, endodermal sinus tumor, embryonal carcinoma, polyembryoma, choriocarcinoma, and teratoma.
- Roughly 70% to 80% of all germ cell tumors occur before age 20 years, and approximately one third of these are malignant. The median age of women diagnosed

with a malignant germ cell tumor is 16 to 20 years. About 50% to 75% of patients with malignant germ cell tumors present with stage I disease. Overall survival rates, including those with advanced disease, are 60% to 80%.

- The most common germ cell tumor is a benign cystic teratoma (dermoid), and the most common malignant tumor is the dysgerminoma.

## Pathology

- Germ cell tumors are derived from the primordial germ cells of the ovary; however, they are a heterogeneous group of tumors. They gradually differentiate to mimic tissues of embryonic origin (ectoderm, mesoderm, endoderm) and extraembryonic origin (trophoblast, yolk sac). They are aggressive tumors, frequently unilateral, and usually curable if treated early.

## Diagnosis

- Clinically, germ cell malignancies grow quickly and are often characterized by acute pelvic pain. The pain can be caused by distention of the ovarian capsule, hemorrhage, necrosis, or torsion. A palpable pelvic mass is a common finding on presentation. Abdominal distention and abnormal vaginal bleeding may also be the presenting complaint. The tumors are often large at presentation, with a median diameter of 16 cm.
- Ovarian masses that are 2 cm or larger in premenarchal girls or >8 to 10 cm in premenopausal patients generally require exploratory surgery.
- **Preoperative workup:** Measurement of serum tumor markers may assist in the diagnosis of germ cell malignancies (Table 48-7). Workup should include measurement of serum human chorionic gonadotropin (hCG), alpha-fetoprotein (AFP) titers, lactate dehydrogenase (LDH) levels, a complete blood count, and liver

| TABLE 48-7 | The Karnofsky Performance Scale | |
| --- | --- |
| Description | % |
| Normal; no complaints; no evidence of disease | 100 |
| Able to carry on normal activity; minor signs and symptoms of disease | 90 |
| Normal activity with effort; some signs and symptoms of disease | 80 |
| Cares for self; unable to carry on normal activity or do work | 70 |
| Requires occasional assistance but is able to care for most personal needs | 60 |
| Requires considerable assistance and frequent medical care | 50 |
| Disabled; requires special care and assistance | 40 |
| Severely disabled; hospitalization indicated although death not imminent | 30 |
| Very sick; hospitalization necessary; requires active support treatment | 20 |
| Moribund; fatal processes progressing rapidly | 10 |
| Dead | 0 |

Originally published by Karnofsky DA, Burchenal JH. The clinical evaluation of chemotherapeutic agents in cancer. In Macleod CM, ed. *Evaluation of Chemotherapeutic Agents.* New York, NY: Columbia University, 1949:199–205.

function tests. A chest radiographic study is important to rule out pulmonary metastases. A preoperative CT scan should be considered to assess for the presence or absence of liver metastases and retroperitoneal lymphadenopathy.

## Germ Cell Tumor Types

- **Dysgerminomas** are the most common malignant germ cell tumor, comprising up to 50%. All dysgerminomas are malignant; however, not all are aggressive. Seventy-five percent of dysgerminomas occur in the second and third decades of life. They are the only germ cell tumor that tends to be bilateral (10% to 15% of cases). The 5-year survival rate for stage IA disease is 95% and for all stages is 85%.
- **Endodermal sinus tumors** (yolk sac tumors) are derived from cells of the primitive yolk sac and are the second most common malignant germ cell tumor, accounting for 20% of cases.
  - Histologically, they are characterized by **Schiller-Duval bodies**. These tumors tend to grow rapidly and aggressively. They secrete AFP. The disease-free survival for all stages is >80%.
- **Embryonal carcinoma** tumors are extremely rare and occur in children and young adults. They may secrete both hCG and AFP. Patients may present with sexual precocity and vaginal bleeding.
- **Polyembryoma** tumors are exceedingly rare and highly malignant. They resemble early embryos and may secrete AFP or hCG.
- **Nongestational choriocarcinoma:** Pure, nongestational choriocarcinoma involving the ovary is very rare and is histologically similar to gestational choriocarcinoma (see Chapter 49). Almost all patients are premenarchal. This tumor often produces remarkably high levels of hCG, which may in turn increase thyroid function. Precocious puberty is seen occasionally, and patients may present with vaginal bleeding. Historically, choriocarcinomas have had a poor prognosis but tend to respond to combination chemotherapy.
- **Immature malignant teratomas** contain tissues resembling those in an embryo. They account for 20% of malignant germ cell tumors and 1% of ovarian malignancies. Half of immature teratomas occur in patients between ages 10 and 20 years. These tumors may secrete AFP. The most important prognostic factor is tumor grade. The 5-year survival rate is 95% for stage I disease and 75% for advanced disease.
- **Mixed germ cell tumors** account for 10% of malignant germ cell tumors and contain elements of two or more of the germ cell tumors discussed previously.

## Management of Germ Cell Tumors

- **Surgical:** Primary treatment for all germ cell tumors is surgical and should include proper surgical staging to rule out the presence of extraovarian microscopic disease. Because most patients are of reproductive age, preservation of fertility is important.
  - Unilateral oophorectomy is performed along with unilateral pelvic and para-aortic lymphadenectomy. A frozen section should be obtained. Bilateral involvement is rare in germ cell tumors, with the exception of dysgerminomas (10% to 15% bilaterality).
  - The contralateral ovary should be inspected, and a biopsy may be performed if there is suspicion of involvement. The ovary should only be removed in a young patient if disease is present. The remaining pelvic organs may be left in situ to preserve fertility.
  - For patients who have completed childbearing, a total abdominal hysterectomy with bilateral salpingo-oophorectomy is reasonable. If metastatic disease is present on initial surgery, cytoreductive surgery is recommended, although data are limited.

| TABLE 48-8 | Serum Markers for Germ Cell and Sex Cord–Stromal Ovarian Tumors | | | | | | | |
|---|---|---|---|---|---|---|---|---|
| Tumor | LDH | AFP | hCG | E$_2$ | Inhibin | Testosterone | Androgen | DHEA |
| Dysgerminoma | ± | − | ± | − | − | − | − | − |
| Embryonal | − | ± | + | − | − | − | − | − |
| Endodermal sinus tumor | − | + | − | − | − | − | − | − |
| Polyembryoma | − | ± | + | − | − | − | − | − |
| Choriocarcinoma | − | − | + | − | − | − | − | − |
| Immature teratoma | − | ± | − | ± | − | − | − | ± |
| Granulosa cell | − | − | − | ± | + | − | − | − |
| Thecoma-fibroma | − | − | − | − | − | − | − | − |
| Sertoli-Leydig | − | − | − | − | ± | + | + | − |
| Gonadoblastoma | − | − | − | ± | ± | ± | ± | ± |

LDH, lactate dehydrogenase; AFP, alpha-fetoprotein; hCG, human chorionic gonadotropin; E$_2$, estradiol; DHEA, dehydroepiandrosterone.

- Surgical therapy alone is recommended for stage IA dysgerminomas and stage IA, grade I immature teratomas. These patients have a 5-year survival of >90%. Approximately 15% to 25% will recur but can be treated successfully at the time of presentation. For endodermal sinus tumors, staging is not always recommended because chemotherapy should be given regardless.
- **Adjuvant therapy:** The decision to administer adjuvant therapy depends on the histologic type of germ cell tumor. Except those with stage IA, grade I immature teratoma and stage IA dysgerminoma, all patients require postoperative chemotherapy. Dysgerminomas are very sensitive to radiation therapy; however, fertility is lost as a consequence of irradiation. Therefore, chemotherapy is the first-line treatment. Combination therapy with three agents (bleomycin, etoposide, and cisplatin [BEP]) is recommended, although in some cases, bleomycin may be omitted due to its significant pulmonary toxicity. Prognosis has significantly improved with platinum-based chemotherapy.
- Ninety percent of patients with germ cell tumors who experience a **recurrence** will do so in the first 2 years after therapy. If initially treated with surgery alone, BEP chemotherapy can be used. Patients who initially received chemotherapy can be treated with a platinum-based agent.

## SEX CORD–STROMAL OVARIAN TUMORS

**Sex cord–stromal tumors** are derived from the sex cords and mesenchyme of the embryonic gonad and account for 5% to 8% of all ovarian neoplasms (Table 48-8). Most of these tumors are hormonally active. Types include the following: granulosa–stromal cell, Sertoli-Leydig, sex cord tumor, and gynandroblastoma.

## Granulosa Cell Tumor

- **Incidence:** The granulosa cell tumor is the most common malignant sex cord–stromal tumor, accounting for 70% of cases. Adult granulosa cell tumors occur primarily in the perimenopausal years, with a mean age of 52 years at presentation. Two forms exist: an adult form (95%) and a much rarer juvenile form (5%). The tumor is bilateral in <10% of cases.
- **Diagnosis and presentation:** In the majority of cases, tumors secrete estrogen and inhibin. Histologically, **Call-Exner bodies** are seen. Patients may present with abnormal vaginal bleeding, abdominal distention, pain, or a mass, usually >10 cm in diameter. Granulosa cell tumors are characteristically hemorrhagic and can present with a hemoperitoneum.
  - The incidence of concurrent endometrial hyperplasia is over 50%, and the incidence of concurrent endometrial adenocarcinoma ranges from 3% to 27%, demonstrating the importance of endometrial biopsy when the diagnosis of granulosa cell tumor is made. The majority (90%) of affected patients present with stage I disease, mainly because the hormonal effects of the tumor cause symptoms early in the disease. In juvenile type, patients present with pseudoprecocious puberty and have elevated serum estradiol.
- **Treatment:** Surgery alone is usually sufficient treatment only for stage IA or IB disease. For all other stages, platinum-based chemotherapy is recommended. Carboplatin and paclitaxel has been increasingly used; however, regimens used for germ cell tumors (BEP) can also be considered. Radiation and/or chemotherapy can be used to treat recurrent disease. If the patient desires to maintain fertility, a unilateral salpingo-oophorectomy is adequate for treating stage IA tumors, and surgical staging should also be performed. With completion of childbearing, a total abdominal hysterectomy and bilateral salpingo-oophorectomy should be performed. If the uterus is left in situ, the patient should undergo dilation and curettage to rule out endometrial hyperplasia or adenocarcinoma. Chemotherapy after surgery has not been shown to reduce the recurrence risk.
- **Prognosis and survival:** Granulosa cell tumors have a propensity for late recurrence, which has been reported as long as 30 years after treatment of the primary tumor. The 10-year and 20-year survival rates are 90% and 75%, respectively.

## Sertoli-Leydig Cell Tumor

- **Incidence:** Sertoli-Leydig cell tumors account for only 0.2% of ovarian neoplasms. The average age at diagnosis is 25 years. These tumors are most frequently low-grade malignancies, and nearly all patients (97%) present with stage I disease.
- **Diagnosis and presentation:** Sertoli-Leydig cell tumors often produce androgens. Patients present with virilization (30% to 50%), menstrual disorders, and symptoms related to an abdominal mass. The average size of these tumors is about 16 cm. They may produce testosterone, androstenedione, or AFP.
- **Treatment:** In young patients, unilateral salpingo-oophorectomy with staging may be performed to preserve fertility. In older patients, a total abdominal hysterectomy and bilateral salpingo-oophorectomy should be performed as well. Treatment of those with higher stage and/or grade typically includes chemotherapy.
- **Prognosis and survival:** Prognosis is related to stage and histologic grade. The 5-year survival rate is 70% to 90%.

## SPECIAL CONSIDERATIONS IN OVARIAN CANCER

- **Metastatic tumors** account for 5% to 20% of ovarian malignancies and are often, but not always, bilateral.
- **Gastrointestinal tract tumors** are the most likely to metastasize to the ovary. Krukenberg tumors of the stomach are usually bilateral and account for 30% to 40% of metastatic tumors to the ovary. These tumors are characterized histologically by signet ring cells, in which the nucleus is flattened against the cell wall by the accumulation of cytoplasmic mucin. In postmenopausal women who undergo evaluation for an adnexal mass, metastatic colon cancer should be ruled out, using colonoscopy if possible.
- **Breast cancer** is the second most likely cancer to metastasize to the ovary.
- **Lymphomas** can also metastasize to the ovary. Burkitt lymphoma may affect children or young adults. Rarely, ovarian lesions are the primary manifestation of disease in lymphoma patients.
- **Metastatic gynecologic tumors** may involve the ovaries. Fallopian tube cancer is the most common malignancy to metastasize to the ovaries and occurs by direct extension. Cervical cancer very rarely spreads to the ovaries without other sites of metastasis. Endometrial cancer may metastasize to the ovaries; however, synchronous endometrioid adenocarcinoma, primary to both the ovary and the endometrium, can also occur.
- Ovarian carcinosarcomas, also known as **malignant mixed mesodermal tumors of the ovary**, are extremely rare. These lesions are very aggressive, and treatment consists of surgical resection followed by combination chemotherapy. They are associated with a low response to treatment and overall poor outcome.
- **Ovarian tumors during pregnancy** are very rare. The incidence of an adnexal mass during pregnancy is approximately 1 in 800. The majority of adnexal masses discovered during the first trimester resolve by the second trimester. However, approximately 1% to 6% of these masses are malignant.
  - Germ cell tumors (primarily dysgerminoma) account for approximately 45% of ovarian malignancies diagnosed in pregnancy.
  - Masses are usually diagnosed during routine ultrasonography or at the time of cesarean section. The majority of patients (74%) are diagnosed with stage I disease.
  - Early-stage disease can be treated with conservative surgery in the second trimester of pregnancy, usually with good maternal and fetal outcomes. Late-stage and high-grade disease should be treated aggressively after appropriate counseling of the patient.

## SUGGESTED READINGS

Armstrong DK, Bundy B, Wenzel L, et al; Gynecologic Oncology Group. Intraperitoneal cisplatin and paclitaxel in ovarian cancer. *N Engl J Med* 2006;354:34–43.

Burger RA, Brady MF, Bookman MA, et al; Gynecologic Oncology Group. Incorporation of bevacizumab in the primary treatment of ovarian cancer. *N Engl J Med* 2011;365:2473–2483.

Hoskins WJ, Perez CA, Young RC, eds. *Principles and Practice of Gynecologic Oncology*, 4th ed. Philadelphia, PA: Lippincott Williams & Wilkins, 2005.

Kauff ND, Domchek SM, Friebel TM, et al. Risk-reducing salpingo-oophorectomy for the prevention of BRCA1- and BRCA2-associated breast and gynecologic cancer: a multicenter, prospective study. *J Clin Oncol* 2008;26(8):1331–1337.

Kurman RJ, Shih IeM. The origin and pathogenesis of epithelial ovarian cancer—a proposed unifying theory. *Am J Surg Pathol* 2010 34(3):433–443.

Vergote I, Trope CG, Amant F, et al; European Organization for Research and Treatment of Cancer-Gynaecological Cancer Group; NCIC Clinical Trials Group. Neoadjuvant chemotherapy or primary surgery in stage IIIC or IV ovarian cancer. *N Engl J Med* 2010;363(10):943–953.

# 49 Gestational Trophoblastic Disease

Lauren Cobb and Robert L. Giuntoli II

**Gestational trophoblastic disease (GTD)** is a heterogeneous group of interrelated but distinct neoplasms derived from the trophoblastic cells of the placenta. Lesions range from the premalignant complete and partial hydatidiform moles to the malignant invasive mole, choriocarcinoma, placental site trophoblastic tumor (PSTT), and epithelioid trophoblastic tumor (ETT). Most women with GTD can be cured with their fertility preserved.

## EPIDEMIOLOGY OF GESTATIONAL TROPHOBLASTIC DISEASE AND TYPES OF TROPHOBLASTIC CELLS

- **Incidence of GTD** varies widely throughout the world, with the highest rates reported in Asia, Africa, and Latin America.
- In the United States, hydatidiform moles are observed in 1 in 600 therapeutic abortions and 1 in 1,000 to 1,200 pregnancies. Approximately 20% of patients require treatment for malignant sequelae after evacuation of hydatidiform mole.
- Gestational choriocarcinoma, by comparison, occurs in about 1 in 20,000 to 40,000 pregnancies.
- Although much less common than hydatidiform mole or choriocarcinoma, PSTT and ETT can develop after any type of pregnancy.

### Risk Factors for Gestational Trophoblastic Disease
- Risks for GTD include:
  - **Extremes of reproductive age:** Women older than age 40 years have a 5.2-fold increased risk, whereas women younger than age 20 years have a 1.5-fold increased risk. Persistent GTD occurs more frequently in older patients.
  - **History of previous hydatidiform mole:** The risk of a subsequent hydatidiform mole rises by 10- to 20-fold. With two previous molar pregnancies, the risk multiplies by 40-fold. Conversely, term pregnancies and live births produce a protective effect.
  - Obstetric **history of spontaneous abortions** doubles the risk of molar gestation.
  - **Race:** Asians and Latin Americans demonstrate a higher risk of being diagnosed with GTD, whereas North Americans and Europeans have lower risk.
  - **Low socioeconomic status** and **dietary factors** such as vitamin A deficiency and low carotene intake may be associated, as well as **cigarette smoking** and **oral contraceptive use**. However, these associations are weak and not demonstrated consistently across all studies.

### Types of Cells and Hormone Secretion
- Trophoblasts are specialized cells of the early blastocyst that play a role in implantation of the embryo and will eventually form the placenta.

643

- Three types of placental trophoblastic cells have been identified: cytotrophoblast, syncytiotrophoblast, and intermediate trophoblast.
- **Cytotrophoblasts** comprise the inner layer of the trophoblast. They are primitive trophoblastic cells that are polygonal to oval in shape. They exhibit a single nucleus and clearly defined borders. Mitotic activity is evident, as these cells behave like stem cells. Implantation of the embryo is dependent on functioning cytotrophoblasts.
  - Cytotrophoblasts do not produce either human chorionic gonadotropin (hCG) or human placental lactogen (hPL).
- **Syncytiotrophoblasts** comprise the outer layer of the trophoblast. They are well-differentiated cells that interface with the maternal circulation and produce most of the placental hormones. No mitotic activity is evident.
  - Syncytiotrophoblasts demonstrate **hCG** production at 12 days of gestation. Secretion rapidly increases and peaks by 8 to 10 weeks, with a decline thereafter. By 40 weeks, hCG is present only focally in syncytiotrophoblasts. At 12 days, **hPL** is also present in syncytiotrophoblasts. Production continues to rise throughout pregnancy.
- **Intermediate trophoblasts** show infiltrative growth into decidua, myometrium, and blood vessels and in a normal pregnancy, they anchor the placenta to maternal tissue. Intermediate trophoblasts characteristically invade the wall of large vascular channels until the wall is completely replaced. Intermediate trophoblasts are the predominant cells of PSTT and exaggerated placental sites.
  - As early as 12 days after conception, **hCG** and **hPL** are present focally in intermediate trophoblasts. However, at 6 weeks, hCG production disappears, whereas secretion of hPL peaks at 11 to 15 weeks' gestation.

## CLASSIFICATION OF GESTATIONAL TROPHOBLASTIC DISEASE

Gestational trophoblastic neoplasms are unique among human neoplastic disorders because they are genetically related to fetal tissues. The molecular pathogenesis of these tumors is an area of active research interest.

### Hydatidiform Mole

- In both partial and complete hydatidiform moles, the placental villi become edematous, forming small grape-like structures. Despite the cytogenetic, pathologic, and clinical differences in these disease processes (Table 49-1), the management of patients is similar.
- Ultrasound establishes the diagnosis, identifying a mixed echogenic pattern as villi and blood clots replace normal placental tissue. Medical complications occur in approximately 25% of patients, being more prominent in those with uterine enlargement >14 to 16 weeks' gestational size.

#### Complete Mole

- **Clinical findings**
  - Presentation is between 11 and 25 weeks' gestation, with an average gestational age of 16 weeks.
  - Vaginal bleeding is the most common presenting symptom, occurring in 97% of cases.
  - Uterine size is often greater than expected for gestational age; however, in approximately one third of patients, the uterus is small for gestational dates. Ovarian enlargement caused by theca lutein cysts occurs in 25% to 35% of cases.

| TABLE 49-1 | Comparison of Complete versus Partial Hydatidiform Mole | |
|---|---|---|
| | **Complete** | **Partial** |
| Karyotype | Most commonly 46,XX or 46,XY | Most commonly 69,XXX or 69,XXY |
| Uterine size | | |
|   Large for gestational age | 33% | 10% |
|   Small for gestational age | 33% | 65% |
| Diagnosis by ultrasonography | Common | Rare |
| Theca lutein cysts | 25%–35% | Rare |
| β-hCG (mIU/mL) | >50,000 | <50,000 |
| Malignant potential | 15%–25% | <5% |
| Metastatic disease | <5% | <1% |

Adapted from Soper JT. Gestational trophoblastic disease. *Obstet Gynecol* 2006;108(1):176–187.

- Levels of β-hCG are generally above 50,000 mIU/mL.
- Severe hyperemesis and pregnancy-induced hypertension can develop in up to 25% of women, with hyperthyroidism in 7% of cases (hCG has weak thyroid-stimulating activity secondary to some homology between the beta subunits of thyroid-stimulating hormone and hCG).
- Ultrasonography often, but not always, shows a classic "snowstorm" appearance.
- **Pathologic features**
  - Gross findings include massively enlarged, edematous villi that give the classic grape-like appearance to the placenta and lack embryonic tissue.
  - Microscopic examination shows hydropic swelling in the majority of villi, accompanied by a variable degree of trophoblastic proliferation. Complete moles have widespread, diffuse immunostaining for hCG; moderately diffuse staining for hPL; and focal staining for placental alkaline phosphatase (PLAP).
- **Chromosomal abnormalities**
  - Most complete moles are diploid, with a 46,XX karyotype; rare examples of triploid or tetraploid moles have been reported.
  - In most cases, all of the chromosomal complements are paternally derived. The XX genotype typically results from duplication of a haploid sperm pronucleus in an empty ovum. Three percent to 13% of complete moles have a 46,XY chromosome complement, presumably as a result of dispermy, in which an empty ovum is fertilized by two sperm pronuclei.

*Incomplete Mole*

- **Clinical findings**
  - Commonly, patients present between 9 and 34 weeks' gestation.
  - These tumors are consistently associated with embryonic/fetal tissue.
  - Patients report abnormal uterine bleeding in about 75% of cases. A clinical diagnosis of a missed or spontaneous abortion is made in 91% of women with incomplete molar pregnancy.
  - Uterine size is generally small for gestational dates; excessive uterine size is observed in less than 10% of patients.

- Serum hCG level is in the normal or low range for gestational age.
- Preeclampsia occurs with lower incidence (2.5%) and presents much later with a partial mole than with a complete mole but can be equally severe.
- **Pathologic features**
  - Gross findings reveal fetal tissue in nearly all instances, although its discovery may require careful examination because early fetal death normally takes place (i.e., 8 to 9 weeks' gestational age).
  - Microscopic examination finds two populations of chorionic villi: one of normal size and the other grossly hydropic. Partial moles show focal to moderate immunostaining for hCG and diffuse staining for hPL and PLAP.
- **Chromosomal abnormalities**
  - Karyotype of partial moles most frequently shows triploidy (i.e., 69 chromosomes), with two paternal and one maternal chromosome complement.
  - The chromosomal complement is XXY in 70% of cases, XXX in 27% of cases, and XYY in 3% of cases. The abnormal conceptus in these cases arises from the fertilization of an egg with a haploid set of chromosomes either by two sperm, each with a set of haploid chromosomes, or by a single sperm with a diploid 46,XY complement.

*Invasive Mole*

- **Invasive mole** is an important complication of hydatidiform mole, representing 70% to 90% of cases of persistent GTD. Other common names include chorioadenoma destruens, penetrating mole, malignant mole, or molar destruens.
- **Pathologic features**
  - Histologically, hydropic chorionic villi migrate into the myometrium, vascular spaces, or outside of the pelvis in 20% of cases to the vagina, perineum, or lungs.
  - Grossly, invasive moles present as erosive, hemorrhagic lesions extending from the uterine cavity into the myometrium. Metastasis can range from superficial penetration to extension through the uterine wall, with subsequent perforation and life-threatening hemorrhage. Molar vesicles are often apparent.
  - Microscopically, the diagnostic feature of invasive mole is the presence of molar villi and trophoblast within the myometrium or at an extrauterine site. Lesions at distant sites are usually composed of *molar villi confined within blood vessels, without invasion into adjacent tissue.*

## Choriocarcinoma

- **Gestational choriocarcinoma** is a highly malignant epithelial tumor that can be associated with any type of gestational event, most often a complete hydatidiform mole. In the United States, choriocarcinoma occurs in 1 in 20,000 to 40,000 pregnancies. Approximately 25% of gestational choriocarcinomas develop after term pregnancies, 50% after molar gestations, and 25% after abortion or ectopic pregnancies. Early systemic hematogenous metastasis often takes place.
- **Clinical findings**
  - Eighty percent of patients with extrauterine disease show pulmonary metastases, whereas approximately 30% demonstrate extension to the vagina. Ten percent of women also exhibit liver and central nervous system involvement.
- **Pathologic features**
  - On gross examination, these tumors appear as dark red, hemorrhagic masses with shaggy, irregular surfaces. Metastatic lesions outside the uterus are well circumscribed.

On microscopic examination, sheets of syncytiotrophoblasts and cytotrophoblasts are seen *without chorionic villi, invading surrounding tissue or permeating vascular spaces.*

## Placental Site and Epithelioid Trophoblastic Tumor

- **PSTT** and **ETT** are rare gestational trophoblastic neoplasms, accounting for 1% of persistent GTD. Both can develop long after prior gestational events. Most cases of PSTT and ETT are benign, especially those tumors that are confined to the uterus, but about 15% to 25% of cases are malignant and present with local invasion and distant metastasis.
- **Clinical features**
  - PSTTs and ETTs usually remain confined to the uterus and metastasize late. In some cases, recurrent or metastatic PSTT/ETTs can occur in patients long after initial treatment.
  - These tumors typically produce only small amounts of β-hCG, despite a large tumor burden. Serum hPL, produced by the intermediate trophoblasts that predominate, serves as a better marker for disease progression or recurrence.
  - Approximately 15% of lesions metastasize to extrauterine sites (e.g., lungs, liver, abdominal cavity, and brain). In contrast to other trophoblastic tumors, these tumors are relatively insensitive to chemotherapy, and surgical excision is usually the best treatment modality.
- **Pathologic features**
  - By contrast to the normal implantation site, where invasion of the extravillous subtype of intermediate trophoblast is tightly regulated and confined to the inner third of the myometrium, tumor cells of PSTT and ETT are invasive and infiltrate deeply into the myometrium.
  - Although PSTT and ETT share similar clinical features, careful examination of tumor histology and gene expression patterns shows that PSTT and ETT are composed of different extravillous trophoblastic cells.
  - Gross lesions may be barely visible or may result in diffuse nodular enlargement of the myometrium. Most tumors are well circumscribed. Microscopically, invasion may extend to the uterine serosa and, in rare instances, extends to adnexal structures.

## DIAGNOSIS AND MANAGEMENT OF MOLAR PREGNANCY

- The **pathologic diagnosis** of hydatidiform mole is typically made following dilation and curettage (D&C) performed for an incomplete abortion or because of suspicion of hydatidiform mole based on clinical findings.
  - The following tests should be performed preoperatively:
    - Quantitative serum β-hCG level
    - Complete blood count
    - Prothrombin time, partial thromboplastin time
    - Comprehensive metabolic panel with renal and liver function tests
    - Blood type and screen
      - Rh-negative patients must be given Rh$_O$ (D) immunoglobulin (RhoGAM)
    - Chest radiograph
- The **primary treatment** for hydatidiform mole is suction D&C.
  - The following steps should be taken before suction D&C:
    - Stabilization of medical complications
    - Full operating room support in a hospital setting
    - Large-bore intravenous (IV) access with possible central line monitoring

○ Induction of regional or general anesthesia

○ Initiation of oxytocin drip (during D&C)

- Uterine evacuation is accomplished with the largest cannula that can be safely introduced through the cervix. IV oxytocin is begun after the cervix is dilated and suction is initiated and is continued postoperatively for several hours.
- Postevacuation **follow-up** should include:
  - β-hCG level 48 hours after evacuation
  - Weekly β-hCG level until three consecutive negative results, then monthly until results are negative for 6 consecutive months (Fig. 49-1)
  - Regular pelvic examinations to monitor involution of pelvic organs and for detection of metastasis
  - Repeat chest radiograph if the β-hCG titer plateaus or rises.
  - Effective contraception for the entire interval of β-hCG follow-up testing. Preventing pregnancy is crucial, as a rising β-hCG titer due to a normal pregnancy cannot be distinguished from persistent GTD.
  - Because of increased risk (1% to 2%) of a second mole in subsequent pregnancies, all future pregnancies should be evaluated by ultrasonography early in their course.
- **Complications** include anemia, infection, hyperthyroidism, pregnancy-induced hypertension or preeclampsia, and theca lutein cysts.

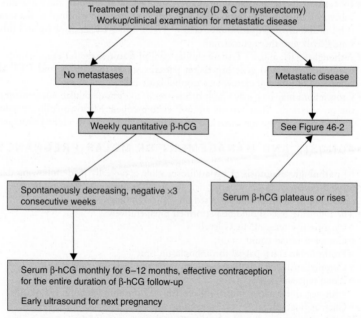

**Figure 49-1.** Follow-up of molar pregnancy. D&C, dilation and curettage; β-hCG, beta-human chorionic gonadotropin. (Adapted from American College of Obstetricians and Gynecologists Committee on Practice Bulletins—Gynecology. ACOG practice bulletin no. 53: diagnosis and treatment of gestational trophoblastic disease. *Obstet Gynecol* 2004;103:1365–1377.)

# DIAGNOSIS AND MANAGEMENT OF PERSISTENT GESTATIONAL TROPHOBLASTIC DISEASE

**Persistent GTD** includes invasive mole, choriocarcinoma, and PSTT. Persistent disease occurs in approximately 20% of cases of complete mole; approximately 15% develop invasive GTD and <5% develop metastatic GTD.

- Over 95% of malignant sequelae occur within 6 months after surgical evacuation. If β-hCG levels plateau or rise, immediate evaluation is required, and treatment for persistent GTD may be indicated.
- **Predictors** for persistent GTD include large-for-dates uterus, ovarian enlargement due to theca lutein cysts, recurrent molar pregnancy, uterine subinvolution, advanced maternal age, significantly elevated β-hCG level, and acute pulmonary compromise. The risk of persistent GTD is considerably lower for partial moles than for complete moles.

## Diagnosis of Persistent Gestational Trophoblastic Disease

- A plateau or rise in β-hCG titers is typically the first indication of persistent GTD. Patients may also present with recurrent vaginal bleeding after D&C.
- Other presenting signs and symptoms are related to the anatomic sites involved with metastatic disease: chest pain, hemoptysis, or persistent cough with pulmonary involvement; bleeding from vaginal extensions; and focal neurologic deficits from cerebral hemorrhage.
- Rarely, the diagnosis of persistent GTD is made via histologic evidence of choriocarcinoma. Given the risk of hemorrhage associated with biopsy, pathologic specimens are usually not obtained.
- **Criteria** for persistent GTD include:
  - hCG level plateau of four measurements ±10% recorded over a 3-week duration (days 1, 7, 14, and 21)
  - hCG level increase of >10% for three measurements over a 2-week duration (days 1, 7, and 14)
  - Detectable hCG for >6 months after molar evacuation
  - Histologic diagnosis of choriocarcinoma
- The diagnosis of persistent GTD is based on the quantitative pattern of serum β-hCG level, D&C findings, presence of metastatic disease, and histology. Both invasive mole and choriocarcinoma are typically detected by a plateau or elevation in the β-hCG titer. It may not be possible to distinguish clinically between these lesions.
  - Obtaining a tissue diagnosis is not necessary (because the treatment for both is the same) and may be associated with significant hemorrhage. PSTTs and ETTs typically demonstrate low β-hCG levels; however, serum hPL level is often elevated and may be a more useful serologic marker.
- All patients suspected of having persistent GTD should undergo the following workup to evaluate the extent of disease (Fig. 49-2):
  - Complete history and physical examination
  - Serum β-hCG level, possibly serum hPL level
  - Liver, thyroid, and renal function tests
  - Complete blood count
  - Pelvic ultrasonography to evaluate for intrauterine pregnancy
  - Chest radiograph
  - Computed tomography of pelvis, abdomen, and brain
  - Stool guaiac test

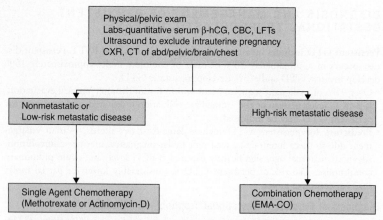

**Figure 49-2.** Management of persistent GTD. β-hCG, beta-human chorionic gonadotropin; CBC, complete blood count; LFT, liver function test; CXR, chest radiograph; CT, computed tomography; EMA-CO, etoposide, methotrexate, actinomycin D, cyclophosphamide (Cytoxan), and vincristine sulphate. (Adapted from American College of Obstetricians and Gynecologists Committee on Practice Bulletins—Gynecology. ACOG practice bulletin no. 53: diagnosis and treatment of gestational trophoblastic disease. *Obstet Gynecol* 2004;103:1365–1377.)

## Treatment of Persistent Gestational Trophoblastic Disease

- **Treatment** depends on the stage of disease (Table 49-2) and risk assessment based on the World Health Organization (WHO) prognostic scoring system (Table 49-3).

*Nonmetastatic Disease and Low-Risk Metastatic Disease*

- Disease falls into the category of low risk based on a WHO prognostic score ≤6.
- **Primary treatment** is with single-agent chemotherapy with either methotrexate (MTX) or actinomycin D.
  - MTX is alternated with folinic acid in most institutions and given with a fixed window of 7 to 14 days between courses. Some evidence suggests that dactinomycin may provide slightly higher remission rates than MTX but is

| TABLE 49-2 | International Federation of Gynecology and Obstetrics Staging System for Gestational Trophoblastic Neoplasia |
|---|---|

| Stage | Description |
|---|---|
| I | Strictly confined to uterus |
| II | Extension outside uterus but limited to pelvic structures |
| III | Extension to lungs |
| IV | All other metastatic sites |

Each stage is divided into high or low risk using the World Health Organization prognostic scoring index. From FIGO Committee on Gynecologic Oncology. Current FIGO staging for cancer of the vagina, fallopian tube, ovary, and gestational trophoblastic neoplasia. *Int J Gynecol Obstet* 2009;105:3–4.

| TABLE 49-3 | International Federation of Gynecology and Obstetrics/ World Health Organization Prognostic Scoring Index for Gestational Trophoblastic Neoplasia | | | |
|---|---|---|---|---|
| Score | 0 | 1 | 2 | 4 |
| Age | <40 yr | ≥40 yr | — | — |
| Antecedent pregnancy | Mole | Abortion | Term | — |
| Time since pregnancy | <4 mo | 4–6 mo | 7–12 mo | >12 mo |
| Initial hCG levels (mIU/mL) | <1,000 | 1,000–9,999 | 10,000–99,999 | ≥100,000 |
| Largest tumor size (in cm, including uterus) | <3 | 3–4 | 5 or more | — |
| Site of metastases | Lung, vagina | Spleen, kidney | Gastrointestinal tract | Brain, liver |
| Number of metastases | 0 | 1–4 | 5–8 | >8 |
| Prior failed chemotherapy | None | | Single drug | ≥2 drugs |

The total score is obtained by adding the scores for individual prognostic factors. Scores from 0 to 6 are categorized as low risk, whereas a score of 7 or higher is high risk.

Adapted from Kohorn EI. The new FIGO 2000 staging and risk factor scoring system for gestational trophoblastic disease: description and clinical assessment. *Int J Gynecol Cancer* 2001;11:73–77.

associated with more toxicity. Pulsed dactinomycin (higher dose administered every 2 weeks) generally is used more frequently than the 5-day regimen.

- Systemic treatments are administered until hCG levels normalize for two or more consecutive assessments. An additional one to three cycles of consolidation chemotherapy can be given after a negative serum hCG is obtained.
- If hCG titers plateau or rise after two courses, the patient is considered resistant to that particular chemotherapeutic agent, and the alternative single-agent chemotherapy is promptly instituted. If no response is seen after both single agents, then combination chemotherapy is required.
- For patients who have completed childbearing, hysterectomy should be considered for refractory disease confined to the uterus.
- For patients with stage I or II PSTT, the primary treatment is hysterectomy, especially given the wide variation in response of PSTT to chemotherapy.
- Patients with nonmetastatic disease are less likely to require second-line therapy than patients with low-risk metastatic disease. Overall, 85% to 95% of patients can be cured with single-agent chemotherapy without hysterectomy. The cure rate for patients with low-risk disease approaches 100% with recurrence rates <5%.

*High-Risk Metastatic Disease*

- Disease may be deemed high risk based on a WHO prognostic score ≥7.
- For patients with high-risk metastatic disease, the recommended **treatment** is combination chemotherapy with etoposide, MTX, actinomycin D, cyclophosphamide (Cytoxan), and vincristine sulfate (EMA-CO). Recurrent or refractory disease,

particularly in cases of chemoresistant PSTT and ETT, may respond better to platinum–etoposide combinations such as etoposide, methotrexate, actinomycin, and cisplatinum (EMA-EP).

- EMA-CO is administered every 2 weeks until remission (negative hCG levels are achieved in 3 consecutive weeks) or until intolerable side effects occur. After the normalization of hCG levels, an additional three courses should be given as consolidation therapy.
- For patients with **complications** of metastatic disease specific to the organ involved, the following interventions can be instituted:
  - **Vaginal involvement:** These lesions can bleed profusely. Bleeding can be controlled with packing for 24 hours. Prompt radiation to the affected region may provide further hemostasis. Although infrequently used, embolization of the pelvic vessels may also be implemented in women with life-threatening or recurrent hemorrhage.
  - **Pulmonary metastases:** These lesions usually respond to chemotherapy. Occasionally, thoracotomy is required to remove a persistent viable tumor nodule. Not all chest lesions clear radiographically due to scarring and fibrosis from the injury and healing process.
  - **Hepatic lesions:** If these lesions fail to respond to systemic chemotherapy, other options include hepatic arterial infusion of chemotherapy or partial hepatic resection to remove resistant tumor. These lesions are usually hypervascular and prone to hemorrhage if biopsied.
  - **Cerebral metastases:** Whole brain irradiation (approximately 3,000 cGy) is initiated as soon as the extent of disease is confirmed. Radiation and chemotherapy reduce the risk of spontaneous cerebral hemorrhage. However, concurrent whole brain radiation and chemotherapy increase treatment-related toxicity, especially leukoencephalopathy (radiographic diffuse white matter changes with symptoms of lethargy, seizures, and dysarthria and rarely ataxia, dementia, memory loss, and death). Alternatively, cerebral metastases can be treated with high-dose EMA-CO with or without intrathecal MTX.
  - **Extensive uterine disease:** Hysterectomy is indicated in cases with large intra-uterine tumor burden, infection, or hemorrhage.
- Following EMA-CO, the overall remission rate is 80% to 90%. Approximately 25% of high-risk patients demonstrate incomplete responses to first-line therapy and relapse. When brain metastases are present, the overall remission rate drops to 50% to 60%. Higher failure rates are also seen with stage IV disease, greater than eight metastatic lesions, and a history of previous chemotherapy.
- For patients with refractory or recurrent disease after EMA-CO treatment, salvage therapies often consist of platinum–etoposide combinations. Bleomycin and ifosfamide (etoposide, ifosfamide, and cisplatin [VIP]; ifosfamide, carboplatin, and etoposide [ICE]) have also been used with limited success. Experimental protocols may be investigated in these patients.

## SUGGESTED READINGS

Berkowitz RS, Goldstein DP. Gestational trophoblastic disease. In Berek JS, ed. *Berek and Novak's Gynecology*, 15th ed. Philadelphia, PA: Lippincott Williams & Wilkins, 2012.

Hoffman BL, Schorge JO, Schaffer JI, et al, eds. Gestational trophoblastic disease. In *Williams Gynecology*, 2nd ed. New York, NY: McGraw-Hill, 2012.

# 50 Chemotherapy and Radiation Therapy

Sonia Dutta and Amanda Nickles Fader

- Treatment of gynecologic cancer typically requires a multidisciplinary and multitreatment approach involving a combination of surgery, **chemotherapy**, and **radiation therapy**. When more than one modality is used, they may be delivered sequentially or at the same time, as with chemoradiation or intraoperative radiation therapy. The sequence of treatment is characterized as "**primary**," referring to initial treatment; "**adjuvant**," referring to secondary treatment for micrometastatic disease after surgical management; "**neoadjuvant**," referring to induction chemotherapy, radiation therapy, or both administered before definitive therapy; and "**salvage**," referring to treatment at time of recurrence.

All methods used to treat gynecologic cancer can cause damage to normal tissue. Therefore, the governing principle of both chemotherapy and radiation therapy is to attain maximal therapeutic cytotoxic effects on cancer cells without extreme toxicity to normal tissues. Unfortunately, it is not always possible to obtain a therapeutic effect without temporarily or permanently altering the functions of other healthy cells, tissues, or organs. The term **therapeutic index** is the ratio of a toxic dose to the curative dose. An optimal treatment goal is to use chemotherapy agents and radiation doses that have a high therapeutic index.

## CELL CYCLE

- Tumor cells grow as a result of deregulation between proliferation and suppression. Our understanding of cancer cell kinetics and the classical cell cycle (Fig. 50-1) has led to the development of several chemotherapy drugs. There are both **cell cycle–specific chemotherapeutic agents** and **cell cycle–nonspecific chemotherapeutic agents**.
  - Cell cycle–specific agents depend on the proliferative capacity of the cell and the phase of the cell cycle for their action. They are effective against tumors with relatively long S phases and rapid proliferation rates.
  - Cell cycle–nonspecific drugs kill cells in all phases of the cell cycle and their effectiveness is not dependent on proliferative capacity. Radiation therapy is not cell cycle dependent.

## CHEMOTHERAPY

### Types of Chemotherapy

- Chemotherapeutic agents commonly used for the treatment of gynecologic cancer may be grouped into the following categories (Table 50-1):
  - **Alkylating agents** are cell cycle–nonspecific. They contain an alkyl group that forms a covalent bond with the DNA helix, preventing DNA duplication. They

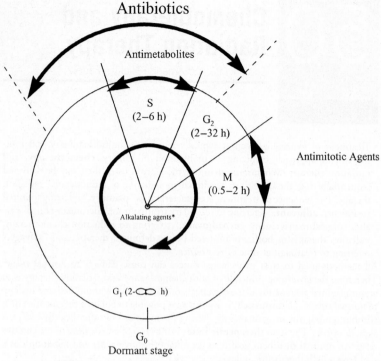

**Figure 50-1.** Phases of the cell cycle, relative time intervals, and sites of action of the various classes of antineoplastic agents. (From Trimble EL, Trimble CL, eds. *Cancer Obstetrics and Gynecology.* Philadelphia, PA: Lippincott Williams & Wilkins, 1999:60, with permission.)

also function by attaching to free guanine bases of DNA thereby prohibiting their action as templates for new DNA formation.

- **Antimetabolites** are similar in chemical structure to compounds required by normal and tumor cells for cell division. These antimetabolites may be incorporated into new nuclear material or combined with enzymes to inhibit cell division.
- **Plant alkaloids** are derived from various plants and trees, including the periwinkle plant (*Vinca rosea*), the mayapple (*Podophyllum peltatum*), and the Pacific yew (*Taxus brevifolia*). They bind to tubules, blocking microtubule formation, and interfering with spindle formation. This leads to the arrest of metaphase and inhibits mitosis.
- **Antitumor antibiotics** have many different modes of action, including increasing cell membrane permeability, inhibiting DNA and RNA syntheses, and blocking DNA replication.
- Biologics target known mutations to oncogenic signal transduction pathways specific to cancer cells. As cancer biology is further elucidated, increasing numbers of biologics are being discovered and tested.
- **Miscellaneous agents** have different modes of action than those previously mentioned.

| TABLE 50-1 | Chemotherapeutic Agents Frequently Used in Gynecologic Cancer and Their Most Common Toxicities |
|---|---|

| Chemotherapeutic Agent | Toxicity |
|---|---|
| **Alkylating agents** | |
| Cyclophosphamide (Cytoxan) | Myelosuppression (WBCs > platelets), hemorrhagic cystitis, bladder fibrosis, alopecia, hepatitis, amenorrhea |
| Ifosfamide | Myelosuppression, hemorrhagic cystitis, CNS dysfunction, renal toxicity, emetogenic |
| **Alkylating-like agents** | |
| Cis-dichlorodiaminoplatinum (Cisplatin) | Nephrotoxicity, emetogenic, tinnitus and hearing loss, myelosuppression, peripheral neuropathy characterized by paresthesia of the extremities<br>• Renal insufficiency is the major dose-limiting toxic effect causing elevations in BUN, serum creatinine, and serum uric acid levels within 2 wk of treatment. Irreversible damage can occur. Prevention with IV hydration and diuretics is important during treatment. A 24-hr creatinine clearance is measured to establish baseline renal function before treatment.<br>• Tinnitus or high-frequency hearing loss may be cumulative and possibly irreversible. Audiograms may be obtained before and during treatment to assess hearing loss. |
| Carboplatin | Less neuropathy, ototoxicity, and nephrotoxicity but more myelosuppression (platelets > WBC) than cisplatin |
| **Antitumor antibiotics** | |
| Actinomycin D (Dactinomycin) | Nausea and vomiting, skin necrosis, mucosal ulceration, myelosuppression, alopecia |
| Bleomycin sulfate | Pulmonary toxicity, fever, anaphylactic reactions, dermatologic reactions, mucositis, alopecia<br>• May cause significant ***pulmonary fibrosis***. Generally, both dose- and age-related but can be idiopathic. Pulmonary function tests are performed to assess baseline pulmonary capacity before the first dose is administered.<br>• Can cause anaphylaxis, skin reactions, fever, and chills. Because of the high incidence of allergic reactions, patients are given a test dose of 2–4 U intramuscularly before the first dose of drug. |

*(Continued)*

| TABLE 50-1 | Chemotherapeutic Agents Frequently Used in Gynecologic Cancer and Their Most Common Toxicities (Continued) |
|---|---|

| Chemotherapeutic Agent | Toxicity |
|---|---|
| Doxorubicin hydrochloride (Adriamycin) | Myelosuppression, cardiac toxicity, alopecia, mucosal ulcerations, emetogenic, cholestasis, hyperpigmentation<br><br>Irreversible cardiomyopathies that involve progressive congestive heart failure, pleural effusions, heart dilation, and venous congestion. These are generally cumulative; therefore, dosages are kept under the maximum. Multiple-gated acquisition (MUGA) scans are commonly obtained before treatment to obtain a baseline ejection fraction and may be repeated as necessary. |
| Liposomal doxorubicin (Doxil) | Myelosuppression, skin and mucosal toxicity, hand-foot syndrome |
| **Antimetabolites** | |
| 5-Fluorouracil (5-FU) | Myelosuppression, emetogenic, anorexia, alopecia, hyperpigmentation, mucosal ulceration, cardiotoxic (MI, angina, arrhythmia) |
| Methotrexate sodium (MTX) | Myelosuppression, mucosal ulceration (stomatitis and mucositis), hepatotoxicity, acute pulmonary infiltrates that respond to steroid therapy, emetogenic, alopecia, peripheral neuropathy |
| Gemcitabine hydrochloride (Gemzar) | Mild myelosuppression, flu-like syndrome, emetogenic |
| **Plant alkaloids** | |
| Vincristine sulfate (Oncovin) | Neurotoxicity (peripheral, central, and visceral neuropathies that are cumulative), alopecia, myelosuppression, cranial nerve palsies |
| Epipodophyllotoxin (etoposide, VP-16) | Myelosuppression, alopecia, hypotension, allergic reaction, emetogenic |
| Paclitaxel (Taxol) | Myelosuppression (WBC > platelets), alopecia, allergic reactions, cardiac arrhythmias, peripheral neuropathies, emetogenic<br><br>• Asymptomatic and transient bradycardia (40–60 beats/min), ventricular tachycardia, and atypical chest pain during infusion. These symptoms resolve with slowing of infusion. |

| TABLE 50-1 | Chemotherapeutic Agents Frequently Used in Gynecologic Cancer and Their Most Common Toxicities *(Continued)* |
|---|---|

| Chemotherapeutic Agent | Toxicity |
|---|---|
| | • Hypersensitivity reactions with characteristic bradycardia, diaphoresis, hypotension, cutaneous flushing, and abdominal pain. Premedications of diphenhydramine hydrochloride, dexamethasone, and ranitidine are given prophylactically. |
| Docetaxel (Taxotere) | Myelosuppression (neutropenia), hypersensitivity; cutaneous reactions, alopecia, mucosal ulcerations, paresthesias |
| **Biologics** | |
| Bevacizumab (Avastin)— monoclonal antibody, anti-VEGF | Hypertension, proteinuria, small risk of bowel perforations |
| Erlotinib, gefitinib— anti-EGFR | Skin rash, diarrhea |
| Rapamycin—anti-mTOR | Unknown side effects, still in clinical trials |
| **Miscellaneous** | |
| Topotecan hydrochloride (Hycamtin; topoisomerase 1 inhibitor) | Myelosuppression (WBC > platelets), mucosal ulcerations, emetogenic, paresthesias |

WBC, white blood cell; CNS, central nervous system; BUN, blood urea nitrogen; IV, intravenous; MI, myocardial infarction; VEGF, vascular endothelial growth factor; EGFR, epidermal growth factor receptor; mTOR, mammalian target of rapamycin.

## Common Side Effects of Chemotherapy

- Hematologic toxicity and myelosuppression is a dangerous effect of chemotherapy that varies in severity depending on the drug administered. A nadir in white cell, red cell, or platelet count is usually observed 7 to 14 days after drug administration. Most agents are readministered every 3 to 4 weeks if the patient has recovered from pancytopenia.
- **Neutropenia** is defined as an absolute neutrophil count (ANC) less than 500/mL. Recombinant human granulocyte colony-stimulating factor (G-CSF) (filgrastim, **Neupogen**) or pegylated filgrastim (Neulasta) is administered to at-risk patients or the cycle after neutropenia is diagnosed as prophylaxis against this reaction in subsequent cycles. Use of G-CSF is contraindicated during the actual administration of chemotherapy or during a neutropenic fever.
  - Neutropenic fever is a medical emergency, as these patients can quickly become septic and decompensate. Common causes of infection include enteric Gram-negative bacteria, Gram-positive bacteria (*Staphylococcus epidermidis*, *Staphylococcus aureus*, and diphtheroids), viruses (herpes simplex and herpes zoster), and

fungi (*Candida* and *Aspergillus* species), although often an offending agent is not identified. Infections are generally due to reduced integrity of the mucous membranes and skin during chemotherapy. Once fever (temperature greater than 38°C) is noted, broad-spectrum antibiotics with antipseudomonal coverage should be initiated immediately.

- **Anemia** can be treated acutely with blood transfusions. Long-term treatment may be accomplished with ferrous sulfate and erythropoietin-stimulating agents (e.g., epoetin α, Epogen, Procrit). The target is a hemoglobin level of 10 g/dL or hematocrit of 30%, although all of these interventions have potentially significant risks that must be considered against their benefits prior to their use.
- **Thrombocytopenia** is treated with platelet transfusion when the platelet count drops below 20,000/mL or if signs of spontaneous bleeding are evident. **Thrombopoietin** (e.g., oprelvekin [Neumega]) may also be given.
  - Gastrointestinal toxicity is commonly seen due to the direct action of chemotherapy on these cell types.
- **Nausea and vomiting** are the most common side effects of chemotherapy due to decreased intestinal motility. The severity and incidence of these symptoms vary greatly but the inability to effectively control them can result in patient refusal to carry out potentially curative treatment. Nausea and vomiting can be
  - *acute*—occurring during or immediately after chemotherapy administration,
  - *delayed*—occurring several days after chemotherapy administration, and
  - *anticipatory*—occurring before the administration of chemotherapy.
- The incidence and severity are related to the emetogenic potential of the drug, the dose, the route and time of day of administration, patient characteristics, and the combination of drugs used. Gastrointestinal obstruction must be considered if abdominal distention or obstipation is present.
- Antiemetic regimens including a combination of serotonin 5-HT3 receptor–blocking agents (e.g., **ondansetron**, **granisetron**), neurokinin receptor antagonists (e.g., aprepitant, fosaprepitant), and dexamethasone have been shown to be particularly effective in reducing acute and delayed emesis.
- **Diarrhea** may occur in association with chemotherapy and is typically not infectious; however, necrotizing enterocolitis must always be considered if diarrhea is watery, bloody, and associated with abdominal pain and fever.
- **Stomatitis and mucositis** occur most commonly following therapy with antimetabolites because these cells are naturally rapidly proliferating. Treatment is with either **Larry's solution** (three equal parts diphenhydramine hydrochloride elixir [Benadryl], magnesium and aluminum oral suspension [Maalox], and viscous lidocaine) or **nystatin** swish and swallow. Severe cases may require hospitalization for nutrition supplementation, intravenous (IV) hydration, and pain management.
- **Dehydration** may occur in the setting of emesis and diarrhea. Patients are encouraged to increase their fluid intake to prevent postchemotherapy dehydration, given the risk of secondary side effects, such as nephrotoxicity or electrolyte disturbances.
- **Hepatic toxicity** including transient elevations in transaminase and alkaline phosphatase levels may occur with chemotherapy. Cholangitis, hepatic necrosis, and hepatic veno-occlusive disease, although rare, must be considered.
- Common **dermatologic toxicities** are alopecia and photosensitivity. Extravasation of chemotherapeutic agents can additionally cause skin necrosis. Once identified, the infusion should be immediately stopped and the patient given topical steroids and hyaluronidase or sodium thiosulfate.

- Acute allergic or infusion reactions may occur with the use of chemotherapeutic agents. For agents that cause **hypersensitivity**, such as paclitaxel, premedication with diphenhydramine hydrochloride, dexamethasone, and ranitidine are given. For agents that may cause **anaphylaxis**, such as bleomycin, a test dose should be performed prior to administration. Platinums are notorious for causing an allergy after several doses of the medication has been administered, and prompt recognition of anaphylaxis is key.

- **Neurologic side effects** of chemotherapy include damage to peripheral nerves as well as subtle changes in cognitive function. Peripheral nerve damage may range from transient paresthesias, such as a "pins-and-needles" sensation, to chronic loss of sensitivity and fine motor control. Changes in cognitive function are generally perceived as difficulties with concentration and short-term memory. To date, there are no interventions proven to prevent or ameliorate this neurologic damage.

- **Fatigue** is commonly reported. The mechanisms causing fatigue are not well understood; however, correction of anemia, good sleep hygiene, and regular exercise can help reduce symptoms.

- Pulmonary toxicity in the form of interstitial pneumonitis with pulmonary fibrosis is classically seen with bleomycin. Once diagnosed, the medication should be stopped and steroids started.

- Cardiac toxicity is rare with chemotherapy because myocytes do not readily divide. However, doxorubicin is classically associated with cardiomyopathy. Additionally, use of bevacizumab (Avastin) has been associated with the development of hypertension.

- Genitourinary toxicity is typically seen in the form of renal tubular toxicity with platinums, especially cisplatin.

- Additionally, **hemorrhagic cystitis** can occur with ifosfamide and cyclophosphamide treatment. Preventive measures include hydration and administration of diuretics. Treatment includes dosage reduction or discontinuation of the drug. **Mesna**, a uroprotector, is administered simultaneously with ifosfamide to protect against bladder toxicity. Mesna acts to detoxify *acrolein*, the common metabolite of both cyclophosphamide and ifosfamide.

## RADIATION THERAPY

- X-rays or gamma rays destroy tumor and normal cells by creation of oxygen-free radicals and a multitude of other reactions ultimately resulting in DNA and cell membrane injury.

- The absorption of energy by tissue is measured in rads. One gray (Gy) is 100 rad and 1 centigray (cGy) is 1 rad. The **inverse square law** states that the dose of radiation at a given point is inversely proportional to the square of the distance from the source of radiation.

### Clinical Radiation Sources

- **Teletherapy** is external beam radiation. During external beam radiation, the patient may be in prone or supine position. The usual total dose to the pelvis ranges from 4,000 to 5,000 cGy given in daily fractions of 180 to 200 cGy over 5 weeks.

- **Brachytherapy** involves placement of a radiation device either within or close to the target tumor volume (i.e., interstitial and intracavitary irradiation); the radiation dose to the tissue is determined largely by the inverse square law.

- The radiation applicators are called **intrauterine tandems** and **ovoids/colpostats**. Intrauterine tandems are placed in the uterine cavity while the patient is under anesthesia and position is confirmed with radiographic studies. Vaginal ovoids are designed for placement in the vaginal vault and support the position of the tandem but they may also be loaded with radioactive sources themselves.

- Vaginal, endometrial, and cervical cancers may be treated by either high- or low-dose-rate intracavitary implants. Replacing low-dose-rate (usually **cesium**) with high-dose-rate intracavitary brachytherapy treatments (usually **iridium-192**) is becoming increasingly common in the United States and Europe. High-dose-rate applications do not require anesthesia nor operating room time and radiation exposure is 10 to 20 minutes for each outpatient visit (usually four to six visits are required), whereas use of low-dose-rate cesium implants require hospitalization for 48 to 72 hours.

- **Interstitial implants** are another form of brachytherapy configured as radioactive wires or seeds and placed directly within tissues. Hollow guide needles are inserted in a geometric pattern to deliver a relatively uniform dose of radiation to a target tumor volume. After the position of the guide needles is confirmed, they can be threaded with the radioactive sources and the hollow guides removed. Interstitial implants are sometimes used in the treatment of locally advanced cervical cancer or for women with pelvic recurrences of endometrial or cervical cancer.

## Common Side Effects of Radiation Therapy

- Dermatologic toxicity such as an acute skin reaction typically becomes evident by the third week of therapy. The reaction is characterized by erythema, desquamation, and pruritus and should resolve completely within 3 weeks of the end of treatment. Topical corticosteroids or moisturizing creams may be applied several times a day for symptomatic relief and to promote healing. If the reaction worsens, treatment is stopped and zinc oxide or silver sulfadiazine is applied to the affected area. The perineum is at greater risk for skin breakdown because of its increased warmth, moisture, and lack of ventilation. Therefore, patients should be instructed to keep the perineal area clean and dry. Additionally, late subcutaneous fibrosis can develop, especially with doses higher than 6,500 cGy.

- **Hematologic toxicity** is dependent on the volume of marrow irradiated and the total radiation dose. In adults, 40% of active marrow is in the pelvis, 25% is in the vertebral column, and 20% is in the ribs and skull. Extensive radiation to these sites may result in the need for blood product transfusions or administration of erythropoietin to support the patient's hematologic function during therapy.

- **Gastrointestinal toxicity** may be either acute or chronic. Nausea, vomiting, and diarrhea commonly occur 2 to 6 hours after abdominal or pelvic irradiation. Supportive therapy with hydration and administration of antiemetics and antidiarrheals are used for first-line therapy. In patients with severe diarrhea, opiates such as opium tincture, paregoric elixir, or codeine may be used to decrease peristalsis, whereas octreotide acetate (Sandostatin) may be given to reduce the volume of persistent high-output diarrhea. Occasionally, a reduction in fraction size or a break in treatment is necessary to control acute gastrointestinal side effects. Chronic diarrhea, obstruction caused by bowel adhesions, and fistula formation are serious complications of irradiation that occur in less than 1% of cases. Small bowel and rectovaginal fistulas can be caused by radiation effects or by recurrent disease. Once recurrence is ruled out as an etiology, the patient may require a temporary or permanent colostomy to allow healing of the affected bowel.

- Genitourinary toxicity typically presents as cystitis where the patient has pain, urgency, hematuria, and urinary frequency. The bladder is relatively tolerant of radiation, but doses higher than 6,000 to 7,000 cGy over a 6- to 7-week period can result in cystitis. The diagnosis of radiation cystitis may be made after a normal urine culture result has been obtained. Hydration, frequent sitz baths, and, possibly, the use of antibiotics and antispasmodic agents may be necessary for treatment. **Hemorrhagic cystitis** may lead to symptomatic anemia that requires blood transfusions and hospitalization. Clot evacuation of the bladder with continuous bladder irrigation is often necessary. Bladder irrigation with 1% alum or 1% silver nitrate can alleviate bleeding. Persistent bleeding on continuous bladder irrigation or significant gross hematuria in the unstable patient requires immediate cystoscopy to localize and control the bleeding.
- **Vesicovaginal fistulas and ureteral strictures** are possible long-term complications of radiation therapy. Placement of nephrostomies, insertion of ureteral stents, and, less commonly, surgical intervention may be necessary.
- **Vulvovaginitis** occurs secondary to erythema, inflammation, mucosal atrophy, inelasticity, and ulceration of the vaginal tissue. Adhesions and stenosis of the vagina are common and can result in pain on pelvic examination and intercourse. Treatment involves vaginal dilation, either by frequent sexual intercourse or with a vaginal dilator. In addition, the use of estrogen creams is useful in promoting epithelial regeneration. Infections, including candidiasis, trichomoniasis, and bacterial vaginosis, may be associated with radiation-induced vaginitis.
- The most common neurologic side effect is fatigue. This may continue for several months after completion of therapy. As with chemotherapy-induced fatigue, correction of anemia, good sleep hygiene, and regular exercise can help decrease fatigue.

## OTHER ANTICANCER AGENTS

- **Hormonal agents** have been studied extensively in gynecologic cancer, including **tamoxifen** (which has both antiestrogenic effects in breast tissue as well as estrogen stimulatory effect in endometrial and myometrial tissues), **medroxyprogesterone acetate** (Provera), and progesterone-releasing intrauterine devices. These agents take advantage of the fact that both normal and well-differentiated neoplastic gynecologic tissues generally have both estrogen and progesterone receptors.
- These receptors are commonly lost as tumors become less well differentiated.

## PRIMARY TREATMENT MODALITIES ACCORDING TO CANCER SITE

### Epithelial Ovarian Cancer

- Women with epithelial ovarian cancer (EOC) need surgical staging to confirm the diagnosis and guide treatment planning. Patients with stage III and IV EOC require optimal surgical cytoreduction (residual tumor implants less than 1 cm in diameter), either at time of initial surgery or after three to four cycles of neoadjuvant chemotherapy. Carcinoma of the fallopian tube and primary peritoneal carcinoma should be managed the same way as epithelial ovarian carcinoma.
- Patients with stage IA and IB, grades 1 to 2, disease do not benefit from adjuvant chemotherapy. Patients with stage IC, all grades, and those with stage IA and IB, grade 3, disease should receive three to six cycles of IV **platinum-based adjuvant chemotherapy**, which has been shown to improve both recurrence-free and overall survival.

- Patients with stages III and IV EOC should be treated with at least six cycles of platinum-taxane–based chemotherapy. As mentioned earlier, neoadjuvant chemotherapy may also be considered for patients unfit for surgery at the time of presentation due to extent of disease, comorbidities, or poor performance status. Women with stage III EOC who have minimal or no residual disease after primary surgery should receive combined IV and intraperitoneal (IP) chemotherapy. Although the combined IV/IP regimens are associated with greater neurologic, metabolic, and hematologic toxicity than IV regimens, there is significant improvement in both progression-free survival and overall survival associated with the combined IV/IP approach.
- EOCs that persist or progress despite surgery and primary platinum-based chemotherapy are termed "platinum refractory." EOCs that recur within 6 months of the last platinum-based treatment are termed "platinum resistant," whereas neoplasms that recur more than 6 months later than the last platinum-based treatment are considered "platinum sensitive." Drugs commonly used for the treatment of women with platinum-refractory or platinum-resistant disease include topotecan, liposomal doxorubicin, docetaxel, gemcitabine, weekly paclitaxel, and bevacizumab. Patients with platinum-sensitive disease are generally treated with a combination of platinum and another active agent.

## Ovarian Germ Cell Cancers

- As with EOC, comprehensive surgical staging is critical for patients with ovarian germ cell cancers. Young patients with stage I pure dysgerminoma and low-grade (grade 1) immature teratoma who wish to preserve fertility are adequately treated with unilateral salpingo-oophorectomy alone. All other patients with stage I to IV disease should undergo adjuvant chemotherapy with three courses of **bleomycin**, **etoposide**, and **cisplatin** after primary surgery. Postoperative radiation is an option for patients with dysgerminoma.

## Cervical Cancer

- Surgery, chemotherapy, and radiation therapy all play a role in the management of women with cervical cancer limited to the pelvis (stages IA to IVA). Treatment options for a woman with stage IA1 cervical cancer include cervical conization and simple hysterectomy. For IA2 to IIA disease, options with similar benefit include radiation therapy and radical hysterectomy with bilateral pelvic lymphadenectomy. Treatment options for women with stage IIB to IVA disease include radiation, platinum-based chemoradiation, and neoadjuvant chemotherapy followed by radical hysterectomy.
- Radiation sensitization with concomitant cisplatin improves both progression-free and overall survival for women with cervical cancer. For women who cannot tolerate platinum, other chemosensitizing agents such as 5-fluorouracil (5-FU) can be considered. It is important to note, however, that patients who undergo both surgery and radiation (or chemoradiation) for the treatment of their cervical cancer will experience more short- and long-term toxicity than those who are treated with one modality alone.
- Treatment for women with stage IVB disease should focus on symptom control, as these patients are not curable with currently available treatment options. Radiation may be used for palliation of central disease and/or distant metastases. Drugs with known activity include cisplatin, ifosfamide, paclitaxel, irinotecan, and the two-drug combinations of cisplatin with ifosfamide, paclitaxel, or gemcitabine. Women

who experience a pelvic recurrence after primary surgery for cervical cancer should be considered for chemoradiation or pelvic exenteration, both of which have cure rates <50%. The same chemotherapeutic agents listed for women with stage IVB disease also may be considered for women with distant recurrent disease.

## Vulvar Cancer

- The goals for treatment of vulvar cancer include efforts to decrease the extent of surgery and preserve normal urinary, rectal, and sexual functions while providing curative therapy. Early vulvar cancer (less than 1 mm deep) is treated with wide local excision. When the lesion is deeper than 1 mm and less than 2 cm from the midline, the patient is offered a radical local excision with bilateral inguinal node dissection. If greater than two lymph nodes return positive, the pelvic nodes are examined and radiation started. Locally advanced disease may be treated with neoadjuvant chemoradiation, radical vulvectomy and lymph node dissection, or exenteration. There is no effective chemotherapy identified for patients with distant metastatic vulvar cancer.

## Vaginal Cancer

- Early vaginal cancer may be treated with either surgery or radiation (intracavitary with or without interstitial radiation). More advanced disease (stage II to IV) is generally treated with radiation alone. Platinum-based chemoradiation is also commonly used.

## Endometrioid Endometrial Carcinoma

- Endometrioid endometrial carcinomas are thought to arise in the hormonal milieu of estrogen excess relative to progesterone. Prolonged progesterone therapy has been shown to induce histologic regression of cancer in about 50% to 78% of women with well-differentiated endometrioid endometrial carcinoma confined to the endometrium. Hormonal therapy, therefore, may be a treatment option among young women who wish to preserve fertility, as well as among patients with multiple comorbidities for whom the operative risks outweigh the benefits.
- Hysterectomy and bilateral salpingo-oophorectomy are the standard of care for women with stage I disease and radical hysterectomy and bilateral salpingo-oophorectomy for women with stage II disease. Pelvic and para-aortic lymphadenectomy are also advocated to complete surgical staging. Pelvic radiation, whether vaginal cuff brachytherapy or external beam radiation, should also be offered. Patients found to have metastatic disease at time of hysterectomy (stages III and IV) will benefit from platinum and taxane chemotherapy. Radiation directed at sites is offered to patients with adequate performance status.
- Patients found to have endometrial cancer recurring in the pelvis may benefit from surgical resection and radiation. Patients with distant metastatic disease should receive the same combination chemotherapy as those with stage III and IV disease. The small subset of women with recurrent grade I disease may benefit from hormonal therapy.

## Uterine Carcinosarcomas

- The primary treatment for uterine carcinosarcomas is total abdominal hysterectomy, bilateral salpingo-oophorectomy, and lymphadenectomy. Adjuvant chemotherapy with ifosfamide and paclitaxel is recommended given improved progression-free and overall survival. Adjuvant pelvic radiation is often offered due to decreased risk of local recurrence, although overall survival is not impacted.

## Uterine Leiomyosarcomas

• The primary treatment for leiomyosarcomas remains total abdominal hysterectomy and bilateral salpingo-oophorectomy. Adjuvant doxorubicin appears to offer a high-response rate for primary treatment, whereas adjuvant pelvic radiation reduces the risk of local recurrence but does not improve overall survival. The most active agents for women with recurrent or metastatic disease include gemcitabine and docetaxel.

## Gestational Trophoblastic Tumors

• Hydatidiform mole is treated with dilatation and curettage, although hysterectomy is advised if childbearing is completed. When persistent disease is suspected (serum human chorionic gonadotropin levels that rise or plateau), women are treated with either methotrexate with leucovorin or single-agent dactinomycin. Those with recurrent gestational trophoblastic tumors (GTT) after primary chemotherapy are treated with a five-drug combination of etoposide, methotrexate, actinomycin D, cyclophosphamide, and vincristine (Oncovin). This combination is commonly abbreviated as **EMA-CO**. Hysterectomy may be indicated for patients with disease that persists after multidrug therapy. Women with recurrent GTT metastatic to the brain should be treated with both whole brain radiation therapy and chemotherapy with ifosfamide, carboplatin, and etoposide. Placental site trophoblastic tumors are not sensitive to chemotherapy; they should be treated with primary hysterectomy.

## SUGGESTED READINGS

American College of Obstetricians and Gynecologists. Clinical management guidelines for obstetricians-gynecologists. ACOG practice bulletin no. 65: management of endometrial cancer. *Obstet Gynecol* 2005;106(2):413–425.

Baekelandt MM, Castiglione M; ESMO Guidelines Working Group. Endometrial carcinoma: ESMO recommendations for diagnosis, treatment and follow-up. *Ann Oncol* 2008;19(suppl 2): ii19–ii20.

Byrd LM, Swindell R, Webber-Rookes D, et al. Endometrial adenocarcinoma: an analysis of treatment and outcome. *Oncol Rep* 2008;20:1221–1228.

Chemotherapy for Cervical Cancer Meta-Analysis Collaboration. Reducing uncertainties about the effects of chemoradiotherapy for cervical cancer: a systematic review and meta-analysis of individual patient data from 18 randomized trials. *J Clin Oncol* 2008;26:5802–5812.

Fiorelli JL, Herzog TJ, Wright JD. Current treatment strategies for endometrial cancer. *Expert Rev Anticancer Ther* 2008;8:1149–1157.

Gershenson DM. Management of ovarian germ cell tumors. *J Clin Oncol* 2007;25:2938–2943.

Greer BE, Koh WJ, Abu-Rustum N, et al. Cervical cancer. *J Natl Compr Canc Netw* 2008;6(1): 14–36.

Haie-Meder C, Morice P, Castiglione M; ESMO Guidelines Working Group. Cervical carcinoma: ESMO recommendations for diagnosis, treatment and follow-up. *Ann Oncol* 2008; 19(suppl 2):ii17–ii18.

Kyrgiou M, Salanti G, Pavlidis N, et al. Survival benefits with diverse chemotherapy regimens for ovarian cancer: meta-analysis of multiple treatments. *J Natl Cancer Inst* 2006;98: 1655–1663.

Morgan RJ Jr, Alvarez RD, Armstrong DK, et al. Ovarian cancer: clinical practice guidelines in oncology. *J Natl Compr Canc Netw* 2008;6:766–794.

Pectides D, Kamposioras K, Papaxoinis G, et al. Chemotherapy for recurrent cervical cancer. *Cancer Treat Rev* 2008;34(7):603–613.

Reed NS. The management of uterine sarcomas. *Clin Oncol (R Coll Radiol)* 2008;20:470–478.

Temkin SM, Fleming G. Current treatment of metastatic endometrial cancer. *Cancer Control* 2009;16:38–45.

# 51 Palliative Care

Lauren Cobb and Teresa P. Díaz-Montes

## DEFINITIONS

### Palliative Care

- Palliative care is specialized medical care for people with serious illnesses. The main focus is to provide patients with relief of distressing symptoms, pain, and the stress of a serious illness, irrespective of the prognosis. Additionally, it focuses on the psychological and spiritual care as well as the development of a support system for the patient and their family and aims to improve their quality of life. The palliative care team is composed of physicians, nurses, and other specialists who work together with the patient's other physicians to provide an extra layer of support. It is appropriate at any age or at any stage in a serious illness and can be provided along with curative treatment. Benefits of palliative care are that it:
  - provides relief from pain, shortness of breath, nausea, and other distressing symptoms;
  - affirms life and regards dying as a normal process;
  - intends neither to hasten nor to postpone death;
  - integrates the psychological and spiritual aspects of patient care;
  - offers a support system to help patients live as actively as possible;
  - offers a support system to help the family cope;
  - uses a team approach to address the needs of patients and their families;
  - enhances quality of life;
  - is applicable early in the course of illness, in conjunction with other therapies that are intended to prolong life, such as chemotherapy or radiation therapy; and
  - can be obtained in the hospital setting (inpatient palliative care unit or consult service), in the outpatient setting, or in hospice.

### Hospice Care (End-of-Life Care)

- Hospice care is end-of-life care provided by health professionals and volunteers. The main goal is to provide medical, psychological, and spiritual support to the patient and their family. Additionally, the primary focus is to assist the dying individual in achieving peace, comfort, and dignity during the process. The caregivers try to control pain and other symptoms so the individual can remain as alert and comfortable as possible. Usually, a hospice patient is expected to live 6 months or less. Hospice care can take place at home, at a hospice center, in a hospital, or in a skilled nursing facility. It serves to:
  - deliver palliative care to patients at the end-of-life and
  - provide psychosocial care, nursing support, respite care, and bereavement support for the patient and their family.
- To obtain Medicare hospice benefits:
  - Physician must certify that the patient has <6-month life expectancy assuming that the disease progresses as expected; there are no penalties for outliving the 6-month limit.

- Patient must qualify for Medicare Part A (insurance for hospital care and skilled nursing facility care).
- Patient selects a Medicare-approved hospice.
- Patient elects hospice care over regular Medicare care. However, Medicare will still cover regular medical expenses when not associated with the terminal illness.
- Physician Medicare benefits are maintained and patients can sign back on to Medicare whenever they wish.
- In general, comfort and quality of life are the primary goals. A "do not resuscitate" order is not necessary.

## ETHICAL CONSIDERATIONS

### Do Not Resuscitate/Do Not Intubate

- Do not resuscitate/do not intubate (DNR/DNI) is often a difficult discussion that patients expect their doctors to initiate. In general, the conversation should address the goals of treatment and the patient's priorities, including prolongation of life and quality of life, preferences for life-sustaining therapies, and goals for pain management.
- A patient can decide to be DNR/DNI but still pursue aggressive treatment; likewise, a patient can decide to pursue palliative treatment and still desire full resuscitation.
- Data show that resuscitation and intubation efforts in oncology patients are rarely successful.
- DNR/DNI discussion is urgently indicated if
  - death is imminent or the patient is otherwise at high risk for intubation or resuscitation (e.g., compromised pulmonary function);
  - the patient expresses a desire to die;
  - the patient or her family wants to discuss hospice options;
  - the patient has been recently hospitalized for progressing illness; or
  - the patient has significant suffering coupled with a poor prognosis.

### Legal Considerations

- The patient's decision may not always be the same as that of her physician or family.
- The principle of autonomy is an important consideration in American medicine.
  - Living wills and DNR orders can ensure that patients' wishes are carried out.
  - Situations in which patients' surrogate decision makers may disagree with previously formulated advance directives are common.
    - Legally and ethically, a surrogate decision maker must clearly follow the advance directive formulated by a competent patient.
- Patients have the right to refuse or to withdraw care.
- Permitting death by not intervening is distinct from the action of killing.
- Physician-assisted suicide (i.e., a doctor provides a patient with the means to commit suicide with knowledge of the patient's intent) is legal only in Oregon and Washington states.
- Voluntary euthanasia (i.e., an intervention to end a patient's life with her consent) is illegal in all states.
- Difficulties can arise when patients and their families request treatments considered futile or inappropriate by their physicians.
  - No legal or societal consensus exists for situations in which patients and families disagree with physicians' recommendations to stop treatment.

- Consultation with an ethics committee or palliative care can be helpful.
- Excellent communication regarding educational, spiritual, and psychosocial needs can often resolve these conflicts.

## END-OF-LIFE CARE: PAIN MANAGEMENT

- One of the most common and frightening symptoms for patients with terminal illness
- Patient surveys have shown that pain associated with advanced illness is often undertreated and that approximately 40% of cancer pain is undertreated.
- Pain should be addressed aggressively with multimodal therapy.
  - The World Health Organization (WHO) pain ladder provides guidelines for pain control escalation (Fig. 51-1).
  - Adjuvants include medicines, interventions, and alternative/complementary approaches designed to reduce fear or relieve anxiety.
  - Pain can be visceral, somatic, or neuropathic; many patients have multifactorial pain.

### Medical Treatments
*Nonsteroidal Anti-Inflammatory Drugs*
- First step in the WHO pain treatment ladder
- Can act synergistically with opioids

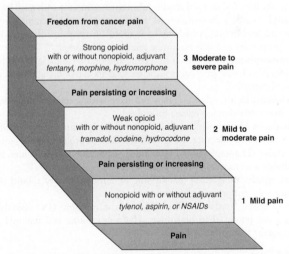

**Figure 51-1.** The WHO three-tier analgesia ladder depicts a rationale for escalating combination pain treatments as necessary to achieve pain control goals. Pain medications should be administered in order (nonopioids, then mild opioids like codeine, then strong opioids like morphine) until pain relief is achieved. Analgesics should be scheduled rather than given as needed. (Adapted from World Health Organization. Cancer pain relief and palliative care: report of a WHO expert committee. Geneva, Switzerland: World Health Organization, 1990:7–21.)

- Should be given around the clock if pain is constant—twice daily options can aid in compliance
- No nonsteroidal anti-inflammatory drug (NSAID) has greater efficacy than another.
- Side effects include platelet inhibition (some nonsteroidals, such as Trilisate, do not inhibit platelets), gastrointestinal (GI) effects, and nephrotoxicity. These can be especially pronounced in older, frail patients.
- Often contraindicated in clinical trials or while receiving chemotherapy. GI prophylaxis is usually indicated for long-term palliative use.
- Acetaminophen is often just as effective and may be safer in some situations.

### Opiates

- Second and third steps in the WHO ladder
- Opioids can be considered first line for terminal patients, especially those with severe pain.
- When pain is constant, escalate to around-the-clock dosing or longer acting narcotics with rescue doses as needed.
- There are various formulations and routes of administration (there is variation in response to these formulations and none are universally preferred over the other):
  - Mu opioid receptors are a subset of opioid receptors that provide anesthesia in response to specific narcotics. Pure mu agonists specifically target these receptors for pain relief: morphine, fentanyl, oxycodone, hydromorphone, and methadone.
    - **Morphine:** Available in oral tablets, solutions, elixirs, suppositories, and injectable formulas. Also available sublingually but is poorly absorbed in that route. Metabolized by the liver and excreted renally. Administer cautiously with renal insufficiency.
    - **Fentanyl:** Available in transdermal, transmucosal, and injectable formulations. No active metabolites, which make it useful in renal insufficiency. Relatively lower propensity to cause histamine release and itching.
    - **Hydromorphone:** Available in injectable and oral formulations and has a short half-life. Also useful in renal insufficiency, as its active metabolite is present in low concentration.
    - **Oxycodone:** In formulations alone or mixed with acetaminophen. Available in immediate- or extended-release formulas.
    - **Methadone:** Mu agonist but also N-methyl-D-aspartate antagonist which helps to reverse opioid tolerance. Long half-life. Risk of prolonging QT interval.
    - Meperidine (Demerol) should be avoided, especially in renal failure, because its metabolite can accumulate and cause seizures.
    - Partial agonist/antagonists (nalbuphine or buprenorphine) should be avoided because they can precipitate withdrawal.
    - Refer to dosing guidelines (Table 51-1), as intravenous (IV) opioids are three times more potent than oral doses. Hydromorphone and fentanyl are much more potent than other opiates.

### Severe Pain Crisis

- Treat with a rapid taper of a fast-acting IV narcotic or with IV patient-controlled analgesia (PCA).
- Once acute pain is controlled, calculate the dose and convert to a long-acting form.

### Side Effects

- To alleviate side effects, decrease the dose, change to a different narcotic, change the route, or treat the symptoms.

| TABLE 51-1 | Opioid Analgesics: Equivalent Dosing for Various Narcotic Formulations | | | |
|---|---|---|---|---|
| Analgesic | Parenteral IM/IV Dose (mg) | Oral Dose (mg) | Half-life[a] (hr) | Peak Effect[a] (hr) |
| Morphine | 10 | 30 | 2–3 | 0.5–1 |
| Hydromorphone | 1.5 | 7.5 | 2–3 | 0.5–1 |
| Meperidine | 75 | 300 | 2–3 | 0.5–1 |
| Fentanyl | 0.1 | Variable | 3–12 | 0.1–0.25 |
| Levorphanol | 2 | 4 | 12–15 | 0.5–1 |
| Oxycodone | NA | 20 | 2–3 | 1 |
| Codeine | 130 | 200 | 2–3 | 1.5–2 |
| Hydrocodone | NA | 30 | 4–6 | 0.5–1 |
| Methadone | 10 | 20 | 12–190 | 0.5–1.5 |

Use rows to convert dosing route and columns to convert between medications.
[a]Parenteral dosing except for oral-only medications.
IM, intramuscularly; IV, intravenously; NA, not available (oral only).
Adapted from Barakat RR, Markman M, Randall ME. *Principles and Practice of Gynecologic Oncology.* Philadelphia, PA: Lippincott Williams & Wilkins, 2009:993.

- See the following text for treatment of nausea and vomiting.
- Constipation is frequently a problem for patients on around-the-clock opioid. A bowel regimen should be prescribed; senna is often the first choice.
- Sedation is common, although tolerance often develops.
- Treat pruritus with Benadryl or low-dose nalbuphine or naloxone.

*Adjuvant Treatment*
- Used to supplement or synergize with other pain medications
- Can be used to reduce narcotic dose and side effects

Neuropathic Pain
- **Corticosteroids (such as dexamethasone)** are often given as first line, especially with advanced cancer pain that exists with other symptoms.
- **Tricyclic antidepressants** are especially good for neuropathic pain.
  - Side effects are related to their anticholinergic properties: sedation, urinary retention, dry mouth, constipation, dysphoria, and blurred vision.
  - Can cause cardiac conduction abnormalities and decrease seizure threshold
- Other types of antidepressants (selective serotonin reuptake inhibitors [SSRIs]) also have some evidence for efficacy. They are particularly helpful in patients with both depression and neuropathic pain.
- **Anticonvulsants** can be used for neuropathic pain.
- **Carbamazepine** can be started at 100 mg orally (PO) twice a day (bid) and titrated up rapidly.
  - Side effects include sedation, vertigo, hyponatremia, bone marrow suppression, and hepatotoxicity.
  - Complete blood count and liver function tests should be followed.

- **Phenytoin** can be loaded as 20 mg/kg or 1,000 mg (whichever is less) IV and then 100 mg three times a day (tid).
  - Side effects include anemia, anorexia, nausea/vomiting, hepatotoxicity, ataxia, bone marrow suppression, and hypersensitivity (fever, rash, hepatitis).
- **Gabapentin/pregabalin** shows good efficacy in some randomized controlled trials for cancer.
  - Must be started at low dose and titrated slowly.
  - Principal side effect is sedation.
- All adjuvants for neuropathic pain generally take weeks for efficacy. Acute pain should be treated with acetaminophen, NSAIDs, and/or opioids.
- **Capsaicin** can be effective for neuropathic pain (especially zoster) but may burn when applied. Mechanism of action is depletion of substance P.

Bone Pain

- **Bisphosphonates** (osteoclast inhibitors) are useful to treat bone metastasis, breast pain, and possibly other cancers. They also prevent skeletal complications.
- **Corticosteroids and NSAIDs** can also be useful with pain from bone metastases.

Other Pain Symptoms

- Visceral crampy abdominal pain may be relieved by treating coexisting constipation or with anticholinergics such as **hyoscyamine**.
- Topical **lidocaine**—for sores or mucositis; lidocaine patch for herpes zoster.

## Nonmedical and Invasive Treatments

- About 30% of cancer patients will have inadequate pain control despite large doses of opiates or will have intolerable side effects at opiate doses that do control pain.
- **Radiation** may be useful for bone metastasis and bulk effects.
- **Chemotherapy** may be useful for tumor effects, such as bowel obstruction.
- **Anesthesia/neurosurgical procedures**
  - Myofascial injections may work for pain from localized muscle contractions.
    - Relief lasts from days to weeks.
  - Neurostimulation (implanted device) has an unclear mechanism of action.
    - Stimulation can be given to the spinal cord or thalamic nuclei.
    - Spinal cord stimulators are electrodes placed in the epidural space. They are very expensive and require patient involvement which may not be ideal for end-of-life.
  - Epidural or spinal PCA can decrease narcotic doses and reduce side effects.
  - Somatic nerve block works for pain localized to a single nerve, plexus, or dermatome.
    - A temporary injection is used to test for effectiveness.
    - A neurolytic block can then be used for longer relief.
    - The block can disrupt motor, sensory, or autonomic pathways.
  - Sympathetic blocks can relieve visceral pain.
    - Do not cause somatosensory or motor dysfunction
    - A celiac plexus block can treat pain from the upper abdomen.
      - Performed under fluoroscopic or computed tomography guidance.
      - Almost all patients have transient hypotension, diarrhea, and back pain.
      - Other complications include unilateral paresis and retroperitoneal bleeding.
    - Superior hypogastric plexus blocks relieve pain from the pelvic viscera.
      - Seventy-nine percent of patients achieve pain relief with a low complication rate.

- **Surgery**
  - May be necessary for the most severe and persistent pain
  - Vertebral body collapse and long bone fractures are treated best with prompt surgical intervention.
- **Psychotherapy support groups, cancer counseling, and spiritual support**
  - Help patients deal with their diagnosis, decrease cognitive dissonance, and assist with coping skills
  - Cognitive behavior techniques (progressive muscle relaxation, focused breathing, and meditation) require an alert patient but can be very helpful.
- Topical warm and cold treatments have few side effects.
  - Can provide relief for muscle pain
- Transcutaneous electrical nerve stimulation and acupuncture
  - No proven effect in randomized trials but virtually no side effects

## END-OF-LIFE CARE: SYMPTOM MANAGEMENT

### Respiratory Symptoms

*Dyspnea*

- **Dyspnea** is the sensation of uncomfortable breathing or shortness of breath.
- Differential diagnosis includes pulmonary embolus, pleural effusion, anemia, lung metastasis, pneumonia, anxiety, and fatigue/weakness.
- Treatment of the underlying cause (e.g., with antibiotics, anticoagulation, blood transfusion, thoracentesis) can provide relief.
- Oxygen and opiates can also relieve the sensation and reduce fear and anxiety.
- Increase opiates about 25% above baseline, just as for escalating pain treatment, for comfort.
- Benzodiazepines, corticosteroids, and bronchodilators may be useful.

### Gastrointestinal Symptoms

*Anorexia/Cachexia*

- Usually a symptom of, not the cause of, functional decline. May be a symptom of the dying process.
- **Anorexia** refers to decreased appetite.
- **Cachexia** implies wasting; seen in cancer patients at the end-of-life.
  - The pathophysiology of cachexia is not completely understood, but it appears to be related to decreased intake and increased cytokine levels.
  - Cachexia does not respond well to nutritional supplements.
- Forced feeding often produces no weight gain and can increase patient discomfort and nausea.
- Treatment
  - Appetite stimulants can restore appetite briefly but have multiple side effects and are not associated with improved survival.
    - Use when appetite is a significant quality of life issue and potential benefits outweigh side effects.
  - Only two classes of drugs are well supported by multiple randomized trials:
    - Dexamethasone 4 mg daily; side effects are those associated with chronic steroid use.
    - Megace 400 to 800 mg daily; liquid and long-lasting forms are available. Significant side effects.

- Artificial nutrition is indicated only for patients who are unable to eat (e.g., bowel obstruction) and have relatively good prognosis (3 months or greater). Substantial adverse effects.

### Nausea/Vomiting

- May result from chemotherapy, opiates, or disease progression.
- The type of nausea may determine treatment strategy:
  - *Acute* (within 24 hours of a treatment or procedure)
  - *Delayed* (after 24 hours)
  - *Anticipatory* (a conditioned response after severe nausea and vomiting in the past)
- Treatment: Around-the-clock dosing with rescue and escalation regimens using drugs from different categories is often successful. Multiple receptor-signaling pathways in the area postrema have been suggested to mediate nausea and vomiting.
- **Anticholinergic** drugs act mainly on muscarinic receptors.
  - Scopolamine 1.5 mg transdermally q72hr
  - Side effects include dry mouth, drowsiness, and visual changes.
- **Antihistamines** have sedation as their greatest side effect.
  - Diphenhydramine (Benadryl) 25 to 50 mg PO q6hr or 10 to 50 mg IV
  - Dimenhydrinate (Dramamine) 50 mg PO q4hr
  - Cyclizine (Marezine) 50 mg PO/intramuscularly (IM) q4hr or 100 mg per rectum (PR) q4hr
  - Meclizine (Antivert) 25 to 50 mg PO daily (qd)
  - Promethazine (Phenergan) 12.5 to 25 mg PO/IM q4hr or PR q12hr
- **Dopamine receptor antagonists**
  - Phenothiazines may lead to extrapyramidal reactions which can be treated with diphenhydramine.
  - Prochlorperazine (Compazine) 5 to 10 mg PO q6hr or 2.5 to 10 IM/IV q3hr or 25 mg PR q12hr
  - Chlorpromazine (Thorazine)
  - Haloperidol (Haldol)
  - Side effects include akathisia, dystonia, and tardive dyskinesia.
  - Metoclopramide (5 to 10 mg PO/IV/IM q6hr) is a modest antiemetic and increases gastric emptying.
- **Serotonin antagonists** are highly efficacious but very expensive. Side effects are mild, including headache and constipation. Granisetron, dolasetron, and palonosetron are in this category and have equivalent efficacy.
- **Neurokinin receptor antagonists** are a newer option.
  - Aprepitant is approved for short-term use only, with highly emetogenic chemotherapy.
- Other antiemetics have unclear mechanisms of action.
  - Corticosteroids are especially effective for chemotherapy-induced nausea.
  - Cannabinoids have modest antiemetic effects.
    - Dronabinol 5 to 10 mg PO q6hr is the legal prescribable form.
  - Benzodiazepines are weak antiemetics but are very good at treating anxiety, which can contribute to nausea.
  - Small studies have shown that acupuncture has some antiemetic effects.
- Prophylaxis
  - The appropriate method depends on the emetogenic property of the chemotherapy.
  - If severe nausea has occurred with a particular regimen, treatment should be escalated.

- Agents with very low emetogenic risk usually require no prophylaxis.
- Low-risk regimens: dexamethasone 20 mg IV or prochlorperazine 10 mg PO once before chemotherapy
- Moderate- to high-risk regimens: serotonin antagonist, such as ondansetron (oral dosing equivalent to IV) plus dexamethasone 8 mg IV prior to chemo, followed by dexamethasone 4 to 8 mg PO bid × 2 more days to prevent delayed nausea
- Extremely high-risk chemotherapy (especially cisplatin): serotonin antagonist plus dexamethasone 8 mg IV plus aprepitant 125 mg PO prior to chemo, followed by dexamethasone 8 mg PO qd × 3 days and aprepitant 80 mg PO qd × 2 days.
- Anticipatory nausea can be treated with alprazolam 0.5 to 2 mg as needed.

## Ascites

- A frequent problem in late-stage ovarian cancer
- Not many treatment options are available.
  - High-dose spironolactone has shown some benefit in small trials.
  - Therapeutic large-volume paracentesis can be performed for acute relief:
    ○ Mean duration of relief is only 10 days.
    ○ Large-volume drainage leads to hypovolemia.
    ○ Repetitive taps increase the risk of infection.
    ○ If more than 5 L are drained, albumin can be given.
  - Permanent catheters (PleurX) are available and may reduce infection risk; patients can drain ascites at home.

## Bowel Obstruction

- Bowel obstruction is frequent in ovarian cancer patients.
- **Small bowel obstruction (SBO)**
  - Usually managed conservatively with bowel rest and decompression (i.e., nasogastric tube) unless bowel ischemia or strangulation is present.
  - Further intervention depends on the clinical situation.
    ○ Surgery should not occur routinely in patients with very poor prognosis (e.g., massive ascites, multiple sites of obstruction, diffuse carcinomatosis, or poor performance status).
    ○ Obstruction can be relieved by surgery, but perioperative morbidity and mortality are high. Reobstruction is common.
  - A percutaneous gastrostomy tube can be placed for venting.
  - Hyoscyamine or octreotide (0.3 to 0.6 mg subcutaneous [SQ]) decreases gastric secretion and slows intestinal motility, thereby decreasing the nausea/vomiting associated with SBO. This is supported by several randomized trials.
- **Colonic obstruction**
  - Less frequent than SBO
  - Surgical correction is indicated.
  - Endoscopic stents may work for palliative treatment.
- **Acute colonic pseudo-obstruction**
  - Mimics anatomic obstruction which must be ruled out by imaging.
  - Follow with serial abdominal exams and daily x-rays.
  - Supportive care with bowel rest is often enough to reverse the pseudo-obstruction.
  - Low magnesium, calcium, and potassium should be replaced.
  - Neostigmine 2 mg IV × 1 can be used; however, some patients experience bradycardia and should be monitored in an intensive care setting with atropine available.

- Endoscopic decompression with placement of a rectal tube may be attempted if neostigmine fails, if evidence of decompensation exists, or if the bowel diameter is >13 cm.
- Surgery should be attempted if the aforementioned measures fail.

*Constipation*

- **Constipation** is common for patients on opiates. Both prophylaxis and treatment are indicated.
- Treatment regimens should incorporate multiple mechanisms of action.
  - Fiber and bulk-forming laxatives are usually contraindicated for palliative care.
  - Hyperosmolar laxatives draw water into the stool (polyethylene glycol 240 to 720 mL a day; lactulose 15 to 30 mL bid; sorbitol 120 mL of 25% solution daily; and glycerine 3 g PR daily or 5 to 15 mL enemas).
  - Saline laxatives are also hyperosmolar (magnesium sulfate 15 g daily, magnesium citrate 200 mL daily).
  - Stool softeners are usually ineffective when used alone (docusate sodium 100 mg PO bid, mineral oil 15 to 45 mL a day).
  - Stimulants increase bowel motility (Bisacodyl 30 mg PO qd or 10 mg PR qd and senna 1 to 4 tsp qd).
- Fecal impaction should be treated aggressively.
  - Can be extremely painful and even lead to mental status changes
  - Mechanical disimpaction is required, followed by enemas. Colonic cleanout with polyethylene glycol is important, and aggressive bowel therapy should be started to prevent a recurrence.

## Constitutional Symptoms

*Fatigue*

- The pathophysiology of **fatigue** from cancer is unclear.
- Can significantly decrease quality of life
- Differential diagnosis includes anemia, chronic stress reaction, inflammation/immune reaction, disrupted circadian rhythm or sleep disturbance, hormonal changes, depression, and direct central nervous system toxicity.
  - Evaluation of reversible causes should be initiated.
- Workup includes evaluation of disease progression, medication effects and interactions, hematocrit, electrolytes, pain assessment, depression risk, and medical comorbidities.
- At the end-of-life, reassurance for the family may be the most appropriate step.
- Treatments:
  - Severe anemia may be treated with red cell transfusion, erythropoietin injection, iron, folic acid, and vitamin $B_{12}$ supplementation.
  - Moderate exercise may reduce fatigue and improve functional status in healthier patients. Energy conservation (including limiting/scheduling activities) is more appropriate in patients with more advanced illness.
  - Sleep hygiene and cognitive behavioral therapy can increase the effectiveness of sleep.
  - Psychostimulant use is not well supported (methylphenidate 5 mg PO every morning and noon to start; modafinil, a nonamphetamine activating agent, 100 to 200 mg every morning and at noon can be used in some situations).
  - Antidepressants may decrease fatigue associated with depression. Nortriptyline has sedative properties but can be useful for insomnia and poor sleep hygiene contributing to fatigue; alternatively, bupropion is more activating.

## Neurologic Symptoms

*Insomnia*

- Often alleviated by treating underlying pain, anxiety, depression, or by addressing psychosocial/spiritual issues. Consider delirium in the diagnosis.
- When initial treatment is ineffective, a hypnotic agent can be used short term.
- In patients already on hypnotics, reduced dosing may restore normal sleep patterns.
- Sleep hygiene is often helpful.

*Delirium/Agitation*

- Mental status changes can be very distressing for families and can complicate home care.
- Workup depends on the patient's status and preferences.
- The mnemonic DELIRIUM can be helpful:
  D: drugs (e.g., anticholinergics, ranitidine, lorazepam, opiates)
  E: electrolytes, emotions (e.g., hyponatremia, hypophosphatemia, hyperammonemia)
  L: low $O_2$, lack of drugs (e.g., pneumonia, pulmonary embolus, withdrawal)
  I: ictal (e.g., stroke, brain metastases, seizure disorder)
  R: retention (e.g., of $CO_2$, urine, or stool)
  I: ischemia, infection (e.g., transient ischemic attack, stroke, meningitis, urosepsis, pneumonia)
  U: uremia (e.g., renal failure)
  M: myocardial (e.g., infarction, arrhythmia, heart failure)
- Rapid sedation with haloperidol 0.5 to 1 mg IV/PO/SQ, repeated as needed and coupled with lorazepam 0.5 to 1 mg PO/IV q1 to 2hr may be helpful.

## Symptoms from Distant Metastases

*Bone Metastases*

- Can be very painful and lead to pathologic fractures
- Localized radiation provides pain relief in 35% to 100% of patients but has toxicity including mucositis, enteritis, dermatitis, and bone marrow suppression.
- Can often be relieved with single treatment (well supported by randomized trials) but may take several weeks for full efficacy
- Hemibody radiation can be used for diffuse metastasis but has complications including radiation pneumonitis.
- Surgical fixation is appropriate for fractures and some impending fractures.
- Bisphosphonates decrease the rate of skeletal complications in breast cancer, but their role in the treatment of bone pain and in other cancers is less clear.
- Consider NSAIDs and steroids.
- Calcitonin has not been shown to relieve bone pain from metastasis.

*Brain Metastases*

- Initial presentation may be seizures, nausea/vomiting, persistent headache, neurologic symptoms, or cognitive/personality changes.
- Magnetic resonance imaging (MRI) is usually necessary for diagnosis.
- Symptomatic patients receive dexamethasone 10 mg then 4 mg PO every 6 hours.
  - Response is usually within 24 to 72 hours.
  - Patients are at risk for opportunistic infections. *Pneumocystis carinii* pneumonia prophylaxis should be initiated.
  - Proton pump inhibitor prophylaxis is appropriate.

- Wean steroids to lowest effective dose.
- Prophylactic seizure medication is not required, but treatment is necessary if seizures persist.
- Radiation can reduce symptoms and improve survival, depending on patient prognosis.

*Spinal Metastases*

- Cause bone pain, cord compression, fractures, leptomeningeal metastasis, and malignant plexopathy
- Epidural spinal cord compression requires rapid diagnosis and treatment to avoid permanent paralysis.
  - Presentation is pain progressing to weakness and hyperreflexia, followed by bowel and bladder dysfunction and paralysis.
  - An MRI should be obtained on all cancer patients with new or worsening back pain.
- Treatment:
  - Steroids relieve pain and decrease the rate of neurologic complications.
    - Low-dose regimen: 10 mg load then 16 mg a day tapered over 2 weeks.
    - High-dose regimen: 100 mg IV load then 24 mg tid for 3 days, tapered over 10 days. There are significant side effects with this dosing regimen.
- Spinal cord compression requires urgent radiation treatment or surgical decompression.
  - Radiation treats pain and stabilizes neurologic function.
  - Eighty percent to 100% of patients who are walking at the time of radiation will retain function; patients who have lost function are unlikely to regain it.

## Other Considerations

*Hydration*

- The decision to begin or continue hydration can be difficult at the end-of-life; treatment should be formulated in consultation with the patient and her family.
- There is no evidence that hydration improves patient comfort.
- Dry mouth is best treated with mouth swabs.
- May prolong death process and increase secretions and edema. IV access may be difficult.
- May decrease electrolyte-induced delirium

*Palliative Sedation*

- Rarely used except for extreme symptom control
- Use of benzodiazepines or phenobarbital at end-of-life should be discussed.
- Palliative care consultation may be helpful before initiating heavy sedation.

*Death Rattle*

- The course rasps at the end-of-life are sometimes described as a "death rattle."
- A scopolamine patch can help decrease these distressing sounds.

*Depression*

- Adjustment reaction to a terminal diagnosis is expected; however, depression should be formally evaluated and treated when diagnosed.
- Counseling and cognitive behavioral therapy are useful adjuncts.
- All antidepressants have side effects, which should be considered in the choice of treatment.
  - Tricyclic antidepressants are sedating and have anticholinergic effects (e.g., dry mouth, constipation, urinary retention).
  - SSRIs are less sedating and less anticholinergic than tricyclics.
  - Bupropion can lower seizure threshold.

*Anxiety*

- Benzodiazepines are the mainstay of acute treatment.
  - Short acting: alprazolam 0.25 to 1 mg PO tid or four times a day; lorazepam 0.5 to 2 mg PO/IV/IM q3 to 6hr
  - Longer acting: clonazepam 1 to 2 mg PO bid; diazepam 2.5 to 10 mg PO/IV/IM q3 to 6hr
- Many antidepressants, especially SSRIs, also have anxiolytic effects.
- Neuroleptics may be used if benzodiazepines are ineffective: thioridazine 10 to 25 mg PO tid; haloperidol 0.5 to 5 mg PO/IV/SQ q2 to 12hr
- Other options include methotrimeprazine 10 to 20 mg IM/IV/SQ q4 to 8hr and chlorpromazine 12.5 to 50 mg PO/IM/IV q4 to 12hr. These are more sedating but are also analgesic.
- Atypical antipsychotics:
  - Olanzapine 2.5 to 10 PO qd and risperidone 0.5 to 4 PO qd may be useful in frail, older patients.
  - Buspirone 10 PO tid may be used for chronic anxiety; takes 5 to 10 days to see any effect.

*Spiritual/Existential Issues*

- Concerns about maintaining personal dignity, lack of closure in relationships, inability to discern meaning in life, and spiritual crisis are often very distressing to patients.
- Counseling and early involvement of a spiritual counselor can often give comfort.

## SUGGESTED READINGS

Chase DM, Monk BJ, Wenzel LB, et al. Supportive care for women with gynecologic cancers. *Expert Rev Anticancer Ther* 2008;8(2):227–241.

Doyle D, Woodruff R. *The IAHPC Manual of Palliative Care*, 2nd ed. Houston, TX: International Association of Hospice and Palliative Care, 2004.

Grant M, Elk R, Ferrell B, et al. Current status of palliative care clinical implementation, education, and research. *Cancer J Clin* 2009;59:327–335.

Sepulveda C, Marlin A, Yoshida T, et al. Palliative care: the World Health Organization's global perspective. *J Pain and Symptom Manage* 2002;24(2):91–96.

# Index

Page numbers followed by *f* indicate a figure; page numbers followed by *t* indicate a table.